Laboratory Procedures for Veterinary Technicians

Laboratory Procedures for Veterinary Technicians

Eighth Edition

Kristin Jean Holtgrew-Bohling, DVM

Veterinary Medicine

Town & Country Veterinary Clinic P.C.

Auburn, Nebraska

ELSEVIER

Elsevier
3251 Riverport Lane
St. Louis, Missouri 63043

Previous editions copyrighted 2020, 2015, 2007, 2002, 1997, 1992, and 1985.

Content Strategist: Melissa Rawe
Senior Content Development Specialist: Betsy McCormac
Publishing Services Manager: Deepthi Unni
Project Manager: Thoufiq Mohammed
Design Direction: Patrick Ferguson

Printed in India

Last digit is the print number: 9 8 7 6 5 4 3 2 1

Working together
to grow libraries in
developing countries

www.elsevier.com • www.bookaid.org

I would like to dedicate this edition to my children.

PREFACE

In recent years, there has been tremendous growth in the number and types of laboratory data that can be obtained in the in-house veterinary practice laboratory. Laboratory procedures remain an important aspect of most veterinary practices, both diagnostically and financially, and a major responsibility of the technician. Performing the tests in the in-house veterinary practice laboratory also provides improved service to both the patient and client and an additional revenue source for the clinic.

This edition is an effort to collect the relevant clinical laboratory information needed by the practicing veterinary technician. Veterinary assistant and veterinary technology students will also find this a valuable everyday reference. Principles and procedures for laboratory diagnostics in clinical chemistry, microbiology, hematology, hemostasis, parasitology, urinalysis, immunology, and cytology are all presented. Information on commonly performed tests done in referral laboratories is also provided to allow greater understanding of the clinical relevance of these tests. Reviews of anatomy and physiology topics are included in many sections to aid in developing an understanding of the rationale for performance of specific tests.

This new edition has been significantly reorganized with the student in mind. The organization should allow the student to easily review material introduced and provide a student-friendly introduction of new materials. Technician tips are interspersed throughout the text to highlight important points. Additional full-color illustrations have been added, including photomicrographs of blood cells, cytology and microbiology samples, and urine sediment. Key points and recommended readings are included in each chapter. The new atlas-style appendices will enhance laboratory exercises and provide an excellent resource as the students move into clinical practice.

Step-by-step procedure boxes for all commonly performed hematology, cytology, and parasitology laboratory tests are included in this new edition. The procedure boxes represent those skills that veterinary technician students must perform during their educational program, as well as additional procedures that are commonly performed by veterinary technicians in private veterinary practice.

ACKNOWLEDGMENTS

I would like to thank all of the wonderful people at Elsevier that helped make this textbook possible: Betsy McCormac (Content Development Specialist), Melissa Rawe (Content Strategist), and Thoufiq Mohammed (Project Manager). Their hard work and dedication are extremely appreciated. I would also like to thank Kassie Wessendorf, DVM for helping me with obtaining images and allowing me to bounce content ideas off of her. Her insight and content specialization made her invaluable.

CONTENTS

The Veterinary Practice Laboratory

Unit Outline

Unit Objectives

Describe the role of the veterinary technician in the clinical laboratory.
List and describe the regulations related to safety concerns in the veterinary practice laboratory.
Describe the components of a quality control program for the veterinary practice laboratory.
Identify, use, and maintain common laboratory equipment.
Use the metric system to perform calculations and measurements.

Veterinarians depend on laboratory results to help establish diagnoses, to track the course of diseases, and to offer prognoses to clients. The veterinary practice laboratory can also be a significant source of income for the practice. The rapid availability of test results improves patient care and client service. Although some veterinary clinics use outside reference laboratories for test results, this may delay the implementation of appropriate treatments for patients. Most diagnostic tests can be performed in house by a well-educated veterinary technician. Veterinary practice laboratories have become increasingly sophisticated. Analytic instruments are affordable and readily available for inclusion in even the smallest veterinary clinic.

The veterinary technician/veterinarian team approach works efficiently in a laboratory situation. A veterinarian is educated in the interpretation of test results, whereas a veterinary technician is educated on generating accurate test results. The consistent generation of reliable laboratory results requires an educated veterinary technician. A veterinary technician must understand the value of quality control in the laboratory.

1

Safety Concerns and OSHA Standards

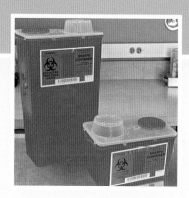

LEARNING OBJECTIVES

After studying this chapter, you will be able to:

- Discuss the requirements of a chemical hygiene plan.
- Identify mechanisms for minimizing exposure to hazards in the veterinary practice laboratory.
- Describe general concerns related to laboratory design.
- Identify, use, and care for personal protective equipment.
- Discuss criteria for evaluating Internet resources.

OUTLINE

KEY TERMS

Biohazard
Bloodborne pathogen
Chemical Hygiene Plan (CHP)
Engineering controls

Safety Data Sheet (SDS)
Occupational Safety and Health Administration (OSHA)
Personal protective equipment (PPE)

Zoonoses

A comprehensive laboratory safety program is essential to ensure the safety of employees in the clinical laboratory area. The safety policy should include procedures and precautions for the use and maintenance of equipment. Safety equipment and supplies—such as eyewash stations (Fig. 1.1), fire extinguishers, spill cleanup kits (Fig. 1.2), hazardous and biohazard waste disposal containers (Fig. 1.3), and protective gloves—must be available.

Emergency showers and eyewash stations provide on-the-spot decontamination. They allow workers to flush away hazardous substances that can cause injury in the event a chemical exposure were to occur within the laboratory. All employees working in the clinical laboratory must be aware of the location of these items and thoroughly trained in their use. The first 10 to 15 seconds after exposure to a hazardous substance, especially a corrosive substance, are critical. Delaying treatment, even for a few seconds, may cause serious injury. The following are recommended times in the event you are exposed to chemicals within the lab:

- 5 minutes for non-irritants or mild irritants
- 15–20 minutes for moderate to severe irritants and chemicals that cause acute toxicity if absorbed through the skin, or unknown substances
- 30 minutes for most corrosives, and
- 60 minutes for strong alkalis (e.g., sodium, potassium, or calcium hydroxide).

Laboratory safety policies must be in writing and placed in an accessible location within the clinical laboratory area. Signs should be posted to notify employees that eating, drinking, applying cosmetics, and adjusting contact lenses in the laboratory are prohibited.

> **TECHNICIAN NOTE** Written laboratory safety policies must be accessible to all employees in the clinical laboratory area.

In the United States, the Occupational Safety and Health Administration (OSHA) mandates specific laboratory practices

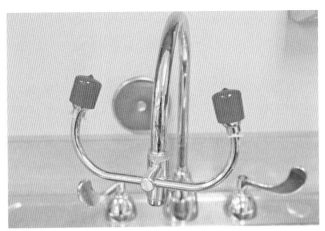

Fig. 1.1 Sink-mounted eyewash station. This type of station is preferable to wall-mounted eyewash bottles that require regular refilling and that may not be of adequate volume to properly flush the eyes.

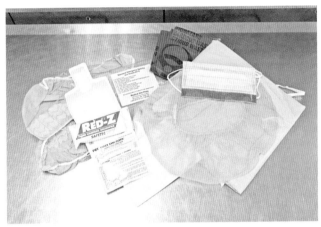

Fig. 1.2 Spill cleanup kit. These kits generally contain biohazard bags, personal protective equipment, absorbent materials, and disinfectants.

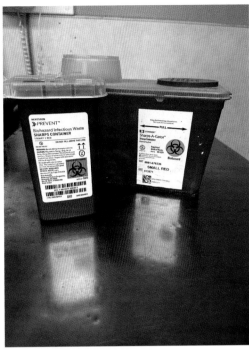

Fig. 1.3 Biohazard waste disposal containers are available in a variety of sizes. This rigid type is generally used for the disposal of sharps (e.g., scalpel blades, hypodermic needles).

that must be incorporated into the laboratory safety policy. Many other countries have similar regulations. The regulations are focused on protecting the health and safety of employees. OSHA is responsible for determining and enforcing protective standards. Some states have regulations that supersede the federal OSHA regulations. In those cases, the state regulations are at least as stringent as the federal ones. Some state and federal regulations also contain exemptions for facilities that have 10 or fewer employees. The regulations specifically include requirements for employers to do the following:

- Comply with all relevant OSHA standards.
- Correct any safety and health hazards in the workplace.
- Educate employees about any potential workplace hazards.
- Provide training to employees regarding health and safety hazards.
- Provide required **personal protective equipment (PPE)** to employees.
- Maintain accurate records of work-related injuries and illnesses.
- Post specific OSHA posters, citations, and injury and illness data (Fig. 1.4).

Depending on the specific types of equipment present and the tests performed in the veterinary practice laboratory, veterinary technicians can be exposed to a variety of potential hazards. These include biologic and physical hazards as well as hazards to the musculoskeletal system related to improper ergonomics.

HAZARD CONTROL

Methods for minimizing potential workplace hazards can be categorized as one of four types.

1. Engineering controls
2. Administrative controls
3. Procedural controls
4. PPE

Engineering controls are focused on changing the work environment to eliminate or minimize exposure to a hazard. An example would be the use of a fume hood when handling hazardous chemicals.

Administrative controls involve the creation of specific protocols to minimize worker exposure to hazards; these protocols include those found in a **Chemical Hygiene Plan (CHP)**, which is discussed in more detail later in this chapter.

Procedural controls involve the development of policies that modify worker behavior. Examples would include the restriction from mouth pipetting and the substitution of less hazardous materials when feasible. When engineering, administrative, and procedural controls are not fully effective for the removal of a hazard, PPE would be required.

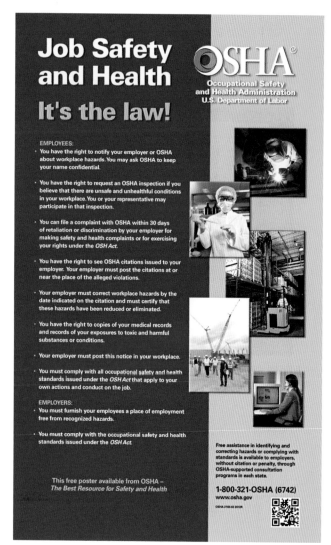

Fig. 1.4 OSHA requires that this Job Safety and Health poster or an equivalent state version be posted in all workplaces. (From United States Department of Labor, Occupational Safety and Health Administration.)

OSHA STANDARDS

There are a large number of specific standards related to veterinary practice contained in the Occupational Safety and Health Act. These standards can be found in the Code of Federal Regulations (CFR) in the section designated as Title 29. Each standard is also designated with a part number. For example, the standard regarding formaldehyde for use in locations other than clinical laboratories is designated as 29 CFR 1910.1048 to indicate Title 29, Part 1910.1048; this standard also has several appendices. The vast majority of the standards that apply specifically to workplace safety are found in Part 1910, which is divided into subparts designated with letters A through Z. Summary information regarding some of the OSHA standards with application to the veterinary practice laboratory is contained in this chapter.

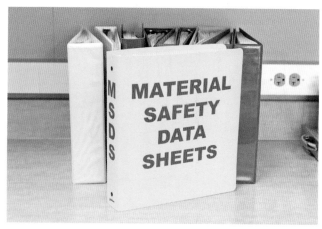

Fig. 1.5 Material Safety Data Sheets must be available to employees.

Occupational Exposure to Hazardous Chemicals in Laboratories Standard

The OSHA standard titled Occupational Exposure to Hazardous Chemicals (29 CFR 1910.1450) is commonly referred to as the Laboratory Standard. This standard requires that each employer designate an employee as the Chemical Hygiene Officer; this individual is responsible for the implementation of the required CHP. The CHP must contain specific details about the chemical hazards present in the workplace, the scope and extent of worker training and documentation of that training, criteria for the use of PPE, precautions for handling hazardous chemicals, monitoring of exposure, and specific actions required when exposure occurs, including the medical care required.

> **TECHNICIAN NOTE** Hazards associated with chemicals are described in Material Safety Data Sheets.

The Hazard Communication Standard

The OSHA Hazard Communication Standard (29 CFR 1910.1200) contains requirements for employers to evaluate potential chemical hazards and to communicate information about those hazards and appropriate protective measures to employees that would be potentially exposed to those hazards. Information must be communicated to employees in writing and must include a list of all hazardous chemicals to which they may be exposed. Worker training programs regarding the use of PPE when dealing with hazardous chemicals are included in this standard. The standard mandates the placement of specific types of labels on containers of hazardous chemicals; it also requires that the employer maintain Safety Data Sheets (SDSs) for all chemicals and that these SDSs be accessible to employees (Fig. 1.5). SDSs are provided by manufacturers of potentially hazardous chemicals, and they must contain specific information. The minimum information required by OSHA is as follows:

BOX 1.1 Components of the Material Safety Data Sheet

Section 1. Chemical Product & Company Information
Section 2. Composition/Information on Ingredients
Section 3. Hazards Identification
Section 4. First Aid Measures
Section 5. Fire Fighting Measures
Section 6. Accidental Release Measures
Section 7. Handling and Storage
Section 8. Exposure Controls/Personal Protection
Section 9. Physical and Chemical Properties
Section 10. Stability and Reactivity
Section 11. Toxicological Information
Section 12. Ecological Information
Section 13. Disposal Considerations
Section 14. Transport Information
Section 15. Regulatory Information
Section 16. Other Information

- Manufacturer's name and contact information
- Hazardous ingredients/identity information
- Physical/chemical characteristics
- Fire and explosion hazard data
- Reactivity data
- Health hazard data
- Precautions for safe handling and use
- Control measures

Additional information may also be present. OSHA recommends the use of a specific 16-section format for SDSs, which is summarized in Box 1.1.

Container Labeling

The Hazard Communication Standard contains detailed information about the proper labeling of containers of chemicals (Fig. 1.6). When chemicals are removed from their primary container and placed in secondary containers for use, the secondary label must also contain specific information. The secondary label is required when the material is not used within the work shift of the person who filled the container, when the person who filled the container leaves the work area, or when the container is moved to a different work area from where it was filled and is not in the possession of the person who filled it. Pictograms are used to communicate some hazard information on secondary containers (Fig. 1.7).

> **TECHNICIAN NOTE** OSHA mandates specific types of labels on containers of hazardous chemicals.

The Bloodborne Pathogens Standard

The Bloodborne Pathogens Standard (29 CFR 1910.1030) includes OSHA mandates to protect workers from infection with infectious agents that are present in the bloodstream; it also incorporates the requirements of another law, the Needlestick

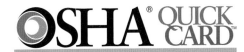

Hazard Communication Standard Labels

OSHA has updated the requirements for labeling of hazardous chemicals under its Hazard Communication Standard (HCS). As of June 1, 2015, all labels will be required to have pictograms, a signal word, hazard and precautionary statements, the product identifier, and supplier identification. A sample revised HCS label, identifying the required label elements, is shown on the right. Supplemental information can also be provided on the label as needed.

For more information:

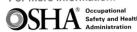 Occupational Safety and Health Administration

(800) 321-OSHA (6742)
www.osha.gov

SAMPLE LABEL

CODE_____
Product Name_____ } Product Identifier

Company Name_____
Street Address_____
City_____ State_____
Postal Code_____ Country_____
Emergency Phone Number_____ } Supplier Identification

Keep container tightly closed. Store in a cool, well-ventilated place that is locked.
Keep away from heat/sparks/open flame. No smoking.
Only use non-sparking tools.
Use explosion-proof electrical equipment.
Take precautionary measures against static discharge.
Ground and bond container and receiving equipment.
Do not breathe vapors.
Wear protective gloves.
Do not eat, drink or smoke when using this product.
Wash hands thoroughly after handling.
Dispose of in accordance with local, regional, national, international regulations as specified. } Precautionary Statements

In Case of Fire: use dry chemical (BC) or Carbon Dioxide (CO_2) fire extinguisher to extinguish.

First Aid
If exposed call Poison Center.
If on skin (or hair): Take off immediately any contaminated clothing. Rinse skin with water.

Hazard Pictograms

Highly flammable liquid and vapor. May cause liver and kidney damage. } Hazard Statements

Signal Word
Danger

Supplemental Information
Directions for Use
_____
_____
_____
_____

Fill weight: _____   Lot Number: _____
Gross weight: _____   Fill Date: _____
Expiration Date: _____

OSHA 3492-02 2012

Fig. 1.6 OSHA requires that specific information be included on all containers of hazardous materials. (From United States Department of Labor, Occupational Safety and Health Administration.)

Safety and Prevention Act of 2001. In the veterinary practice laboratory, exposures to human bloodborne pathogens could potentially occur during the handling of certain biological control materials used in quality control programs. However,

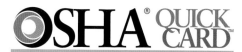

Hazard Communication Standard Pictogram

As of June 1, 2015, the Hazard Communication Standard (HCS) will require pictograms on labels to alert users of the chemical hazards to which they may be exposed. Each pictogram consists of a symbol on a white background framed within a red border and represents a distinct hazard(s). The pictogram on the label is determined by the chemical hazard classification.

HCS Pictograms and Hazards

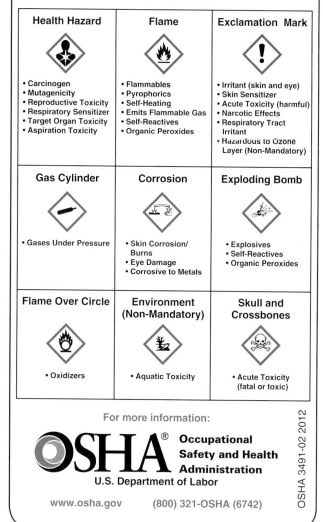

Health Hazard	Flame	Exclamation Mark
• Carcinogen • Mutagenicity • Reproductive Toxicity • Respiratory Sensitizer • Target Organ Toxicity • Aspiration Toxicity	• Flammables • Pyrophorics • Self-Heating • Emits Flammable Gas • Self-Reactives • Organic Peroxides	• Irritant (skin and eye) • Skin Sensitizer • Acute Toxicity (harmful) • Narcotic Effects • Respiratory Tract Irritant • Hazardous to Ozone Layer (Non-Mandatory)
Gas Cylinder	Corrosion	Exploding Bomb
• Gases Under Pressure	• Skin Corrosion/Burns • Eye Damage • Corrosive to Metals	• Explosives • Self-Reactives • Organic Peroxides
Flame Over Circle	Environment (Non-Mandatory)	Skull and Crossbones
• Oxidizers	• Aquatic Toxicity	• Acute Toxicity (fatal or toxic)

For more information:

OSHA Occupational Safety and Health Administration
U.S. Department of Labor

www.osha.gov   (800) 321-OSHA (6742)

OSHA 3491-02 2012

Fig. 1.7 Pictograms allow for the rapid communication of specific hazard information. (From United States Department of Labor, Occupational Safety and Health Administration.)

the majority of such control material is no longer manufactured as human-based products. As with the chemical standard, the training of those who will potentially be exposed is required. Mechanisms to control and minimize exposure must be established and communicated in writing.

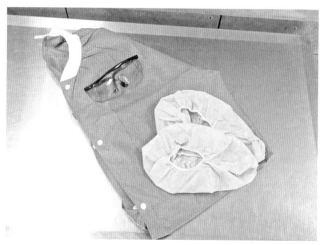

Fig. 1.8 Examples of personal protective equipment include gloves, goggles, and shoe covers.

Other Potentially Infectious Materials

Although exposure to most human bloodborne pathogens is not a common problem in the veterinary practice laboratory, a variety of other infectious agents may be encountered. Zoonoses are diseases that can be transmitted between animals and humans. The agents of zoonotic diseases may be present in samples of body fluids, feces, skin scrapings, and other types of samples presented for analysis. Regulations related to these other potentially infectious materials (OPIM) are less specific than for the bloodborne pathogens, except when they have the potential to cause serious threats to public health and safety (e.g., bacterial organisms that cause anthrax, botulism, or plague). Veterinary technicians may encounter such materials either by contact with infected animals or during the course of collecting and handling samples for analysis. Protocols must be in place to prevent exposure and must also include the proper disposal of potentially infectious materials. These protocols generally focus on the use of PPE, the proper disinfection of materials and work surfaces, and mechanisms such as autoclaving infectious materials before disposal or disposal by incineration.

The Personal Protective Equipment Standard

The Personal Protective Equipment Standard (29 CFR 1910.132) requires that employers provide, pay for, and ensure the use of appropriate PPE when needed to avoid hazards associated with chemicals and other hazards capable of causing injury through absorption, inhalation, or physical contact. Depending on the types of hazards present, PPE may include eye protection, protective clothing, shields, and barriers (Fig. 1.8). Employers are required to provide training for workers that documents that the workers know what PPE is required, how to use that PPE, and how to properly care for the PPE. Additional mandates related to PPE are included in the Eye and Face Protection Standard (29 CFR 1910.133), the Respiratory Protection Standard (29 CFR 1910.134), and the Hand Protection Standard (29 CFR 1910.138).

Other PPE that may be needed includes chemical fume hoods and biosafety cabinets. Both chemical fume hoods and biosafety cabinets are specialized types of laboratory equipment. Chemical fume hoods and biosafety cabinets look similar, and both protect laboratory workers from laboratory hazards—their purpose, function, and operation differ significantly.

A chemical fume hood is designed to remove chemical fumes and aerosols from the work area while a biosafety cabinet is designed to provide both a clean work environment and protection for employees who create aerosols when working with infectious agents or toxins. A chemical fume hood protects the user while a biosafety cabinet protects the user, the environment, and the material. Biosafety cabinets have high-efficiency particulate air (HEPA) filters while chemical fume hoods do not. The HEPA filter in the exhaust system of a biosafety cabinet will effectively trap all known infectious agents and ensure that only microbe-free exhaust air is discharged from the cabinet (i.e., 99.97% of particles 0.3 μm in diameter and 99.99% of particles of greater or smaller size).

> **TECHNICIAN NOTE** Employers are required to provide necessary PPE to employees.

Biosafety Hazard Considerations

Special considerations are given to hazards that are unique to the biomedical industry. Biohazards are biological substances (e.g., used hypodermic needles, patient samples that contain infectious agents) that pose a threat to human health as well as those substances that are harmful to animals. Containers that hold biohazardous material are marked with a specific symbol (Fig. 1.9). The Centers for Disease Control and Prevention is a U.S. government agency that has established precise guidelines for the safe handling and management of infectious agents in the biomedical industry. Biosafety levels are graded as 1, 2, 3,

and 4 or I, II, III, and IV; the higher the number, the greater the risk. Brief summaries of the precautions for each biosafety level are included in the following sections. Requirements for each level increase and requirements for lower levels are automatically included in higher levels.

Biosafety Level I

The agents in biosafety level I are those that ordinarily do not cause disease in humans. It should be noted, however, that these otherwise harmless substances may affect individuals with immune deficiency.

Examples of products and organisms found in biosafety level I include most soaps and cleaning agents, vaccines that are administered to animals, and species-specific infectious diseases (e.g., infectious canine hepatitis).

There are no specific requirements for the handling or disposal of biosafety level I materials other than the normal sanitation that would be used in a home kitchen. This always includes the complete washing of counters, equipment, and hands.

Biosafety Level II

The agents in biosafety level II are those that have the potential to cause human disease if handled incorrectly. The hazards included in this level may result from mucous membrane exposure, possible oral ingestion, and puncture of the skin. Examples of organisms in this level are the bacterial agents that cause toxoplasmosis and salmonellosis. Substances in this group generally have a low potential for aerosol contamination.

Although precautions will vary with specific substances, these are the general requirements for biosafety level II:
- Limited access to the area, including signs that warn of biohazards
- The wearing of gloves, laboratory coats, gowns, and face shields and the use of Class I or Class II biosafety cabinets to protect against splash potential or aerosol contamination
- Appropriate use of sharps containers
- Specific instructions for the disposal and decontamination of equipment and potentially dangerous materials, including the monitoring and reporting of contamination problems
- Physical containment devices and autoclaving, if needed

Biosafety Level III

Agents in biosafety level III are substances that can cause serious and potentially lethal diseases. The potential for aerosol respiratory transmission is high. An example of an organism in this category is *Mycobacterium tuberculosis*. At this level, primary and secondary barriers are required to protect personnel. General requirements at this level are as follows:
- Controlled access
- Decontamination of waste
- Decontamination of cages, clothing, and other equipment

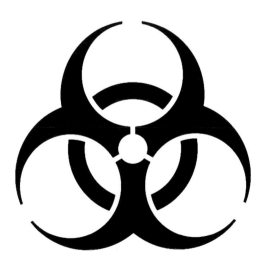
Fig. 1.9 The universal biohazard symbol.

- Testing of personnel to evaluate possible exposure
- Use of Class I or Class II biosafety cabinets or other physical containment devices during all procedures
- Use of PPE by all personnel

Biosafety Level IV

It is unlikely that persons with limited experience handling biohazards will ever encounter substances that are included in biosafety level IV. Agents found in this category pose a high risk of causing life-threatening diseases. Included in this level are the Ebola and Marburg viruses and other dangerous and exotic agents. Facilities that handle these substances exercise maximum containment. Personnel follow shower-in and shower-out procedures and dress in full body suits that are equipped with a positive air supply. Individuals who plan to work in these facilities will undergo extensive training to ensure their safety.

Shipping Hazardous Materials

Some veterinary practices ship diagnostic specimens to outside laboratories for analysis. Regulations related to the safe shipment of potentially hazardous or infectious materials in the United States are mandated by the U.S. Department of Transportation and enforced by the Federal Aviation Administration. The U.S. Department of Transportation considers any materials that are reasonably expected to contain microorganisms that can cause disease in animals or humans to be potentially hazardous or infectious. Infectious materials are classified as either Category A or Category B, depending on the degree of risk associated with exposure to the materials.

Category A poses a higher degree of risk than Category B. Category A includes those materials that are known or likely to contain an infectious agent in a form that could cause permanent disability, life-threatening disease, or fatal disease in healthy humans or animals if exposed to the material. Examples include cultures known to contain agents such as *Bacillus anthracis, Coccidioides immitis, Mycobacterium tuberculosis,* and West Nile virus.

Category B includes materials that contain an infectious agent that is not in a form that could cause permanent disability, life-threatening disease, or fatal disease in healthy humans or animals exposed to the material. Most diagnostic samples from veterinary patients sent to outside laboratories for analysis fall into Category B. Infectious agents that do not meet the criteria for inclusion in Category A will generally fall into Category B, unless they are exempt from the regulations. Exemptions include the following:

- Specimens in which pathogens have been inactivated
- Specimens or samples known to not contain infectious agents
- Specimens or samples that contain only nonpathogenic microorganisms
- Dried blood and fecal occult blood samples

The shipping of materials in either category requires specific packaging and labeling before they are presented to a transportation carrier (e.g., FedEx, U.S. Postal Service).

In general, specimens must be packaged correctly for shipping.

1. Place each specimen within two sealable containers (i.e., a primary plastic bag or container and a secondary plastic bag or container sealed securely to contain any fluid).
2. Attach identification matching the submission form information to the outside of each double-enclosed specimen. This is essential if more than one specimen per package.
3. Place double-enclosed specimen(s) inside an inner container, such as a Styrofoam box.
4. Use absorbent packing material, such as newspaper or paper towels, to cushion the specimen(s) and to absorb condensation or potential leaks.
5. Place frozen cold packs in the inner container if the sample is to be kept cool during shipping. Ensure samples are completely surrounded and will remain cold for at least 48 hours. Do not use dry ice! If wet ice is used (not recommended), double bag and seal securely to prevent leakage.
6. Close the inner container and secure the outer container with packing tape.

The shipping carton must also carry the appropriate substance labels and other identifying markers as specified in the regulations.

LABORATORY DESIGN
General Considerations

The veterinary clinical laboratory should be located in an area that is separate from other hospital operations (Fig. 1.10). The area must be well lit as well as large enough to accommodate laboratory equipment and to provide a comfortable work area. Countertop space must be sufficient so that sensitive equipment such as chemistry analyzers and cell counters are physically separated from centrifuges and water baths. Room temperature controls should provide a consistent environment that in turn provides for optimal quality control. A draft-free area is preferable to one with open windows or with air conditioning or heating ducts blowing air on the area. Drafts can carry dust, which may contaminate specimens and interfere with test results. Although each veterinary practice is unique, every practice laboratory has certain components, including a sink, storage space, an electrical supply, and Internet access.

Sink

The laboratory area needs a sink and a source of running water to provide a place to rinse, drain, or stain specimens and reagents and to discard fluids. In every veterinary practice, caution should be paramount; the handling and disposing of hazardous laboratory materials bear legal and ethical responsibilities that have increased substantially in recent decades. Certain basic laboratory practices are essential for the protection of workers and the environment. Some of these practices are simply good laboratory hygiene, whereas federal, state, and local regulations have mandated others. A thorough understanding of the laws is at the foundation of proper laboratory practices that involve hazardous

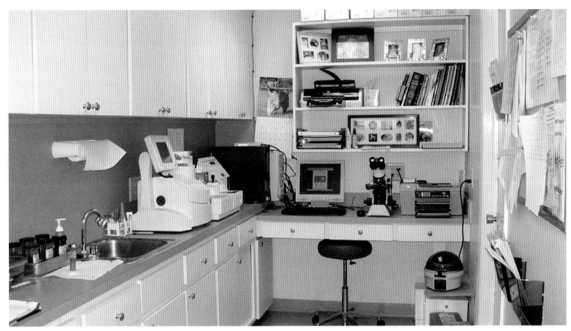

Fig. 1.10 The clinical laboratory should be separate from the main traffic flow in the clinic.

chemicals and specimens. When in doubt, the veterinary technician should never dispose of unknown reagents or chemicals down any sink drain.

Storage Space

Adequate storage space must be available for reagents and supplies to avoid clutter on the laboratory counter space. Drawers and cabinets should be available so that needed supplies and equipment are conveniently located near the site where they will be used. Some reagents and specimens must be kept refrigerated or frozen. A refrigerator and freezer should be readily available. A compact countertop refrigerator is sufficient for most practice laboratories. Frost-free freezers remove fluid from frozen samples, thus making them more concentrated if they are left in the freezer too long. For the long-term storage of fluid samples (e.g., serum, plasma), a chest freezer or freezer that is not self-defrosting should be used.

Electrical Supply

The placement of electrical equipment requires careful consideration. Sufficient electrical outlets and circuit breakers must be available. Circuits must not be overloaded with ungrounded three-prong adapters or extension cords. Veterinary technicians should avoid working with fluids around electrical wires or instruments. An uninterruptible power supply may be necessary if sensitive equipment will be used or if the practice is located in an area that is subject to frequent power outages or fluctuations.

Internet Access

The diagnostic laboratory of the progressive veterinary clinic should have Internet access in the laboratory or at another location within the veterinary clinic. Many reference laboratories use e-mail or fax to report the critical results of submitted diagnostic tests. These reference labs may also have the capability of integrating with your practice software and reporting the results directly back to the patient's chart. In a veterinary clinic that has access to a digital camera attachment for the compound microscope, the veterinarian and the veterinary technician should use the Internet as a diagnostic aid. Photographic images such as scanned microscopic images of blood smears and urine sediments may be sent as e-mail attachments to an outside reference laboratory for diagnostic assistance.

> **TECHNICIAN NOTE** A computer with Internet access is a vital component of the veterinary practice laboratory.

The Internet also may be a valuable resource for veterinary medical information. However, information on the Internet may be oversimplified, incomplete, or inaccurate. The veterinary technician should use Internet sources for supplemental information in addition to consultation with the veterinarian. The veterinarian and the technician should carefully examine all Internet resources together to determine the quality of each website.

Two basic determinants are used to assess website quality. First, high-quality Internet sites are unbiased: the group providing the information should not have a vested interest (e.g., selling a product) in slanting the information a certain way. Second, sources should be staffed by recognized experts in the field, such as those from a government agency, a college or university diagnostic laboratory, or the American Veterinary Medical Association.

Other signs of the quality of a website include the following:

- Funding and sponsorship are clearly shown.
- Timeliness indicators (i.e., date of posting, revising, and updating) is clear and easy to locate.
- Information about the source (e.g., the organization's mission statement) is clear and easy to find.
- Authors and contributors to references on the site are clearly identified.
- References and sources of information are listed.
- Experts have reviewed the site's content for accuracy and completeness.
- Box 1.2 summarizes some important criteria for the evaluation of Internet resources.

BOX 1.2   Evaluation Criteria for Internet Sources

Authority: Who is the author? Does the author list his or her occupation and credentials?
Affiliation: What company or organization sponsors the site?
Currency: When was the information created or updated?
Purpose: What is the purpose of the site (inform, persuade, explain)?
Audience: Who is the intended audience?
Comparison: How does the information compare with other similar works?
Conclusion: Is this site appropriate for research?

KEY POINTS

- A comprehensive laboratory safety program must be implemented in the practice laboratory to ensure the safety of employees.
- SDSs must be available for all chemicals and accessible to all potentially exposed staff members.
- Regulations related to laboratory safety involve multiple government agencies.

- Personnel must be provided with appropriate PPE when required.
- Chemical container labels communicate specific hazardous information.
- Secondary chemical containers must be properly labeled.

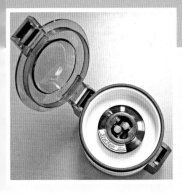

2

General Laboratory Equipment

LEARNING OBJECTIVES

After studying this chapter, you will be able to:
- List the types of equipment commonly found in the veterinary practice laboratory.
- Differentiate between horizontal- and angled-head centrifuges.

- Describe the proper use and care of the centrifuge.
- Discuss the selection and proper use of pipettes.
- Define the term refractive index, and describe the proper use of a refractometer.

OUTLINE

KEY TERMS

Centrifuge
Incubator

Pipette
Refractive index

Refractometer
Supernatant

A variety of general laboratory equipment is needed for the in-house clinical laboratory. The size of the veterinary practice and the tests that are routinely performed in the laboratory determine the equipment and instrumentation needed. Minimal equipment includes a microscope, a refractometer, a microhematocrit centrifuge, and a clinical centrifuge. Additional instrumentation that may be needed—including blood chemistry analyzers, cell counters, water baths, and incubators—depends on the type and size of the practice, the geographic locale of the practice, and the special interests of practice personnel. Test tubes, pipettes, heat blocks, and aliquot mixers are also commonly found in veterinary practices. The proper use and maintenance of this equipment are essential to ensure accurate test results and safety of personnel.

TEST TUBES

Test tubes that are used in the veterinary practice laboratory may be made of glass or plastic, and they are available in many sizes. Microhematocrit tubes, which are primarily used for evaluation of packed cell volume, may be plain or contain anticoagulant. If you are using microhematocrit tubes you will need clay tube

sealant as well. Blood collection tubes are generally made of glass and have color-coded caps to indicate whether any additives are present (Fig. 2.1). Further discussion of the color-coded caps and what they indicate is covered in Chapter 7. Test tube racks are also commonly found in practice. The racks have openings of various sizes to accommodate a specific tube diameter or a range of tube diameters and securely hold tubes on benchtops or in water baths, incubators, or refrigerators. Test tube racks have various configurations and can be stackable, have grips for inversion, be angled, or have alphanumeric labels. Test tube rack shapes and sizes vary and they can be made from a variety of materials, including plain or epoxy-coated metal, wood, foam, and various acrylics and plastics.

Conical tubes have a narrow base and are most often used to centrifuge substances such as urine, which contain solid material within the solution (Fig. 2.2). Blood collection and conical tubes are available in a large number of sizes.

CENTRIFUGE

Centrifuges are vital instruments with many uses in the veterinary practice laboratory. The centrifuge is used to separate

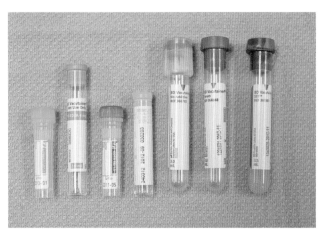

Fig. 2.1 Blood collection tubes are available in a variety of sizes and color coded to identify the presence or absence of specific additives and anticoagulants.

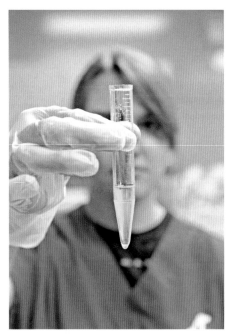

Fig. 2.2 Conical centrifuge tube. This type of tube is used to centrifuge substances that contain solid material in solution.

substances of different densities that are in a solution. The centrifuge spins samples at high speeds, which pushes the most dense components in the sample to the bottom of the tube. Liquid components are layered above the solid components, also according to their densities. When solid and liquid components are present in the sample, the liquid portion is referred to as the supernatant, and the solid component is referred to as the sediment. The supernatant (e.g., plasma or serum from a blood sample) can be removed from the sediment and stored, shipped, or analyzed. Centrifuges vary in size, capacity (i.e., the number of tubes that can be spun at one time), and speed capabilities. Veterinary practice laboratories often have more than one type of centrifuge. A microhematocrit centrifuge is designed to hold capillary tubes, whereas a clinical centrifuge

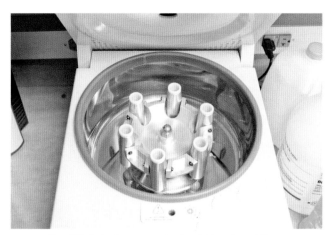

Fig. 2.3 Swinging-arm or horizontal-head centrifuge.

accommodates test tubes of varying sizes. Larger referral practices and reference laboratories may have additional types of centrifuges. A refrigerated centrifuge is used when materials must be kept cool during centrifugation (e.g., processing of blood components for transfusion therapy).

> **TECHNICIAN NOTE** Centrifuges separate substances according to their densities.

Clinical centrifuges that are used in veterinary laboratories are one of two types, depending on the style of the centrifuge head. A horizontal centrifuge head, which is also known as the "swinging-arm" type, has specimen cups that hang vertically when the centrifuge is at rest (Fig. 2.3). During centrifugation, the cups swing out to the horizontal position. As the specimen is centrifuged, centrifugal force drives the particles through the liquid to the bottom of the tube. When the centrifuge stops, the specimen cups fall back to the vertical position.

The horizontal head centrifuge has two disadvantages. At excessive speeds (i.e., greater than 300 revolutions/min), air friction causes heat buildup, which can damage delicate specimens. In addition, some remixing of the sediment with the supernatant may occur when the specimen cups fall back to the vertical position when the centrifuge head stops spinning.

The second type of centrifuge head that is available is the angled centrifuge head. The specimen tubes are inserted through drilled holes that hold the tubes at a fixed angle, usually of approximately 52 degrees. This type of centrifuge rotates at higher speeds than the horizontal-head centrifuge, without excessive heat buildup. The angled centrifuge head is usually configured to accommodate just one tube size. Smaller-sized tubes require the use of an adapter unless a small-capacity centrifuge is available (Fig. 2.4). Microhematocrit centrifuges are a type of angled centrifuge. The microhematocrit centrifuge is configured to accommodate capillary tubes. In veterinary practice, the microhematocrit centrifuge is used for evaluation of the packed cell volume in a whole blood sample. Centrifuges that combine the features of more than one type of centrifuge are also available (Fig. 2.5).

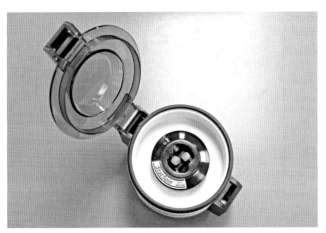

Fig. 2.4 The StatSpin Centrifuge. This angled-head centrifuge is specifically designed for small sample volumes.

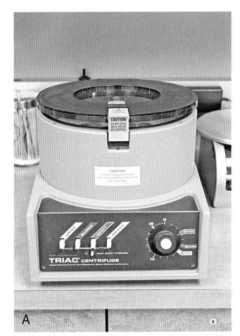

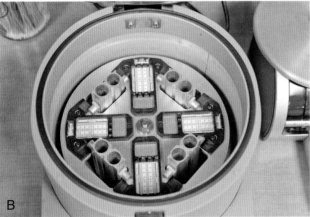

Fig. 2.5 This centrifuge is capable of accommodating both centrifuge tubes and hematocrit tubes. The tube adapters are removed when the centrifuge is used to spin microhematocrit tubes. **A,** Outside of typical centrifuge. **B,** Inside of centrifuge.

In addition to a standard on/off switch, most centrifuges have a timer that automatically turns the centrifuge off after a preset time. A tachometer or dial to set the speed of the centrifuge is also usually present. Some centrifuges do not have a tachometer and always run at maximal speed. Most centrifuges have speed dials that have been calibrated in revolutions per minute (rpm) times 1000. Thus, a dial setting of 5 represents 5000 rpm. Some laboratory procedures require that a specific relative centrifugal force (RCF) or G-force be used. The calculation of RCF requires measurement of the radius of the centrifuge head (r), measured from the center to the axis of rotation. The RCF is then calculated as follows:

$$RCF = \left(1.118 \times 10^{-5}\right) \times r \times rpm^2$$

A centrifuge may also have a braking device to rapidly stop it. The brake should only be used in cases of equipment malfunction, when the centrifuge must be stopped quickly. The centrifuge must never be operated with the lid unlatched. Always load the centrifuge with the open ends of the tubes toward the center of the centrifuge head. Tubes must be counterbalanced with tubes of equal size and weight placed directly opposite from each other. Water-filled tubes may be used to balance the centrifuge. This ensures that the centrifuge will operate correctly without wobbling and that no liquid is forced from the tubes during operation. Incorrect loading of the centrifuge can cause damage to the instrument and injury to the operator. The centrifuge should be cleaned immediately if anything is spilled inside it. Tubes sometimes crack or break during centrifugation. Pieces of broken tubes must be removed when the centrifuge stops. If these are not removed, they could permanently damage the centrifuge. Box 2.1 contains general rules for centrifuge operation.

The operator's manual should list maintenance schedules for the different components of the centrifuge. Some centrifuges require periodic lubrication of the bearings, and most need the brushes to be checked or replaced regularly. Periodic verification that the centrifuge timer is operating correctly can be performed with a stopwatch. Run the centrifuge at several speeds, and repeat each test run at least twice to ensure reproducibility. A tachometer can be used to verify that the centrifuge is reaching the appropriate speeds. A regular maintenance schedule prevents costly breakdowns and keeps the centrifuge running at maximal efficiency.

> **TECHNICIAN NOTE** Centrifuges must always be balanced with tubes of equal size and weight placed opposite each other.

BOX 2.1 General Rules for Centrifuge Use

Verify that the load is properly balanced, with tubes of equal size and weight placed across from each other.

Ensure that the lid is tightly closed before operation.

Do not open the lid until the centrifuge has come to a complete stop.

Clean all spills immediately, and thoroughly remove any broken glass.

Specimens must be centrifuged for a specific time at a specific speed for maximal accuracy. A centrifuge that is run too fast or for too long may rupture cells or destroy the morphologic features of cells in the sediment. A centrifuge may not completely separate the specimen or concentrate the sediment if it is run too slowly or for less than the proper time. Information about the speed and time of centrifugation should be developed for all laboratory procedures and strictly followed for maximal accuracy. I recommend posting a sign on the centrifuge itself with the time and speed needed for each type of sample to ensure consistency of specimen sample preparation between staff members.

REFRACTOMETER

A refractometer, or total solids meter, is used to measure the refractive index of a solution (Fig. 2.6). Refraction is the bending of light rays as they pass from one medium (e.g., air) into another medium (e.g., urine) that has a different optical density. The degree of refraction is a function of the concentration of solid material in the medium. Refractometers are calibrated to a zero reading (zero refractive index) with distilled water at a temperature of between 60° F and 100° F. The most common uses of the refractometer are for the determination of the specific gravity of urine or other fluids and the protein concentration of plasma and other fluids.

The refractometer has a built-in prism and calibration scale (Fig. 2.7). Although refractometers can measure the refractive index of any solution, the scale readings in the instrument have been calibrated in terms of the specific gravity ratio and protein concentrations (g/dL). The specific gravity or protein concentration of a solution is directly proportional to its concentration of dissolved substances. Because no solution can be more dilute or have a lower concentration of dissolved substances than distilled water, the scale calibration and readings (either specific gravity or protein concentration) are always greater than zero. The refractometer is read on the scale at the distinct light–dark interface.

Various refractometer models are available. Most are temperature compensated between 60° F and 100° F. As long as the temperature remains between these two extremes, even as the refractometer is held in the hands, the temperature fluctuation will not affect the accuracy of the reading. Refractometers are available that are calibrated for canine, feline, and equine samples. The refractive index of some species correlates to a unique urine specific gravity so these veterinary-specific refractometers are calibrated to account for those differences. Newer refractometers are digital and contain a microprocessor that provides automatic calibration and temperature monitoring (Fig. 2.8).

Care and Maintenance

The procedure for the use of the refractometer is given in Procedure 2.1. The refractometer should be cleaned after each

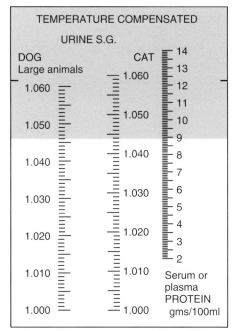

Fig. 2.7 Refractometer scale. The reading is taken at the light–dark interface. In this image, if the sample was serum or plasma the protein would be read as 9.1. If the sample was dog urine, it would be read as S.G. 1.046. If it was cat urine, the S.G. would be read as 1.044. (Courtesy B. Mitzner, DVM.)

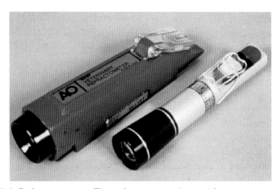

Fig. 2.6 Refractometers. The refractometer is used for measurement of urine specific gravity and total solids in plasma.

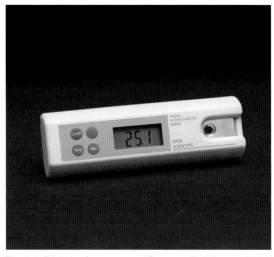

Fig. 2.8 Digital refractometer. (Courtesy B. Mitzner, DVM.)

PROCEDURE 2.1 Use and Care of the Refractometer

1. Inspect and clean the prism cover glass and cover plate.
2. Place a drop of sample fluid on the prism cover glass, and close the cover.

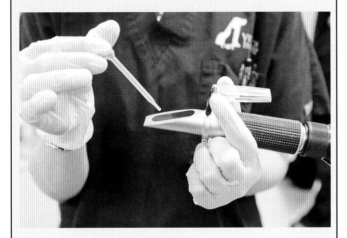

3. Point the refractometer toward bright artificial light or sunlight.

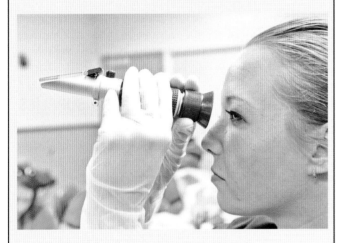

4. Bring the light—dark interface line into focus by turning the eyepiece.
5. Read and record the result with the appropriate scale (e.g., specific gravity, protein).
6. Clean the refractometer according to the manufacturer's recommendations.

PROCEDURE 2.2 Calibration of the Refractometer

1. Distilled water at room temperature should be placed on the refractometer.
2. The refractometer should have a zero refractive index and therefore read 1.000 on the specific gravity scale.
3. If the light—dark boundary deviates from the zero mark by more than one-half of a division, the refractometer is adjusted by turning the adjusting screw as directed by the manufacturer.

NOTE: The refractometer should NOT be used if it is not calibrated to zero with distilled water.

PIPETTES

Although most test kits and analyzers contain their own specific pipettes and pipetting devices, some additional pipettes and pipetting devices may be needed in the veterinary practice laboratory. The primary types of pipettes used in the practice laboratory are transfer pipettes and graduated pipettes. Transfer pipettes are used when critical volume measurements are not needed. These pipettes may be plastic or glass, and some can deliver volumes by drops. Graduated pipettes may contain a single volume designation or have multiple gradations. Pipettes with single gradations are referred to as volumetric pipettes and are the most accurate of the measuring pipettes. It is important that the pipette be used correctly to ensure that the desired volume is measured. Always hold the pipette vertically, not tipped to the side. Larger volumetric pipettes are usually designated as TD pipettes, which means that the pipette is designed "to deliver" the specific volume. A small amount of liquid should remain in the tip of the pipette after the volume has been delivered. Volumetric pipettes that have been designed to deliver microliter volumes are designated as TC pipettes, which means that the pipette is designed "to contain" the specified volume. These pipettes must only be used to add specified volumes of substances to other liquids. The pipette then must be rinsed with the other liquid to deliver the specified volume accurately. The small volume of fluid left in the tip of the pipette is then blown out of the pipette. Pipettes that contain multiple gradations are marked as either "TD" or "TD with blow out," depending on whether the fluid remaining in the tip of the pipette should remain or be blown out. TD with blow out pipettes usually contain a double-etched or frosted band at the top.

The pipette chosen for a specific application should always be the one that is the most accurate and that measures volumes closest to the volume needed. For example, if 0.8 mL is needed, a 1-mL pipette rather than a 5-mL pipette should be chosen. Pipettes are also designed for measuring liquids at specified temperatures, most commonly room-temperature liquids. Liquids that are significantly colder or warmer will not measure accurately. Pipetting devices must also be used correctly, and fluid must not be allowed to enter the pipetting device. The pipette must be held vertically without tilting to the side when transferring liquids. Never pipette any fluid by placing your mouth directly on the pipette.

use and the prism cover glass and the cover plate wiped dry. Lens tissue should be used to protect the optical surfaces from scratches. Some manufacturers suggest cleaning the cover glass and plate with alcohol. The manufacturer's cleaning instructions should be consulted.

The refractometer should be calibrated regularly (i.e., weekly or daily, depending on use). See Procedure 2.2.

TECHNICIAN NOTE Calibrate the refractometer with distilled water on at least a weekly basis.

TEMPERATURE-CONTROLLING EQUIPMENT

Incubators

A variety of microbiology tests require the use of an incubator. Incubators for the in-house veterinary practice laboratory are available in a variety of sizes and configurations. The incubator must be capable of sustaining a constant 37° C, which is the temperature at which the majority of pathogenic organisms grow. The incubator should be fitted with a thermometer, or one should be placed inside the chamber to monitor the temperature (Fig. 2.9). Heat should be provided by a thermostatically controlled element. A small dish of water should also be placed inside to maintain proper humidity. Some incubators have built-in humidity controls, but this type of equipment tends to be expensive. Larger laboratories may have incubators that automatically monitor temperature and humidity as well as carbon dioxide and oxygen levels.

Refrigerators

Many reagents and test kits that are used in the in-house veterinary clinical laboratory require refrigeration, and some may require storage in the freezer. Samples such as blood and urine may also require refrigeration. A basic tabletop refrigerator can be used for most items. This refrigerator may not contain any food for human consumption. Facilities that perform blood-banking services or transfusions must also have a special blood-bank refrigerator.

Water Baths and Heat Blocks

Some clinical chemistry assays, coagulation tests, and blood-banking procedures may require the use of a water bath or heat block that is capable of maintaining a constant temperature of 37° C. A variety of types of water baths are available, including simple standard water baths, circulating water baths, and waterless bead baths. A rack must be placed inside the standard and circulating types to hold materials in place. Bead baths do not require a rack and have little need for maintenance. Heat blocks are generally designed to accommodate just one tube size, although some have multiple adapters that can be used for a variety of tube sizes (Fig. 2.10).

> **TECHNICIAN NOTE** All temperature-controlling equipment, including refrigerators, should have a secondary thermostat placed inside to ensure the equipment is operating correctly. It is best practice to keep a daily log of the equipment temperatures.

AUTOMATED ANALYZERS

A large number of automated analyzers are available for use in the in-house veterinary practice laboratory. These include hematology, clinical chemistry, electrolyte, immunology, coagulation, fecal, cytology, and urine analyzers. The units may run single tests, or they may be capable of running multiple tests on the same sample. Analyzers vary considerably in test principle, and each one has specific advantages and disadvantages. Detailed information about analyzers that are available for specific types of testing is provided in their respective chapters.

MISCELLANEOUS EQUIPMENT AND SUPPLIES

Slide dryers can be a useful addition to the busy veterinary practice laboratory. The dryer minimizes the time required to prepare samples such as blood cell films. Aliquot mixers can also be helpful by keeping items well mixed and ready for use (Fig. 2.11). Slides are commonly utilized in practice. The major difference between slides is if they are frosted or not. There are slides that are frosted, where you can write on the end of the slide to identify it, and slides that don't have frosted edges. You will need to also have available in your laboratory coverslips and immersion oil.

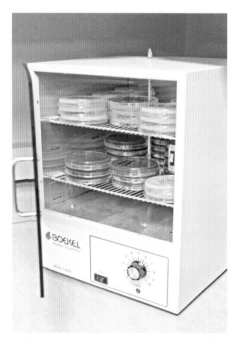

Fig. 2.9 Small incubator for use in the veterinary practice laboratory.

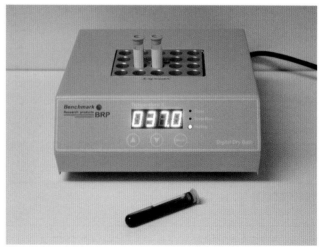

Fig. 2.10 Heat block.

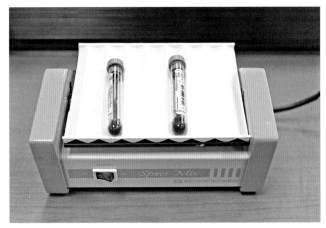

Fig. 2.11 Aliquot mixer.

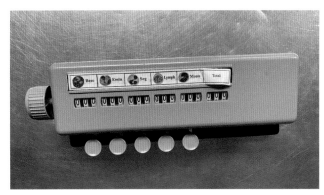

Fig 2.12 Cell counter.

Cell counters are utilized for manual differential counts, and for semen testing they allow you to count and categorize the types of cells before the machine produces an audible "Ding," telling you when you have evaluated 100 cells (Fig 2.12). There are also handheld counters that allow you to count one type of cell.

Other types of cell counting devices include the hemocytometer and McMaster slides. A hemocytometer (also known as a haemocytometer or a cell counting chamber) is a tool used for manual cell counting. The McMaster counting slides are widely used for performing fecal worm egg counts (FECs). Fecal worm egg counts are performed on feces samples mainly from large animals such as horses, sheep, and cattle.

There are numerous stain types that are utilized within veterinary medicine to perform multiple types of tests; examples of commonly used stains include Wright's stains and Gram stains. Discussion on the types of stains needed will be covered with each procedure.

Purchasing Equipment

When evaluating the need to purchase equipment for a practice it is important to evaluate the potential return on investment of the item being purchased. It is important to remember that veterinary clinics are businesses, and despite the extreme advancements in laboratory testing it may not be financially feasible to purchase all of the equipment available on the market. If you do decide to purchase equipment for your facility, there are four very important things to consider before deciding on the company or type of equipment you need.

1. What type of after-purchase support does the company provide?
2. What are the terms of the contract you will be asked to sign, if any, when purchasing the new piece of equipment?
3. Will the purchase be an outright purchase or a lease?
4. Does the equipment integrate with your practice software?

KEY POINTS

1. Clinical centrifuges are used to prepare samples for analysis.
2. Periodic calibration of the centrifuge is needed to ensure that it is reaching the required speeds.
3. The refractometer is used for several types of tests and must be calibrated on a regular basis to ensure diagnostic-quality results.
4. A variety of additional supplies and equipment may be needed in the veterinary practice laboratory, depending on the specific tests performed.
5. Pipettes may be of several types, and each is handled somewhat differently.
6. Proper pipette use ensures accurate measurement of substances.

3

The Microscope

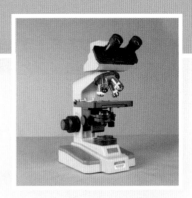

LEARNING OBJECTIVES

After studying this chapter, you will be able to:
- List the parts of the microscope.
- Describe the functions of the parts of the microscope.
- Describe the proper use of the fine and coarse adjustment knobs.
- List the steps in examining a microscope slide.
- Discuss the use, care, and maintenance of the microscope.

OUTLINE

KEY TERMS

Binocular
Compound light microscope
Condenser
Dark field microscope

Fluorescent microscope
Numerical aperture
Objective lenses
Ocular

Phase-contrast microscope
Planachromatic
Resolution

Different types of microscopes are available for clinical use, but the in-house veterinary laboratory generally has just one type.

Electron microscopes, which use an electron beam to create magnified images of objects, are primarily found in research settings and large human medical facilities.

Light microscopes are those that utilize a visible, ultraviolet, or laser light source and include four types.
1. Compound light microscopes
2. Fluorescent microscopes
3. Phase-contrast microscopes
4. Dark field microscopes

Phase-contrast, fluorescent, and dark field microscopes are used primarily in reference laboratories, especially for viewing of unstained specimens. In the veterinary practice laboratory, a high-quality binocular compound light microscope is essential (Fig. 3.1). This microscope may be used to evaluate blood, urine, semen, exudates, and transudates; other body fluids; feces; and other miscellaneous specimens. It may also be used to detect internal and external parasites and to initially characterize bacteria. The practice should ideally maintain two microscopes. One should be used for performing routine parasite studies and procedures that involve the use of corrosive or damaging materials. The second microscope should be reserved for use with cytology and hematology evaluations.

A compound light microscope is so named because it generates an image by using a combination of lenses. Compound light microscopes have many components and a light path. The optical tube length is the distance between the objective lens and the eyepiece. In most microscopes, this distance is 160 mm. The mechanical stage holds a glass slide to be evaluated. The microscope should have a smoothly operating mechanical stage to allow easier manipulation of the sample (Fig. 3.2). Left- or right-handed stages are generally available. Coarse (Fig. 3.3) and fine focus (Fig. 3.4) knobs are used to focus the image of the object being viewed.

The compound light microscope consists of two separate lens systems: the ocular system and the objective system. The ocular lenses are located in the eyepieces and most often have a magnification of 10×. This means that the ocular lens magnifies an object 10 times. A monocular microscope has one eyepiece, whereas a binocular microscope, which is the most commonly used type, has two eyepieces. The two eyepieces can be adjusted to match the interpupillary distance of the user.

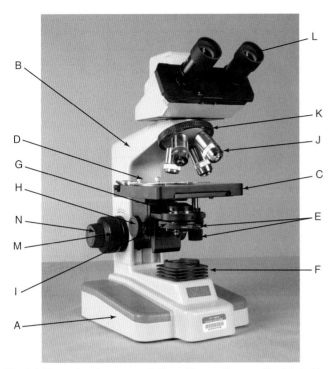

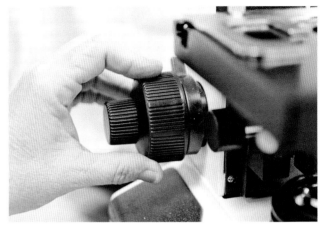

Fig. 3.3 The coarse focus adjustment knob.

Fig. 3.1 Parts of a microscope. **A,** Base; **B,** arm; **C,** stage; **D,** slide holder; **E,** mechanical slide controls; **F,** light source; **G,** condenser; **H,** condenser adjustment; **I,** diaphragm lever; **J,** low-power objective; **K,** nosepiece; **L,** ocular lens; **M,** coarse focus objective; and **N,** fine focus adjustment. (From Garrels M: *Laboratory and diagnostic testing in ambulatory care: a guide for health professionals*, ed 3, St Louis, 2015, Saunders.)

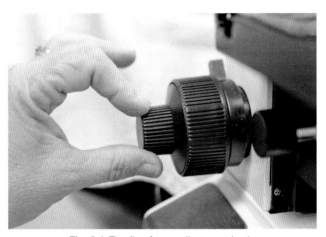

Fig. 3.4 The fine focus adjustment knob.

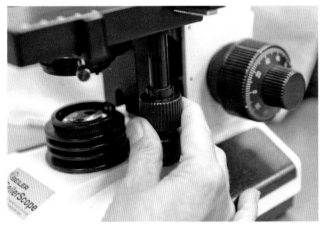

Fig. 3.2 The mechanical stage controls move the stage back and forth, and left to right.

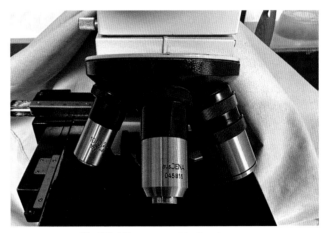

Fig 3.5 Microscope objective lenses.

Most compound light microscopes have three or four objective lenses (Fig 3.5), each with a different magnification power. The most common objective lenses are 4× (scanning), 10× (low power), 40× (high dry), and 100× (oil immersion). The scanning lens is not found on all microscopes. An optional fifth lens, a 50× (low oil immersion), is found on some microscopes. Some microscopes may also have phase-contrast lenses. It is important that only immersion oil designed for microscopy be used on the microscope. Other oils may be damaging to the optics.

Total magnification of the object being viewed is calculated by multiplying the ocular magnification power and the objective magnification power (Fig 3.6). For example, an object

Objective Lens Type	Objective Lens Magnification	Ocular Lens Magnification	Total Magnification	Image Example
Scanning Power	4x	10x	40x	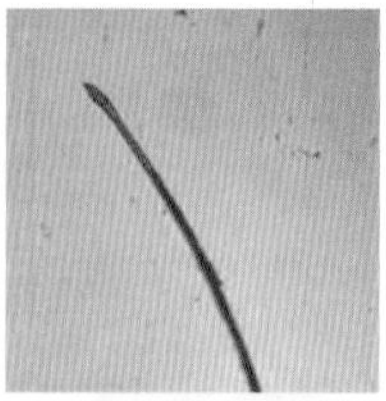
Low Power	10x	10x	100x	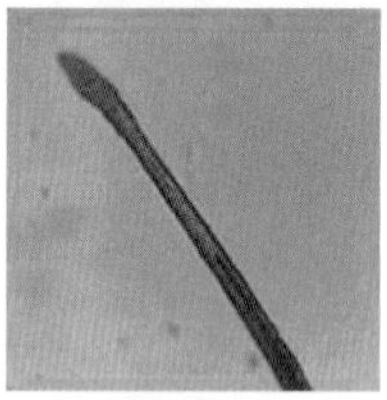
High-Dry Power	40x	10x	400x	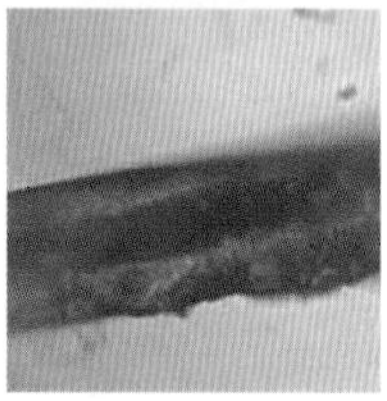
Oil Immersion	100x	10x	1000x	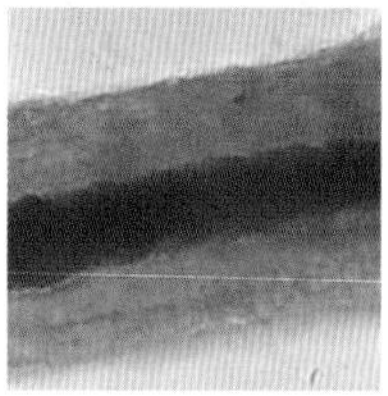

Fig 3.6 Microscopic magnification.

viewed through the 40× objective lens and the 10× ocular lens is 400 times larger in diameter than the unmagnified object:

$$10 \times \text{(ocular lens)} \times 40 \times \text{(objective lens)}$$
$$= 400 \times \text{(total magnification)}$$

> **TECHNICIAN NOTE** Multiply the magnifications of the ocular and objective lenses to obtain the total magnification of the object that you are viewing.

The microscope head supports the ocular lenses and may be straight or inclined. A microscope with an inclined head has ocular lenses that point back toward the user. This minimizes the need to bend over the microscope to look through the lenses. A binocular head is needed for nearly all routine laboratory evaluations. Trinocular heads are also available and can be used for training purposes or client education. The nosepiece holds the objective lenses. It should always rotate easily and provide ready access to the objective lenses for cleaning. The ocular lenses must be compatible with the objective lenses in use, so be cautious about buying objectives and oculars from different sources. Wide-field objective lenses provide a larger visual field area than the standard type and are recommended

when the user spends long periods looking through the microscope, because they tend to reduce fatigue. High-eyepoint ocular lenses are for individuals who need or prefer to keep their eyeglasses on while using the microscope; however, those who do not wear eyeglasses may find these lenses to be advantageous as well.

The most important components of the microscope are the objective lenses. Objective lenses are characterized as one of three types: achromatic, semi-apochromatic, and apochromatic. The latter two are primarily used in research settings and for photomicrography. A type of achromatic lens known as planachromatic lens is also available. This lens type, which is also referred to as flat field lens, provides a more uniform field of focus from the center to the periphery of the microscopic image. However, high-quality achromatic lenses are also acceptable for most routine veterinary uses.

The resolving power of the microscope is an indicator of image quality and is described with the term numerical aperture (NA). The most common type of condenser is the two-lens Abbe type. The NA of the condenser should be equal to or greater than the NA of the highest power objective. The NA or resolving power of the lens system will be no greater than the NA of the highest power objective. This is especially important for objectives with NA greater than 1.0. To obtain the highest resolution from these objectives, a condenser of 1.0 or greater must be used, and the condenser must be raised so that it makes contact with the bottom of the slide. Otherwise, air—which has an NA of 1.0—will be part of the system, thereby relegating the system to a maximal resolution of 1.0.

When viewed through a compound light microscope, an object appears upside down and reversed. The actual right side of an image is seen as its left side, and the actual left side is seen as its right side. Movement of the slide by the mechanical stage also is reversed. Travel knobs are used to move the glass slide and thus the object (or portion of the object) to be moved. When the stage is moved to the left, the object appears to move to the right.

The substage condenser consists of two lenses that focus light from the light source on the object being viewed. Light is focused by raising or lowering the condenser (Fig. 3.7). Without a substage condenser, halos and fuzzy rings appear around objects. The aperture diaphragm is usually an iris type, which consists of a number of leaves that are opened or closed to control the amount of light illuminating the object (Fig. 3.8).

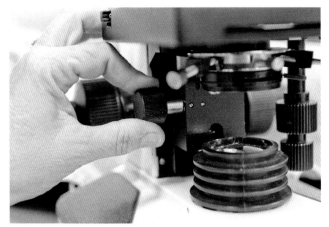

Fig. 3.7 The substage condenser control is used to raise and lower the stage to allow light to be focused through the sample.

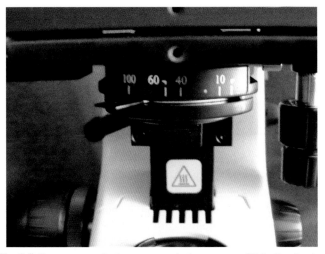

Fig. 3.8 The aperture diaphragm controls the amount of light illuminating the object.

In modern microscopes, the light source is contained within the microscope. The most common light sources found on compound light microscopes are low-voltage tungsten lamps, higher-quality quartz-halogen lamps, and light-emitting diode (LED) light. The light source can be in the base or separate, and it should have a rheostat to adjust intensity. Many older clinical microscopes that are currently in use contain filament light sources (generally halogen or tungsten) and are configured for Köhler illumination. To obtain high-quality images, the microscope must be adjusted for proper Köhler illumination (Box 3.1). Koehler illumination is a process that provides optimum contrast and resolution by focusing and centering the light path and spreading it evenly over the field of view.

Microscope prices vary depending on their quality and the accessories included. The best microscope for a typical practice is most often neither the most expensive nor the least expensive one. Accessories such as dual-viewing options, phase-contrast or darkfield capabilities, digital cameras, and lighted pointers add to the price but also increase the versatility of the microscope (and the diagnostic laboratory). Reconditioned microscopes are sometimes available through medical or optical equipment suppliers and are an economical alternative to the purchase of a new microscope.

CARE AND MAINTENANCE

Regardless of the features of the individual microscope, care must be taken to follow the manufacturer's recommendations for use and routine maintenance (Procedure 3.1). Only high-quality lens tissue should be used to clean the lenses. If a cleaning solvent is needed, methanol can be used, or a specially formulated lens-cleaning solution can be purchased. Excess oil may require the use of xylene for cleaning. However, xylene

---

BOX 3.1 Adjusting the Microscope for Köhler Illumination

1. Secure the slide on the microscope stage.
2. Adjust the light source to approximately half of its total brightness.
3. Place the 10× ocular lens in position.
4. Verify that the eyepiece is at the correct interpupillary distance and that it is focused.
5. Focus on the specimen using the coarse adjustment knob.
6. Close the field diaphragm and condenser until a small ring of light is visible in the field of view through the specimen.
7. If needed, adjust the condenser screws until the light is centered in the field of view.
8. Open the diaphragm until the circle of light just touches the edge of the circumference of the field of view.
9. Adjust the condenser until the light is in sharp focus. This may make the image darker, so adjust the brightness to compensate.
10. Repeat the procedure for each of the ocular objectives.

NOTE: For dry mounted slides like cytology and blood smears, adjust the condenser as high as it will go and set the aperture diaphragm to 100×; use a bright light for best visualization. For wet mounted slides with a coverslip (urine sediment, fecal exams), lower the condenser a bit and set the aperture diaphragm to 4× with lower light. This will increase your contrast and allow you to see more.

PROCEDURE 3.1   Operating the Microscope

1. Lower the stage to its lowest point.
2. Turn on the light.
3. Inspect the eyepieces, the objective lenses, and the condenser lens, and clean them as necessary. (Consult the manufacturer's operating manual for any special cleaning instructions.)
4. Place the slide on the stage, with the appropriate side facing up.
5. Move the 10× objective lens into position by turning the nosepiece turret (rather than the objective lens).

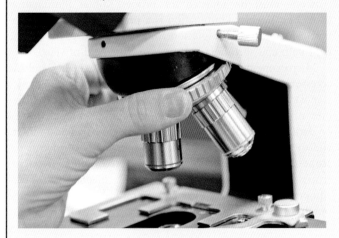

6. While looking through the eyepieces, adjust the distance between them so that the two fields appear to be nearly identical and can be viewed as one.

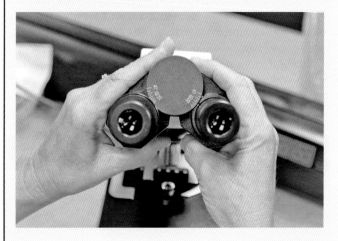

7. Use the coarse and fine focus knobs to bring the image into focus.
8. Adjust the condenser and diaphragm in accordance with the manufacturer's instructions. This allows one to take full advantage of the microscope's resolving power.
9. When using the 40× (high-dry) objective lens:
   - Look for a suitable examination area using the 10× (low-power) objective lens.
   - Rotate the nosepiece to move the high-dry objective lens into place.
   - Use the fine adjustment knob to focus on the image.
   - Do not use oil on the slide when using the high-dry objective lens.
   - Do not use the coarse adjustment knob to focus on the specimen while the high-power lens is in place.

   NOTE: If you are unable to focus the microscope at this magnification after success at lower magnifications, check to see if your microscope slide is upside down. Your sample should be on facing the objective, not the stage.
10. When using the 100× (oil-immersion) objective lens:
    - Locate a suitable examination area using the 10× (low-power) objective lens.
    - Rotate the nosepiece to move the high-power objective lens into place, and refocus on the area with the fine adjustment knob.
    - Rotate the nosepiece so that it is halfway between the high-power and oil-immersion objective lenses.
    - Place a drop of immersion oil on the slide.
    - Rotate the nosepiece to bring the oil-immersion lens into place.
    - Use the fine adjustment knob to focus on the image.
    - Do not use the coarse adjustment knob to focus on the specimen while the oil-immersion lens is in place.
11. When finished:
    - Turn the light off.
    - Lower the stage completely.
    - Rotate the nosepiece to move the low-power objective lens into place.

    NOTE: Do NOT drag lower magnification lens through oil.
    - Remove the specimen from the stage.
    - Clean the oil-immersion lens, if necessary.
    - Cover the microscope.

may also dissolve some of the adhesives that are used to secure the objective lenses and must therefore be used sparingly. Note that methanol and xylene are flammable and toxic. The microscope should be wiped clean after each use and kept covered when not in use. A dirty field of study may be caused by debris on the eyepiece. The eyepieces should be rotated one at a time while the technician looks through them. If the debris also rotates, it is located on the eyepiece. The eyepiece is cleaned with lens paper. Cleaning and adjustment by a microscope professional should be performed at least annually.

> **TECHNICIAN NOTE** Always move objectives into place by turning the nosepiece of the microscope rather than the lenses.

Extra light bulbs should be available. Changing a light bulb requires turning off the power and unplugging the microscope. When the defective bulb has cooled, it should be removed and replaced with a new bulb according to the manufacturer's instructions. Replacement bulbs should be identical to those that they are replacing. Avoid touching the replacement bulb directly, because oils from the skin can shorten the life of some types of bulbs.

Locate the microscope in an area where it is protected from excessive heat and humidity. With proper care, a high-quality microscope can last a lifetime. The microscope should be placed in an area where it cannot be moved frequently, jarred by vibrations from centrifuges or slamming doors, or splashed with liquids. It must be kept away from sunlight and drafts. The microscope is carried with both hands, with one hand securely under the base and the other holding the supporting arm.

CALIBRATION OF THE MICROSCOPE

The size of various stages of parasites is often important for their correct identification. Some examples are the eggs of *Trichuris vulpis* versus the eggs of *Capillaria* species and the microfilariae of *Dirofilaria immitis* versus the microfilariae of *Dipetalonema reconditum*. Calibration of the microscope lenses should be performed on every microscope that is used in the laboratory. Each objective lens must be individually calibrated (Procedure 3.2).

The stage micrometer is a microscope slide etched with a 2-mm line marked in 0.01-mm (10-μm) divisions (Fig. 3.9); 1 micrometer (μm) equals 0.001 mm. The stage micrometer is used only once to calibrate the objectives of the microscope. After the ocular micrometer within the compound microscope has been calibrated at 4×, 10×, and 40×, it is calibrated for the service life of the microscope; the stage micrometer is never

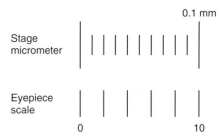

Fig. 3.9 The stage micrometer is a microscope slide etched with a 2-mm line marked in 0.01-mm (10-μm) divisions. (From Samples OM, et al: *McCurnin's clinical textbook for veterinary technicians and nurses,* ed 10, St. Louis, 2022, Elsevier.)

used again. The stage micrometer should therefore be borrowed from a university or other diagnostic laboratory rather than purchased.

The ocular micrometer is a glass disk that fits into one of the microscope eyepieces. It is sometimes referred to as a reticle. The disks impose an image of a net, scale, or crosshairs over the viewing area. The reticle should be mounted in a separate ocular lens that can be removed and replaced with a nonreticle assembly for times when the scale is not needed. The disk is etched with 30 hatch marks that are spaced at equal intervals. The number of hatch marks on the disk may vary, but the calibration procedure does not change. The stage micrometer is used to determine the distance in micrometers between the hatch marks on the ocular micrometer for each objective lens of the microscope being calibrated. This information is recorded and labeled on the base of the microscope for future reference.

DIGITAL MICROSCOPY

Digital microscopes use optics and a camera to capture images and display them on a computer screen or monitor. There are a large number of models available that vary widely in quality and price. The most inexpensive models have small monitors in place of the eyepieces of the microscope. These also tend to have the poorest image quality. Microscopes that connect to a computer via a USB cable incorporate digital imaging technology similar to that of a standard digital camera and tend to provide high-quality images.

Capturing Digital Images

Digital microscopy can greatly enhance practice record keeping and become a valuable tool for client education and staff training. Obtaining photomicrographs of abnormalities seen on blood films or tissue cytology preparations, parasite evaluations, urine sediment evaluations, and similar diagnostic tests can be used to document findings in a patient medical record.

Photomicrographs can also be added to electronic patient records as a simple way to permanently document diagnoses. Digital images can be used to share patient information during consultations with other veterinary professionals and to create a library of images for teaching purposes.

PROCEDURE 3.2 Calibrating the Microscope

1. Start at low power (10×), and focus on the 2-mm line if using the stage micrometer. The 2-mm mark equals 2000 μm.
2. Rotate the ocular micrometer within the eyepiece so that its hatch-mark scale is horizontal and parallel to the stage micrometer (see Fig. 3.9).
3. Align the 0 points on both scales.
4. Determine the point on the stage micrometer that is aligned with the 10 hatch mark on the ocular micrometer. (In Fig. 3.9, this point is at 0.100 mm on the stage micrometer.)
5. Multiply this number by 100. In this example, 0.100 × 100 = 10 μm. This means that, at this power (10×), the distance between each hatch mark on the ocular micrometer is 10 μm. Any object may be measured with the ocular micrometer scale; the chosen distance is measured by multiplying the number of ocular units by a factor of 10. For example, if an object is 10 ocular units long, then its true length is 100 μm (10 ocular units × 10 μm = 100 μm).
6. Repeat this procedure at each magnification.
7. For each magnification, record this information and place it on a label on the base of the microscope for future reference. The ocular micrometer within the microscope is now calibrated for the duration.

Objective distance between hatch marks (micrometers):
    4×: 25 μm
    10×: 10 μm
    40×: 2.5 μm

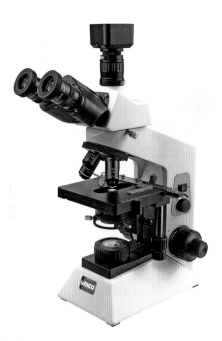

Fig. 3.10 A trinocular head microscope (UNICO Microscope) with an attached digital camera. (Courtesy VetLab Supply, Palmetto Bay, FL.)

> **TECHNICIAN NOTE** Photomicrographs can be added to the patient's record to document findings.

Digital microscopy has become more affordable for even a small practice. Common types of digital systems include those incorporated into a digital microscope, those that attach to the third eyepiece of a trinocular microscope (Fig. 3.10), and those that replace one of the eyepieces on a standard binocular microscope. Some of the systems incorporate a small viewing screen in addition to the ability to interface with a computer screen or monitor. Although it is possible to obtain adapter attachments for a microscope eyepiece that allow a standard handheld digital camera to be used to obtain photomicrographs, some newer cameras cannot be used in this way, and the cost of the adapters may make this method prohibitive. Computer software is also included with digital microscopy systems that allow images to be categorized and archived. The systems are capable of capturing the images in standard image formats (e.g., .jpg, .bmp, .tiff). Some of these programs are capable of directly exporting the images to a photo-editing program.

Regardless of the type used, these systems are nearly all capable of capturing video in addition to still images. Most of the systems also have the flexibility to allow for projection of the images in real time onto a computer screen or monitor. This can also serve as a training tool for new staff members by allowing multiple individuals to view the microscopic images as the veterinary technician is performing a microscopic evaluation. Real-time streaming of these images on the Internet may also be possible, and this can greatly enhance consultations with other veterinary professionals.

Resolution

Digital microscopy systems vary with regard to their image resolution capabilities. The term resolution refers to the degree of detail visible in the images and the clarity of the image. Resolution is measured in pixels, with the highest resolution number providing the greatest detail and clarity. The greater the number of pixels, the greater the degree of detail and clarity and the more the image can be enlarged without loss of clarity. There are two primary types of digital imaging methods, and these use different types of image sensors. The charge-coupled device (CCD) and the complementary metal–oxide–semiconductor (CMOS) image sensors vary in the degree of sharpness of the images that they produce. CCD cameras are recommended because they tend to provide a higher-quality image than a comparable CMOS camera at the same resolution. In addition, a CMOS camera may not allow for the smooth projection of images in real time. The resolution of a particular image is limited by the resolution of the output device used, such as the computer screen or monitor being used to display the image. A resolution of 2 megapixels is generally sufficient for printing images up to 5" × 7" without any loss of clarity. A higher resolution will be needed for images that will be published.

Types of Systems

Digital microscopes that incorporate a digital camera and include software to download and save images to a computer are generally compatible with Windows operating systems. These integrated systems tend to be a great deal more costly than purchasing a separate camera to attach to a standard binocular or trinocular clinical microscope. However, they do have the advantage of always being ready, and they generally capture images quickly. The very busy practice laboratory may find the higher cost worthwhile. A variety of less expensive types of digital cameras are available for photomicroscopy and can be added to a standard clinical microscope. Digital cameras attached to trinocular microscopes are the most efficient. The camera attachment is mounted to the third eyepiece, and the system is attached to a computer, most often via a USB attachment. Some systems will instead contain an integrated media device (e.g., an SD card) that can be removed for the transfer of images to a computer. When the veterinary technician encounters an abnormality to be photographed, these systems can perform the needed functions very quickly.

Eyepiece cameras that attach to a binocular microscope usually involve the removal of one of the microscope eyepieces and replacing it with the eyepiece camera for the capturing of images directly onto a computer (Fig. 3.11). These systems are highly cost-effective, but they tend to take slightly longer to use.

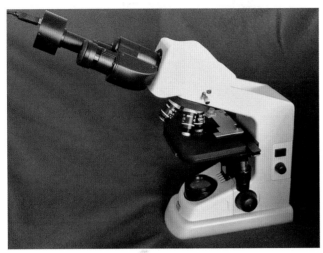

Fig. 3.11 A digital eyepiece camera in place on a clinical microscope.

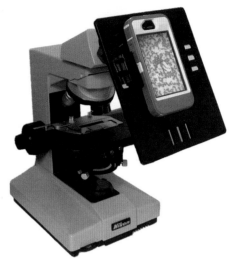

Fig. 3.13 The miPlatform system for obtaining photomicrographs using a smartphone or tablet. (Courtesy VetLab Supply, Palmetto Bay, FL.)

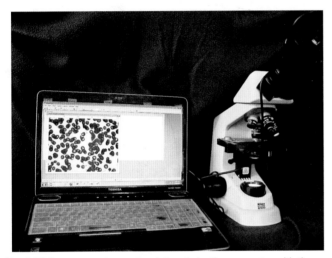

Fig. 3.12 Images can be captured directly by the computer with the use of the software provided by the camera manufacturer.

evaluation. Attachments are also available that can allow a smartphone or tablet to be attached to an eyepiece for the capture of photomicrographs (Fig. 3.13).

Quality

It is important that the microscope used to obtain photomicrographs has high-quality optics. The overall quality of digital photomicrographs is greatly influenced by the quality of the microscope optics. The microscope should have planachromatic (flat field) objective lenses. If the microscope requires Köhler illumination, be sure to adjust this before attempting to capture images. Without proper illumination and adjustments, the image may appear to be unevenly illuminated, and this may result in bright and dark areas or shadows on the image. Newer clinical microscopes that make use of LED light sources tend to produce the highest-quality images as a result of the enhanced color balance and greater stability of the light output achievable with these light sources. Regardless of the type of microscope used, it is essential that the microscope be professionally serviced at least annually.

When the veterinary technician encounters an image to be recorded, one of the microscope eyepieces is removed, the camera is put in its place, and the image is captured by the computer (Fig. 3.12). The technician then removes the camera and replaces the eyepiece to continue the remainder of the

▋ KEY POINTS

- The clinical laboratory must have at least one high-quality binocular compound light microscope.
- The clinical microscope should have a focusable substage condenser and a mechanical stage.
- The proper care and use of the microscope are essential to ensure accurate results.

- The calibration of the microscope is needed to allow for the accurate measurement of cells or organisms that may be present in samples.
- Digital microscopy can enhance the veterinary practice's record keeping, client education, and staff training.

4

The Metric System and Lab Calculations

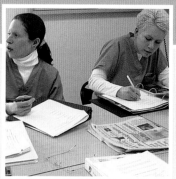

Photo from Bassert JM, McCurnin DM: *McCurnin's clinical textbook for veterinary technicians*, ed 7, St Louis, 2010, Saunders.

LEARNING OBJECTIVES

After studying this chapter, you will be able to:
- Explain basic mathematical principles, such as decimals, multiplication, division, and ratios.
- Perform calculations related to dilutions.
- Describe and utilize metric units and the International System of Units.
- Perform calculations to convert between Fahrenheit and Celsius measurements.

OUTLINE

KEY TERMS

Dilutions
Gram
International System of Units

Liter
Metric system
Ratio

Serial dilution

Veterinary technicians require knowledge and skill at performing a variety of calculations in the clinical laboratory. Reagent solutions may need to be prepared or diluted, samples must be measured and sometimes diluted, and results must be calculated. All of these mathematical operations require that the veterinary technician have a thorough understanding of the metric system as well as a strong background in basic algebra.

NUMBERING SYSTEMS

Abstract numbers are those with no unit designations. Concrete numbers have a specific unit value, such as dollars or pounds. A number without a designation (unit) is an abstract or pure number. A number that designates a specific value (e.g., grams) is a concrete or denominate number. Numbers of different denominations cannot be used together in mathematical operations. When numbers of different denominations must be manipulated mathematically, you must convert all of the numbers to the same designation. Numbers may be whole numbers, fractions, or mixed numbers.

The Metric System

Although several systems of measurement are used in veterinary medicine, most of the calculations performed in veterinary practice involve the units of the metric system. The metric system uses powers of 10 as a base for different units in the system.

The metric system is a decimal system of notation with only three basic units for weight, volume, and length. Various values can be expressed in the metric system by adding prefixes to the basic units that designate multiples or fractions of the basic units. To work in the metric system, some of the more commonly used prefixes and their abbreviations must be memorized.

TABLE 4.1 Prefixes for the Multiples and Submultiples of Basic Units

Power of 10	Prefix	Symbol
10^{12}	tera-	T
10^{9}	giga-	G
10^{6}	mega-	M
10^{3}	kilo-	K
10^{2}	hecto-	h
10^{1}	deca- or deka-	da
10^{-1}	deci-	d
10^{-2}	centi-	c
10^{-3}	milli-	m
10^{-6}	micro-	mc or μ
10^{-9}	nano-	n
10^{-12}	pico-	p
10^{-15}	femto-	f
10^{-18}	atto-	a

The three basic units of measure are summarized here:

Measurement	Unit	Symbol
Length	Meter	m
Mass	Gram	g
Volume	Liter	l or L

The metric system uses multiples or powers of 10 to describe magnitudes that are more or less than the basic units of meter, gram, and liter. The prefixes for the multiples and submultiples of the basic units are provided in Table 4.1. For example, 1 kilogram is 1000 grams, and a milligram is $^1/_{1000}$ of a gram. In addition, 100 centimeters is 1 meter, and 1000 meters is 1 kilometer. With regard to volume, there are 10 deciliters in 1 liter, 10 liters in 1 decaliter, and 10 decaliters in 1 hectoliter. Consistency is important in all use of numbers, but especially in the metric system. Although the unit gram may be abbreviated as gm or Gm, the correct use is g.

> **TECHNICIAN NOTE** The basic units of the metric system are the gram, the meter, and the liter.

To minimize errors and the misinterpretations of numbers, a few general rules for the use of the metric system must be learned. The one rule that is most often encountered is the unit equivalence of the cubic centimeter and the milliliter. In the metric system, these two units are both used for volume, and they designate the same volume. This is because the metric measure of a liter is defined as a volume of 1000 cubic centimeters (cc) or a volume of 10 cm × 10 cm × 10 cm. Although the terms *milliliter* and *cubic centimeter* are often used interchangeably, milliliter is the correct designation for use in medicine.

Any decimal number that has no whole number to the left of the decimal point must have a zero inserted as a placeholder.

Zeroes should not be added after decimal numbers, to avoid confusion in medication orders. Fractions are not written in the metric system. Always use decimal numbers to express numbers that are less than 1.

> **TECHNICIAN NOTE** Decimal numbers that have no whole number to the left of the decimal point must have a zero inserted as a placeholder to the left of the decimal.

The International System of Units

The National Institute of Standards and Technology is a U.S. government agency that promotes the use of the International System of Units. This system is derived from the French Le Système International d'Unités and is abbreviated SI. SI units are designated for seven different types of measurements: length, mass, time, electric current, temperature, luminosity, and quantity. In the veterinary clinical laboratory, the SI units of importance are those for mass, temperature, and quantity. The SI unit of mass is the kilogram; temperature is reported in kelvins and quantity as moles. The Clinical and Laboratory Standards Institute is an international agency that publishes guidelines for the use of SI units. It is important to know the units in which a particular test result is reported. For example, we have traditionally reported serum glucose results in mg/dL, and a normal value for dogs could be 90 mg/dL. The Clinical and Laboratory Standards Institute guidelines designate the reporting of glucose results in mmol/L, and a normal value could be 5 mmol/L.

Dilutions

The veterinary technician may be asked to prepare dilutions of reagents or patient samples in the clinical laboratory. Concentrations of dilutions are usually expressed as ratios of the original volume to the new volume. A ratio is the amount of one thing relative to another or the number of parts relative to a whole. Ratios may be written in a number of ways; for example, $^1/_2$, 1 : 2, and 0.5 are all equivalent. These terms express the ratio that means "one in two," "one to two," or "one half." All three ratios are equal. The terms of a ratio are either abstract numbers (i.e., no units) or of the same units. The only ratio that is usually expressed as a decimal in veterinary technology is specific gravity. Specific gravity is a ratio expressed in decimal form that represents the weight of a substance relative to the weight of the same volume of water.

To prepare a 1 : 10 dilution of a patient sample, combine 10 microliters (μL) of the sample with 90 μL of distilled water. This represents a dilution that is 10 : 100, which reduces mathematically to 1 : 10. Results from any tests involving this 1 : 10 dilution must then be multiplied by 10 to yield the correct result for the undiluted sample.

> **TECHNICIAN NOTE** Ratios indicate the amount of one thing relative to another or the number of parts relative to a whole.

Serial dilutions are sometimes needed when performing certain immunologic tests or when preparing manual calibration curves for some equipment. The dilutions are prepared as described previously, and the concentrations of substances in each dilution are calculated. For example, if a standard solution of bilirubin contains 20 mg/dL and is diluted 1:5, 1:10, and 1:20, then the concentration of each dilution would be 4 mg/dL, 2 mg/dL, and 1 mg/dL, respectively.

Scientific Notation

Scientific notation is a method of handling very large or very small numbers. The manipulation of numbers with the use of scientific notation is sometimes easier when the numbers have many decimal places. Certain laboratory tests are reported with results given in scientific notation. Scientific notation involves the use of exponents to represent powers of 10 for a given number.

> **TECHNICIAN NOTE** Very large or very small numbers are usually written in scientific notation.

Powers of 10 may mean multiplying or dividing by 10:

$$10^0 = 1$$
$$10^1 = 10$$
$$10^2 = 10 \times 10 = 100$$

The steps that are used to convert a number into its exponential form for scientific notation are as follows:
1. Move the decimal point so that the first term is more than 1 and less than 10.
2. The second term is a power of 10 that is equal to the number of times that the decimal point was moved.
3. The sign (+ or −) determines the direction in which to move the decimal. The use of + means that the decimal point was moved to the left; the use of − means that the decimal point was moved to the right.

For example, to convert 6,097,000 to scientific notation, the following steps occur:
1. Move the decimal point to the left so that is behind the 6.
2. Record the first term as 6.097.
3. Count the number of places that the decimal point was moved.
4. Record the number of places as the exponent.
5. The correct answer would be given as 6.097×10^6.

To convert a number from scientific notation, simply move the decimal point the number of places indicated by the exponent. For example, to convert 32.3×10^2, move the decimal place two spaces to the right to get 3230. For negative exponents, the decimal place would be moved to the left. For example, 32.3×10^{-2} would be 0.323.

pH and Logarithms

Logarithmic notation is related to scientific notation, and it has some applications in veterinary medicine. Certain laboratory tests (e.g., pH) and some clinical chemistry analyzers involve the use of logarithmic notation. Like scientific notation, logarithmic notation is used to simplify the manipulation of very large or very small numbers. Logarithmic notation expresses numbers as powers of 10. For example, the number 150 is expressed as $10^{2.1761}$, and it can also be written as log 150, because log 150 = 2.1761.

The pH scale is an example of a practical application of logarithmic notation. pH is defined as the negative logarithm of the hydrogen ion (H^+) concentration of a solution. A solution with an H^+ concentration of 10^{-6} has a pH of 6. A solution with an H^+ concentration of 10^{-7} has a pH of 7 and is considered a neutral solution. A pH of less than 7 indicates an acid solution; a pH of more than 7 indicates an alkaline or basic solution. Note that the difference between any two consecutive numbers on the pH scale represents a power of 10 difference in H^+ concentration. Another common application of logarithms is the Richter scale. This scale is used to characterize the intensity of earthquakes, and each consecutive number on the scale represents a power of ten difference in the intensity or strength of the earthquake.

> **TECHNICIAN NOTE** A pH of 7 is neutral. A pH of less than 7 is acidic, and a pH of more than 7 is alkaline.

Temperature Conversions

The most used temperature measurement system in the veterinary clinical laboratory is the Celsius scale. However, many items (e.g., test kits) may provide critical temperature measurements using the Fahrenheit or Kelvin systems, including such information as proper storage temperatures for reagents or the correct temperature for performing a particular test.

There are several different calculations that may be used for conversions among the various temperature scales. All of these calculations are based on the fact that there are points of equivalence among the three systems.

Points of Equivalence
1. Absolute zero K = −273° C = −459.4° F
2. −40° C = −40° F
3. 0° C = 32° F

In the Fahrenheit scale, water freezes (or ice melts) at 32° and boils at 212°. In the Celsius scale, the difference between the freezing (melting) and boiling points is 100°. Therefore, each degree in the Celsius scale is equivalent to 1.8 or ⁹⁄₅ degrees in the Fahrenheit scale. By using the points of equivalence, it is possible to derive a number of different equations that will allow for the conversion of a thermometer reading from one scale to another. You may use whichever method you find easiest.

$$1. \quad \frac{(C + 273)}{(F + 459.4)} = \frac{5}{9}$$

This equation can be used to convert a value to either Celsius or Fahrenheit, provided that the other is known.

These equations are based on the point of equivalence of −40 in both systems:

2. $F = \frac{9}{5}(C + 40) - 40$

   $C = \frac{5}{9}(F + 40) - 40$

These equations are based on the point of equivalencies of 0° C and 32° F:

3. $C = \frac{5}{9}(F - 32)$

   $F = 32\frac{9}{5}C$

The Kelvin scale begins at absolute zero and so has no negative numbers. Converting to kelvins is accomplished by adding 273 to the temperature in Celsius. Temperatures reported as kelvins do not involve the use of the term degrees; rather, only the letter K is used. For example, 30° C = 303 K.

KEY POINTS

- Metric system units are used in clinical laboratory measurements.
- Laboratory results are reported in either metric system units or SI units.
- Temperature measurements are made in degrees Fahrenheit, degrees Celsius, or kelvins.

- Very small or very large numbers are written with scientific notation.
- Concentrations of dilutions are usually expressed as ratios of the original volume to the new volume.
- The terms of a ratio are either abstract numbers (i.e., no units) or of the same units.

5

Quality Control and Record Keeping

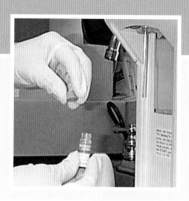

KEY TERMS

Accuracy
Controls
Hemolyzed
Icteric

Lipemic
Preanalytic variables
Precision
Quality assurance

Reliability
Standard operating procedures
Standards

The term quality assurance refers to the procedures established to ensure that clinical testing is performed in compliance with accepted standards and that the processes and results are properly documented. Unlike human medical laboratories, veterinary facilities are not subject to regulations that require quality assurance programs. However, without a comprehensive quality assurance program, the accuracy and precision of laboratory test results cannot be verified. A comprehensive quality assurance program addresses all aspects of the operation of the clinical laboratory. These aspects include the qualifications of laboratory personnel; standard operating procedures (SOPs) for the care and use of all supplies and equipment; sample collection and handling procedures; the methods and frequency of the performance of quality control assays; and record-keeping procedures.

ACCURACY, PRECISION, AND RELIABILITY

Accuracy, precision, and reliability are terms that are frequently used to describe quality control, and they are the standards for any quality control program. Accuracy refers to how closely results agree with the true quantitative value of the constituent. Precision is the magnitude of random errors and the reproducibility of measurements. Reliability is the ability of a method to be accurate and precise. Factors that affect accuracy and precision are test selection, test conditions, sample quality, technician skill, electrical surges, and equipment maintenance.

The term test selection refers to the principle of the test method. Many of the tests used in veterinary laboratories were adapted from human medical laboratory tests. In addition, the clinical significance of test results may vary among different species. Regardless of the test method used, care must be taken to follow the analytic procedure exactly; any deviation can seriously affect the accuracy of results. Sample quality also greatly affects the quality of test results. Samples that are lipemic, icteric, or hemolyzed may require special handling before use with most clinical analyzers. The collection of blood samples from properly fasted animals using appropriate techniques and equipment will minimize this significant source of error.

> **TECHNICIAN NOTE** Careful attention to proper sample collection methods will help to ensure accurate hematology results.

Although they are not an obvious source of error, electrical power surges and dropouts can significantly alter equipment function. Repeated surges shorten the life of light sources in diagnostic equipment. All electrical equipment should be connected to a device designed to protect it from surges and electrical dropouts. Human error is perhaps the most difficult testing parameter to control. Personnel responsible for the performance of clinical testing must be appropriately trained in test principles and procedures. Mechanisms should be in place to provide for the continual education of all clinical laboratory personnel. The maintenance of equipment must also be included in quality control programs. A regular written schedule of equipment maintenance allows for changes in equipment function to be detected before obvious errors occur. Always follow the manufacturer's recommendations for the routine maintenance of instruments and equipment. The manufacturer will also provide information regarding calibration procedures that may be needed. Standards are nonbiological materials used for calibrating equipment.

ANALYSIS OF CONTROL MATERIALS

Control serum is used for technician and instrument assessment. The production of valid results with control materials ensures that the procedure was performed correctly and that all components (e.g., reagents, equipment) are functioning correctly. Controls are handled exactly as patient test samples are, and they should be regularly assayed (i.e., with each test batch, daily, or weekly) at the same time that patient serum samples are assayed (Fig. 5.1). The frequency of control testing depends on the laboratory's goals. To ensure reliability, control samples must be tested when a new assay is set up, when a new technician runs the test, when a new lot number of reagents is used, or when an instrument is known to perform erratically.

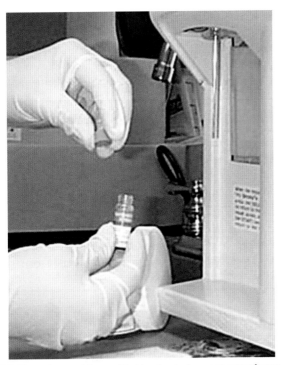

Fig. 5.1 Control materials provided by the instrument manufacturer are assayed in the same manner as a patient sample.

Ideally, a control sample will be tested with each batch of patient samples. A problem with a particular assay may require an increase in the frequency of control testing.

> **TECHNICIAN NOTE** The regular analysis of control materials helps to verify the accuracy of test results.

After the assay is completed, the control value should fall within the manufacturer's reported range. If it does not, the assays of the patient and control samples must be repeated. The results of the analysis of the control serum are recorded on a chart or log for each assay (Fig. 5.2). The values for tests performed on control serum should not vary significantly each time the tests are performed. Data may be analyzed in two ways: via the detection of shifts or trends and via the determination of whether results for control samples are within the range established by the manufacturer. If a control serum result does not fall within the range, it should be retested. If it still fails to fall in the range, the reagents, instruments, and techniques must be checked. When control values are successively distributed on one or the other side of the mean, the mean has shifted, and a systematic error is involved.

Depending on the chemistry analyzer or electronic cell counter in the laboratory, an individual quality control program will involve the use of a number of solutions. Control serum consists of pooled, freeze-dried serum from many patients (usually human) that must be accurately rehydrated before use. Assayed control serum has been analyzed repeatedly for each of the many constituents present in serum (e.g., glucose, urea nitrogen, calcium). Data are statistically analyzed, and a range of acceptable values for each constituent is established. The accepted ranges are specific for each test method and equipment manufacturer. The manufacturer of the control serum provides a chart that lists the range (i.e., the lowest acceptable value to the highest acceptable value obtained during the many assays) and the mean (i.e., the average value) for each constituent.

> **TECHNICIAN NOTE** Controls must be assayed regularly to help verify the accuracy of test results.

Controls with both normal and abnormal concentrations of constituents should be evaluated, because an assay method may not perform the same at all concentrations tested by a particular method. Normal control serum has constituent concentrations that approximate the levels that are normal for that constituent. Abnormal control serum has constituent concentrations that are either higher or lower than normal. These abnormal concentrations represent concentrations that are seen clinically with various disease conditions. If an abnormal concentration of a constituent is found in a patient sample, the results may be trusted if the abnormal control serum concentration was assayed as "in range."

Individual laboratories may produce their own control serum. Serum samples obtained from at least 20 clinically healthy animals of one species are pooled and analyzed

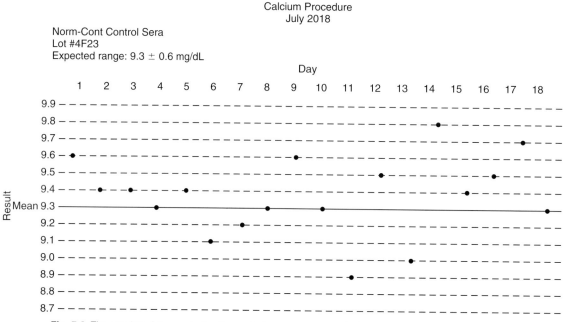

Fig. 5.2 The results of the analysis of a control serum are recorded on a chart or log for each assay.

numerous times in the laboratory. Data collected from these tests can be statistically analyzed to establish appropriate ranges and mean values. This procedure is time consuming, especially for smaller laboratories. For this reason, the purchasing of commercial control sera is much more convenient.

Some manufacturers provide a quality control service in which test samples are sent to many laboratories for assay each month. The results from all of the laboratories are collected and compared. From these results, the manufacturer can identify laboratories with accuracy problems.

ERRORS

Many factors other than disease influence the results of laboratory tests. These factors may be preanalytic, analytic, or postanalytic in nature. Postanalytic factors are primarily related to data entry and record keeping.

Preanalytic Variables

Preanalytic variables may be biologic or nonbiologic. Biologic variables are factors that are inherent to the patient, such as breed, age, and gender. Because these cannot be controlled, they must be considered by the veterinarian when test results are being evaluated. Other biologic variables involve factors that can be controlled when drawing the blood sample, such as ensuring that the animal is properly fasted. Nonbiologic variables are those related to clerical errors as well as sample collection and handling errors. Clerical errors are avoidable and include incorrect labeling, delays in transporting samples, incorrect calculations, transcription errors, and sampling the wrong patient. A well-trained and conscientious staff produces few clerical errors. Some of the most common problems related to sample handling are mislabeling and incomplete or incorrect requisition forms. All tubes, slides, and sample containers should be labeled

with the owner's last name in addition to the patient's name, species, identification number (if available), and date.

Analytic Variables

Analytic variables affect the procedure by which the analyte is measured by the instrument. The specific impact on a test result will differ among laboratories, depending on the type of instrumentation. Improperly maintained instruments can cause errors that are evident as shifts or trends in results obtained with a specific assay method. These errors often result in gradual changes that cause the mean value of results to shift in one direction (i.e., to be elevated or decreased). Some factors that cause systematic errors include inaccurate standard sera, reagent instability, and method nonspecificity (i.e., using a test method that is unsuitable for the constituent being assayed).

> **TECHNICIAN NOTE** The proper maintenance of equipment minimizes analytic errors.

Random errors are caused by variations found in glassware and pipettes, electronic and optic variations of instruments, and variations in temperature controls and timing. These errors occur in all parts of a system and increase the variability of results.

> **TECHNICIAN NOTE** Taking care of laboratory equipment is important and vital to quality results. Read the manuals to ensure proper quality control procedures are performed, daily, weekly, monthly and yearly.

APPLIED QUALITY CONTROL

Instrument maintenance is required to prolong the life of the instrument and to prevent expensive downtime. All instruments are accompanied by an owner's manual. If the manual has been misplaced, the manufacturer should be contacted for a replacement. The manual lists the instrument components that must be inspected and attended to regularly. A notebook that lists a schedule with the types of maintenance required for each instrument facilitates instrument maintenance. A page is dedicated to each instrument and includes the following information:

- Instrument name
- Serial number
- Model number
- Purchase date
- Points to be checked
- Frequency of checks
- Record of test readings
- Changes made to restore the accuracy and precision of readings
- Cost and time associated with necessary repairs and restoration
- Name or initials of the person performing the maintenance Results obtained with control serum are recorded and kept in a permanent record. The veterinary technician should graph results so that changes or trends can be visually detected.

If attention is paid to detail and if as many sources as possible of the three types of errors can be eliminated, then the laboratory can provide reliable results. Sloppy and inattentive work habits can lead to diagnostic and therapeutic disasters that may result in the death of an animal. Careful attention to detail ensures that the veterinarian has all of the correct information needed to make a proper diagnosis, prescribe appropriate treatment, and offer an educated prognosis. Most major manufacturers have carefully constructed manuals for troubleshooting laboratory equipment within the clinic and provide excellent service support when troubleshooting of the equipment is needed.

> **TECHNICIAN NOTE** Poorly maintained equipment with improper quality control is a major cause of in-house laboratory testing not being a trusted source of data in veterinary medicine.

LABORATORY RECORDS

Laboratory records are divided into internal and external record systems. Complete and up-to-date records are necessary for both systems. Numerous computer systems are now available for almost all of the records generated in the veterinary clinic or hospital. Patient information, inventory, ordering information, sales records, and laboratory data can be stored on a computer. Clinics that use computer systems should be sure to keep backup records in case of computer failure or damage from computer viruses.

Internal Records

By using internal records, the laboratory tracks assay results and obtains methods. The records consist of SOPs and quality control data and graphs. The SOPs contain the instructions for all analyses run in the laboratory. Each procedure is described on a separate page. The easiest way to maintain the SOP book is to insert the instruction sheets that accompany each commercial test kit in a three-ring binder along with pages for any other procedures performed in the laboratory. Each procedure not performed with commercial kits is described on a separate page that includes the name of the test, synonyms (if any) for the test, the rationale for the test, the reagent list, and step-by-step instructions for a single analysis. Individual pages can be inserted into plastic overlays for protection. The SOP book is reviewed periodically and updated as needed. Those who keep an SOP book on a computer should make sure that an up-to-date hardcopy backup is available. An excellent format for any SOP is as follows:

- Title — The name of the procedure
- Purpose — Clinical relevance for the procedure
- Specimen — The type of specimen needed along with acceptable preservatives or anticoagulants
- Equipment/Reagents/Supplies — All necessary supplies to complete the procedure
- Quality Control — Detail the quality control materials and appropriate use
- Procedure — Ensure it is a step by step format
- Results — Provide the raw data analysis or calculations used to derive the result
- References — Include any references

External Records

Laboratory personnel communicate with people throughout the veterinary clinic or hospital and in other laboratories through the use of external records. These consist of request forms that accompany the sample to the laboratory, report forms for assay results, laboratory log books with individual test results, and a book that contains pertinent information about samples sent to reference laboratories. In a clinic or hospital with an internal computer network, all personnel can access much of this information as needed.

Information provided on a request form includes the patient's full identification information (including an identification number, if available) as well as the presenting signs, the date, the method used to obtain the sample, the pertinent history, the tests desired, any special notes regarding sample handling, and to whom and by what method (e.g., telephone, fax, e-mail, written report) results are to be reported.

The report form should include complete patient identification and presenting signs, test results (including appropriate units), and the notation of any extraordinary observations or explanatory comments, if applicable. For additional backup, the laboratory staff should keep a logbook to record test results. This way, if the original laboratory report form is lost in transit, the results are retrievable.

> **TECHNICIAN NOTE** It is also important to remember that you should conduct quality control tests on all technical staff as well. It is advisable to monthly confirm the results of their work with other technicians, doctors, or even assayed controls. This can be done by having technicians read samples in house and then send the same samples out to be read by an external company.

KEY POINTS

- Proper quality control procedures are essential to the production of diagnostic quality laboratory results.
- Factors that affect accuracy and precision are test selection, test conditions, sample quality, technician skill, electrical surges, and equipment maintenance.
- The collection of blood samples from properly fasted animals with the use of appropriate techniques and equipment will minimize errors in test results.
- To ensure reliability, control samples must be tested when a new assay is set up, when a new technician runs the test, when a new lot number of reagents is used, or when an instrument is known to perform erratically.
- SOPs and quality control data and graphs are components of the internal records of the clinical laboratory.
- The SOP manual contains the instructions for all analyses run in the laboratory.
- Errors in test results may involve preanalytic, analytic, or postanalytic variables.

Hematology

Unit Outline

Unit Objectives

List and describe the hematology evaluations that are commonly performed in veterinary practice.
Describe the components of blood.
Describe the development of the formed elements in blood.
Describe the appearance of normal blood cells and platelets.
Describe the appearance of commonly seen abnormal blood cells.
List the tests that comprise the complete blood count.
List and describe the equipment needed to perform a complete blood count.
Discuss aspects of quality control related to hematology testing.

Hematology is the science involved with the study of blood cells and their formation. Hematology testing represents an important role of the veterinary technician: providing accurate and reliable clinical laboratory test results to the veterinarian. An understanding of the principles of the various hematology tests and the methods used to ensure the accuracy of results is vital. The recent focus on the economic health of the veterinary clinic has also provided an opportunity for veterinary technicians to perform additional diagnostic testing, to improve overall animal care, and to provide an additional source of revenue for the clinic.

A complete hematology profile is indicated for the diagnostic evaluation of disease states, well-animal screening (e.g., geriatric), and as a screening tool before surgery. The complete blood count includes red and white blood cell counts, hemoglobin concentration, packed cell volume (PCV), a differential white blood film examination, and calculation of absolute values and erythrocyte indices. Additional tests that may be needed include reticulocyte counts, measurement of total solids, and thrombocyte (platelet) estimates. For some patients, additional information about the hematopoietic system is needed, and bone marrow evaluation must be performed. Specific indications include unexplained nonregenerative anemia, leukopenia, thrombocytopenia, and pancytopenia (i.e., decreased numbers of all cell lines). Bone marrow evaluation is also used to confirm certain infections (e.g., ehrlichiosis) and to diagnose hematopoietic neoplasms (e.g., lymphoproliferative disorders).

Please note that normal values are affected by a variety of factors, including the following:

- Testing methods used
- Type of equipment used
- Patient age
- Patient gender
- Breed
- Reproductive status

Laboratories should determine reference ranges for the tests performed in the clinic for the species that are commonly seen.

6

Hematopoiesis

KEY TERMS

Agranulocytes
Erythropoiesis
Erythropoietin
Granulocytes
Hematopoiesis
Left shift

Leukemia
Leukemoid response
Leukocytosis
Leukopoiesis
Lymphopenia
Pancytopenia

Pluripotent stem cell
Thrombocytes
Thrombopoiesis
Thrombopoietin

HEMATOPOIESIS

The term hematopoiesis refers to the production of blood cells and platelets. The body must continuously produce new cells as old cells are used up in the body's processes or age and die.

Whole blood is composed of fluid and cells. The fluid component is plasma. The cellular component is made up of:
- Red blood cells (RBCs), which are also called erythrocytes
- White blood cells (WBCs), also called leukocytes, which can be differentiated into:
  - Granulocytes
    - Neutrophils
    - Eosinophils
    - Basophils
  - Agranulocytes
    - Lymphocytes
    - Monocytes
- Platelets, which are also called thrombocytes (Fig 6.1)

WBCs are further differentiated based on the presence or absence of granules that stain in specific ways. The agranulocytes are the lymphocytes and monocytes. These cells may sometimes contain granules, but only in very small numbers. They are also commonly referred to as mononuclear leukocytes. Granulocytes include the neutrophils, eosinophils, and basophils. The granulocytes are also commonly referred to as polymorphonuclear leukocytes (PMNs), a term that refers to the segmentation or lobulation of the nucleus. However, this term applies specifically to mammals. Nuclear segmentation is less prominent in birds and reptiles.

Blood cells are constantly being produced and have a finite life span (Table 6.1). They must be continually replaced. The life span of blood cells varies among different types of cells and different species of animals. An understanding of the overall process for the production of these components will aid in their evaluation. The process begins during early embryonic life and involves a number of complex chemical pathways and various

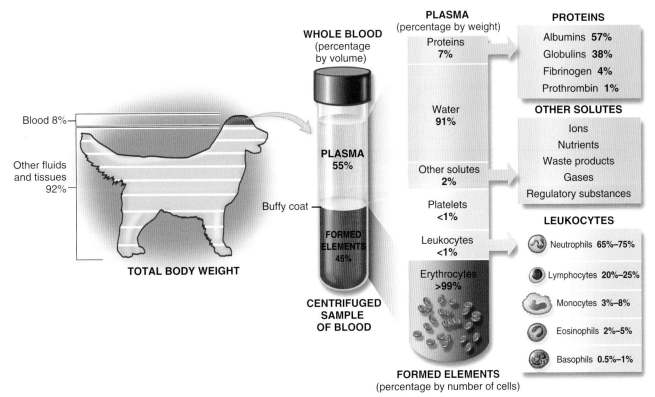

Fig. 6.1 Blood components and the approximate values for the components of blood in a typical, healthy adult. (From Kevin T. Patton, et al: *The human body in health & disease*, ed 8, 2024, Elsevier.)

TABLE 6.1 **Average Life Spans of Blood Cells in Mammals**	
Cell Type	**Life Span in Circulation***
Neutrophils	4–6 hours
Eosinophils	30 minutes
Basophils	4–6 hours
Monocytes	2–3 days
Lymphocytes	Months to years
Erythrocytes	2–5 months
Platelets	4–6 days

*Some species have values that are outside of the averages listed.

organs. Some variations in the process exist between juvenile and adult animals. Hematopoietic activity in the prenatal animal occurs in a variety of organs, including the liver, spleen, thymus, and red bone marrow. Red bone marrow is found in nearly every bone in the fetus and young animal, and it is the primary site for the production of blood cells in the neonatal and juvenile animal.

In the adult animal, the red bone marrow is the primary site for the production and maturation of all of the blood cells and platelets. However, fewer bones contain red bone marrow in adults. In some of the bones, the red marrow is converted to yellow bone marrow, which does not actively produce cells. The marrow is yellow in appearance due to the presence of yellow fat cells. Red marrow is retained primarily in the long bones

(e.g., femur, tibia, humerus, ulna) and the hips, sternum, and ribs. During periods of hematopoietic stress, the liver and spleen may revert to their fetal role and produce blood cells in the adult.

Erythropoiesis (the production of erythrocytes), leukopoiesis (the production of leukocytes), and thrombopoiesis (the production of platelets) involve different pathways and chemical messengers. However, all of the blood cells arise from the same pluripotent hematopoietic stem cells (HSCs). A pluripotent stem cell is capable of developing into various types of cells. Pluripotent HSCs can develop into any of the blood cells. HSCs are capable of regeneration; the numbers of HSCs in bone marrow are relatively small but constant. HSCs initially differentiate into the hematopoietic progenitor cells, which consist of the common myeloid progenitors and the common lymphoid progenitors. The development pathway is determined by interactions with various chemical messengers, which are referred to as cytokines. Specific cytokines are involved in producing each of the types of blood cells. Further differentiation in response to additional cytokines results in commitment to the formation of specific cell types. Nearly two dozen different cytokines have been identified.

TECHNICIAN NOTE Pluripotent HSCs give rise to all of the blood cells.

The common lymphoid progenitors eventually give rise to specific progenitors that develop into the various populations of lymphocytes. A common myeloid progenitor will either

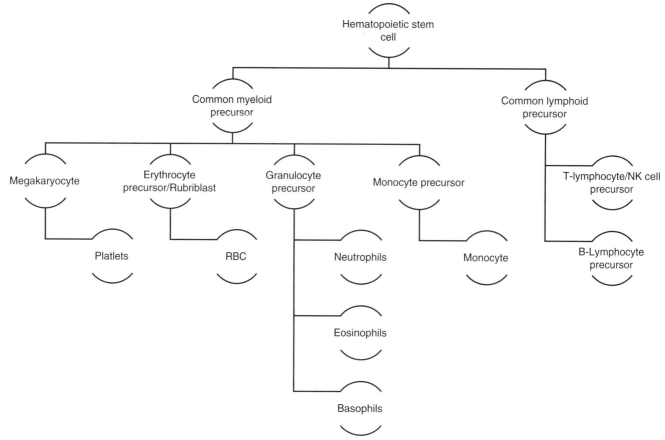

Fig. 6.2 Blood cells arise from pluripotent hematopoietic stem cells.

develop into a megakaryocyte/erythrocyte progenitor or a granulocyte/monocyte progenitor. The megakaryocyte/erythrocyte progenitor then differentiates into either rubriblasts, which give rise to the erythrocytes, or megakaryoblasts, which give rise to platelets. The granulocyte/monocyte progenitor differentiates into either the myeloblast, which gives rise to the granulocytic leukocytes, or the monoblast, which gives rise to the monocytes (Fig. 6.2). Some references refer to the early progenitor lines as colony-forming units and the later stages as blast-forming units. Myeloid cells are relatively large and pale-staining cells, whereas erythroid cells are smaller and have clumped basophilic nuclei.

ERYTHROPOIESIS

The primary cytokine responsible for the production of RBCs is erythropoietin (EPO). EPO is predominantly produced by certain cells in the kidney in response to decreased oxygen tension in the blood. Those kidney cells then produce EPO, which circulates in the blood to the bone marrow. Severe kidney dysfunction can cause anemia due to low EPO production. Lesser amounts of EPO are also produced in hepatocytes. The EPO binds to receptors on the surface of the erythroid precursor cells in the bone marrow, which causes them to divide and mature. After it has been stimulated to develop into an erythrocyte, the cell undergoes additional differentiation into the rubriblast. The rubriblast contains a small round nucleus, one or more nucleoli, and a small amount of basophilic cytoplasm. These cells continue to divide and mature into prorubricytes, then rubricytes, and then metarubricytes. Prorubricytes are smaller than rubriblasts, with a slightly more condensed nucleus and intensely blue cytoplasm. The nucleoli are no longer visible. Cells in the rubricyte stage initially have basophilic cytoplasm and moderate clumping of the nucleus. As the cell matures, the morphologic characteristics of rubricytes are distinguished by marked nuclear clumping and pink cytoplasm because of the incorporation of hemoglobin, which begins during this stage

> **TECHNICIAN NOTE** Erythropoietin is involved in the stimulation of RBC production.

Metarubricytes are the smallest cells in the erythroid series and have a condensed nucleus and deep red cytoplasm. Metarubricytes are not capable of cell division, and hemoglobin formation is completed during this stage. The cell will eventually extrude its nucleus and mature into a reticulocyte. Reticulocytes are immature erythrocytes that contain ribosomal material that is lost as the cell matures (Fig. 6.3). These organelles account for the diffuse blue-gray or polychromatophilic staining of immature cells with Wright's stain. When stained with a supravital stain (e.g., new methylene blue), early reticulocytes demonstrate

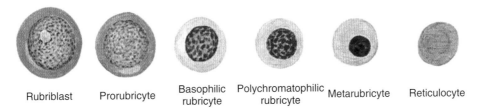

Rubriblast   Prorubricyte   Basophilic   Polychromatophilic   Metarubricyte   Reticulocyte
                                  rubricyte   rubricyte

Fig. 6.3 Maturation of erythrocytes. (Drawing by Perry Bain. In Harvey J: *Veterinary hematology*, St Louis, 2012, Saunders.)

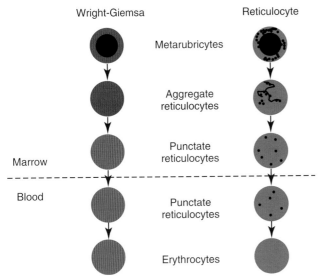

Fig. 6.4 Cat erythroid cells demonstrating reticulocyte release into the blood as it occurs in most normal cats. Note that punctate reticulocytes do not appear polychromatophilic when stained with Wright-Giemsa stain. (From Harvey J: *Veterinary hematology*, St Louis, 2012, Saunders.)

a network or reticulum that appears as aggregated material. This represents the ribosomal material. As the reticulocyte undergoes further maturation, this material decreases and subsequently appears as small dark blue spots. These cells are referred to as punctate reticulocytes (Fig. 6.4). An increase in reticulocytes on a blood smear would then indicate the patient is capable of erythropoiesis and the bone marrow is functioning normally. To summarize the stages of erythropoiesis, they follow the following path:

- Erythroid Precursor Cells
  - Rubriblast
    - ○ Prorubricytes
- Rubricytes
  - Metarubricytes
    - ○ Reticulocyte
- RBC

THROMBOPOIESIS

The stimulus for the production of thrombocytes involves the hormone thrombopoietin as well as numerous additional cytokines. Thrombopoietin is primarily produced in liver endothelial cells, but it is also released from cells in the kidney and other sites. The progenitor cell develops into the megakaryoblast, which contains a single nucleus and dark blue cytoplasm. The cell then develops into the promegakaryocyte, which is a large cell that contains two to four nuclei. The nucleus continues to replicate, and the cell becomes progressively larger until it develops into the megakaryocyte. The mature megakaryocyte has numerous nuclear lobes, and the cytoplasm has reddish granules. The cells are very large (i.e., 50 to 200 μm in diameter), and the cytoplasm extends into marrow sinuses, where it is sheared off by the flow of blood. These sheared fragments are referred to as proplatelets; they eventually fragment further into platelets that are in circulation. To summarize the stages of thrombopoiesis, they are as follows:

- Progenitor Cell (Common Myeloid Precursor)
  - Megakaryoblast
    - ○ Promegakaryocyte
- Megakaryocyte
  - Proplatelets
    - ○ Platelets

TECHNICIAN NOTE Platelets are fragments of the cytoplasm of megakaryocytes.

GRANULOPOIESIS

The stimulus for the production of granulocytes involves the hormone leukopoietin as well as numerous additional cytokines. Cells in the granulocyte series are divided into the proliferation pool, which represents cells that are capable of mitosis, and the maturation pool, which represents cells that are no longer capable of mitosis. The proliferation pool includes myeloblasts, promyelocytes, and myelocytes. The maturation pool includes metamyelocytes and band cells. Myeloblasts are larger than rubriblasts and have a round to oval nucleus, a prominent nucleolus, and pale gray-blue cytoplasm. A few reddish granules may be evident in the cytoplasm. The promyelocyte is a large, pale-staining cell with prominent reddish cytoplasmic granules and no prominent nucleoli. Myelocytes are smaller cells with round nuclei. Granules that are characteristic of the mature neutrophil, eosinophil, and basophil begin to appear during the myelocyte stage. The metamyelocyte is similar in appearance to the myelocyte except that the nucleus is indented. These cells are no longer capable of mitosis. Band cells have horseshoe-shaped nuclei with parallel

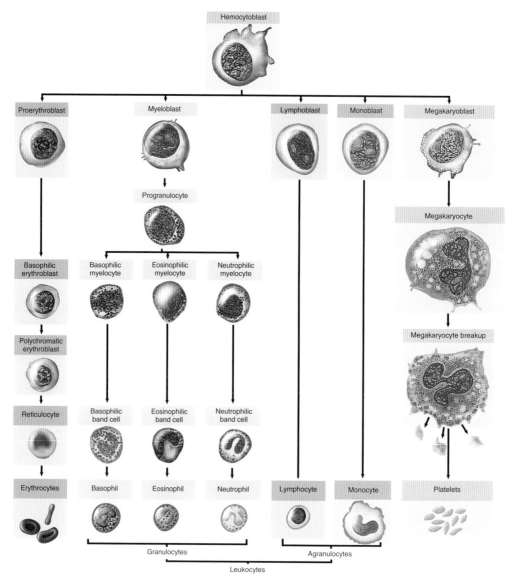

Fig. 6.5 Formation of blood cells. The hematopoietic stem cell serves as the original stem cell from which all formed elements of the blood are derived. Note that all five precursor cells are derived from a stem cell called a hemocytoblast. (From Shiland BJ: Medical assistant: urinary, blood, lymphatic and immune systems with laboratory procedures—Module E, Elsevier Inc. 2005.)

sides. The final stage of maturation produces the mature segmented granulocyte. Nuclei of these cells contain two or more lobes (Fig. 6.5). To summarize the stages of granulopoiesis, they are as follows:
- Myeloblast
  - Promyelocyte
    ○ Myelocyte
    ○ Metamyelocyte
  - Band
    ○ Neutrophils, Basophils, Eosinophils

MONOPOIESIS

Monocyte developmental stages include the monoblast, the promonocyte, and the monocyte. Monoblasts appear similar to myeloblasts except that the nucleus has an irregular shape. Promonocytes appear similar to myelocytes and metamyelocytes. Monocytes may develop into macrophages when

they are exposed to a specific cytokine. However, macrophages are also derived from other sources. To summarize the stages of monopoiesis, they are as follows:
- Monoblast
  - Promonocyte
    ○ Monocyte

TECHNICIAN NOTE Macrophages may be derived from monocytes that are exposed to specific cytokines.

LYMPHOPOIESIS

The production of the various populations of lymphocytes (i.e., T lymphocytes, B lymphocytes, and natural killer [NK] cells) arises from the common lymphoid progenitor and proceeds through the lymphoblast and prolymphocyte stages. The cell is initially differentiated into either a B-lymphocyte precursor or a

T-lymphocyte/NK precursor. Production involves certain cytokines as well as specific antibodies. Juvenile B lymphocytes mature primarily in the bone marrow or in specialized ileal Peyer's patches in dogs, pigs, and ruminants, as well as in the bursa of Fabricius in birds. T lymphocytes mature in the thymus. NK cells mature in the bone marrow, but they may also develop in the thymus and other lymphoid tissues. To summarize the lymphopoieses stages, they are as follows:

- Lymphoid Stem Cells
  - Lymphoblast
    - Prolymphocyte
- B Lymphocytes
- T Lymphocytes/NK Precursor
  - NK Cells

DEFINITIONS

The following are definitions of the hematologic terms used in this unit:

-penia: Decreased number of cells in the blood. For example, neutropenia refers to decreased numbers of neutrophils in the blood. Lymphopenia describes decreased numbers of lymphocytes in the blood, whereas pancytopenia refers to a decrease in the number of all blood cell types.

-philia or -cytosis: Increased number of cells in the blood. For example, neutrophilia refers to increased numbers of neutrophils in the blood. Leukocytosis refers to increased numbers of leukocytes in the blood.

Left shift: Increased numbers of immature neutrophils in the blood.

Leukemia: Neoplastic cells in the blood or bone marrow. Leukemias are often described with the terms *leukemic, subleukemic,* or *aleukemic,* thereby indicating the variation in the tendency for neoplastic cells to be released in the blood.

Leukemoid response: Condition that can be mistaken for leukemia. The leukemoid response is characterized by marked leukocytosis (i.e., >50,000/mL), and it is usually the result of inflammatory disease.

KEY POINTS

- Hematopoiesis refers to the production of blood cells and platelets.
- Erythropoiesis (the production of erythrocytes), leukopoiesis (the production of leukocytes), and thrombopoiesis (the production of platelets) involve specific cytokines.
- Red bone marrow is the primary site for the production and maturation of all of the blood cells and platelets in adult animals.
- All blood cells are derived from pluripotent HSCs.
- The erythrocyte developmental stages are the rubriblasts, the prorubricytes, the rubricytes, the metarubricytes, and the reticulocytes.
- Platelet production proceeds through the megakaryoblast, the promegakaryocyte, and the megakaryocyte stages.
- Mature segmented granulocytes are produced through the myeloblast, the promyelocyte, the myelocyte, the metamyelocyte, and band cell precursors.
- T lymphocytes, B lymphocytes, and NK cells develop through the lymphoblast and prolymphocyte stages.

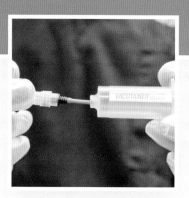

7

Sample Collection and Handling for Hematology

COLLECTION AND HANDLING OF BLOOD SAMPLES

When preparing to collect blood, the technician should first determine what specific test procedures will be needed. This will determine, in part, the equipment and supplies needed and the choice of a particular blood vessel from which to collect the sample. The sample must be drawn before the initiation of any medical treatment. If treatments have been given, these must be noted on the blood sample collection record. Some test methods cannot be accurately performed after the patient has received certain pharmaceutical therapies or hasn't fasted.

The preferred blood source is almost always venous blood. Jugular blood collection is most appropriate in common veterinary species. In some exotic species, there are no readily accessible veins, so it may be necessary to collect peripheral or capillary blood samples in those cases. Commonly used blood collection sites are summarized in Table 7.1. The blood collection site must be cleaned and swabbed with alcohol before collection. The alcohol should be allowed to dry before proceeding with the sample collection. The animal must be restrained, preferably with minimal manual restraint. Every effort should be made to minimize stress in the patient, because it often compromises the sample.

> **TECHNICIAN NOTE** Venous blood is preferred for most blood cell testing.

Collection Equipment

Traditionally, samples have been collected by using a needle and syringe. When this method is used, the needle chosen should always be the largest one that the animal can comfortably accommodate. The syringe chosen should be one that is closest

TABLE 7.1 Commonly Used Blood Collection Sites	
Dog	Cephalic vein Jugular vein Saphenous vein
Cat	Cephalic vein Jugular vein
Horse	Jugular vein
Cattle	Coccygeal vein Jugular vein
Sheep & Goats	Jugular vein
Llama & Alpaca	Jugular vein
Swine	Lateral auricular vein Coccygeal vein Cranial vena cava Jugular vein Orbital sinus Cephalic vein
Bird	Jugular vein Medial metatarsal vein
Rabbit	Ear vein
Rodent	Tail vein

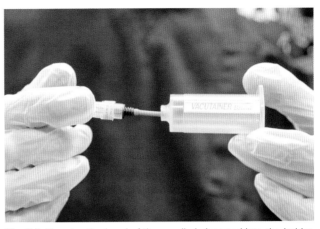

Fig. 7.2 The sheathed end of the needle is inserted into the holder.

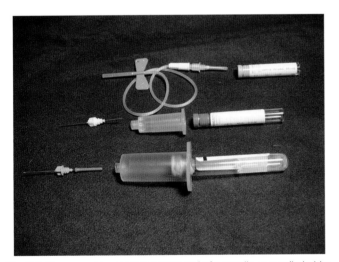

Fig. 7.1 The vacuum system is composed of a needle, a needle holder, and collection tubes.

to the required sample volume. The use of a larger syringe could collapse the patient's vein. The preferred method of blood collection is the use of a vacuum system (Vacutainer) (Fig. 7.1). This system is composed of a needle, a needle holder, and collection tubes. The sheathed end of the needle is inserted into the holder (Fig. 7.2). The sheath prevents blood from entering the holder when the venipuncture is made. The cap of the blood collection tube is penetrated with the needle after the needle is within the lumen of the blood vessel. The collection tubes may be plain sterile tubes, or they may contain

anticoagulants. The tubes are available in sizes that range from a few microliters to 15 mL. The correct-sized tube must be used to minimize damage to the sample or the possibility of collapsing the vein. The tubes should be allowed to fill to the correct volume (based on the strength of the vacuum pressure in the tube) to ensure the appropriate ratio of anticoagulant and blood. An advantage of this system is that multiple samples can be collected directly into the collection tubes without multiple venipuncture procedures. Sample quality is best when samples are collected with vacuum tubes using proper techniques, because this minimizes the potential for platelet activation.

> **TECHNICIAN NOTE** The Vacutainer system is preferred for blood sample collection.

Whole Blood

The veterinary technician obtains a whole blood sample by withdrawing the blood into a suitable container with the proper anticoagulant to prevent clotting. As soon as the blood is collected, the blood and the anticoagulant are mixed with a gentle rocking motion. Shaking the sample vigorously causes hemolysis, which in turn can affect the results of the assays when chemicals that are normally found within the erythrocytes are released into the plasma.

Plasma and Serum

Plasma is the fluid portion of whole blood in which the cells are suspended. It is composed of approximately 90% water and 10% dissolved constituents, such as proteins, carbohydrates, vitamins, hormones, enzymes, lipids, salts, waste materials, antibodies, and other ions and molecules. Serum is plasma from which fibrinogen, a plasma protein, has been removed. During the clotting process, the soluble fibrinogen in plasma is converted to an insoluble fibrin clot matrix (Fig. 7.3). When

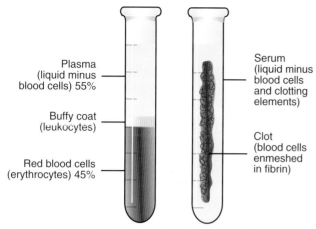

Plasma (liquid minus blood cells) 55%

Buffy coat (leukocytes)

Red blood cells (erythrocytes) 45%

Serum (liquid minus blood cells and clotting elements)

Clot (blood cells enmeshed in fibrin)

Fig. 7.3 The difference between blood plasma and blood serum. Plasma is whole blood minus the cells; serum is whole blood minus the cells and the clotting elements. (From Thibodeau GA, Patton KT: *Anatomy & physiology,* ed 5, St Louis, 2003, Mosby.)

blood clots, the fluid that is squeezed out around the cellular clot is serum.

Anticoagulants

Hematology testing primarily involves the use of whole blood samples. Hemostatic testing uses both whole blood and blood plasma. Anticoagulants are required when whole blood or plasma samples are needed. An anticoagulant is a chemical that, when added to a whole blood sample, prevents or delays clotting (coagulation) of the sample. The choice of a particular anticoagulant should be made on the basis of the tests needed. Some anticoagulants may affect assays, so the test procedure should be consulted for the proper anticoagulant. Some anticoagulants can interfere with certain coagulation tests. Regardless of the anticoagulant chosen, the sample and the anticoagulant must be well mixed by gentle inversion before use. Samples that are not tested within 1 hour of collection should be refrigerated. Refrigerated samples must be brought back to room temperature and

remixed by gentle inversion before analysis. Whole blood should not be frozen, because blood cells lyse during the freezing and thawing processes. Table 7.2 summarizes commonly used anticoagulants.

> **TECHNICIAN NOTE** Samples collected into tubes that contain anticoagulants must be mixed by gentle inversion.

Heparin

Heparin is a suitable anticoagulant for most tests that require plasma samples, particularly blood chemistry analyses. Heparin anticoagulant should never be used for differential blood film analysis, because the anticoagulant interferes with the staining of white blood cells (WBCs). Heparin is available as a sodium, potassium, lithium, or ammonium salt. Heparin acts by preventing the conversion of prothrombin to thrombin during the clotting processes. Because heparin can cause clumping of WBCs and platelets and interferes with the normal staining pattern of the WBCs, it should not be used for analyses of WBC morphology.

Heparin should be used at a ratio of 20 U/mL of blood to be collected. For small sample volumes, a convenient method for using heparin is to coat the inside walls of a syringe with liquid heparin before the sample is drawn from the patient. Vacuum collection tubes that contain the proper amount of heparin are commercially available. These tubes are most convenient when many heparinized samples are needed.

Ethylenediaminetetraacetic Acid

Ethylenediaminetetraacetic acid (EDTA) is the preferred anticoagulant for hematologic studies, because it does not alter cell morphology when it is used in the proper ratio for samples to be analyzed soon after collection. It should not be used if plasma samples are to be used for chemical assays. EDTA is available as sodium or potassium salt, and it prevents clotting by forming an insoluble complex with calcium, which is

TABLE 7.2   Commonly Used Anticoagulants

Name	Mode of Action	Advantages	Disadvantages	Uses
Heparin	Antithrombin	Reversible, nontoxic	Clumps white blood cells, expensive	Critical red blood cell measurements
Ethylenediaminetetraacetic acid (potassium, sodium)	Chelates calcium	Best preservation	Irreversible, shrinks cells	Hematology
Oxalates (potassium, sodium, lithium)	Chelates calcium	Temporary	Variable effects	Coagulation
Citrates (sodium, lithium)	Chelates calcium	Nontoxic, reversible	Interferes with blood chemistry	Coagulation, transfusions
Fluorides (sodium)	Chelates calcium	Inhibits cell metabolism	Interferes with enzymatic tests	Preserves blood glucose

necessary for clot formation. EDTA tubes are available in either liquid or powder forms. The liquid form creates some dilution of the sample. To prevent clotting, EDTA is added at 1 to 2 mg/mL of blood to be collected. Vacuum collection tubes that contain the proper amount of EDTA are commercially available. Excess EDTA causes cells to shrink and invalidates most cell counts performed with automated analyzers.

> **TECHNICIAN NOTE** EDTA is the preferred anticoagulant for most hematology tests.

Oxalates and Citrates

Oxalates are available as sodium, potassium, ammonium, or lithium salts. Citrates are available as sodium or lithium salts. These substances prevent clotting by forming insoluble complexes with calcium, which is necessary for clot formation. Potassium oxalate is the most commonly used oxalate salt. To prevent clotting, it is used at 1 to 2 mg/mL of blood to be collected. Sodium citrates are also commonly used, especially in transfusion medicine. Vacuum collection tubes that contain the proper amount of oxalate and citrate anticoagulants are commercially available. Unfortunately, oxalates may also bind metallic ions necessary for enzyme activity. Potassium oxalate may inhibit lactate dehydrogenase and alkaline phosphatase activity. In addition, because it is a potassium salt, it cannot be used with blood samples to be assayed for potassium. Sodium citrates similarly interfere with sodium assays as well as with many of the commonly performed blood chemistry tests. Note that different laboratories may have tubes with differing concentrations of citrate, which may affect certain coagulation tests.

Sodium Fluoride

Sodium fluoride, which is best known as a glucose preservative, also has anticoagulant properties. As an anticoagulant, it is used at 6 to 10 mg/mL of blood to be collected. Vacuum collection tubes that contain the proper amount of sodium fluoride for anticoagulation are commercially available. Sodium fluoride may also be added to other samples as a glucose preservative, even if a different anticoagulant is present. For glucose preservation, sodium fluoride is used at 2.5 mg/mL of blood. Sodium fluoride interferes with many of the enzymatic tests performed on blood serum.

SAMPLE VOLUME

It is important to remember that you can take 1% of a patient's body weight in blood per blood draw, but no more than 10% of their body weight per week. This is important when performing blood transfusions or with neonates. The amount of blood collected from an animal also depends on the quantity of serum

or plasma required for the assay and the hydration status of the patient. For example, a well-hydrated animal with a packed cell volume of 50% should yield a blood sample that is 50% cells and 50% fluid. A 10-mL blood sample should yield 5 mL of fluid. In dehydrated animals, hemoconcentration results in a smaller ratio of fluid to cells. A dehydrated animal with a packed cell volume of 70% yields a blood sample that is 70% cells and 30% fluid. This means that only 3 mL of fluid is obtained from a 10-mL blood sample.

Ideally, enough blood should be collected to yield enough serum, plasma, or whole blood to run all of the planned assays three times. This allows for technician error, instrument failure, or the need to dilute a sample without having to collect another sample from the animal.

Blood samples must be adequately mixed before the performance of any tests; inadequate mixing results in erroneous data. For example, red blood cells from horses start to settle within seconds, and a packed cell volume performed on an unmixed sample may be erroneous. Tubes of blood may be mixed by gentle inversion 5 to 10 times by hand or by placing the tube on a commercially available tilting rack or rotator.

COLLECTION PROCEDURE

After the volume needed has been determined and the specific types of testing required have been identified, prepare equipment and obtain the appropriate number and types of blood collection tubes. Perform venipuncture with the least tissue injury possible to minimize contamination with tissue fluid and to minimize hemolysis. If a Vacutainer is used, allow the tube to fill to capacity to ensure the proper blood-to-anticoagulant ratio. Restraint is necessary to prevent movement that may result in laceration of a blood vessel or another organ and serious complications. For most small animals, the patient is placed in sternal recumbency. Hair should be shaved from the venipuncture site to minimize the contamination of the sample and the introduction of bacteria from the skin and hair into the patient. The restrainer occludes the vessel or applies a tourniquet distal to the venipuncture site. The tourniquet is placed tight enough to distend the vein without occluding blood flow. Hemoconcentration can occur if the tourniquet is left in place for an excessive amount of time. The technician who is collecting the sample should first locate the vessel and then clean the venipuncture site with alcohol. Do not touch the site with bare fingers after the site has been cleaned. Stabilize the vein and insert the needle with the bevel facing up at approximately a 30-degree angle to enter the vein in one smooth motion. If using a syringe, aspirate blood into the syringe. When the proper volume has been obtained, remove the needle and immediately apply gentle pressure to the venipuncture site to ensure hemostasis. Remove the needle from the syringe before transferring the blood to the vial, because forcing blood through the needle may result in hemolysis. If the vacuum system is used, the needle is inserted into the vessel as described previously, and then the holder is stabilized and the tube gently pushed onto the sheathed end of the needle within the holder. After the tube fills completely, it can be removed and another tube inserted. The sheath prevents blood from dripping into the holder when changing tubes.

All blood samples collected in a tube that contains anticoagulant should be gently inverted several times immediately after collection to distribute the anticoagulant. It is vital that the sample be labeled immediately after collection. The tube should be labeled with the date and time of collection, the owner's name, the patient's name, and the patient's clinic identification number. If the sample is to be submitted to a laboratory,

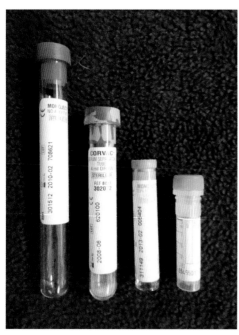

Fig. 7.4 From left to right: red-top plain blood collection tube, tiger-top tube, ethylenediaminetetraacetic acid tube, and heparin tube.

include a request form with the sample that includes all necessary sample identification and a clear indication of which tests are requested.

Order of Draw

When multiple types of samples are required, the samples should always be collected with the vacuum system, and they must be collected in a specific order. The vacuum system ensures that an appropriate volume of each sample type is obtained. However, the tubes need to be collected in a specific order to avoid the potential contamination of samples with additives from other tubes. Tubes that contain citrate additives are drawn first. These tubes usually require that a small amount of sample first be taken in a plain tube that is discarded. If no citrate tube is needed, the plain red-top tube is drawn first (Fig. 7.4). Table 7.3 summarizes the usual order of draw for tubes that are commonly used in veterinary practice. Note that some individuals prefer to collect the red-top tube before the citrate tube rather than using a discard tube. This is acceptable provided that the red-top tube contains no gel additives, which could potentially contaminate the citrate tube.

Fear-Free Venipuncture

When working with any animal it is now commonly accepted to utilize fear-free methods to try and make visits to veterinary clinics and the commonly performed procedures more acceptable to the patients we perform them on. Some of the methods we utilize to help decrease the fear animals experience from veterinary visits include allowing them to explore the environment on their own time, using all of their senses. Have another person offer small frequent treats to the patient while they stand at attention as the venipuncturist attempts to pull blood or prep the area. Condition the patient to the sights, smells, sounds, and vibrations associated with clippers or disinfectants before quickly applying them. Slowly allow the patient to explore them on their own.

TABLE 7.3	**Order of Draw for Commonly Used Blood Collection Tubes**			
Order of Draw	**Cap Color**		**Additive**	**Primary Use**
First		Light blue	Sodium citrate	Coagulation studies
		Red	Glass: no additive Plastic: silicon-coated	Serum for blood chemistry
		Red/gray, gold, or red/black "tiger-top"	Gel separator and clot activator	
		Green or tan	Heparin	Plasma for blood chemistry
		Lavender, royal blue, or tan	EDTA	Hematology
Last		Gray	Potassium oxalate or sodium fluoride	Coagulation testing Glucose testing

KEY POINTS

- Sites for blood collection vary in different species, but the jugular vein is the vessel of choice for blood collection from most mammals.
- The preferred method of blood collection is the Vacutainer system.

- The preferred anticoagulant for hematology testing is EDTA; the preferred anticoagulant for coagulation testing is citrate.
- Plasma is whole blood minus the cells; serum is whole blood minus the cells and the clotting elements.

8

Hemoglobin, PCV, and Erythrocyte Indices

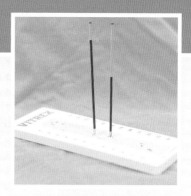

LEARNING OBJECTIVES

After studying this chapter, you will be able to:

- Describe the procedure for performing a packed cell volume test with the microhematocrit method.
- Describe the procedure for calibrating the centrifuge for optimum microhematocrit spin time.
- List the layers in the centrifuged microhematocrit tube in order from bottom to top.

- Explain the significance of reddish, yellow, and cloudy plasma colors in the centrifuged microhematocrit tube.
- Differentiate among oxyhemoglobin, methemoglobin, and sulfhemoglobin.
- List the calculations used to obtain the mean corpuscular volume, the mean corpuscular hemoglobin, and the mean corpuscular hemoglobin concentration.

OUTLINE

KEY TERMS

Buffy coat
Erythrocyte indices
Hemoglobin
Icteric
Lipemic

Mean corpuscular hemoglobin
Mean corpuscular hemoglobin
  concentration
Mean corpuscular volume
Methemoglobin

Microhematocrit
Oxyhemoglobin
Packed cell volume

The complete blood count (CBC) provides a minimum set of values that may be determined reliably and cost effectively in the hospital setting. The tests included in the CBC can be performed manually or by automated analyzers. A variety of procedures are available for both methods.

The CBC should consist of the following basic information:

- Total red blood cell (RBC) count
- Packed cell volume (PCV)
- Plasma protein concentration
- Total white blood cell (WBC) count
- Blood film examination: differential WBC count, erythrocyte and leukocyte morphology, and platelet estimation
- Reticulocyte count when the patient is anemic
- Hemoglobin concentration
- Erythrocyte indices

PACKED CELL VOLUME

- Elevated in
  - Dehydration
  - Polycythemia
  - Splenic contracture
- Decreased in
  - Anemia

The PCV is the percentage of the whole blood that is composed of erythrocytes or RBCs. Although this test is included in the CBC, it is also frequently ordered as a single test. The commonly performed version of the test is referred to as the microhematocrit (mHct) or hematocrit (Hct). The test is performed by placing anticoagulated whole blood into a 75-mm capillary tube. Heparinized tubes are also available and are

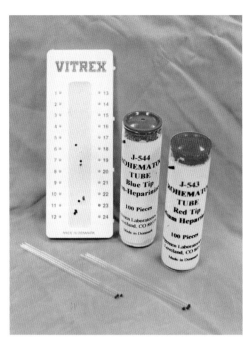

Fig. 8.1 Microhematocrit tubes and clay sealant.

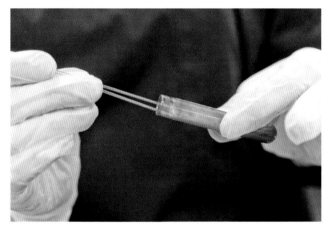

Fig. 8.2 Two tubes can be filled from the same sample at the same time so that they can be placed opposite each other in the centrifuge.

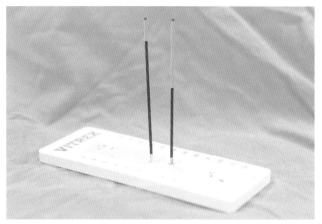

Fig. 8.3 Microhematocrit tubes that have been sealed with clay. These tubes were filled to different volumes and could not be centrifuged without balance tubes of equal size and weight.

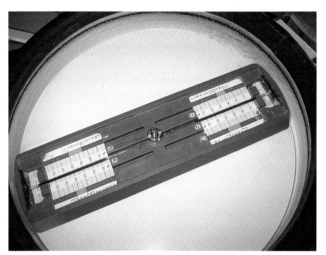

Fig. 8.4 Microhematocrit tubes are placed with the clay plug toward the outside of the centrifuge. Two tubes placed opposite each other are required to balance the centrifuge.

identified by the red ring around the top of the tube. Plain microhematocrit tubes are identified with a blue ring (Fig. 8.1). Microhematocrit tubes should be filled approximately three-fourths full. Usually two tubes are filled from one sample at the same time so that they can be centrifuged together (Fig. 8.2). After a tube has been filled to an appropriate volume, one end is plugged with clay sealant (Fig. 8.3). The tube is then placed in a centrifuge with the plugged end facing outward and then centrifuged in a microhematocrit centrifuge for 2 to 5 minutes, depending on the type of centrifuge used (Fig. 8.4). Small-capacity centrifuges that use 40-mm tubes are also available (Fig. 8.5). See Procedure 8.1 for how to calibrate a microhematocrit centrifuge.

Of the blood cells, RBCs have the highest specific gravity. They gravitate to the bottom of the tube during centrifugation and appear as a dark red layer. A whitish-gray layer just above

the RBC layer is called the buffy coat, and it consists of WBCs and platelets. The height of the buffy coat layer can provide a rough estimate of the total WBC count. The presence of increased numbers of nucleated RBCs imparts a reddish tinge to the buffy coat. The plasma is the clear to pale yellow fluid at the top (Fig. 8.6). Plasma obtained by this method can be used to determine the plasma protein concentration by refractometry. Plasma color and transparency may be helpful for the determination of a diagnosis and should be recorded. Normal plasma is clear (transparent) or a pale straw-yellow color (Fig. 8.7). Serum that appears cloudy is described as lipemic. This may be the result of a pathologic condition, or it may be seen as an artifact if the patient was not properly fasted before blood collection. A reddish-tinged plasma layer is described as hemolyzed. This may also be an artifact if the blood sample was not properly collected and handled, or it may be evidence of a pathologic condition (e.g., hemolytic anemia). Plasma that is deep yellow is described as icteric, and it can be seen in animals

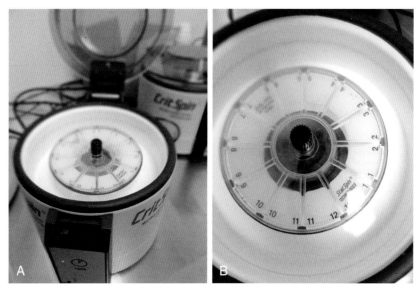

Fig. 8.5 **A** and **B,** A microhematocrit centrifuge designed for small-capacity tubes.

PROCEDURE 8.1   Calibration of the Microhematocrit Centrifuge

1. Use a stopwatch to verify the centrifuge timer operation. Run several tests at different time intervals, and repeat each at least twice to verify reproducibility.
2. Use a tachometer to check the centrifuge speed.
3. Verify the minimum time required to obtain an accurate packed cell volume.
4. The minimum time needed to achieve optimal packing of the red cells should be checked with the following procedure:
   a. Choose two fresh ethylenediaminetetraacetic-acid–anticoagulated blood samples; one sample should have a hematocrit level of more than 50%.
   b. Fill 10 to 12 microhematocrit tubes for each sample.
   c. Perform duplicate microhematocrit determinations at increasing times, beginning at 2 minutes. Centrifuge times should be increased by 30-second intervals. Record duplicate values at each time interval.
   d. Continue to increase the centrifuge time until the value remains the same for two consecutive time intervals.
   e. Centrifuge two more samples for an additional 30 and 60 seconds beyond that interval.
   f. Plot the results on a graph. The plateau point is the first point on the curve after the curve flattens out (see figure below). This is the optimum spin time.
   g. Repeat the procedure periodically, because brushes and motors can wear, thereby reducing the speed of the centrifuge.

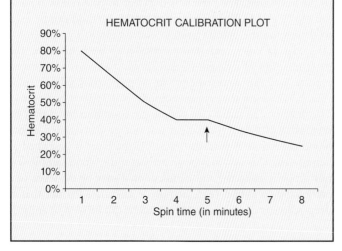

HEMATOCRIT CALIBRATION PLOT

y-axis: Hematocrit (0% to 90%)
x-axis: Spin time (in minutes) (1 to 8)

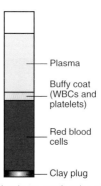

Fig. 8.6 Diagram of a microhematocrit tube after centrifugation. (From Bassert J, Colville T: *Clinical anatomy and physiology for veterinary technicians,* ed 2, St Louis, 2008, Mosby.)

Labels: Plasma; Buffy coat (WBCs and platelets); Red blood cells; Clay plug

with liver disease or hemolytic anemia. Abnormal plasma colors must be noted, because the color can interfere with the chemical analyses if photometric methods are used for the evaluation of plasma constituents. Any measuring device (e.g., a ruler) can be used to determine the PCV.

> **TECHNICIAN NOTE** The PCV evaluates the percentage of whole blood that is composed of RBCs.

Special hematocrit tube reader cards are available, many of which have a linear scale, so the amount of blood in the tube need not be exact. The bottom of the RBC layer should be at the zero line and the top of the plasma on the top line. The percentage can then be read as the line that is level with the top of the RBC layer (Fig. 8.8). To obtain the PCV using a ruler, measure the height of the RBC column and the total height from the top of the clay plug to the top of the plasma column. Divide the height of the RBC column by the total height and multiply by 100 to obtain the percentage. An estimate of the RBC counts may be obtained by dividing the PCV by 6. For example, if the PCV is 36, the estimated RBC count is 36 divided by 6, which is equal to 6 and which represents 6 million RBCs/μL.

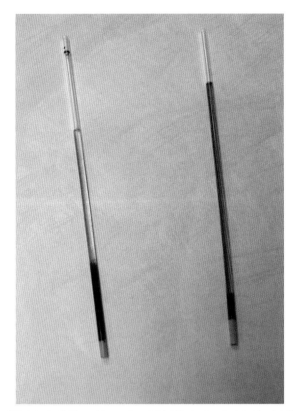

Fig. 8.7 Icteric *(left)* and hemolyzed *(right)* plasma in a packed cell volume tube.

TABLE 8.1 Normal Packed Cell Volume Values for Common Species	
Species	**Packed Cell Volume (%)**
Canine	37–55
Feline	30–45
Equine	32–57
Bovine	24–42
Ovine	25–45
Caprine	21–38
Porcine	32–43

excess anticoagulant may over-dilute the sample and yield erroneous results. If the venipuncturist failed to obtain a free-flowing blood sample from the skin puncture this can cause excess tissue fluid that may produce results similar to excess anticoagulant. If centrifugation is not performed at the appropriate duration or speed the results can be erroneous. Other causes can include failure to mix the blood adequately and failure to read the sample correctly. Remember, the buffy coat should not be included as part of the erythrocyte volume. Finally, irregularity of the inside diameter of the capillary tube can cause erroneous results; ensure you buy your capillary tubes from a reliable vendor. Normal PCV values for common domestic species are listed in Table 8.1.

> **TECHNICIAN NOTE** An increased PCV is commonly due to dehydration.

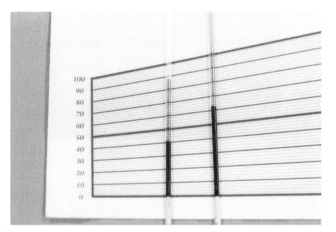

Fig. 8.8 The packed cell volume is determined by aligning the top of the clay plug on the zero line and locating the intersecting line where the packed red cells and the buffy coat meet.

Plasma Protein Concentration

- Elevated in
  - Dehydration
  - Hyperglobulinemia
  - Error
    - Hemolysis
    - Lipemia
- Decreased in
  - Hemorrhage
  - Hypoalbuminemia
  - Liver failure
  - External plasma loss
  - GI fluid loss
  - Malassimilation
  - Starvation
  - Overhydration
  - Glomerular loss
  - Cancer

The macrohematocrit method for determining PCV is not commonly performed, because it requires a large amount of blood, generally a minimum of 10 mL. The blood is placed in a Wintrobe tube and centrifuged for 10 minutes at 18,000 rpm. The scale on the Wintrobe tube is read at the level of the packed RBCs, and that number is multiplied by 10 to determine the PCV.

Sources of error when performing the PCV can occur when excessive anticoagulant is present in the blood sample. The

Although it is not specifically considered a hematologic test, the materials needed for the plasma protein concentration are already available as a result of performing the PCV. Plasma protein concentration estimation by refractometry is an important component of the CBC in all species. The principle of this test is based on the fact that proteins in solution cause a change in refractive index that is proportional to protein concentration.

The plasma that is used to determine the PCV is collected by breaking the hematocrit tube just above the buffy coat—plasma interface. The plasma is allowed to flow onto the refractometer prism (see Unit 1, Procedure 2.1). The refractometer is then held to a bright light, and the reading is made at the dividing line between the bright and dark fields. The protein value (in g/dL) is read directly from a scale inside the refractometer. Lipemic plasma contains chylomicrons that cause the light to diffract in many different directions and usually results in a false increase in the total protein reading. It is important to remember that extreme variations in room temperature can cause erratic readings so temperature-compensated refractometers are ideal. The sample can also be erroneous if the sample is hemolytic or icteric. Abnormally high concentrations of glucose, urea, sodium, or chloride may falsely increase the plasma protein readings. Remember that fresh serum contains all the plasma proteins except fibrinogen, Factor V, and Factor VIII; these are the factors consumed in clot formation. Therefore, serum proteins measured by refractometry will be lower than that of plasma.

HEMOGLOBIN TESTING

- Elevated in
  - Dehydration
  - Polycythemia
  - Splenic contracture
- Decreased in
  - Anemia

The protein molecule hemoglobin is the functional unit of the erythrocyte. The molecule consists of two main components: the heme portion, which contains iron, and the globin portion, which is composed of paired chains of amino acids. The synthesis of hemoglobin occurs during the maturation of the RBCs in the bone marrow. After entering the circulation, different forms of hemoglobin can exist. Hemoglobin that is bound to oxygen is referred to as oxyhemoglobin. When the oxygen is delivered to the tissues by the RBCs, carbon dioxide binds in place of the oxygen. The carbon dioxide is then replaced again by oxygen during respiration. Other forms of hemoglobin that may also be present include methemoglobin and sulfhemoglobin. Both of these forms are inefficient when it comes to oxygen transport. Sulfhemoglobin results from normal RBC aging processes. Methemoglobin occurs naturally both in plasma and within RBCs, but it can be converted to hemoglobin and used for oxygen delivery. Carboxyhemoglobin results from exposure to carbon monoxide. Hemoglobin and methemoglobin have a much higher affinity for carbon monoxide than for oxygen or carbon dioxide. Therefore, the reaction that creates carboxyhemoglobin is irreversible.

A variety of methods are available for the determination of hemoglobin. The oldest methods involve color matching of lysed RBCs (Fig. 8.9). Some automated analyzer types provide

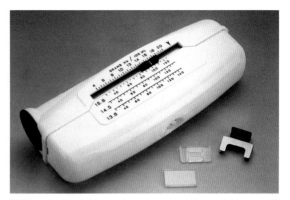

Fig. 8.9 The hemoglobinometer uses a color-matching method to determine the hemoglobin concentration in a sample of lysed red blood cells.

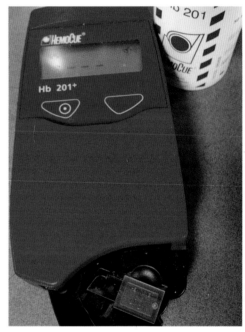

Fig. 8.10 The HemoCue is a type of photometer that is used to measure hemoglobin concentration.

only an estimate of the hemoglobin concentration on the basis of the RBC count. Most automated analyzers determine hemoglobin concentration by mixing a small amount of blood with a solution to lyse the blood cells and then comparing the color of the sample with a standard. Exposure to cyanide converts all forms of hemoglobin to cyanmethemoglobin. Lysing solutions that contain small amounts of cyanide function convert all forms of hemoglobin to cyanmethemoglobin and therefore provide a measure of all forms of hemoglobin in the sample. A number of automated and semiautomated analyzers are dedicated to hemoglobin measurement. Most of these use a modification of the cyanmethemoglobin photometric procedure, and they are quite accurate if properly maintained. Small dedicated analyzers are also available (Fig. 8.10); some of these provide results only for oxyhemoglobin and use simple color-matching technology. Other types use a cyanide-free

TABLE 8.2 Normal Hemoglobin Values for Common Species

Species	Hemoglobin Value (g/dL)
Canine	12—20
Feline	11—16
Equine	11—18
Bovine	8—14
Ovine	8—16
Caprine	8—13
Porcine	10—16

hemoglobin—hydroxylamine method and photometric procedures that are calibrated to approximate the cyanmethemoglobin procedure. Normal hemoglobin values for common domestic species are located in Table 8.2.

> **TECHNICIAN NOTE** Erythrocyte indices can be used to help classify types of anemia.

ERYTHROCYTE INDICES

The determination of erythrocyte indices is helpful for the classification of certain types of anemia. The erythrocyte indices include the mean corpuscular volume (MCV), the mean corpuscular hemoglobin (MCH), and the mean corpuscular hemoglobin concentration (MCHC). The indices can provide an objective measure of the size of the RBCs and their average hemoglobin concentration. The accuracy of the calculation depends on the accuracy of the individual measurements of total RBC count, PCV, and hemoglobin concentration. Values for erythrocyte indices should always be compared with the morphologic features of the cells on the blood smear. For example, a low value for the MCH level should be evident as erythrocytes that appear more pale than normal (hypochromic) on the blood smear.

Mean Corpuscular Volume

- Elevated in
  - Macrocytosis
    - Regeneration
    - FELV
    - FIV
    - Poodles
    - Dyserythropoiesis
    - Swelling of RBCs secondary to prolonged storage in EDTA tubes
- Decreased in
  - Microcytosis
    - Iron deficiency
    - Portosystemic shunt
    - Polycythemia
    - Akitas, Shar-peis, and Shiba Inus

MCV is the measure of the average size of the erythrocytes. MCV is calculated by dividing the PCV by the RBC concentration and multiplying by 10. The unit of volume is the femtoliter (fL).

For example, if a dog has a PCV of 42% and an RBC count of 6.0 million/mL, the MCV is 70 fL.

Many of the automated hematology analyzers determine the MCV electronically and use that measurement to calculate the PCV.

Mean Corpuscular Hemoglobin

> **TECHNICIAN NOTE** The MCHC is more useful than the MCH.

MCH is the mean weight of hemoglobin (Hb) contained in the average RBC, which is measured in picograms (pg). It is calculated by dividing the hemoglobin concentration by the RBC concentration and multiplying by 10:

$$MCH\ (pg) = \frac{Hb\ (g/dL)}{RBC\ (\times 10^9/mL)} \times 10$$

Mean Corpuscular Hemoglobin Concentration

- Elevated in
  - Hyperchromic
    - Hemolysis
    - RBC shape changes like Heinz bodies and spherocytes
  - Lipemia
- Decreased in
  - Hypochromic
    - Reticulocytosis
    - Iron deficiency

MCHC is the concentration of hemoglobin in the average erythrocyte (or the ratio of the weight of hemoglobin to the volume in which it is contained). The MCHC (in g/dL) is calculated by dividing the hemoglobin concentration (in g/dL) by the PCV (percentage) and multiplying by 100.

$$MCHC\ (\%) = \frac{Hb\ (g/dL)}{PCV\ (\%)} \times 100$$

For example, if a dog has a hemoglobin concentration of 14 g/dL and a PCV of 42%, the MCHC is 33.3 g/dL. The normal range for the MCHC is 30 to 36 g/dL for all mammals, with the exception of some sheep and all members of the family *Camelidae* (i.e., camels), which have MCHC values of 40 to 45 g/dL.

KEY POINTS

- PCV is a commonly performed hematology test.
- PCV can be increased as a result of dehydration or polycythemia.
- Decreased PCV may indicate anemia.
- The microhematocrit test uses capillary tubes that are filled with blood and centrifuged.
- The layers in the microhematocrit tube are the packed RBCs, the buffy coat, and the plasma.
- Plasma color must also be evaluated and recorded when performing the PCV.
- Hemoglobin testing can be performed with automated analyzers or with handheld meters.
- Erythrocyte indices are calculated values that provide a measure of the size of the RBCs and their average hemoglobin concentration.

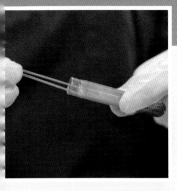

Evaluating the Blood Smear

PREPARATION OF BLOOD SMEARS

The blood smear is used to perform the differential white blood cell (WBC) count, to estimate platelet numbers, and to evaluate the morphologic features of WBCs, red blood cells (RBCs), and platelets. Peripheral blood smears can be prepared with the use of either a wedge smear technique or a coverslip technique. The wedge smear is the most commonly used type of preparation. The coverslip technique is often used to prepare smears from blood samples obtained from avian and exotic animal species.

To prepare a blood smear, a drop of blood is withdrawn from the ethylenediaminetetraacetic-acid (EDTA)–anticoagulated blood collection tube. The drop can be obtained either with a plastic transfer pipette or by placing two wooden applicator sticks into the blood tube (Fig. 9.1). When the sticks are held together and withdrawn, a drop of blood of the appropriate size will be between them. The blood drop is placed toward the frosted end of a clean glass microscope slide (Fig. 9.2). The patient information can be written directly on the frosted area with a pencil. The end of a second slide is placed against the surface of the first slide at a 30-degree angle and drawn back into the drop of blood (Fig. 9.3). The angle of the second slide can be modified to account for changes in the consistency of blood from an anemic patient (Fig. 9.4 and Procedure 9.1). When the blood has spread along most of the width of the spreader slide, it is then pushed forward with a steady, even, rapid motion. The slide should be gently waved in the air to allow it to air dry quickly. A properly prepared blood smear is thin, with an even distribution of cells.

Coverslip smears are made by putting one drop of blood in the center of a clean square coverslip. Place a second coverslip diagonally on top of the first, causing the blood to spread evenly between the two surfaces. Then pull the coverslips apart in a

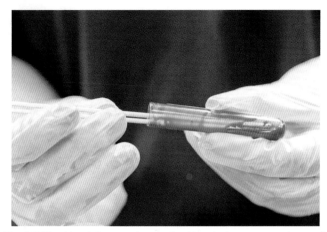

Fig. 9.1 The blood drop can be obtained by placing two wooden applicator sticks into the tube and holding them together when withdrawing them from the tube.

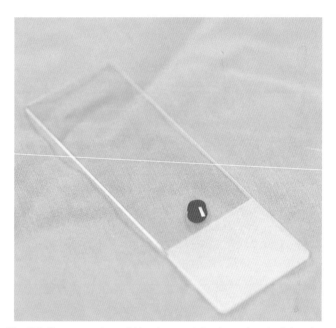

Fig. 9.2 Place one drop of blood toward the frosted end of the glass slide.

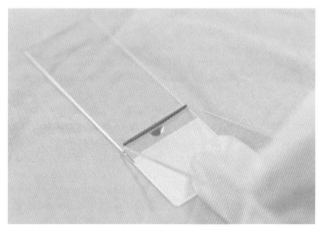

Fig. 9.3 Hold the top (spreader) slide at approximately 30 degrees, and draw it back into the blood drop.

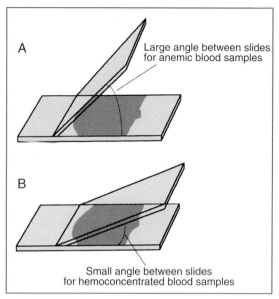

Fig. 9.4 The difference in slide angle necessary for making blood smears from anemic or hemoconcentrated blood. **A,** A large angle is used for anemic blood. **B,** A small angle is used for hemoconcentrated blood.

PROCEDURE 9.1   Making a Wedge Smear

1. Place a small drop of blood at the end of a clean glass slide using a micro-hematocrit tube or the end of a wooden applicator stick. Place this slide on a flat surface, or suspend it in midair between the thumb and the forefinger.
2. Hold a second slide (the spreader slide) at a 30-degree angle, and pull it back into contact with the drop of blood, spreading the blood along the edge of the spreader slide. Push the spreader slide forward in a rapid, steady, even motion to produce a blood smear that is thick at one end and that tapers to a thin, feathered edge at the other. The blood smear should cover about three quarters of the length of the slide.

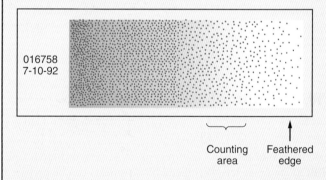

016758
7-10-92

Counting area   Feathered edge

A blood smear showing the label area, the monolayer counting area, and the feathered edge. (From Sirois M: *Principles and practice of veterinary technology,* ed 3, St Louis, 2011, Mosby.)

3. Air dry the smear by waving the slide in the air. This fixes the cells to the slide so that they are not dislodged during staining.
4. Label the slide at the thick end of the smear. If the slide has a frosted edge, the label may be written there.
5. After drying, stain the smear with Wright's stain or a Romanowsky-type stain, which is available in commercial kits (e.g., Wright's Dip Stat #3 [Medi-Chem, Santa Monica, CA]). Follow the directions for the staining kit. Smears typically must be immersed in each solution for 5 to 10 seconds.
6. After staining, rinse the slide with distilled water. Allow the slide to dry upright, with the feathered edge pointed upward; this allows the water to drip off of the slide and away from the smear.

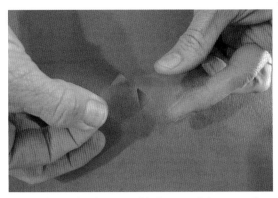

Fig. 9.5 Preparing a blood smear with the use of the coverslip method.

PROCEDURE 9.2 Preparation of Coverslip Blood Smear

1. Place a small drop of blood in the center of a clean, square coverslip.
2. Place a second coverslip diagonally on top of the first.
3. Allow the blood to spread evenly between the two surfaces until the blood almost fills the area between the coverslips.
4. Pull the coverslips apart in a single smooth motion.
5. Wave the coverslips gently to allow them to air dry.

single smooth motion before the blood has completely spread (Fig. 9.5 and Procedure 9.2). Wave the smears gently in the air to promote drying.

TECHNICIAN NOTE The wedge smear is the most common technique for preparing a blood smear for the differential WBC count.

Staining Blood Smears

After they air dry, the blood smears must be stained to clearly distinguish the individual cells and to identify any abnormal cellular characteristics. Blood smears can be stained with any of the Romanowsky-type stains. The commonly available Romanowsky stains include Wright's stain and Wright-Giemsa stain. Romanowsky stains are available in either one-step or three-step formulations. The components of the stain may vary somewhat, but they usually include a fixative and buffered solutions of eosin and methylene blue. The fixative used is usually 95% methanol. The eosin component is buffered at an acidic pH, and it stains the basic components of the cells, such as hemoglobin and eosinophilic granules. The methylene blue component is buffered to an alkaline pH, and it stains the acidic components of the cell, such as leukocyte nuclei. A three-step stain that gives acceptable results is Diff-Quik (Siemens USA, Palo Alto, CA). When a three-step stain is used, the slide may be rinsed with distilled water between each of the three components. Care must be taken to avoid dripping water into any of the stain components, or the stain will become degraded. A

final rinse with distilled water should be done on all slides and then the slides allowed to dry before microscopic examination of the smear.

The best stain quality is achieved when slides are fixed in methanol for at least 60 seconds before staining. The length of time to stain the slide is variable and affected by a number of factors, such as the age of the stains. For three-step stains, an average time to immerse the slide is 30 seconds for each component. It is not necessary to dip slides in and out of stain jars.

Table 9.1 lists problems related to staining. Cells appear dark if they are overstained, whereas extensive rinsing may cause them to look faded. Changing stains regularly is necessary for consistent results and for the prevention of stain precipitation on the smear. Stains can also be filtered to remove excess debris. Refractile artifacts on RBCs are another common problem. These are usually caused by moisture in the fixative solution, which may be the result of water dripping off of slides and into the jars or from jars being left uncovered when not in use. Take care to not confuse these artifacts with cellular abnormalities.

Some common problems that occur with staining blood smears include having an excessive pink color; this occurs when the nuclei are pale gray or pale blue, the RBCs appear bright red or orange, and the eosinophils appear bright red. This occurs for several reasons including the stain, buffer, or water being too acidic or if insufficient stain was used. Another reason this can occur is prolonged washing of the slide. To correct these problems ensure you are replacing stains as needed, adjust the amount of time you are staining your slides, or perform the washing procedures.

Another common problem is when the stain is excessively blue. In this situation nuclear chromatin is blue to black, the RBCs appear blue or green, and the eosinophilic granules are deep gray or blue. This can occur due to the stains being to alkaline. Ensure you are changing the stains as needed. Other causes of this can be prolonged staining, inadequate washing, or the smear being too thick. Try adjusting your staining technique times or make your smears thinner to correct this problem.

If all the cells are pale when you are evaluating your smear this is often due to understaining or excessive washing. Try adjusting your technique times.

If stain precipitate is present you are inadequately washing your smear. Try washing your slides longer or using link-free slides to correct the problem.

If there are refractile areas on your red blood cells this is due to water artifact, which is caused by your stain being diluted. To correct this problem again ensure you are changing your stains regularly. Depending on the number of blood smears you are performing in clinic, this can vary from daily to weekly.

White Blood Cells

Mature and immature neutrophils, lymphocytes, monocytes, eosinophils, and basophils make up the leukocytes (WBCs)

TABLE 9.1   Troubleshooting Staining Problems

Problem	Solution
Excessive Blue Staining (Red Blood Cells May Stain a Blue-Green Color)	
Prolonged stain contact	Decrease staining time
Inadequate wash	Wash longer
Specimen too thick	Make thinner smears, if possible
Stain, diluent, buffer, or wash water too alkaline	Check with pH paper and correct pH
Exposure to formalin vapors	Store and ship cytologic preparations separate from formalin containers
Wet fixation in ethanol or formalin	Air dry smears before fixation
Delayed fixation	Fix smears sooner, if possible
Surface of the slide was alkaline	Use new slides
Excessive Pink Staining	
Insufficient staining time	Increase staining time
Prolonged washing	Decrease duration of wash
Stain or diluent too acidic	Check with pH paper and correct pH; fresh methanol may be needed
Excessive time in red stain solution	Decrease time in red stain solution
Inadequate time in blue stain solution	Increase time in blue stain solution
Mounting coverslip before preparation is dry	Allow preparation to dry completely before mounting coverslip
Weak Staining	
Insufficient contact with one or more of the stain solutions	Increase staining time
Fatigued (old) stains	Change stains
Another slide covered specimen during staining	Keep slides separate
Uneven Staining	
Variation of pH in different areas of slide surface (may be caused by slide surface being touched or slide being poorly cleaned)	Use new slides; avoid touching their surface before and after preparation
Water allowed to stand on some areas of the slide after staining and washing	Tilt slides close to vertical to drain water from the surface or dry with a fan
Inadequate mixing of stain and buffer	Mix stain and buffer thoroughly
Precipitate on Preparation	
Inadequate stain filtration	Filter or change the stain(s)
Inadequate washing of slide after staining	Rinse slides well after staining
Dirty slides used	Use clean, new slides
Stain solution dries during staining	Use sufficient stain; do not leave it on slide too long
Miscellaneous	
Overstained preparations	Destain with 95% methanol and restain; Diff-Quik—stained smears may have to be destained in the red Diff-Quik stain solution to remove the blue color; however, this damages the red stain solution
Refractile artifact on red blood cells with Diff-Quik stain (usually caused by moisture in the fixative)	Change the fixative

From Valenciano AC, Cowell RL: *Cowell and Tyler's diagnostic cytology and hematology of the dog and cat*, ed 4, St Louis, 2014, Mosby.

found in the blood of most mammals. Each type of cell plays an important role in the body's defense system, and the total concentration of each type is extremely valuable for the diagnosis of various diseases. Functions of the WBCs include phagocytosis, the release of substances that modulate the immune system, and the production of antibodies. Fig 9.6 is a WBC comparison chart to help you quickly compare the identifying characteristics of WBCs seen in blood smears.

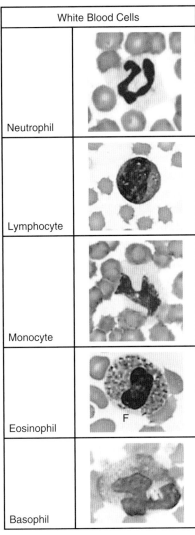

White Blood Cells	
Neutrophil	
Lymphocyte	
Monocyte	
Eosinophil	
Basophil	

Fig 9.6 WBC comparison chart.

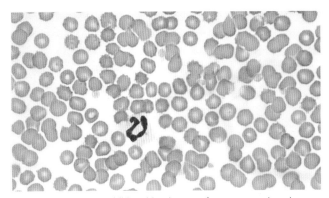

Fig. 9.7 A neutrophil in a blood smear from a normal canine.

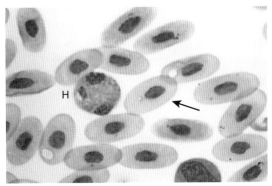

Fig. 9.8 Nucleated erythrocytes in a blood smear from a reptile. A heterophil *(H)* is also present.

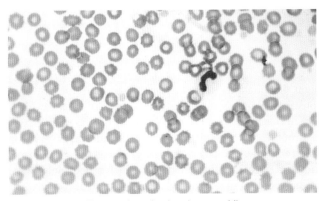

Fig. 9.9 A canine band neutrophil.

Morphologic Features of Mammalian Leukocytes in the Peripheral Blood

Neutrophil. Neutrophils are the most abundant WBCs in the peripheral blood of most mammals. The nucleus of the neutrophil is irregular and elongated, and true filaments between nuclear lobes are rare (Fig. 9.7). The presence of three to five nuclear lobes is characteristic of mammalian neutrophils in the peripheral circulation. The nucleus of equine neutrophils has heavily clumped, coarse chromatin. The cytoplasm stains pale pink, with fine, diffuse granules. Bovine neutrophils have darker-pink cytoplasm. The primary function of neutrophils is phagocytosis. Increased numbers of neutrophils usually indicate infection or inflammation.

> **TECHNICIAN NOTE** Mature neutrophils in the peripheral blood contain three to five nuclear lobes.

In avian, reptile, some fish, and some small mammal species (e.g., rabbits, guinea pigs), the cell that is functionally equivalent to the neutrophil is referred to as a heterophil. Heterophils have distinct eosinophilic granules in their cytoplasm (Fig. 9.8).

The function of a neutrophil is to transmigrate through the vascular endothelium. They serve as the first line of defense against microbial invasion. Neutrophils are responsible for both phagocytosis and microbiocidal action, which includes chemotaxis followed by ingestion and degranulation, ultimately leading to microbial death. This action is not limited to bacteria as fungi, yeasts, algae, viruses, and parasites may be damaged or destroyed by neutrophils as well.

Band neutrophil. The nucleus of band neutrophils is horseshoe-shaped, with large round ends (Fig. 9.9). Although

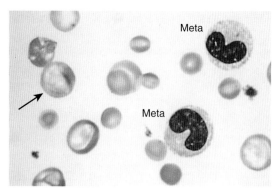

Fig. 9.10 Metamyelocytes on a blood smear from a dog with regenerative anemia. Polychromatophilic red blood cells *(arrow)* are also present, along with several spherocytes.

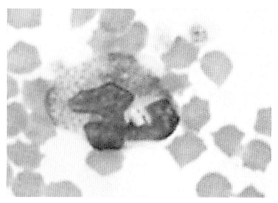

Fig. 9.12 Normal feline basophil.

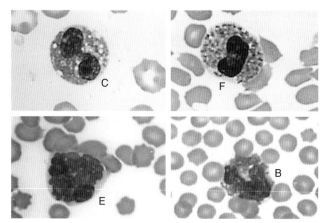

Fig. 9.11 Canine *(C)*, feline *(F)*, equine *(E)*, and bovine *(B)* eosinophils that demonstrate the variable size, shape, and color of granules in different species.

slight indentations may be present in the nucleus, if the constriction makes up more than one third of the width of the nucleus, the cell is usually classified as a segmented neutrophil. The designation of a neutrophil as a band or a mature segmented cell is somewhat subjective. Each facility should clearly state the criteria for which a neutrophil will be designated a band and apply those criteria consistently to all samples. If in doubt about whether a particular cell is a band or a mature segmented cell, the cell is best classified as a mature cell. More immature neutrophils (e.g., myelocytes, metamyelocytes) are not common in peripheral blood (Fig. 9.10). They may be seen in response to infection.

Eosinophil. Eosinophils contain a nucleus that is similar to that of neutrophils, but the chromatin is usually not as coarsely clumped. The shape of the eosinophilic granules varies considerably among species (Fig. 9.11). The granules in canine eosinophils often vary in size with small and large granules within the same cell, and they stain less intensely than those of other species; they are usually dark red and round. Feline eosinophils contain granules that are small, rod-shaped, and numerous. Equine eosinophil granules are large and round to

oval, and they stain an intense orange-red color. Eosinophil granules in cattle, sheep, and pigs are round and much smaller than those found in horses, and they stain an intense pink. Eosinophils are capable of phagocytosis, but their primary function is in the modulation of the immune system. They possess both phagocytic and bactericidal properties, but they are less effective in these processes than neutrophils. Eosinophils attach to and kill parasites and are attracted by chemical mediators liberated by mast cells during allergic and anaphylactic reactions. Increased numbers of eosinophils are commonly seen in patients with allergic reactions and parasite infections or infestations.

> **TECHNICIAN NOTE** The size, color, shape, and number of granules present in eosinophils vary among species.

Basophil. The nuclei of basophils are similar to those of monocytes. Basophil granules in dogs are few in number and stain a purple to blue-black color. Equine and bovine basophil granules are usually more numerous, they tend to stain a blue-black color, and they may completely pack the cytoplasm. Feline basophil granules are round, and they stain a light lavender color (Fig. 9.12). Basophils are involved in the mediation of the immune system. They are the source of mediators of inflammation. If they are even present it will be in small numbers within the peripheral blood. Basophils can increase in numbers with a variety of inflammatory and infectious conditions.

> **TECHNICIAN NOTE** Basophils are not commonly seen on the blood smear.

Lymphocyte. Lymphocytes are present in a variety of sizes in the peripheral blood. They are the most abundant WBCs in samples from ruminant patients. Small lymphocytes are approximately 7 to 9 μ in diameter in dogs and cats, and they have slightly indented nuclei (Fig. 9.13). The chromatin is coarsely clumped, and the cytoplasm is light blue and quite

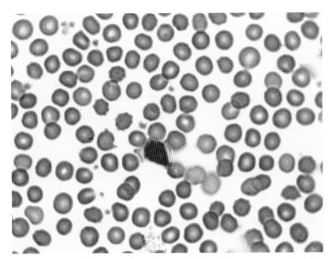

Fig. 9.13 A small, mature lymphocyte in blood from a normal canine.

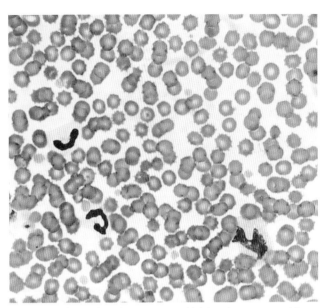

Fig. 9.14 Normal canine monocyte *(right)* and two neutrophils.

scanty. Chromocenters, which are areas of condensed chromatin, should not be confused with nucleoli; chromocenters appear as dark clumps within the nucleus. Medium-size to large lymphocytes are 9 to 11 μ in diameter, with more abundant cytoplasm. The cytoplasm may contain pink-purple granules. Normal bovine lymphocytes may contain nucleolar rings, and they are large and difficult to distinguish from monocytes or neoplastic lymphoid cells. A major function of lymphocytes is the production of antibody. There are essentially two types of lymphocytes: T cells and B cells. T cells circulate throughout the blood and lymph systems. B cells typically reside in in the lymph nodes. You cannot differentiate T cells from B cells by looking at their morphology. Increased numbers of lymphocytes often indicate a viral infection.

> **TECHNICIAN NOTE** A variety of sizes of lymphocytes are usually present in the peripheral blood.

Monocyte. Monocytes are the largest of the WBCs in the peripheral blood, and they contain variably shaped nuclei (Fig. 9.14). The nucleus is occasionally the shape of a kidney bean, but it is often elongated, lobulated, or amoeboid. The nuclear chromatin is more diffuse in monocytes than in neutrophils, in which it is coarsely clumped. The cytoplasm of monocytes is a blue-gray color, and it may contain vacuoles and small, fine, pink granules. Monocytes may be difficult to distinguish from band neutrophils, large lymphocytes, or metamyelocytes that are toxic. If a left shift is not present, the cells in question are probably monocytes. The major function of monocytes is phagocytosis. They digest foreign material, cellular debris, and dead cells. They are less efficient phagocytes than neutrophils. Increased numbers of monocytes are seen in a variety of chronic infections. Once monocytes are distributed to the surrounding tissue, they

transform to macrophages that contain more proteolytic enzymes and granules than the precursor monocyte. Macrophages are rarely encountered in blood but may be observed in capillary blood smears where certain diseases are present.

> **TECHNICIAN NOTE** Monocytes are the largest WBCs in the peripheral blood.

Morphology of Normal Erythrocytes in the Peripheral Blood

Normal erythrocyte morphologic features vary among different species of domestic animals. Normal canine erythrocytes have a biconcave disc shape and a distinct area of central pallor (Fig. 9.15). Feline erythrocytes are round, with little or no central pallor. Unlike mammalian RBCs, RBCs of avian, reptile, amphibian, and fish species are nucleated (see Fig. 9.8). Oval, elliptical, and elongated erythrocytes may be seen with various types of anemia; these are sometimes referred to as pencil cells. In the llama and other members of the camel family, these are the predominant cell type, and they do not indicate a pathologic condition (Fig. 9.16). Normal goat and sheep blood may also contain oval-shaped erythrocytes. Hemoglobin pigment may appear evenly disbursed throughout the cell or concentrated at each end of the oval, with a central area of pallor.

> **TECHNICIAN NOTE** Normal canine erythrocytes have a biconcave disc shape.

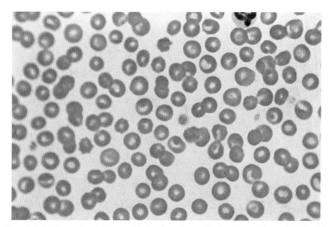

Fig. 9.15 Normal canine red blood cells and platelets. (From Sirois M: *Principles and practice of veterinary technology*, ed 2, St Louis, 2004, Mosby.)

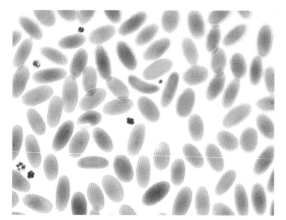

Fig. 9.16 Elliptocytes in blood from a normal llama (Wright-Giemsa stain). (From Harvey J: *Veterinary hematology*, St Louis, 2012, Saunders.)

Performing the Differential Cell Count

Although most veterinary hematology analyzers provide at least a partial differential WBC count, a blood smear must still be prepared and evaluated. A large number of abnormalities will not be routinely reported by automated analyzers, including nucleated RBCs, toxic granulation, platelet clumps, target cells, and hemoparasites.

Examining the slides the same way each time is important to avoid making mistakes when counting cells or missing important observations. Always begin the examination by scanning the slide under low-power magnification (100×). A general assessment of overall cell numbers can be obtained.

The entire slide should then be scanned for the presence of platelet clumps, large abnormal cells, and microfilariae. Locating the feathered edge and the monolayer is performed next, at high-power magnification (Fig. 9.17). The feathered edge area of the blood smear contains cells that are usually greatly distorted and erratically distributed. The monolayer is the area of the blood smear where the cells are evenly and randomly distributed and not distorted. After these two areas

are identified, the technician focuses on one microscopic field in the monolayer just adjacent to the feathered edge. The differential count is performed in the smear monolayer by using oil-immersion (1000×) magnification. A minimum of 100 WBCs are counted, identified, and recorded during this count. Because 100 WBCs are counted, the number of each WBC type observed is recorded as a percentage. This is called the relative WBC count. Various counting devices are available to help perform the differential WBC count (Fig. 9.18).

> **TECHNICIAN NOTE** The differential blood leukocyte count provides the relative percentage of each type of WBC present in the peripheral blood.

Absolute Values

After the relative percentages of each cell type have been determined, the absolute value of each cell type must be calculated. Calculation of absolute values is accomplished by multiplying the total WBC count by the percentage of each cell type. For example, if 80% neutrophils were counted on the blood smear and the total WBC count was 6000/µL, then the absolute value for neutrophils is 80% of 6000 or 4800 neutrophils/µL of blood.

The relative percentage of each cell type from the differential count may be misleading, especially when evaluating samples in which the total WBC count or the relative percentages of the differential count are not in the normal range. For example, consider that the normal range of segmented neutrophils on a canine blood smear is 60% to 70%, with an absolute value of 3000 to 11,300/µL, and that the normal ranges for lymphocytes are 12% to 30%, with an absolute value of 1400 to 8000/µL. If a canine patient has a relative neutrophil count of 88% and 12% lymphocytes, this would appear to be neutrophilia with a normal lymphocyte count. However, if the patient has a total WBC count of 11,000 (within the normal range), the absolute value for neutrophils is 9680/µL (a normal level), and the absolute value for lymphocytes is 1320/µL (a low level); the patient actually has a mild lymphopenia. Similarly, a patient with a relative lymphocyte count of 7% would appear to have a lymphopenia. However, if the patient's total WBC count was 30,000/µL, then the absolute value for lymphocytes for that patient is 2100/µL, which is a normal absolute value.

Platelet Estimate

Platelets (thrombocytes) are an important component of hemostasis. One procedure for platelet evaluation is the examination of the blood smear. When platelet numbers appear to be decreased, determining platelet concentration by a more quantitative procedure is appropriate. Platelet numbers should be evaluated in the counting area of the blood smear. The numbers of platelets in a minimum of 10 1000× microscopic fields should be counted. The size of the oil-immersion field depends on the type of microscope used. An average of 7 to 10

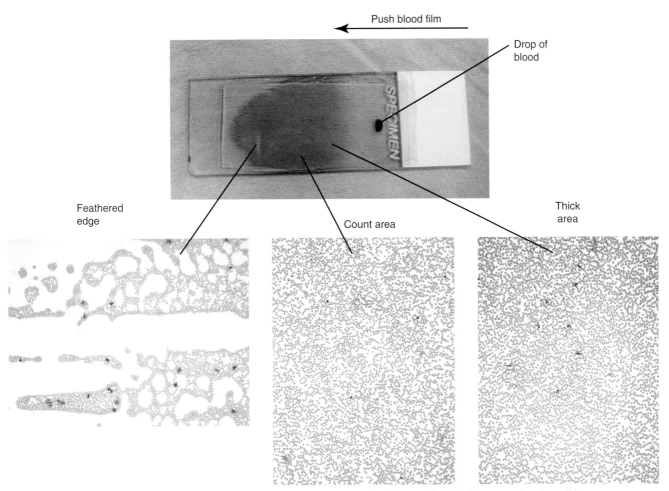

Fig. 9.17 Gross and microscopic views of different areas on a blood smear. The blood smear on the glass slide at the top was made by pushing the blood from the drop *(Drop of blood)* at the right to the left *(large arrow)*. The three major areas of the blood smear *(Feathered edge, Count area,* and *Thick area)* are indicated by the lines connected to the respective microscopic views. (From Valenciano A, et al: *Canine and feline blood smear analysis: a practical atlas,* St Louis, 2014, Mosby.)

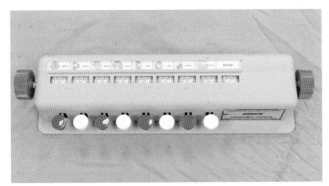

Fig. 9.18 A standard mechanical counter used for the differential leukocyte count.

platelets per oil-immersion field are more common in normal patients. Platelet estimates can also be reported as the average number seen in 10 microscopic fields or as the range seen in 10 fields. Multiplying the estimated platelet number (as averaged from 10 fields) by 20,000 is also used as an indirect measure of the platelet count. An alternative method for the indirect measurement of the platelet number involves counting the number of platelets seen per 100 WBCs on the blood smear. This number is then used to calculate the platelet estimate with the following equation:

$$\text{Thrombocytes per 100 Leukocytes} \times \text{WBC Count per } \mu\text{L}$$
$$= \text{Thrombocytes per } \mu\text{L}$$

Platelet clumping is common among mammals. If clumps are observed (Fig. 9.19), platelets are probably adequate in number. The presence of unusually large platelets (i.e., mega-thrombocytes) (Fig. 9.20) may suggest the early release of platelets from the bone marrow and should be noted. Platelets, especially in cats, may be larger than erythrocytes. The presence of these megaplatelets may affect the total RBC and platelet counts, depending on the type of analyzer used. If decreased platelet numbers are suspected on the basis of the blood smear examination, a platelet count is indicated.

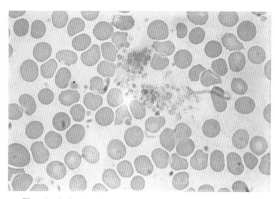

Fig. 9.19 A platelet clump in a canine blood smear.

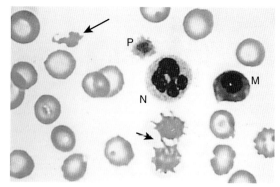

Fig. 9.20 A megathrombocyte *(P)*, an acanthocyte *(short arrow)*, and a schistocyte *(long arrow)* on a canine blood smear. *N,* Neutrophil; *M,* Lymphocyte.

KEY POINTS

- The wedge smear is the most common technique used to prepare the differential blood cell count.
- Differential blood cell smears are usually stained with a Romanowsky stain.
- Blood cell smears are used to determine estimated platelet numbers.
- A minimum of 100 WBCs are counted and classified when performing the differential WBC count.
- The differential WBC count provides the relative percentage of each WBC type present in a sample.

- Absolute values are recorded by multiplying the relative percentage of each cell type by the total WBC count.
- Eosinophilic granules vary in size, color, shape, and number of granules present among species.
- Monocytes tend to have an amoeboid nucleus, and they are the largest of the WBCs in circulation.
- Neutrophils are the largest of the granulocytes, and they contain a nucleus with three to five lobes.
- Basophils are not commonly seen on the blood cell smear.

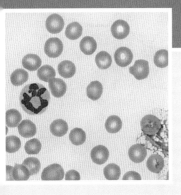

10

Morphologic Abnormalities of Blood Cells

LEARNING OBJECTIVES

After studying this chapter, you will be able to:

- Describe methods for semiquantifying morphologic changes.
- Describe the types of morphologic changes seen in white blood cells.
- Describe the types of morphologic changes seen in red blood cells.
- Discuss what is meant by the term toxic change.
- List and describe the terms used to describe abnormal changes in red blood cell size.
- List and describe the terms used to describe abnormal changes in red blood cell shape.
- List and describe the terms used to describe abnormal changes in red blood cell arrangement.
- List and describe the terms used to describe abnormal changes in red blood cell color.
- List and describe the parasites that may be seen on a blood smear.

OUTLINE

KEY TERMS

Acanthocyte
Anisocytosis
Anulocyte
Apoptosis
Atypical lymphocyte
Autoagglutination
Basophilic stippling
Codocyte
Dacryocyte
Döhle body
Drepanocyte
Echinocyte
Heinz body

Howell-Jolly body
Hyperchromatophilic
Hypersegmented
Hypochromasia
Hyposegmentation
Karyolysis
Karyorrhexis
Keratocyte
Leptocyte
Macrocytosis
Microcytosis
Nucleated erythrocyte
Pelger-Huët anomaly

Poikilocytosis
Pyknosis
Reactive lymphocyte
Rouleaux
Schistocyte
Smudge cell
Spherocyte
Stomatocyte
Target cell
Torocyte
Toxic granulation

In addition to enumerating each type of white blood cell (WBC) and estimating the platelet count, the differential blood cell count requires that the morphologic features of the cells be evaluated. The presence of any abnormal cells or toxic changes should be semiquantified.

QUANTIFYING MORPHOLOGIC CHANGES

Two methods are commonly used to assess the degree of morphologic changes. One method uses a scale of 1+, 2+, 3+, and 4+ to indicate the relative percentage of cells with the morphologic change. The designation 1+ generally equates to 5% to 10% of the cells being affected; 2+ indicates 10% to 25%, 3+ indicates approximately 50%, and 4+ indicates that more than 75% of the cells are affected. These are subjective assessments. Another method uses the designations "slight," "moderate," or "marked" to indicate approximately 10%, 25%, and more than 50% of cells as being affected, respectively.

MORPHOLOGIC ABNORMALITIES SEEN IN WHITE BLOOD CELLS

Nuclear Hyposegmentation

Pelger-Huët anomaly is a congenital hereditary defect that is characterized by the hyposegmentation of all granulocyte nuclei. Nuclear chromatin appears condensed but unsegmented, and the cytoplasm of affected cells appears normal (Fig. 10.1). Eosinophils and basophils may also be affected. The anomaly is believed to result from an autosomal-dominant trait, and it is most common in Australian shepherd dogs. Animals that are homozygous for the trait generally suffer from skeletal abnormalities and die shortly after birth. Hyposegmentation may simply reflect the early release of band neutrophils. Pseudo–Pelger-Huët anomaly has been reported and is either a variant of a normal inflammatory response or an idiosyncratic drug reaction. In general, with pseudo–Pelger-Huët anomaly, fewer neutrophils are hyposegmented than are seen with the congenital anomaly.

Nuclear Hypersegmentation

Canine and feline neutrophils with more than five lobes are considered hypersegmented (Fig. 10.2). This is usually attributable to the aging of neutrophils, either in vivo (as would be seen with endogenous or exogenous glucocorticoids, which prolong the half-life of circulating neutrophils) or in vitro (as a result of the prolonged storage of blood before blood smears are made). Hypersegmented neutrophils also are seen in the blood smears of poodles with poodle macrocytosis.

> **TECHNICIAN NOTE** Nuclear hypersegmentation of neutrophils is a commonly encountered morphologic abnormality.

Toxic Change

The most common disease-induced cytoplasmic changes in neutrophils are referred to as toxic changes and are associated with conditions such as inflammation, infection, and drug toxicity. These changes are more significant when they occur in dogs. If they are severe, they often suggest bacterial infection. However, toxic changes are quite common in cats that are not severely ill. Types of toxic change include cytoplasmic basophilia, Döhle bodies, vacuoles or "foaminess" (Fig. 10.3), and, rarely, intensely stained primary granules referred to as toxic granulation (Fig. 10.4). Affected cells may also appear much larger than normal segmented neutrophils (Fig. 10.5). These toxic changes are thought to be caused by a decreased length of time of neutrophil maturation within the marrow. Criteria for evaluating the degree of toxicity are presented in Box 10.1.

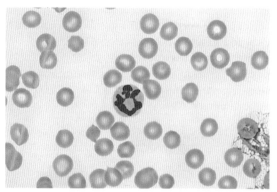
Fig. 10.2 A canine neutrophil with a hypersegmented nucleus.

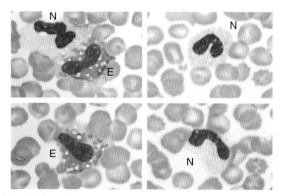
Fig. 10.1 Nuclear hyposegmentation in neutrophils (N) and eosinophils (E) from a dog with Pelger-Huët anomaly. (Wright's stain.)

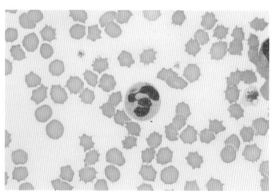
Fig. 10.3 A toxic neutrophil showing cytoplasmic basophilia and a large Döhle body. The red blood cells are crenated.

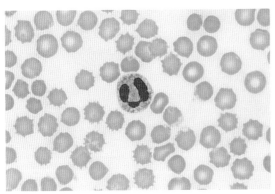

Fig. 10.4 A neutrophil with toxic granulation.

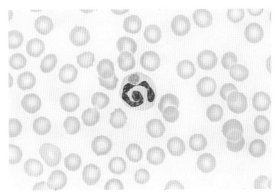

Fig. 10.6 A canine neutrophil that contains an *Ehrlichia* morula.

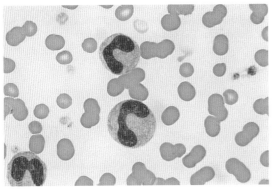

Fig. 10.5 A giant neutrophil adjacent to a normally proportioned feline neutrophil.

BOX 10.1 Semiquantitative Evaluation of Toxic Changes in the Cytoplasm of Neutrophils

Neutrophils With Toxic Changes	
Few	5-10%
Moderate	11-30%
Many	>30%
Severity of Toxic Changes in Cytoplasm	
Döhle bodies*	1+
Mildly basophilic	1+
Moderately basophilic with Döhle bodies	2+
Moderately basophilic and foamy†	3+
Basophilic with toxic granules†	3+

*One or two Döhle bodies are sometimes seen in a few neutrophils from cats that do not exhibit signs of illness.
†May also contain Döhle bodies.
From Harvey JW: *Veterinary hematology*, St. Louis, 2012, Saunders.

TECHNICIAN NOTE Toxic changes include giantism, cytoplasmic basophilia, Döhle bodies, and toxic granulation.

Intracytoplasmic Inclusions in Infectious Diseases

Canine distemper inclusions may appear in red blood cells (RBCs) or neutrophils, and they stain a pale blue to magenta color. The morulae of rickettsial organisms (i.e., *Ehrlichia* and *Anaplasma* species) may be seen within the cytoplasm of neutrophils (Fig. 10.6). Other infectious agents that may be demonstrated as inclusions within neutrophils or monocytes include *Histoplasma capsulatum*, *Francisella philomiragia*, *Mycobacterium*, gametocytes of *Hepatozoon canis*, and amastigotes of *Leishmania infantum*.

Atypical and Reactive Lymphocytes

Azurophilic granules in the cytoplasm of lymphocytes (Fig. 10.7) are often associated with chronic antigenic stimulation, especially with canine ehrlichiosis. Azurophilic granules may be present in normal bovine lymphocytes. Atypical lymphocytes may also have basophilic cytoplasm and cleaved nuclei, and they may show evidence of asynchronous maturation of the nucleus and the cytoplasm. Reactive lymphocytes (Fig. 10.8) have increased basophilia in the cytoplasm; they may have more abundant cytoplasm, and they sometimes contain a larger and more convoluted nucleus. These changes are usually caused by antigenic stimulation secondary to vaccination or infection. Reactive lymphocytes are also referred to as immunocytes.

Lysosomal Storage Disorders

With this group of rare inherited diseases, a substance is abnormally stored within cells, usually as a result of an intracellular enzyme deficiency. Numerous types of these conditions have been reported in animals. Clinical signs vary depending on the specific enzyme deficiency. Most types involve either skeletal abnormalities or progressive neurologic disease. Because most cells of the body are affected, the stored substance may be seen in leukocytes (usually monocytes, lymphocytes, or neutrophils). The appearance of the leukocytes varies depending on the type of lysosomal storage disease. Lymphocytes may be vacuolated, or they may contain granules; neutrophils may also contain granules (Fig. 10.9).

Birman Cat Neutrophil Granulation Anomaly

Neutrophils from cats affected by Birman cat anomaly contain fine eosinophilic to magenta granules (Fig. 10.10). This anomaly is inherited as an autosomal-recessive trait. Neutrophil function is normal, and affected cats are healthy. This

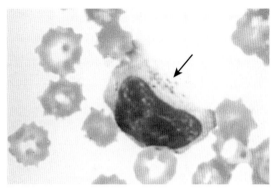

Fig. 10.7 An atypical lymphocyte that contains azurophilic granules in a canine blood smear.

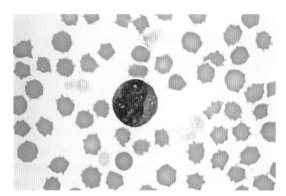

Fig. 10.8 A reactive lymphocyte in a canine blood smear. Numerous acanthocytes are also present.

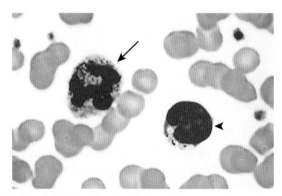

Fig. 10.9 A feline lymphocyte that contains vacuoles and granules *(arrowhead)* as well as a neutrophil with toxic granulation *(arrow)*.

granulation must be distinguished from toxic granulation and the granulation seen in the neutrophils of cats with mucopolysaccharidosis and GM_2 gangliosidosis, which are two of the lysosomal storage disorders.

Chédiak-Higashi Syndrome

Neutrophils in animals with the inherited disorder Chédiak-Higashi syndrome have large, fused 0.5- to 2-mm lysosomes within the cytoplasm and stain lightly pink or eosinophilic (Fig. 10.11). Approximately one in three or four neutrophils

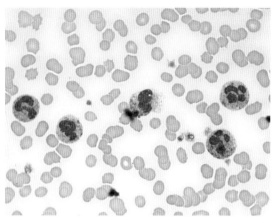

Fig. 10.10 Cytoplasmic granules associated with Birman cat anomaly. (From Valenciano A, Cowell C, Rizzi T, Tyler R: *Atlas of canine and feline peripheral blood smears*, St Louis, 2013, Mosby.)

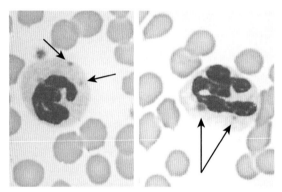

Fig. 10.11 Blood smear from a cat with Chédiak-Higashi syndrome. Note the large pink granules *(arrows)*.

contains fused lysosomes. Granules of eosinophils appear slightly plump and large. Affected animals have a slight tendency to bleed, because their platelet function is abnormal. Although neutrophil function is also abnormal, affected animals are generally healthy. The syndrome has most often been reported in Persian cats, but it has also been demonstrated to occur in cattle, foxes, and other species.

Siderotic Granules

Granules of hemosiderin may be present in the neutrophils and monocytes of animals with hemolytic anemia. They appear similar to Döhle bodies, but they can be differentiated with the use of Prussian blue stain. Döhle bodies do not stain with Prussian blue. Siderotic inclusions can also occur in erythrocytes; affected cells would be referred to as siderocytes.

Smudge Cells

Smudge cells, which are sometimes referred to as basket cells, are degenerative leukocytes that have ruptured (Fig. 10.12). Their presence is not considered significant unless large numbers are seen on the blood smear. Small numbers of smudge cells can be produced as an artifact when blood is held too long before a smear is made or if excess pressure is used when making the smear. Large numbers of smudge cells are associated with leukemia.

Karyolysis, Pyknosis, and Karyorrhexis

Karyolysis is a degenerative change to the nucleus that is characterized by the dissolution of the nuclear membrane. It usually affects neutrophils, and it is associated with the presence of septic exudates. The term karyorrhexis refers to the fragmentation of the nucleus after cell death (i.e., apoptosis); the term pyknosis refers to the condensing of the nucleus as the cell dies (Fig. 10.13).

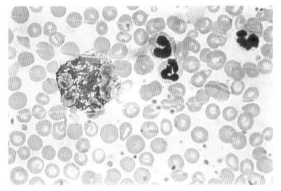

Fig. 10.12 A smudge cell and several neutrophils in a canine blood smear.

MORPHOLOGIC ABNORMALITIES SEEN IN RED BLOOD CELLS

The morphologic characteristics of erythrocytes can be categorized according to cell arrangement on the blood smear and the size, color, shape, and presence of structures in or on erythrocytes.

Variations in Cell Arrangement

Rouleaux

Rouleaux formation involves the grouping of erythrocytes in stacks (Fig. 10.14). Increased rouleaux formation is seen with increased fibrinogen or globulin concentrations. Rouleaux formation is accompanied by an increase in the erythrocyte sedimentation rate. Marked rouleaux formation is seen in healthy horses, and it may also be present on blood smears from healthy cats and pigs. Rouleaux may be seen as an artifact in blood that is held too long before a blood smear is prepared and in blood that has been refrigerated.

Autoagglutination

The agglutination of erythrocytes must be distinguished from rouleaux formation (Fig. 10.15). Autoagglutination occurs in immune-mediated disorders in which antibody coats the erythrocyte, resulting in the bridging and clumping

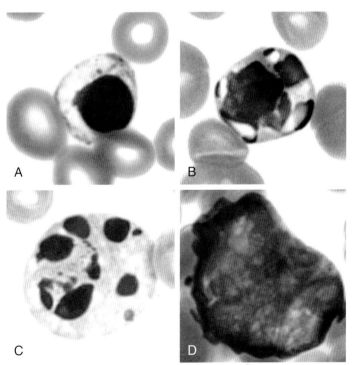

Fig. 10.13 Pyknotic and karyorrhexic cells in blood. **A,** Pyknotic cell with condensed chromatin in blood from a dog with a toxic left shift. **B,** Pyknosis and karyorrhexis of a cell in blood from a dog with dirofilariasis. **C,** Pyknosis and karyorrhexis of a cell in blood from a dog with acute monocytic leukemia (AML-M5). **D,** Pyknosis and karyorrhexis of a cell in blood from a cow with leukemic lymphoma. (Wright-Giemsa stain.) (From Harvey JW: *Veterinary hematology*, St Louis, 2012, Saunders.)

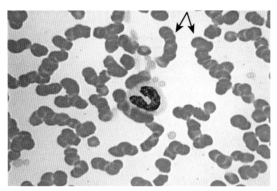

Fig. 10.14 Marked rouleaux formation in a normal equine blood smear. A neutrophilic band cell is also present.

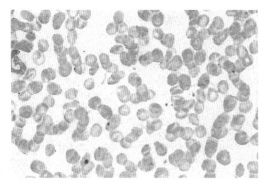

Fig. 10.15 Autoagglutination in a canine blood smear.

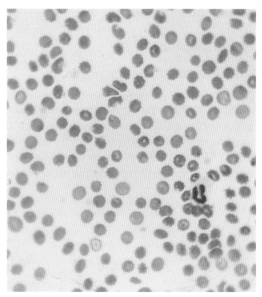

Fig. 10.16 Mixed anisocytosis in a canine blood smear. A neutrophil is also present.

of RBCs. It is sometimes observed macroscopically and microscopically. To differentiate rouleaux from agglutination, add a drop of saline to a drop of blood, and examine the sample microscopically for agglutination. Rouleaux formation will disperse in saline.

> **TECHNICIAN NOTE** Autoagglutination will not disperse when RBCs are mixed with saline.

Variations in Cell Size
Anisocytosis

Anisocytosis is a variation in the size of RBCs (Fig. 10.16), and it may indicate the presence of macrocytes (i.e., large cells), microcytes (i.e., small cells), or both. Anisocytosis is a common finding in normal bovine blood. Macrocytes are RBCs that are larger than normal, with an increased mean corpuscular volume (MCV). Macrocytes are usually young, polychromatophilic erythrocytes (i.e., reticulocytes). Microcytes are RBCs with a diameter that is smaller than that of normal erythrocytes, with a decreased MCV. Microcytic cells may be seen with iron deficiency.

> **TECHNICIAN NOTE** Anisocytosis may involve microcytes or macrocytes, or it may be a mixture of both.

Variations in Cell Color
Polychromasia

The term polychromasia refers to erythrocytes that exhibit a bluish tint when stained with Romanowsky-type stain (e.g., Wright's stain) (Fig. 10.17). The blue tint is a result of the presence of organelles that remain within the cytoplasm; therefore, these are young cells. When stained with new methylene blue or brilliant cresyl blue, these cells usually appear as reticulocytes.

Hypochromasia

Hypochromasia is a decreased staining intensity that is caused by an insufficient amount of hemoglobin within the cell (Fig. 10.18). The cell will normally appear more darkly stained along the periphery, and this gradually tapers to a much paler central region. Iron deficiency is the most common cause, although macrocytic erythrocytes often appear hypochromic because of their large diameter. Hypochromic cells should be distinguished from bowl-shaped cells (i.e., anulocytes) or "punched-out" cells (i.e., torocytes), which are generally considered artifacts that result from improper smear technique (Fig. 10.19). Animals with true hypochromasia almost always have microcytosis, which is determined by a decreased MCV. Normochromia is a normal staining intensity.

> **TECHNICIAN NOTE** True hypochromic cells have a gradual tapering of chromic material from the center of the cell to the cell's periphery.

Hyperchromatophilic

The word hyperchromatophilic refers to cells that appear to be more darkly stained than normal cells. This gives the appearance

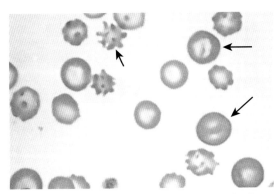

Fig. 10.17 Macrocytic polychromatophilic red blood cells *(long arrows)* and acanthocytes *(small arrow)* are present in this canine blood smear.

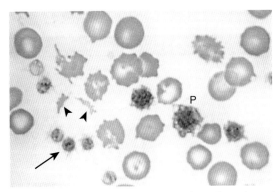

Fig. 10.20 Schistocytes *(arrowheads)*, platelets *(arrow)*, and giant platelets *(P)* are seen on this blood smear from a dog with iron-deficiency anemia.

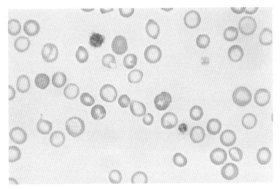

Fig. 10.18 Hypochromasia in a smear from a dog with iron deficiency. Note the increased central pallor. Several polychromatophils are also present. (From Sirois M: *Principles and practice of veterinary technology,* ed 2, St Louis, 2004, Mosby.)

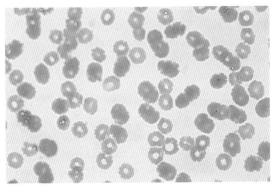

Fig. 10.19 The punched-out appearance of many of these red blood cells is an artifact caused by inadequate drying of the blood smear.

a specific diagnosis or provide information regarding the cause of the shape change. The origin of the abnormal shape depends in part on the species being examined. Shape and color changes are considered important when they are associated with specific disorders. The term poikilocytosis should be used only when the morphologic abnormalities cannot be described with the use of more specific terms.

Schistocytes

Schistocytes (Fig. 10.20), which are RBC fragments, are usually formed as a result of the shearing of the RBC via intravascular trauma. Schistocytes may be observed with disseminated intravascular coagulopathy (DIC) when erythrocytes are broken by fibrin strands, with vascular neoplasms (e.g., hemangiosarcoma), and with iron deficiency. Animals with DIC usually have concurrent thrombocytopenia.

Acanthocytes

Acanthocytes, which are also called spur cells, are irregular, spiculated RBCs with a few unevenly distributed surface projections of variable length and diameter (Fig. 10.21). They are seen in patients with altered lipid metabolism (e.g., cats with hepatic lipidosis, dogs with hemangiosarcoma of the liver). The presence of acanthocytes in middle-aged to old large-breed dogs with concurrent regenerative anemia is suggestive of hemangiosarcoma.

Echinocytes

Echinocytes, which are also called burr cells, are spiculated cells with numerous short, evenly spaced, blunt to sharp surface projections of uniform size and shape (Fig. 10.22). Echinocyte formation can be an artifactual, in vitro process associated with the slow drying of blood smears or prolonged storage of a sample. The common term for this abnormality is crenation. Echinocytes can also be produced as an artifact if the ethylenediaminetetraacetic acid tube is underfilled. Echinocytes have also been seen with renal disease and lymphosarcoma in dogs;

that the cells are oversaturated with hemoglobin. Because an RBC has a fixed maximum capacity for hemoglobin, oversaturation cannot occur. These cells are usually microcytes or spherocytes.

Variations in Cell Shape
Poikilocytes

Abnormally shaped erythrocytes are called poikilocytes. However, this terminology is not helpful, because it does not suggest

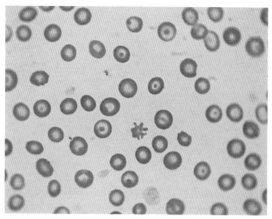

Fig. 10.21 An acanthocyte in the blood of a cat with hepatic lipidosis (Wright-Giemsa stain.) (From Harvey JW: *Veterinary hematology*, St Louis, 2012, Saunders.)

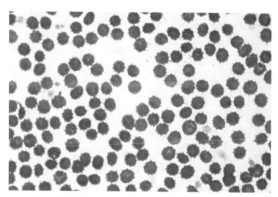

Fig. 10.22 Echinocytes in a feline blood smear.

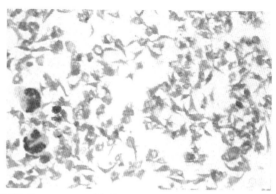

Fig. 10.23 Drepanocytes (sickle cells) in a blood smear from a normal deer.

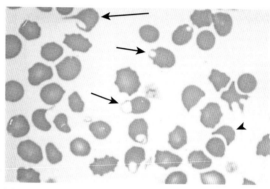

Fig. 10.24 Numerous keratocytes *(arrows)* and a schistocyte *(arrowhead)* are present in this blood smear from a cat with iron-deficiency anemia.

after exercise in horses; and in samples from normal, healthy pigs. They have also occurred after rattlesnake, coral snake, water moccasin, and asp viper envenomation in dogs.

TECHNICIAN NOTE Echinocytes are commonly produced as artifacts when slides are dried too slowly or when a sample is not mixed with the appropriate ratio of anticoagulant.

Drepanocytes

Drepanocytes, which are also called sickle cells, are observed in the blood of normal deer and angora goats. This is thought to be an in vitro phenomenon that is caused by high oxygen tension (Fig. 10.23).

Keratocytes

Keratocytes are commonly referred to as helmet cells, blister cells, or bite cells. The presence of keratocytes has been associated with hemangiosarcoma, neoplasia, glomerulonephritis, and various hepatic diseases. The cell may appear to contain a vacuole. Keratocytes are believed to form from intravascular trauma that involves the bisection of the cell by fibrin strands.

The opposing sides of the cell may then adhere to each other and form a pseudovacuole (Fig. 10.24). Keratocytes have also been demonstrated in blood from patients with anemia, liver disorders, and myelodysplastic syndrome.

Spherocytes

Spherocytes are darkly staining RBCs with reduced or no central pallor (Fig. 10.25). Spherocytes are not easily detected in species other than dogs. They have a reduced amount of membrane surface area as a result of partial phagocytosis by macrophages, which occurs in response to the presence of antibody or complement on the surface of the RBC. Spherocytes are significant in that they suggest the immune-mediated destruction of RBCs, resulting in hemolytic anemia. They also may be seen after transfusion with mismatched or improperly stored blood, after snake envenomation, in association with RBC parasites, and with zinc toxicity. Immune-mediated hemolytic anemia is usually a regenerative anemia, with marked polychromasia and a high reticulocyte count. However, in some instances, the anemia is nonregenerative as a result of antibodies against RBC precursors within the bone marrow. In these cases, spherocytes are often difficult to detect, because the presence of large polychromatophilic cells facilitates the

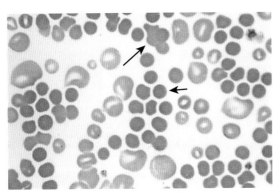

Fig. 10.25 Anisocytosis and spherocytes *(short arrow)* are present in this canine blood smear. A cluster of agglutinated cells *(long arrow)* is also present.

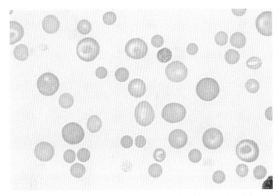

Fig. 10.26 Several target cells are present in this canine blood smear. Mixed anisocytosis and polychromasia is also present.

recognition of the small spherocytes. Although spherocytes have a decreased diameter and appear to be small, their volume is normal. In addition, dogs with immune-mediated hemolytic anemia do not have a decreased MCV.

Leptocytes

These cells are characterized by an increased membrane surface area relative to cell volume, and the affected cells may take a variety of shapes. Target cells, which are also referred to as codocytes, are leptocytes with a central area of pigment surrounded by a clear area and then a dense ring of peripheral cytoplasm (Fig. 10.26). A few may be seen in normal blood smears, and they may also be associated with anemia, liver diseases, and some inherited disorders. Leptocytes may also appear as folded cells and stomatocytes. Folded cells have a transverse, raised fold that extends across the center of the cell as well as a clear, slitlike pale region in the center of the cell (Fig. 10.27). Folded cells and stomatocytes are considered artifacts if the areas of pallor are all perpendicular to the feathered edge. Barr cells are also referred to as knizocytes. This type of leptocyte appears to have a bar of hemoglobin across the center of the cell.

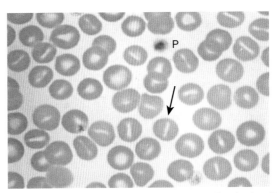

Fig. 10.27 Folded cells and stomatocytes *(arrow)* and a platelet *(P)* on a canine blood smear.

> **TECHNICIAN NOTE** Target cells are a type of leptocyte.

Elliptocytes (Ovalocytes)

Erythrocytes from camelid species and nonmammals are normally oval or elliptical in shape (see Fig. 9.16). In other species, these cells are associated with lymphoblastic leukemia, hepatic lipidosis, portosystemic shunts, and glomerulonephritis.

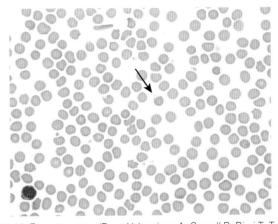

Fig. 10.28 Eccentrocytes. (From Valenciano A, Cowell R, Rizzi T, Tyler R: *Atlas of canine and feline peripheral blood smears*, St Louis, 2013, Mosby.)

Eccentrocytes

Eccentrocytes have been described in patients with diabetic ketoacidosis or neoplasia, with *Babesia canis* infections, and after the ingestion of oxidants such as garlic, onions, and acetaminophen. The cells appear to have their hemoglobin primarily pushed to one side (Fig. 10.28).

Dacryocytes

Dacryocytes are teardrop-shaped cells that are seen with myelofibrosis and certain other myeloproliferative diseases. They have also been identified in blood from llamas and alpacas that are iron deficient. These cells may be produced as artifacts, but they can be identified by the direction of their elongated

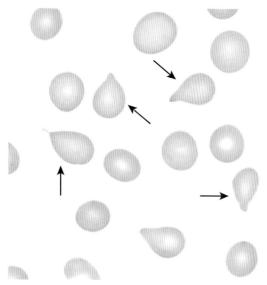

Fig. 10.29 Dacryocytes *(arrows)*. (From Turgeon ML: *Linne and Ring-srud's clinical laboratory science: the basics and routine techniques,* ed 6, St Louis, 2012, Mosby.)

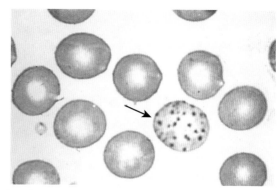

Fig. 10.30 Basophilic stippling of a red blood cell *(arrow)* from a dog with lead poisoning.

tails; dacryocytes that have been produced as artifact have their tails pointing in the same direction (Fig. 10.29).

Inclusions
Basophilic Stippling

Basophilic stippling—or the presence of small, dark-blue bodies within the erythrocyte—is observed in Wright-stained cells and represents residual RNA. It is common in immature RBCs of ruminants and occasionally in those of cats during a response to anemia. It is also characteristic of lead poisoning (Fig. 10.30).

Howell-Jolly Bodies

Howell-Jolly bodies are basophilic nuclear remnants that are seen in young erythrocytes during the response to anemia (Fig. 10.31). As cells that contain nuclear remnants pass through the spleen, phagocytic cells remove the remnants. Consequently, increased numbers may be seen after the removal of the spleen or with splenic disorders.

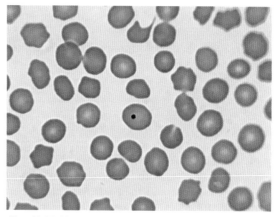

Fig. 10.31 Howell-Jolly bodies on a canine blood smear.

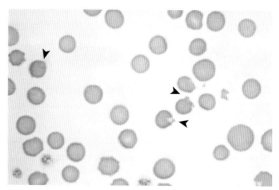

Fig. 10.32 Heinz bodies *(arrowheads)* on a feline blood smear. (Wright's stain.)

Heinz Bodies

Heinz bodies are round structures that represent denatured hemoglobin and that are caused by certain oxidant drugs or chemicals. The denatured hemoglobin becomes attached to the cell membrane and appears as a pale area with Wright's stain (Fig. 10.32). When stained with new methylene blue with the same technique used for reticulocytes, the Heinz bodies appear blue (Fig. 10.33). In dogs, Heinz bodies are 1 to 2 mm in diameter. Unlike other domestic animals, normal cats have Heinz bodies in as many as 5% of their RBCs, and Heinz bodies are often increased in concentration with diseases such as

lymphosarcoma, hyperthyroidism, and diabetes mellitus in cats.

Nucleated Erythrocytes

In mammals, nucleated erythrocytes represent the early release of immature cells during anemia, but they may also be occasionally observed in nonanemic animals (Fig. 10.34). All RBCs of nonmammalian species (e.g., birds, reptiles) contain nuclei. Nucleated RBCs (nRBCs) are included in the total WBC count performed by hemocytometers and electronic cell counters.

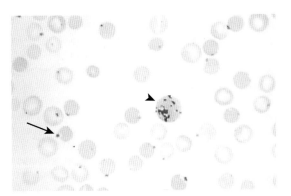

Fig. 10.33 Heinz bodies *(arrow)* on a feline blood smear. A reticulocyte *(arrowhead)* is also present. (New methylene blue stain.)

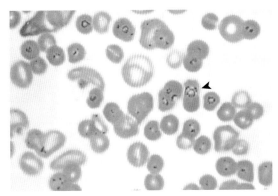

Fig. 10.35 Drying artifacts. These will appear refractile under the microscope.

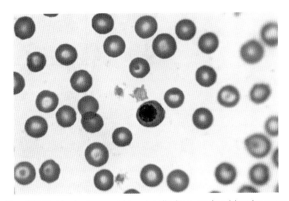

Fig. 10.34 Nucleated red blood cells in a canine blood smear.

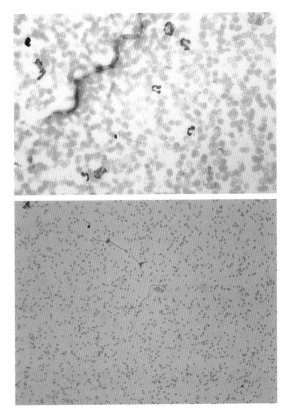

Fig. 10.36 Microfilaria of *Dirofilaria immitis* in a canine blood smear.

When performing a differential cell count, nRBCs may be counted separately and reported as nRBCs/100 WBCs. The number of nRBCs encountered while counting 100 WBCs is incorporated into the following equation to calculate a corrected leukocyte count:

$$\text{Corrected leukocyte count} = \frac{(\text{measured leukocyte count} \times 100)}{(100 + \text{nRBC})}$$

Parasites

Parasites may be present in or on erythrocytes. Stain precipitate and drying artifacts are sometimes confused with RBC parasites. Drying artifact usually appears to be refractile (Fig. 10.35). The most commonly seen blood parasites in small animals are *Ehrlichia* and *Mycoplasma*. Occasionally, a microfilaria of *Dirofilaria immitis* may be seen on a peripheral blood smear (Fig. 10.36). Other parasites that may be encountered include *Eperythrozoa, Anaplasma, Cytauxzoon,* and *Babesia*. Additional information on parasites that may infect blood cells is in Unit 6.

Mycoplasma haemofelis is a fairly common parasite of feline erythrocytes. The disease that it causes is referred to as hemobartonellosis or feline infectious anemia. The organisms appear as small (i.e., 0.2 to 0.5 mm), coccoid, rod-shaped, or ringlike structures that stain dark purple with Wright's stain

(Fig. 10.37). They most frequently appear as short rods on the periphery of RBCs. The parasitemia is cyclic; if hemobartonellosis is suspected, the blood should be examined several times at different times of the day before the infection is ruled out. Whole blood that has not been in contact with anticoagulant is preferred when evaluating a sample for suspected hemobartonellosis. The organisms often detach from the surface of the RBC when in anticoagulant. *Haemobartonella canis* infection is rare in dogs, and it is usually observed only in splenectomized or immunosuppressed dogs. The organism most commonly appears as a chain of small cocci or rods that stretch across the surface of the erythrocyte. These chains may also appear to branch.

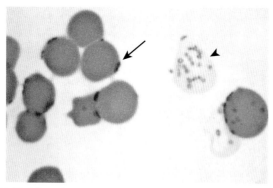

Fig. 10.37 *Mycoplasma* organisms on the periphery of erythrocytes *(arrow)*. Ring forms are visible in the lysed erythrocyte *(arrowhead)*.

A variety of species of *Ehrlichia* and *Anaplasma* are capable of infecting dogs. *Anaplasma platys* (previously *Ehrlichia platys*) affects only platelets and causes infectious cyclic thrombocytopenia. Other *Ehrlichia* species may infect any of the leukocytes. *Ehrlichia canis* commonly infects monocytes and neutrophils (Fig. 10.38). The organisms are transmitted by tick vectors; they appear as small clusters (i.e., 3 to 6 mm) called morulae in the cytoplasm. *Anaplasma marginale* is an intracellular blood parasite that causes anaplasmosis in cattle and wild ruminants. It appears as small, dark-staining cocci at the margin of the RBCs, and it must be differentiated from Howell-Jolly bodies, because their sizes are similar. Early during the course of the disease, as many as 50% of RBCs may contain parasites. By the time the anemia is severe, usually less than 5% of RBCs are affected.

Anaplasma and *Ehrlichia* parasites belong to a group of rickettsial organisms. The nomenclature of the various species has changed significantly during recent years as additional information about the biochemistry of the organisms has been uncovered. The disease may result in neutropenia, thrombocytopenia, and anemia. Chronically affected animals may be severely anemic, with marked leukopenia and thrombocytopenia, but sometimes the only hematologic abnormality is lymphocytosis. The total plasma protein level is usually increased. The organisms are best demonstrated during the acute phase, but they are usually present in small numbers. Smears made from the buffy coat may help with diagnosis. However, in most cases, organisms are not seen, and the diagnosis is made by immunologic testing.

Eperythrozoonosis in swine, cattle, and llamas is quite similar to hemobartonellosis; the organisms are closely related. *Eperythrozoa* appear as small (i.e., 0.8 to 1.0 mm) cocci, rods, or rings on the RBC surface or free in the plasma. The ring form is the most common (Fig. 10.39).

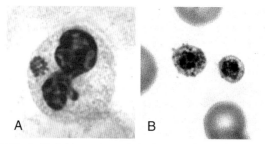

Fig. 10.38 A, *Ehrlichia equi* morula in the cytoplasm of a neutrophil. **B,** Two platelets that contain *Ehrlichia platys* morulae. (From Harvey JW: *Atlas of veterinary hematology: blood and bone marrow of domestic animals*, St Louis, 2001, Saunders.)

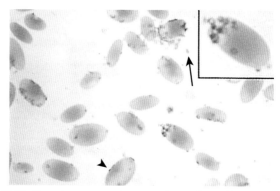

Fig. 10.39 *Eperythrozoa* organisms on the surface of red blood cells *(arrowhead)* and free in the plasma *(arrow)* in a blood smear from a camel. Note the oval red blood cells, which are normal in this species.

Cytauxzoon felis is a rare cause of hemolytic anemia in cats. The organism appears as small (i.e., 1 to 2 mm), irregular ring forms within erythrocytes, lymphocytes, and macrophages (Fig. 10.40).

Babesiosis of cattle is caused by *Babesia bigemina* and *B. bovis.* The disease is also called Texas fever, red water fever, and cattle tick fever. *Babesia* spp. appear as large (i.e., 3 to 4 mm), pleomorphic, teardrop-shaped intracellular organisms that are frequently seen in pairs (Fig. 10.41). Babesiosis in horses (i.e., piroplasmosis) is caused by *B. equi* and *B. caballi,* which are similar to *B. bigemina.* Babesiosis is rare in horses, and the few cases that have been reported in the United States have been seen in the South (especially Florida). Babesiosis in dogs is caused by *B. canis* and *B. gibsoni.* These organisms are similar in appearance to *B. bigemina,* but *B. gibsoni* is slightly smaller, and it appears as rings. Only a small percentage of erythrocytes may be affected. The organisms are more commonly observed in RBCs at the feathered edge.

Stain Precipitate Artifact

Stain precipitate appears as variably sized purple granules (Fig. 10.42). These granules can be concentrated in one area of the smear or may be randomly distributed throughout the smear. To avoid this artifact ensure you are changing your stains regularly.

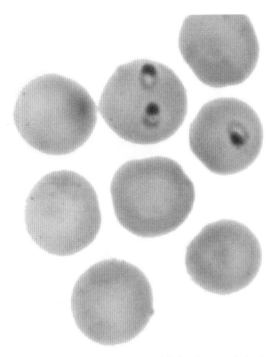

Fig. 10.40 Feline erythrocytes infected with the characteristic signet-ring shaped *Cytauxzoon* piroplasms. The clear nuclear area in the parasite allows the organism to be differentiated from hemotropic *Mycoplasma* organisms. (Wright-Giemsa, ×330.) (From Little S: *The cat*, St Louis, 2011, Saunders.)

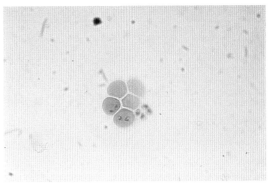

Fig. 10.41 *Babesia* organisms in bovine red blood cells.

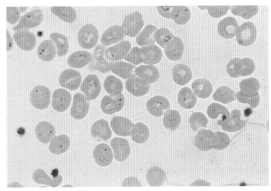

Fig. 10.42 Stain precipitate artifact. (From Valenciano AC, Cowell RL: *Cowell and Tyler's diagnostic cytology and hematology of the dog and cat*, ed 5, 2020, Elsevier Inc.)

▌ KEY POINTS

- Changes in leukocyte morphologic features may affect the nucleus or the cytoplasm or involve inclusions within the cell.
- Changes in erythrocyte morphologic features affect cells' size, shape, color, and arrangement.
- Morphologic changes that are seen on a blood smear must be semiquantified.
- Nuclear changes to leukocytes include hyposegmentation, hypersegmentation, pyknosis, karyolysis, and karyorrhexis.

- Inclusions that are seen in leukocytes include lysosomes, a variety of abnormal granules, and blood parasites.
- Changes in erythrocyte size can involve microcytes, macrocytes, or both.
- Alterations in erythrocyte behavior include rouleaux formation and autoagglutination.
- Inclusions seen in erythrocytes include Howell-Jolly bodies, Heinz bodies, basophilic stippling, and a variety of blood parasites.

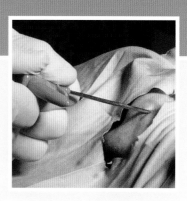

11

Additional Hematological Tests

RETICULOCYTE COUNT

Reticulocytes are immature erythrocytes that contain organelles (ribosomes) that are lost as the cells mature (Fig. 11.1). These organelles account for the diffuse blue-gray or polychromatophilic staining of immature cells with Wright's stain. Romanowsky stain does not stain these cellular components. A supravital stain, such as new methylene blue or brilliant cresyl blue, must be used. Supravital stains contain no fixatives. When reticulocytes are stained with supravital stain, the organelles clump into visible granules that are referred to as reticulum. This reticulum is present as aggregates or chains of blue granules. The stain must be fresh, and it should be filtered before use; this will help to minimize artifacts such as stain precipitate and bacteria that are present in these supravital stains.

Some automated analyzers that use laser-based methods can provide a reticulocyte count. Several manual methods can be used to prepare reticulocyte smears. Special reticulocyte kits are

available, or blood can be stained by placing a few drops of blood and an equal number of drops of new methylene blue or brilliant cresyl blue stain in a small test tube. The mixture is allowed to stand for approximately 15 minutes. A drop of the mixture is then used to prepare a conventional air-dried blood smear, which can then be examined or counterstained with Wright's stain. Because the test is generally performed on anemic patients, the blood drop used should be larger and the smear made a bit more thickly than a standard blood smear. Alternatively, the stain can also be added to a drop of blood directly on a glass slide. The stain and blood should be well mixed and allowed to stand for several minutes before the blood smear is created. The staining intensity of reticulocytes may be enhanced by placing the prepared reticulocyte slide in 95% methanol for a few seconds and following this with placement in the methylene blue component of the Diff-Quik kit (Siemens USA, Palo Alto, CA) for 5 seconds.

Cats, unlike other species, have two morphologic forms of reticulocytes. The aggregate form contains large clumps of

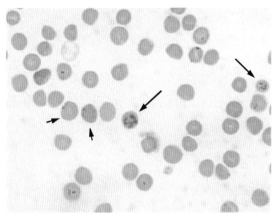

Fig. 11.1 Feline blood smear with both punctate *(short arrows)* and aggregate *(long arrows)* reticulocytes.

TABLE 11.1 Reticulocyte Maturation Index	
Patient Packed Cell Volume	**Maturation Time**
45%	1
35%	1.4
25%	2
15%	2.5

reticulum, it is similar to reticulocytes in other species, and it represents the same cell that stains polychromatophilic with Wright's stain. The punctate form, which is unique to cats, contains two to eight small, singular, basophilic granules. These cells do not stain polychromatophilic with Wright's stain. In normal, nonanemic cats, approximately 0.4% of the red blood cells (RBCs) are aggregate reticulocytes, whereas 1.5% to 10% of the RBCs are punctate reticulocytes. For a meaningful reticulocyte count in cats, only the aggregate form of reticulocytes should be counted.

A reticulocyte count is an expression of the percentage of RBCs that are reticulocytes. The percentage of reticulocytes per 1000 erythrocytes is determined with the use of an oil-immersion lens. A reticulocyte count should be performed on the blood of all anemic domestic animals except horses, which do not release reticulocytes from the bone marrow, even in the face of regenerative anemia. Reticulocyte concentration is useful for assessing the bone marrow's response to anemia.

Reticulocyte counts should be interpreted according to the degree of anemia, because fewer mature erythrocytes are present in anemic animals, and reticulocytes are released earlier and persist longer than they do in normal animals. Higher percentages may be seen in hemolytic anemia as compared with hemorrhagic types of anemia. Although reticulocyte results are often reported as a percentage, a more useful method is to calculate a corrected reticulocyte count and a reticulocyte production index.

A corrected reticulocyte count is calculated by multiplying the observed reticulocyte percentage by the observed packed cell volume (PCV) divided by the normal PCV. For dogs, 45% is used as the normal PCV; 35% is used for cats. For example, if a dog has a PCV of 15% and an observed reticulocyte count of 15%, then the corrected reticulocyte count is obtained as follows:

$$15\% \times \frac{15\%}{45\%} = 5\%$$

Some practitioners may prefer to use the reticulocyte production index. The reticulocyte production index is calculated by dividing the corrected reticulocyte percentage by the maturation time of the reticulocyte for the observed patient's PCV. Maturation time values are based on the patient's PCV (Table 11.1). For the previous example, if the dog's corrected reticulocyte count is 5% with a PCV of 15%, then the reticulocyte production index is $5/2.5 = 2$, which indicates that the patient is producing reticulocytes at a rate that is 2 times greater than normal.

BONE MARROW EVALUATION

Bone marrow evaluation is a valuable tool for diagnosis and prognosis in specific cases. The need for bone marrow evaluation is usually determined by the findings of the differential count from a peripheral blood cell sample. When the differential leukocyte count from the peripheral blood smear demonstrates ambiguous or unexplained abnormal results, bone marrow evaluation is usually needed to provide sufficient detail for the diagnostician. Specific indications for bone marrow evaluation include persistent unexplained pancytopenia, neutropenia or thrombocytopenia, and nonregenerative anemia. Less-common indications for bone marrow evaluation include the presence of cells with abnormal morphologic features or the unexplained presence of immature cells on the differential blood cell count. (e.g., nucleated RBCs, left shift). Bone marrow evaluation is also used to stage neoplastic disease and to diagnose specific parasitic diseases (e.g., leishmaniasis, ehrlichiosis). Bone marrow evaluation may be contraindicated in some cases, particularly when certain hemostatic defects are present.

Collection of Bone Marrow Samples

Samples may be collected by aspiration or removal of a bone marrow core. Proper restraint is crucial for biopsy of the bone marrow in dogs and cats, and sedation or local anesthesia is needed. General anesthesia may be used, but this is complicated, because patients undergoing bone marrow evaluation are usually compromised and represent a significant anesthetic risk. Aseptic technique is vital throughout the procedure.

All necessary equipment and supplies should be gathered before beginning the procedure. To collect bone marrow aspirate samples, prepare syringes with ethylenediaminetetraacetic acid (EDTA) solution by drawing 0.5 mL of saline into the syringe and dispensing it into an empty small EDTA blood collection tube. Withdraw the mixture, and then repeat the procedure; this creates a diluted EDTA flush to use on the

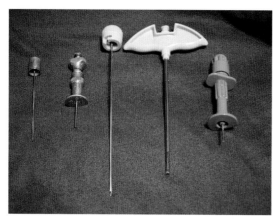

Fig. 11.2 Bone marrow needles *(left to right):* Rosenthal stylet, Rosenthal needle, Jamshidi needle, Jamshidi stylet, and Illinois needle.

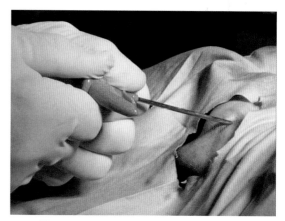

Fig. 11.3 Bone marrow aspiration technique.

syringe and bone marrow needle. Gather the necessary slides, and set them on an incline. Usually, about 12 slides should be prepared. Other equipment that is needed includes a no. 11 scalpel blade, sterile skin preparation supplies, and suture material, if appropriate. Special bone marrow needles are preferred, although an 18-gauge hypodermic needle may be used for collection from puppies and kittens. Bone marrow needles have a stylet that serves to prevent the occlusion of the needle with bone and surrounding tissue as it is inserted into the marrow cavity. Needle types that are used for bone marrow collection include the Rosenthal, Illinois sternal, and Jamshidi needles (Fig. 11.2). Bone marrow needles are available as disposable products.

Aspiration Biopsy

Several sites can be used for an aspiration biopsy, including the head of the humerus and the femoral head. The site must be aseptically prepared and draped. A stab incision is made at the site with a sterile scalpel blade, and the needle is inserted with the stylet in place (Fig. 11.3). Slight pressure should be placed on the side of the needle against the stylet to avoid blockage of the needle with bony material. A slight caudoventral angle introduces the needle into the head of the humerus. The needle and stylet are advanced until the cortex of the humerus is reached. The needle is then rotated while slight forward pressure is applied; this allows the needle to penetrate the cortical bone, and it keeps the needle in place. The stylet is then removed, and a syringe is attached. A large syringe (i.e., 10–20 mL) is usually preferred to allow for greater negative pressure. The syringe plunger is rapidly and vigorously withdrawn until a few drops of blood enter the hub of the needle. As soon as a few drops of material are present in the hub of the needle, pressure should be released to minimize the hemodilution of the sample. Ideally, the stylet should be replaced and the needle left in place until smears are prepared to ensure that an adequate sample has been obtained. A small suture may be needed to close the site. Bone marrow aspirate samples clot rapidly, so smears must be made immediately or the sample

mixed with 0.5 mL of 2% to 3% EDTA in saline. Even when smears are made immediately, placing a small amount of EDTA in the syringe and needle before beginning the collection procedure may be helpful.

Core Biopsy

In most situations, better-quality samples and greater diagnostic information are obtained if a core sample of marrow is collected in addition to an aspiration biopsy. Always use different sites for each collection when collecting both an aspirate and a core sample to ensure that the procedures do not introduce artifact into the next sample. Core samples allow the architecture of the tissue to remain intact, although the morphologic features of individual cells may be more difficult to assess than with an aspiration sample. If present, parasites may be visible within macrophages of the bone marrow, and these will be more easily seen with a core biopsy. The overall cellularity of the marrow is most accurately determined with a core sample, because it is not diluted with blood. The procedure is similar to that used for aspiration biopsy. After the needle is introduced into the cortical bone, the stylet is removed, and the needle is advanced approximately 1 inch and rotated back and forth to cut the piece of bone from the cortex. The needle is then removed and the stylet used to expel the core sample through the proximal (hub) end of the needle. Forcing the sample back through the narrow distal end of the needle introduces pressure artifact into the sample. An imprint should be made from the sample before it is placed in formalin. Never place smears from aspirate samples near formalin-preserved specimens, because formalin fumes interfere with the staining of cytology specimens (see Unit 7).

Preparing Marrow Smears

Smears of bone marrow samples must be made immediately if they are not mixed with EDTA at the time of collection. If EDTA has been used, smears must be made within 1 hour of collection. Marrow smears of aspirate samples can be prepared in a similar manner to smears of peripheral blood. Two to 12 slides are prepared so that samples are available if additional testing (e.g., immunofluorescence assay, special staining) is needed. Aspiration samples should be pushed out of the hub of the needle with the use of pressure from the syringe. Bone marrow samples are thicker than blood and should contain particles or spicules. Excess blood or EDTA in the sample can be removed by tilting the slide to allow it to run off. Alternatively, the sample can be expelled into a Petri dish and the bone marrow spicules removed with a small plastic pipette or a capillary tube.

Line smears, starfish smears, and compression smears can also be used for bone marrow samples. A modified compression technique may provide the most useful sample. The compression prep method has been widely used for many years for the preparation of cytology specimens (see Unit 7). The technique is similar to that used for the coverslip preparation of peripheral blood smears. Bone marrow smears must be rapidly air dried and stained, usually with a Romanowsky-type stain. Staining time must be increased in accordance with the cellularity and thickness of the sample. Smears to be sent to reference laboratories will usually be stained with Prussian blue to identify iron particles in the marrow sample. Hematoxylin—eosin stain is often used for core biopsy samples, although Giemsa stain may also be used. Recent advances in cytochemistry and immunochemistry have also provided a large number of additional staining techniques. These techniques involve the use of special stains that can bind with surface molecules that are unique to specific cell types. They have simplified the definitive identification of cells in the bone marrow.

Evaluation of Bone Marrow Smears

A systematic approach should be used when evaluating a bone marrow smear. Bone marrow status should never be evaluated without the results of a differential white blood cell count from a concurrent peripheral blood smear. Stained bone marrow smears must first be examined at low-power (100×) magnification. This initial examination is used to evaluate the adequacy of the preparation. If the sample is not stained properly or if the cells are not easily distinguished, another slide should be obtained. Assuming that the preparation is adequate, the low-power examination can provide an indication of the overall cellularity of the bone marrow. In adult animals, normal bone marrow generally contains approximately 50% nucleated cells and 50% fat. Marrow samples from juvenile mammals are usually 25% fat, whereas geriatric animals usually have marrow that consists of approximately 75% fat. The marrow sample is described as acellular (i.e., aplasia), hypercellular (i.e., hyperplasia), or hypocellular (i.e., hypoplasia) on the basis of the proportion of nucleated cells versus the amount of fat present. The adipocytes are dissolved during the fixation of samples, which results in large clear areas. Samples are then further characterized by describing the types of cells present (e.g., hypoplasia, myeloid). Neoplasia is a possibility if all of the cells look alike. A systematic approach to bone marrow evaluation is summarized in Procedure 11.1.

PROCEDURE 11.1 Evaluating Bone Marrow Aspirates

Low-Power Examination
1. Evaluate the adequacy of the preparation.
2. Determine the relative percentages of nucleated cells and adipocytes.

High-Power Examination
1. Determine the relative percentages of erythroid and myeloid cells using the method preferred:
   a. Count 500 cells, classify all cell types, and calculate the ratio of myeloid cells to erythroid cells; or
   b. Categorize 500 cells, and calculate the erythroid and myeloid maturation index; or
   c. Categorize 200 cells, and calculate the myeloid and erythroid left shift indexes.
2. Evaluate for the presence of hemosiderin.
3. Describe the cellular morphology.

Cells in Bone Marrow

After the overall cellularity is determined, the sample is examined at higher magnification (i.e., 400× to 450×) to determine the relative percentages of erythroid and myeloid cells. One method requires counting and classifying 500 cells. Mature segmented neutrophils, eosinophils, and basophils are also present in small numbers (Fig. 11.4).

Rubricytes and metarubricytes usually comprise 80% to 90% of the erythroid cells. Metamyelocytes, bands, and segmented myeloid cells comprise approximately 80% to 90% of the myeloid cells. The ratio of myeloid cells to erythroid cells (M:E ratio) is determined by counting 500 nucleated cells and classifying them as erythroid or myeloid. Normal M:E ratios should be between 0.75:1.0 and 2.0:1.0. Normal values for the differential counting of bone marrow cells vary considerably among different species. Because the complete differential count of a marrow smear is time consuming, several modifications to the differential cell count are used. Some laboratories use a system that classifies cells into one of eight categories:
1. Immature myeloid
2. Mature myeloid
3. Immature erythroid
4. Mature erythroid
5. Eosinophilic
6. Monocytoid
7. Lymphocytic
8. Plasma cells

In this classification scheme, immature cells include the myeloblasts, promyelocytes, rubriblasts, and prorubricytes. Several alternate systems for the evaluation of bone marrow cells are used. One system involves classifying cells into groups and then calculating the erythroid maturation index and the myeloid maturation index. An additional system is used that calculates a left shift index for both myeloid and erythroid cell lines. The erythroid left shift index involves counting and

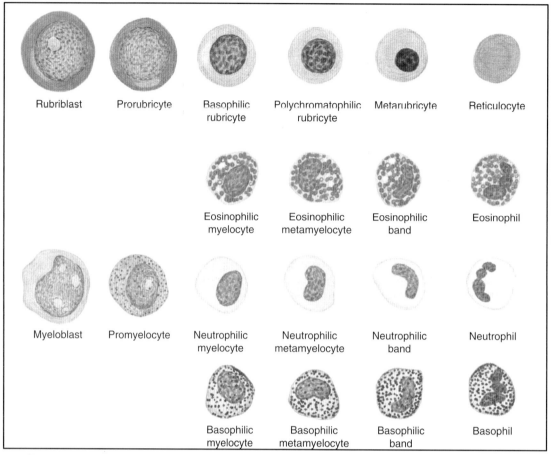

Fig. 11.4 Maturation of myeloid and erythroid cells. (Drawing by Dr. Perry Bain. From Meyer DJ, Harvey JW: *Veterinary laboratory medicine: interpretation and diagnosis,* ed 3, St Louis, 2004, Saunders.)

classifying 200 cells as either immature (i.e., rubriblasts, prorubricytes, and early rubricytes) or mature (i.e., late rubricytes and metarubricytes) and dividing the percentage of immature by mature erythroid cells. The myeloid left shift index is calculated by dividing the percentage of all immature granulocytes (i.e., myeloblast through band cell) by the percentage of mature granulocytes in a 200-cell count differential.

Megakaryocytes are not evenly distributed in a bone marrow aspirate. These are very large cells that contain multiple fused nuclei and that are often seen in clusters, particularly at the edges of the slide (Fig. 11.5). Megakaryocytes may number 8 to 10 per low-power field, although 2 to 3 per low-power field is more common. Generally, more than 10 per low-power field would indicate an increase in this cell line.

Other cell types that are present in bone marrow samples include macrophages, lymphocytes, plasma cells, mast cells, osteoblasts, and osteoclasts. Osteoblasts appear similar to plasma cells except that they are much larger and contain paler-appearing nuclear material. They also tend to be found in clusters when they are seen in samples collected by aspirate techniques. Plasma cells are slightly larger than lymphocytes, with a greater nucleus-to-cytoplasm ratio. Plasma cells often have a perinuclear clear area around the eccentrically located nucleus, and they have distinctly basophilic cytoplasm

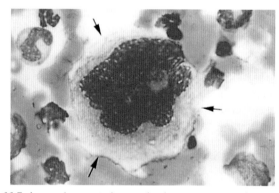

Fig. 11.5 A megakaryocyte in a canine bone marrow aspirate sample.

(Fig. 11.6). Inclusions that contain immunoglobulin are often present. These inclusions are commonly referred to as Russell bodies, and a cell that contains such inclusions is referred to as a Mott cell. Osteoclasts contain multiple nuclei and may appear somewhat fused and similar in appearance to megakaryocytes, except that the megakaryocyte nucleus is multilobed. Osteoclasts are seen most often in samples from young, actively growing animals. The cytoplasm is blue, and it may contain granular material of variable sizes that stains a deep red. Macrophages in bone marrow samples often contain

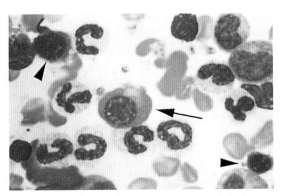

Fig. 11.6 A plasma cell *(arrow)* in a bone marrow aspirate from a normal dog. Rubricytes *(arrowheads)* are also present. The remaining cells are granulocytic precursors.

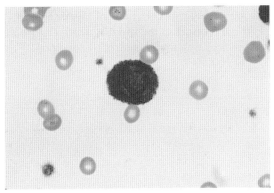

Fig. 11.7 A mast cell in a feline blood smear. (From Valenciano AC, Cowell RL: *Cowell and Tyler's diagnostic cytology and hematology of the dog and cat,* ed 4, St Louis, 2014, Mosby.)

phagocytized material that may aid in diagnosis. In core biopsy samples, macrophages are seen in the center of clusters of erythropoietic areas. These erythropoietic "islands" are usually disrupted during aspiration biopsy. Lymphocytes are produced in the bone marrow, but they are usually present in low numbers. Immature stages (i.e., lymphoblasts and prolymphocytes) are difficult to distinguish from rubriblasts and prorubricytes. Reactive lymphocytes and normal mature lymphocytes may also be present and appear as they would if they were seen in peripheral blood samples. Mast cells are characterized by the presence of abundant, small, metachromatic cytoplasmic granules (Fig. 11.7).

Hemosiderin is present in macrophages in bone marrow, and it is also found free of cells. It is easily identifiable as small gray to black granules when traditional blood smear stains are used. Prussian blue stain may also be used to demonstrate the presence of this iron store. Hemosiderin is almost always absent in bone marrow preparations from cats. A decrease or absence of hemosiderin is significant in most other species.

Reporting of Results

The results of bone marrow evaluation include, at a minimum, the overall cellularity and the M : E ratio, the maturation index, or the left shift index. If a complete differential count of

marrow cells is not possible, the sample is usually described in narrative form, and any unique patterns or morphologic abnormalities are described. When present, stainable iron (i.e., hemosiderin); the increased presence of mitotic figures; the increased presence of osteoblasts, osteoclasts, and mast cells; and the presence of phagocytized material and metastatic cells from other organs should also be recorded. The data are then reported along with the concurrent differential count from a peripheral blood smear.

ERYTHROCYTE SEDIMENTATION RATE

The rate at which erythrocytes fall in their own plasma will be altered in some disease states. These alterations are usually the result of changes in the chemical structure of the erythrocyte membrane, which then alter the physiology of the membrane. Generally, this results in a tendency for the erythrocytes to aggregate more readily.

The erythrocyte sedimentation rate (ESR) can be determined in a variety of ways. Automated analyzers are available to perform the test, although these are not commonly encountered in veterinary practices or referral laboratories. The evaluation of the tendency for erythrocytes to aggregate can also be accomplished by direct measurement of plasma proteins (e.g., globulins, fibrinogen).

Manual methods for performing ESR testing involve the use of a calibrated tube. Depending on the type of tube used, pretreatment of the sample may be required. Several manufacturers provide the tubes and the needed diluents in kit form. The tube is filled with fresh EDTA-anticoagulated blood to the upper calibration mark. It is then placed in a rack that has been designed to hold the tube perpendicular to the table. The tube is allowed to sit undisturbed at controlled room temperature. Manual ESR tests will be affected by vibrations on the lab table and variations in temperature in the room. After 60 minutes (or 20 minutes for equine samples), the level of the top of the RBC column is recorded.

ERYTHROCYTE OSMOTIC FRAGILITY

The osmotic fragility (OF) test provides a measure of the RBCs' ability to withstand hemolysis in varying concentrations of saline solution. The OF test measures the amount of hemolysis that occurs in varying concentrations of saline solution as compared with a normal control solution. This test may provide some useful information for differentiating among some forms of anemia in the dog and cat and with the diagnosis of hereditary spherocytosis. It is not routinely performed in veterinary medicine except at veterinary research and referral centers. OF may be measured by creating serial dilutions of saline ranging from 0.1% to 0.9%. The EDTA-anticoagulated blood sample is added to each dilution and the samples centrifuged. Each dilution is then evaluated with a spectrophotometer to determine the percentage of hemolysis in each solution. Results are plotted to create an erythrocyte fragility curve. The mean OF is expressed as the concentration of saline in which 50% hemolysis occurs. Although the exact relationship between the OF result and the cell's ability to survive in vivo is not well characterized, a relationship exists between abnormal OF test results and decreased survival time for red cells. Increased resistance to hemolysis is noted with a variety of conditions that cause an increase in the surface-to-volume ratio of the red cell (e.g., some forms of liver disease, iron deficiency). Reticulocytes are also more resistant to hemolysis because of their greater surface area. Decreased resistance to hemolysis is seen in patients with autoimmune hemolytic anemia and parasitic infections such as hemobartonellosis, babesiosis, and infection with hookworms.

KEY POINTS

- Reticulocytes are immature RBCs that require staining with a supravital stain for identification.
- Bone marrow samples may be collected via core sampling or aspiration techniques.
- A variety of techniques can be used to prepare bone marrow samples, with the compression smear being the most common method.
- When examining bone marrow samples, evaluate cellular morphologic characteristics to determine the relative percentages of nucleated cells and adipocytes, the relative percentages of erythroid and myeloid cells, and the M : E ratio.
- Prussian blue stain is used to evaluate bone marrow samples for the presence of hemosiderin.
- The results of bone marrow evaluation include, at a minimum, the overall cellularity and the M : E ratio, the maturation index, or the left shift index.
- Erythrocyte OF refers to the ability of RBCs to withstand hemolysis in varying concentrations of saline solution.
- The ESR is a measure of the speed at which erythrocytes fall in their own plasma under controlled conditions.

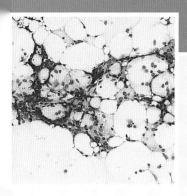

12

Hematopoietic Disorders and Classification of Anemia

LEARNING OBJECTIVES

After studying this chapter, you will be able to:
- Describe the types of abnormalities seen in bone marrow samples.
- Use proper terminology to describe bone marrow samples.
- Describe the procedures for the evaluation of bone marrow samples.

- Discuss the classification of anemias according to erythrocyte indices.
- Discuss the classification of anemias according to etiology.
- Discuss the classification of anemias according to bone marrow response.

OUTLINE

KEY TERMS

Aplastic
Chronic granulomatous
  inflammation
Chronic inflammation

Chronic pyogranulomatous
  inflammation
Fibrinous inflammation
Hypercellular
Hypocellular

Lymphoproliferative disease
Myeloproliferative disease
Nonregenerative anemia
Regenerative anemia

Hematologic abnormalities can be primary diseases, or they may be secondary to other disorders. Specific blood cells or all blood cell types can be affected. These diseases may manifest with alterations in tests of peripheral blood or of the bone marrow. A general understanding of the types of disorders and diagnostic test results that are characteristic of the various disorders will help the veterinary technician to provide diagnostic-quality test results. Disorders related to blood coagulation are presented in Unit 3.

DISORDERS OF THE BONE MARROW

Abnormalities seen in bone marrow samples can be classified as changes in cell numbers or in cell morphologic features and maturation. Samples can be characterized as either increased (hypercellular) or decreased (hypocellular) cellularity of all cell types or increased or decreased cellularity of one cell type (Fig. 12.1). When all blood cell types are decreased or absent,

the marrow is described as aplastic. In addition, abnormal hematopoiesis when cellularity is normal can also occur. A glossary of terms that can be used to describe these abnormalities is presented in Box 12.1.

Inflammatory conditions may also be evident when examining a bone marrow aspirate. These conditions are classified according to the primary cell types, which present as one of four types: fibrinous, chronic, chronic granulomatous, and chronic pyogranulomatous. Fibrinous inflammation typically involves the infiltration of the bone marrow with fibrin exudate without the presence of inflammatory cells. Chronic inflammation is a hyperplastic condition that is characterized by increased numbers of plasma cells, mature lymphocytes, and mast cells. Chronic granulomatous inflammation is characterized by increased numbers of macrophages. If both macrophages and neutrophils are present, the condition is described as chronic pyogranulomatous inflammation.

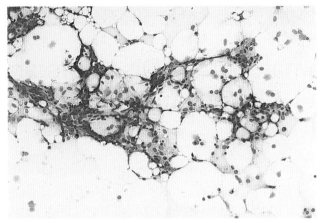

Fig. 12.1 Hypocellular bone marrow from a dog with chronic ehrlichiosis. Marrow flecks are extremely hypocellular and nearly devoid of developing hematopoietic cells. The flecks contain mostly fat cells, capillaries, and stromal cells. (Wright's stain, original magnification 50×.) (From Valenciano AC, Cowell RL: *Cowell and Tyler's diagnostic cytology and hematology of the dog and cat,* ed 4, St Louis, 2014, Mosby.)

BOX 12.1 **Terminology of Bone Marrow Aspirate**

Aplasia: Less than 25% myeloid cells

Basophilic hyperplasia: Basophilia in bone marrow and peripheral blood

Dyserythropoiesis: Abnormal erythrocyte maturation

Dysgranulopoiesis (dysmyelopoiesis): Abnormal granulocyte maturation

Dysmegakaryopoiesis (dysthrombopoiesis): Abnormal megakaryocyte or thrombocyte maturation

Eosinophilic hyperplasia: Eosinophilia in bone marrow and peripheral blood

Erythroid hyperplasia: Normal or increased cellularity with a normal or increased absolute neutrophil count and a low M : E ratio

Erythroid hypoplasia: Normal or decreased cellularity with a normal or decreased absolute neutrophil count and a high M : E ratio

Granulocytic hyperplasia: Normal or increased cellularity with a normal or increased PCV and a high M : E ratio

Hyperostosis: Thickening of cortical bone

Hypocellular: Decrease in overall cellularity

Megakaryocyte emperipolesis: Presence of intact, viable blood cells within the cytoplasm of megakaryocytes

Megakaryocytic hyperplasia: Increase in numbers of megakaryocytes in bone marrow

Monocytic hyperplasia: Increased presence of precursor cells of the monocyte series

Myelodysplasia: Atypical cells with less than 30% blast cells present

Myelofibrosis: Increased presence of fibrous tissue that displaces hematopoietic tissue

Neoplasia: Atypical cells with more than 30% blast cells present

Neutrophilic hyperplasia, effective: Neutrophilia in bone marrow and peripheral blood

Neutrophilic hyperplasia, ineffective: Neutrophilia in bone marrow concurrent with neutropenia in peripheral blood

Osteosclerosis: Thickening of trabecular bone

Reactive macrophage hyperplasia: Increased presence of active macrophages, often containing phagocytized material

---

Neoplasia

Neoplastic disorders of hematopoiesis are classified as either lymphoproliferative or myeloproliferative disease. The common term used to describe the presence of neoplastic blood cells in bone marrow and peripheral blood is leukemia, and it is characterized by a predominance of blast cells in the bone marrow. A comprehensive oncology text should be consulted for more details about the classification of hematopoietic neoplasia.

CLASSIFICATION OF ANEMIA

The function of red blood cells (RBCs) is to transport and protect hemoglobin, which is the oxygen-carrying pigment. The daily production of erythrocytes equals the daily loss from the destruction of aged cells in a healthy animal. If RBC production is decreased or if destruction or loss is increased, anemia results. Anemia is a condition that involves reduced oxygen-carrying capacity of erythrocytes. It may result from a reduced number of circulating RBCs, reduced packed cell volume (PCV), or a reduced concentration of hemoglobin. Anemia may be classified according to bone marrow response as either regenerative or nonregenerative or according to RBC size and hemoglobin concentration (i.e., mean corpuscular volume [MCV] or mean corpuscular hemoglobin concentration [MCHC]). Such classifications help the clinician to identify the cause of the anemia. The veterinarian will interpret the results of laboratory testing, other diagnostics (e.g., imaging), and the patient's history and physical examination to identify the cause of the anemia and to determine the treatment needed. The specific laboratory tests that are generally evaluated to determine the cause of anemia are the reticulocyte count, the erythrocyte indices, RBC morphology, plasma color and turbidity, and the total plasma protein concentration. Additional laboratory diagnostics that are sometimes required included serum iron measurement, serum bilirubin measurement, and bone marrow evaluation.

Classification by Bone Marrow Response

This type of classification is most clinically applicable because it distinguishes between regenerative and nonregenerative anemia. For common domestic animal species other than equine, the bone marrow responds to anemia by increasing erythrocyte production and releasing immature erythrocytes. These immature RBCs are polychromatophilic RBCs or reticulocytes that can be observed on the blood film and enumerated with the reticulocyte count to provide an indication that the marrow is responsive or regenerative. The ability of bone marrow to respond indicates that the cause of the anemia is probably either blood loss (hemorrhage) or blood destruction (hemolysis). In general, most animals exhibit signs of regeneration within about 4 to 7 days from the triggering cause of the anemia. An adequate bone marrow response is indicated when the percentage of reticulocytes is equal to or greater than the expected percentage for the corresponding PCV (Table 12.1).

TABLE 12.1	Expected Reticulocyte Count Relative to Packed Cell Volume in Dogs and Cats With Adequately Regenerative Anemias			
CANINE		**FELINE**		
Packed Cell Volume (%)	Reticulocyte (%)	Packed Cell Volume (%)	Aggregate Reticulocyte (%)	Punctuate Reticulocyte (%)
45	<1.0	45	—	—
35	≥1.0	35	≤0.5	≤10
25	≥4.0	25	0.5-2.0	>10
20	≥6.0	20	2.0-4.0	>10
10	≥10.0	10	>4.0	>10

From Cowell R: *Diagnostic cytology and hematology of the dog and cat,* ed 3, St. Louis, 2008, Mosby.

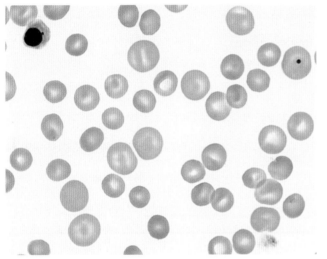

Fig. 12.2 Regenerative anemia in a dog with increased polychromasia and anisocytosis. A metarubricyte is present in the upper left of the image, and a Howell-Jolly body is present in an erythrocyte in the upper right. (Wright-Giemsa stain.) (From Meyer D, Harvey JW: *Veterinary laboratory medicine: interpretation and diagnosis,* ed 3, St Louis, 2005, Saunders.)

Other findings likely to be present when viewing a blood cell film that is indicative of a regenerative response include increased macrocytosis, increased polychromasia, and Howell-Jolly bodies (Fig. 12.2).

Because horses rarely release reticulocytes from the bone marrow, bone marrow evaluation is generally needed to classify anemia. Bone marrow reticulocyte counts of greater than 5% indicate a regenerative response in horses.

In patients with nonregenerative anemia, the bone marrow is unable to respond to the anemic state, and reticulocytes are absent on blood films, which suggests bone marrow dysfunction. A bone marrow aspiration biopsy is then indicated after common endocrine and metabolic causes of nonregenerative anemia are excluded. Common causes of nonregenerative anemia include iron deficiency, ehrlichiosis, drug toxicity, histoplasmosis, hypothyroidism, and renal insufficiency.

Classification by Red Blood Cell Size and Hemoglobin Concentration

Erythrocyte indices can be used to help classify anemia as either normocytic (i.e., RBCs of normal size), macrocytic (i.e., RBCs that are larger than normal), or microcytic (i.e., RBCs that are smaller than normal). Normocytic anemia is characterized by RBCs of normal size, and it occurs secondary to a variety of acute and chronic disorders. In domestic animals, the most common cause of macrocytic anemia is the transitory increase in RBC size seen with regenerative anemia (i.e., reticulocytosis).

- MCV Increased-Macrocytic
- MCV Decreased-Microcytic
- MCHC Increased-Hyperchromic
- MCHC Decreased-Hypochromic

Microcytic anemia is almost always the result of iron deficiency. The division of immature erythrocytes stops when a critical concentration of hemoglobin is reached. With inadequate iron for hemoglobin synthesis, extra division may occur and result in smaller erythrocytes. Although chronic blood loss is the most common cause of iron deficiency in adult animals, inadequate dietary iron results in iron-deficiency anemia in young nursing animals such as kittens and baby pigs.

Anemia may be hypochromic (i.e., with a reduced hemoglobin concentration) or normochromic (i.e., with a normal hemoglobin concentration). A hyperchromic state is not possible, because erythrocytes have a fixed maximum capacity for hemoglobin. Newly released polychromatophilic erythrocytes (i.e., reticulocytes) are hypochromic, because the full concentration of hemoglobin is not yet attained. Macrocytic hypochromic anemia suggests regeneration. Iron deficiency also results in hypochromic anemia and microcytosis (Fig. 12.3). Most other types of anemia are normochromic. A summary of anemias classified by erythrocyte indices is located in Box 12.2.

Classification by Etiology

Anemia can also be classified by cause as hemolytic or hemorrhagic, or it may be the result of decreased or defective RBC production.

Hemolytic

Hemolytic anemias are the result of erythrocyte destruction within the blood, and they are usually regenerative. During the initial stages, this type of anemia is usually normocytic and normochromic, but it becomes macrocytic as a result of the bone marrow's release of reticulocytes. Common causes of hemolytic anemias are located in Table 12.2.

Hemorrhagic

Hemorrhagic anemia can result from acute or chronic blood loss. The patient's history and clinical signs can often help with the determination of the cause of the anemia. Common causes

of hemorrhagic anemia include trauma, parasites, coagulopathy, neoplasia, cystitis, and gastrointestinal ulceration.

Iron Deficiency

Iron deficiency can be the result of a nutritionally deficient diet, or it may result from chronic blood loss. Erythrocytes are generally microcytic and hypochromic. Low MCHC values

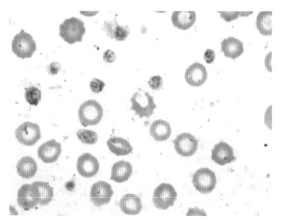

Fig. 12.3 Hypochromic red blood cells in a blood film from a dog with iron-deficiency anemia.

TABLE 12.2 Common Causes of Hemolytic Anemia

Cause	Examples
Immune-mediated destruction	Autoimmune hemolytic anemia Neonatal isoerythrolysis Blood transfusion incompatibility
Erythrocyte parasites	*Anaplasma* *Mycoplasma* *Babesia* *Cytauxzoon felis* *Theileria* spp.
Bacterial and viral agents	*Leptospira* *Sarcocystis* Feline leukemia virus
Toxic exposure	Onions Methylene blue Zinc Acetaminophen Copper

BOX 12.2   Classification of Anemias by Erythrocyte Indices

Normocytic Normochromic
1. Hemolytic anemia if reticulocyte response is mild or if sufficient time has not elapsed for a prominent reticulocyte response to occur
2. Hemorrhage if reticulocyte response is mild or if sufficient time has not elapsed for a prominent reticulocyte response to occur
3. Early iron-deficiency anemia before microcytes predominate
4. Chronic inflammation and neoplasia (sometimes slightly microcytic)
5. Chronic renal disease
6. Endocrine deficiencies
7. Selective erythroid aplasia
8. Aplastic and hypoplastic bone marrows
9. Lead toxicity (may not be anemic)
10. Cobalamin deficiency

Macrocytic Hypochromic
1. Regenerative anemias with marked reticulocytosis
2. Hereditary stomatocytosis in dogs (often with slight reticulocytosis)
3. Abyssinian and Somali cats with increased erythrocyte osmotic fragility (a reticulocytosis is usually present)
4. Spurious with prolonged storage of the blood sample

Macrocytic Normochromic
1. Regenerative anemias (decreased MCHC is not always present)
2. Feline leukemia virus infections with no reticulocytosis (common)

3. Erythroleukemia (AML-M6) and myelodysplastic syndromes
4. Nonregenerative immune-mediated anemia and myelofibrosis in dogs
5. Poodle macrocytosis (healthy miniature poodles with no anemia)
6. Hyperthyroid cats (slight macrocytosis without anemia)
7. Folate deficiency (rare)
8. Congenital dyserythropoiesis of Hereford calves
9. Spurious with erythrocyte agglutination
10. Spurious in cats and dogs with persistent hypernatremia (may be hypochromic)

Microcytic Normochromic/Hypochromic*
1. Chronic iron deficiency (months in adults, weeks in nursing animals)
2. Portosystemic shunts in dogs and cats (often not anemic)
3. Anemia of inflammatory disease (usually normocytic)
4. Hepatic lipidosis in cats (usually normocytic)
5. Normal Akita and Shiba Inu dogs (not anemic)
6. Prolonged recombinant erythropoietin treatment (mild)
7. Copper deficiency (rare)
8. Drugs or compounds that inhibit heme synthesis
9. Myeloid neoplasms with abnormal iron metabolism (rare)
10. Pyridoxine deficiency (experimental)
11. Familial dyserythropoiesis of English Springer spaniel dogs (rare)
12. Hereditary elliptocytosis in dogs (rare)
13. Spurious when platelets are included in erythrocyte histograms
14. Spurious in dogs with persistent hyponatremia (not typically anemic)

*The presence of a low MCHC with a low MCV strongly suggests iron-deficiency anemia.
From Harvey J: *Veterinary hematology*, St. Louis, 2012, Saunders.

are present. The definitive diagnosis of iron-deficiency anemia may require the evaluation of hemosiderin in the bone marrow.

Production Disorders

Reduced rates of erythropoiesis or defective erythropoiesis (i.e., dyserythropoiesis) generally result in a normocytic anemia.

Conditions that result in reduced or defective erythropoiesis include chronic renal disease, hypothyroidism, hypoadrenocorticism, bracken fern poisoning, iron and copper deficiency, parvovirus, and lead toxicity.

KEY POINTS

- Abnormalities that are seen in bone marrow samples can be classified as changes in cell numbers or in cell morphologic features and maturation.
- Inflammatory conditions evident on the examination of bone marrow aspirate are classified as fibrinous, chronic, chronic granulomatous, or chronic pyogranulomatous.
- Neoplastic disorders of hematopoiesis are classified as either lymphoproliferative or myeloproliferative.
- Anemia is generally considered regenerative when the percentage of reticulocytes in the peripheral blood is equal to or greater than the expected percentage for the corresponding PCV.

- Blood films from patients with regenerative anemias may show evidence of increased macrocytosis, increased polychromasia, and Howell-Jolly bodies.
- Common causes of nonregenerative anemia include iron deficiency, ehrlichiosis, drug toxicity, histoplasmosis, hypothyroidism, and renal insufficiency.
- Anemia can be classified as normocytic, macrocytic, or microcytic in addition to being normochromic or hypochromic.
- Anemia can also be classified by its cause as hemolytic or hemorrhagic, or it may be the result of decreased or defective RBC production.

13

Automated Analyzers for Hematology

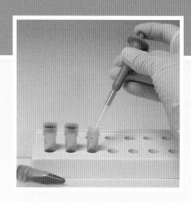

LEARNING OBJECTIVES

After studying this chapter, you will be able to:

- List the types of hematology analyzers available for use in the veterinary practice.
- Describe the principle of the electrical impedance analyzer.
- Describe the laser flow cytometry test principles.
- Describe the principle of quantitative buffy coat analysis.
- Describe the care and maintenance of automated hematology analyzers.
- Describe the procedures for the manual counting of cells.
- Define histogram and explain the use of histograms.

OUTLINE

KEY TERMS

Anemia
Complete blood count
Histogram

Impedance analyzer
Laser flow cytometry
Neubauer rulings

Polycythemia
Quantitative buffy coat analysis
Red cell distribution width

Instrumentation designed for veterinary hospital use is available to facilitate the generation of hematologic data for the complete blood count (CBC). Options are cost-effective and convenient for situations in which at least several CBCs are performed per day. The benefits of instrumentation include a reduced labor investment, more complete information, and the improvement of data reliability.

CELL COUNTS

The counting of erythrocytes (red blood cells [RBCs]) and leukocytes (white blood cells [WBCs]) is a routine part of the CBC. Cell counts are usually performed by automated methods. The total WBC count is one of the most useful values determined in a CBC. Total RBC and platelet (thrombocyte) counts are also performed by automated methods. Manual cell count methods are not routinely performed, except in some avian and exotic animal practices. Since many automated analyzers do not provide accurate platelet counts, these may also be performed with manual methods in some facilities.

An increase in the number of circulating red blood cells is termed polycythemia or erythrocytosis. It is accompanied by an increased packed cell volume and hemoglobin concentration. Such increases can be the result of primary or secondary pathology, or they may be a relative polycythemia. Relative polycythemia is seen with conditions such as splenic contraction (which releases large numbers of erythrocytes into circulation) and dehydration. Primary polycythemia, which is also called polycythemia vera, is a myeloproliferative disorder that is characterized by the proliferation of erythroid precursor cells. Secondary causes of polycythemia include a variety of renal and lung disorders and conditions that lead to increased erythropoietin levels (e.g., chronic hypoxia).

The term anemia refers to a decrease in the oxygen-carrying capacity of the blood, usually as a result of decreased numbers of circulating RBCs. The causes of anemia are further explored in Chapter 12.

TYPES OF HEMATOLOGY INSTRUMENTS

Hematology instrumentation for the veterinary hospital falls into three general categories:

1. Impedance analyzers
2. Laser flow cytometry analyzers
3. The quantitative buffy coat analysis systems

Some manufacturers now provide analyzers that combine several of these methods for performing a CBC. One commonly available system involves the use of impedance methods for the enumeration of cells, as well as laser-based methods for performing the differential WBC count (Fig. 13.1). Some hematology analyzers also contain photometric capabilities for the evaluation of hemoglobin. Each method has specific advantages and disadvantages. Regardless of which analyzer is used, an understanding of the testing principles of the specific analyzer is essential. Knowing the limitations of the analytic system enhances the validity of the test results. Regular quality control is also essential for ensuring the accuracy of the test results.

Impedance Analyzers

A number of electronic cell counters used in human medical laboratories have been adapted for veterinary use (Fig. 13.2). Adaptation was necessary because of the variation in blood cell size among different animal species. Some companies have developed dedicated veterinary multispecies hematology systems that count cells and determine the hematocrit, the hemoglobin concentration, and the mean corpuscular hemoglobin concentration. Some also provide a partial WBC differential count.

Electronic cell counters that use the impedance method are based on the passage of electric current across two electrodes separated by a glass tube with a small opening or aperture (Fig. 13.3). Electrolyte fluid on either side of the aperture conducts the current. Counting occurs by moving a specific volume of cells in the electrolyte solution through the aperture with the use of vacuum or positive pressure. Because cells are relatively poor conductors of electricity as compared with the electrolyte fluid, they impede the flow of current while it passes through the aperture. These transient changes in current may

be counted to determine the blood cell concentration. In addition, the volume or size of the cell is proportional to the change in current, thereby allowing the system to differentiate cell types based on their sizes. Size information may be displayed in a graphical format (histogram) of the cell population. Leukocytes, erythrocytes, and platelets may be enumerated with these systems. However, samples from cats may not be accurately evaluated as a result of the similarity in size of both feline erythrocytes and feline platelets.

Impedance analyzers are calibrated to count cells in specified size ranges as defined by threshold settings (which prevents the erroneous interpretation of small debris and electronic noise as cells) and to properly separate cell populations in the same dilution (e.g., platelets, erythrocytes). Because cell populations vary in size among species, some of the threshold settings are

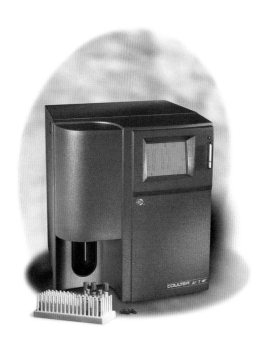

Fig. 13.2 The Coulter AcT hematology analyzer (Beckman Coulter, Brea, CA), which is supplied with software designed specifically for animal species, makes use of impedance technology.

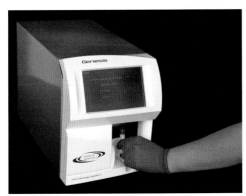

Fig. 13.1 The Genesis hematology analyzer (Oxford Science, Oxford, CT) combines impedance and laser-based methods.

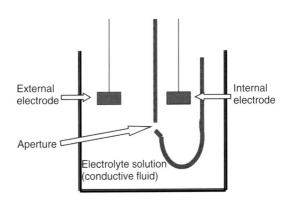

Fig. 13.3 The principle of impedance analysis for cell counts.

species specific. These settings are established by the manufacturer and they are usually set automatically by system software when the user selects the species for analysis in a software menu. Comprehensive hematology systems designed specifically for veterinary applications are now commonly used in veterinary facilities. These systems incorporate the advantages of individual cell analysis that provides sophisticated quantitative information about blood cell populations.

> **TECHNICIAN NOTE** Impedance analyzers classify cells based on their sizes.

The blood sample must be diluted to count cells. For WBCs, a dilution is treated with a lytic agent that destroys cell membranes, leaving only nuclei for counting. Erythrocytes may be analyzed with the use of systems that count the RBCs and that provide cell size information by using a much greater blood dilution to which no lytic agent is added. Erythrocyte analysis on automated systems provides diagnostic information about cell volume and an alternative method for determining the packed cell volume (PCV), which is also referred to as the hematocrit (Hct). The mean corpuscular volume (MCV) may be directly measured from the analysis of the erythrocyte volume distribution. The hematocrit is then calculated by multiplying the MCV by the erythrocyte concentration. On more sophisticated systems, the volume distribution curve of the erythrocyte population is displayed. With some analyzers, the red cell distribution width (RDW) may also be provided. This value is determined by mathematic analysis of the distribution, and it functions as an index of erythrocyte volume heterogeneity. Abnormally high values indicate increased volume heterogeneity and an underlying disturbance of the erythron. When it is used in conjunction with the MCV value, the RDW may alert the veterinarian to diseases of erythrocytes that alter RBC size. In more advanced systems, the same counting and sizing functions exist for evaluating platelets.

Many automated hematology systems provide a complete analysis of platelet, erythrocyte, and WBC populations, including WBC differential count information. Most provide graphic displays of cell population size analysis. Differential information is calculated from the WBC population size distribution. Many of these systems provide an estimate of the relative percentage of granulated and nongranulated WBCs. This value has limited application for the evaluation of patients with a pathologic condition. Variations in the size of the cells introduce error into this measurement. In addition, numerous morphologic abnormalities can be present and may not be identified with this partial differential count. A thorough examination of a blood smear must also be included when evaluating patients.

Impedance analyzers are composed of numerous pumps, tubes, and valves that must be maintained. Diluting fluid and dusty glassware may be contaminated with particles that are large enough to be erroneously counted as cells. A daily "background count" is generally required. This involves running the electrolyte solution through the analyzer so that any small particles may be identified and subsequently not counted by the analyzer. The aperture may become partially or totally obstructed and require cleaning. The threshold setting may be improperly set on a counter with a variable threshold control. Cold agglutinins may cause a decreased RBC count as a result of RBC clumping. Before processing, refrigerated blood samples must be warmed to room temperature. Fragile lymphocytes, which are seen with some forms of lymphocytic leukemia, may rupture in the lysing solution that is used to lyse RBCs; this rupturing can result in a decreased WBC count. The presence of spherocytes (i.e., abnormally small, round RBCs) may alter the MCV, thereby reducing the calculated hematocrit. Elevated serum viscosity may interfere with cell counts. Platelet counts that are obtained with impedance counters are affected by platelet clumping and the presence of nucleated red blood cells, and they are often inaccurate. Small clumps of platelets, large platelets, and nucleated red blood cells may be counted as erythrocytes.

Quantitative Buffy Coat System

The quantitative buffy coat system (Drucker Diagnostics, Port Matilda, PA) uses differential centrifugation and staining to provide an estimation of cellular elements. Measurements are made using an expanded buffy coat layer in a specialized microhematocrit tube. This provides a hematocrit value as well as estimates of leukocyte concentration and platelet concentration. It extrapolates tube volumes to an estimated concentration that is based on fixed cell volumes. Partial differential count information is provided in the form of total granulocytes and lymphocyte and monocyte categories. One limitation of these leukocyte groupings is that abnormalities (e.g., left shift, lymphopenia) may be undetected unless the blood smear is examined as defined for the minimum CBC. These systems are best used as screening tools, because they provide an estimation of cell numbers rather than actual cell counts.

> **TECHNICIAN NOTE** Quantitative buffy coat analyzers provide estimated cell counts.

Laser-Based Flow Cytometer Analyzers

Laser flow cytometer analyzers involve the use of focused laser beams to evaluate the size and density of solid components. Cells scatter light differently depending on the shape and volume of the cell and the presence or absence of granules and nuclei. The laser beam is directed at a channel through which cells in the sample flow in single file. The degree and direction of light scatter from the individual cells allows for the enumeration of monocytes, lymphocytes, granulocytes, and erythrocytes. When certain dyes are added to the sample, variations in laser light scatter can also allow for the enumeration of mature and immature erythrocytes (Fig. 13.4). These systems usually also provide the erythrocyte indices, the RDW, and the platelet parameters (e.g., mean platelet volume, platelet

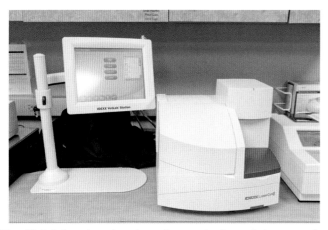

Fig. 13.4 A laser-based analyzer for use in the veterinary practice laboratory.

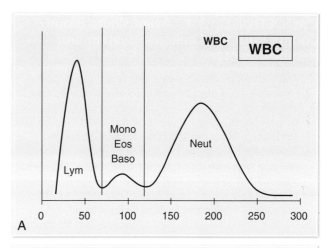

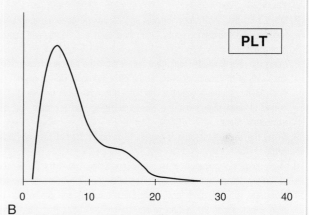

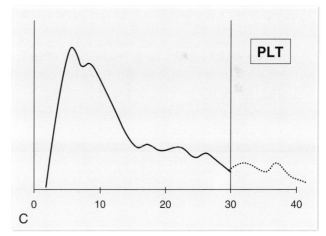

Fig. 13.5 Histograms. **A,** Normal white blood cell histogram. **B,** Platelet histogram. **C,** Platelet histogram with evidence of platelet aggregates.

distribution width, plateletcrit). More information about platelet parameters is presented in Unit 3.

> **TECHNICIAN NOTE** Laser flow cytometry analyzers count and classify cells based on their size and density.

Histograms

Many automated analyzers offer histograms of the cell and platelet counts. A histogram is a graph that provides a visual report of the sizes (on the x-axis) and numbers (on the y-axis) of the various cellular components. Another version of histogram is in the form of a scatter plot, where each dot represents a specific cell. The histogram can be used to verify results of the differential blood cell smear and to provide an indication of any problem with test results. For example, when megathrombocytes or platelet aggregates are present, the WBC count performed on most automated analyzers will be falsely elevated, because those large platelets are usually counted as leukocytes. The histogram can provide evidence of this anomaly, because the WBC curve on the histogram will be altered (Fig. 13.5).

> **TECHNICIAN NOTE** Histograms provide a visual representation of the number and sizes of cell types present in a sample.

Manual Cell Counts

The counting of erythrocytes and leukocytes is a routine part of the CBC. Cell counts are not generally performed with manual methods except in avian and exotic animal practices. Manual WBC count methods for exotic animal samples can be performed with the use of the Leukopet system. This system includes a pipette that holds a predetermined amount of blood and a reservoir that contains a diluting and lysing agent. Procedure 13.1 describes the method for the counting of avian leukocytes using the Leukopet system (Fig. 13.6).

The Leukopet system uses a premeasured volume of phloxine as a diluent. When the dilution tube is filled with the appropriate volume of blood and mixed, a small amount of the blood–diluent mixture is placed on a hemocytometer. The hemocytometer contains an optical quality cover glass and a measured grid that contains a specific volume.

Hemocytometers are counting chambers that are used to determine the number of cells per microliter (i.e., μL, mm³) of

PROCEDURE 13.1   Avian White Blood Counts With the Leukopet System and Hemocytometer

1. Attach a clean, unused disposable pipette tip to the 25-μL pipettor.
2. Unscrew the cap of one of the prefilled phloxine tubes, and place it in a tube rack.
3. Using the pipettor, aspirate 25 μL of freshly drawn anticoagulated blood. Carefully wipe excess sample from the outside of the pipette.
4. Dispense the blood sample into the tube of phloxine, and rinse the pipette tip **thoroughly** by aspirating and dispensing the phloxine—blood solution at least six times. It is critical that all of the blood be rinsed from the pipette tip to ensure a proper dilution. Depending on the viscosity of the sample, this may require additional rinsing of the tip.
5. Cap the tube and mix well by inverting it several times. Do not shake.
6. Allow the tube to incubate for at least 10 minutes but for no longer than 1 hour.
7. Make sure that the hemocytometer and its special coverslip are clean and free of dirt and fingerprints. Clean them with lens cleaner and paper, if needed.
8. Using the rinsed pipette, aspirate a sample from the tube and charge (fill) each side of the hemocytometer at the etched groove. Do not overfill or underfill the counting chamber, because this can cause uneven distribution of cells throughout the Neubauer ruling and contribute to an inaccurate count.
9. Allow the sample to stand for up to 10 minutes so that the cells can settle.
10. Place the hemocytometer on the microscope stage. Lower the condenser of the microscope to increase contrast so that the cells are easier to see.
11. Using the 10× objective lens, count the heterophils and eosinophils in both chambers of the Neubauer hemocytometer. Cells that touch the lines between two squares are considered as within that square if they touch the top or the left-center lines. Cells that touch the bottom or right lines are not counted with that square. All squares from each side (grid) of the hemocytometer are counted, and the total number from both sides of the hemocytometer are used to calculate the total leukocyte count as follows:

Total WBC/μL

$$= \frac{\text{Total Heterophil} + \text{Eosinophil (both chambers)} \times 1.1 \times 16 \times 100}{\% \text{ Heterophils} + \% \text{ Eosinophils (from differential count)}}$$

From Sirois M: *Principles and practice of veterinary technology*, ed 3, St. Louis, 2011, Mosby.

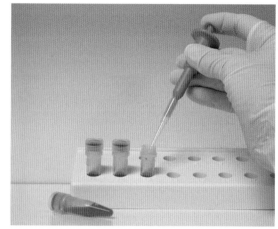

Fig. 13.6 The Leukopet system used for the counting of avian white blood cells. (From Sirois M: *Principles and practice of veterinary technology*, ed 3, St Louis, 2011, Mosby.)

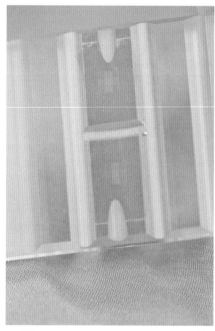

Fig. 13.7 The hemocytometer contains two grid areas.

blood (Fig. 13.7). Several models are available, but the most common type used has two identical sets of fine grids of parallel and perpendicular etched lines called Neubauer rulings (Fig. 13.8). Each grid is divided into nine large squares. The 4 corner squares are divided into 16 smaller squares, and the center square is divided into 400 tiny squares (i.e., 25 groups of 16 each). The area of each grid (i.e., each Neubauer ruling) is designed to hold a precise amount of sample (0.9 μL). Knowing the number of cells in set parts of the grid and the amount of sample in that area is the basis for calculating the number of cells per microliter of blood. Mechanical counters are available to manually keep track of the number of cells observed (Fig. 13.9).

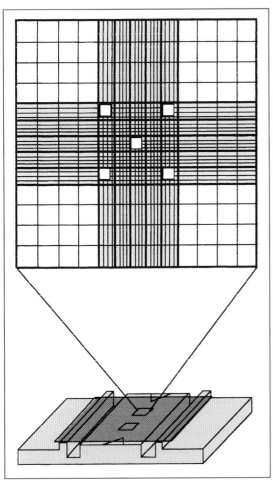

Fig. 13.8 Neubauer Hemocytometer. (From Sirois M: *Principles and practice of veterinary technology,* ed 3, St Louis, 2011, Mosby.)

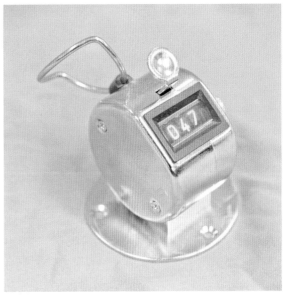

Fig. 13.9 The hand tally counter is used to keep track of numbers of cells counted.

KEY POINTS

- Most cell counters for use in the veterinary practice laboratory involve either impedance or laser-based technology.
- Buffy coat analyzers provide estimates of cell counts.
- Impedance analyzers work by measuring the change in current as cells in electrolyte solution pass through an aperture.
- Impedance analyzers classify cells according to their sizes.
- Laser flow cytometers classify cells on the basis of their size and density as they pass through a focused laser beam.
- Histograms provide a visual representation of the numbers and sizes of the cells present in a sample.
- Manual cell counts are performed with a hemocytometer.

UNIT 3

Hemostasis

Unit Outline

Unit Objectives

Describe the processes and pathways that lead to the clotting of blood.
List the components of the blood-clotting systems.
Describe the proper collection and handling of samples for coagulation testing.
Discuss the methods for the evaluation of platelets.
List and describe the coagulation tests commonly performed in the veterinary practice laboratory.
List and describe the coagulation tests commonly performed in the veterinary reference laboratory.
List and describe common inherited coagulopathies.
List and describe common acquired coagulopathies.

Hemostasis (i.e., blood clotting) involves multiple complex and interrelated processes. A variety of coagulation disorders can be seen in veterinary practice. A basic understanding of the processes involved in blood clotting is essential to ensure accurate test results.

A number of tests can be performed in the veterinary practice laboratory, and many of these tests do not require specialized equipment. Coagulation analyzers are also available for some tests and can be cost effective for the veterinary practice laboratory.

14

Principles of Blood Coagulation

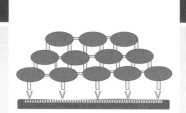

OVERVIEW OF BLOOD COAGULATION

Hemostasis is the ability of the body's systems to maintain the integrity of the blood and blood vessels. It involves a number of complex pathways, platelets, and coagulation factors. Any alteration in these parameters can result in a bleeding disorder. In the simplest terms, the coagulation of blood proceeds through a mechanical phase and a chemical phase. The mechanical phase is initiated when a blood vessel is ruptured or torn. The exposed blood vessel subendothelium is a charged surface, and platelets are attracted to this surface. As platelets congregate at the site, they undergo morphologic and physiologic changes. These changes cause the platelets to adhere to each other as well as to the blood vessel endothelium. The adhesion of platelets to each other and to the endothelium also requires von Willebrand factor, which serves to stabilize the platelet plug (Fig. 14.1). The adhesion and aggregation of platelets also cause the platelets to release the initiating factor for the chemical phase of hemostasis.

Coagulation Cascade

The chemical phase is referred to as the coagulation cascade, and it involves a number of coagulation factors (Table 14.1).

The classical view separates the chemical phase into the intrinsic/induced pathway and extrinsic/tissue factor pathway. Each factor participates in a chemical reaction that serves to initiate the next reaction in the pathway. The end result of the coagulation cascade is the formation of a mesh of fibrin strands that forms the clot. The final phase of hemostasis involves the degradation of the fibrin clot.

Intrinsic/Induced Pathway

It is important to note that the coagulation pathways are interrelated, interdependent, and at least partly cell-based. The intrinsic surface-induced pathway starts with cell damage. The initial mechanical phase is initiated by interactions of negatively charged phospholipid surfaces of cells and platelets or microparticles. Microparticles are membrane-bound cytoplasmic fragments that are released from platelets, leukocytes, and endothelial cells that serve to increase the surface area on which coagulation complexes can form. Tissue factor binds to Factor VIII in the plasma to initiate the coagulation reactions, and Factors I through XI serve to amplify the cascade. The extrinsic pathway actually serves to help initiate the intrinsic pathway. A small amount of thrombin is generated during the initial

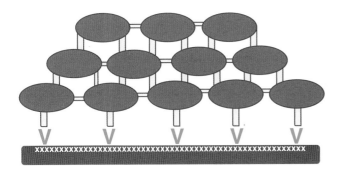

(ellipse)	Platelet
xxxxxxxx	Damaged area of blood vessel
V	von Willebrand factor
⌷	Intra-platelet bridge

Fig. 14.1 Diagram of a stabilized platelet plug.

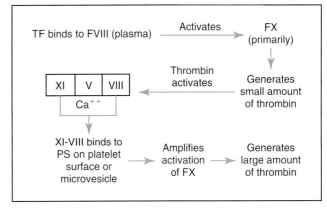

Fig. 14.2 The initial reactions of the chemical phase of hemostasis.

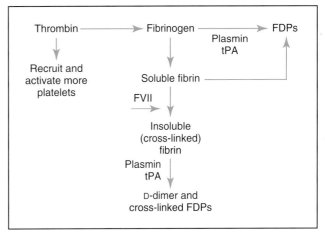

Fig. 14.3 Functions of thrombin during the later stages of chemical hemostasis and the breakdown of fibrin.

TABLE 14.1	**Blood Coagulation Factors**
Designation	**Synonym**
Factor I	Fibrinogen
Factor II	Prothrombin
Factor III	Tissue factor
Factor IV	Calcium
Factor V	Proaccelerin
Factor VI	(There is no Factor VI.)
Factor VII	Proconvertin
Factor VIII	Antihemophilic factor
Factor IX	Christmas factor, plasma thromboplastin
Factor X	Stuart factor
Factor XI	Plasma thromboplastin antecedent
Factor XII	Hageman factor
Factor XIII	Fibrin-stabilizing factor, prekallikrein

phase, and this also recruits and activates platelets and inhibits fibrinolysis. When platelets are activated, phosphatidylserine (PS) is exposed on the outer surface of the membrane. Platelets also release small vesicles from their surface during activation. These microparticles are enriched in PS. PS acts as a binding site for the complexes of the coagulation cascade, which activate Factor X and prothrombin (Factor II), respectively.

Extrinsic/Tissue Factor Pathway

The tissue factor pathway often starts with endotoxemia, neoplasia, etc. The extrinsic pathway involves initiation by Factor III (i.e., tissue factor) and its interaction with Factor VII. The pathway then continues down the common pathway.

Common Pathway

The activation of Factor X results in the generation of a large amount of thrombin (Fig. 14.2). That thrombin continues to recruit and activate more platelets and triggers the conversion of fibrinogen to fibrin. The generation of fibrin proceeds through two phases, with a soluble form being generated initially, followed by the creation of an insoluble form that consists of cross-linked fibrin strands. The coagulation process is also modulated by and its resulting clots broken down through a series of interrelated reactions. In the presence of tissue plasminogen activator (tPA) and plasmin, the soluble fibrin is also broken down into fibrin degradation products (FDPs). Plasmin and tPA also act on the insoluble fibrin to produce a cross-linked version of FDPs and D-dimers (Fig. 14.3). Although the brief description given here seems complex, the actual processes are a great deal more complicated and involve numerous additional serum proteins. The reader

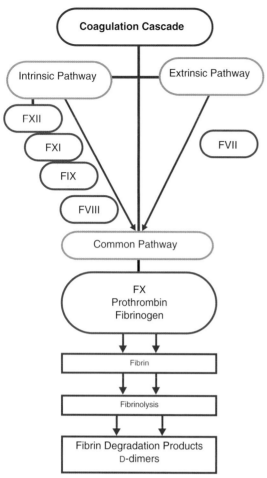

Fig. 14.4 A simplified summary of the chemical phase of hemostasis.

TECHNICIAN NOTE The formation of a stable platelet plug requires an adequate number of functional platelets in addition to von Willebrand factor.

TECHNICIAN NOTE Activated platelets expose phosphatidylserine on their outer membrane.

TECHNICIAN NOTE Fibrinolysis produces ᴅ-dimers and FDPs.

COAGULATION TESTING

Various coagulation tests have been developed to evaluate specific portions of the hemostatic mechanisms. Some tests measure just the mechanical phase of hemostasis, whereas others can measure specific parts of the chemical phase. All patients should be evaluated for coagulation defects before undergoing surgery. Most coagulation tests can be completed with minimal time and equipment and are relatively inexpensive.

Zoetis offers a table top machine for in-clinic use to aid in coagulation testing. This machine is called the VETSCAN® VSpro Coagulation Analyzer, enabling canine and feline PT (prothrombin time) and aPTT (activated partial thromboplastin time) testing and equine fibrinogen testing.

should refer to the recommended readings for more in-depth discussions of hemostasis. Fig. 14.4 summarizes the classical view of the chemical phase of the blood coagulation process.

KEY POINTS

- Hemostasis requires platelets, a number of coagulation factors, and complex reaction pathways.
- Hemostasis proceeds through mechanical and chemical pathways.
- The term mechanical hemostasis refers to the aggregation and adhesion of platelets to exposed blood vessel endothelium.
- The mechanical and chemical phases of hemostasis are interrelated and interdependent.
- Activated platelets expose phosphatidylserine on their surface and release microparticles that also contain phosphatidylserine.

- Coagulation complexes attach to phosphatidylserine on the surfaces of microparticles and platelets.
- Thrombin serves to enhance the recruitment and activation of platelets.
- Fibrinogen is converted first to a soluble form and then to an insoluble form.
- The breakdown of fibrin requires plasmin and tPA.
- Fibrin is broken down into soluble FDPs, insoluble FDPs, and D-dimers.

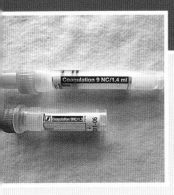

15

Sample Collection and Handling for Hemostasis Analysis

LEARNING OBJECTIVES

After studying this chapter, you will be able to:

- Describe proper sample collection procedures for coagulation testing.
- List the anticoagulants that are used for blood coagulation tests.
- Describe the method used to determine the proper ratio of blood to citrate anticoagulant.
- Discuss proper sample handling of samples for coagulation testing.
- Describe the instrumentation available for coagulation testing in veterinary practices and referral laboratories.

OUTLINE

KEY TERMS

Fibrometer
Hypercoagulable

Hypocoagulable
Monovette

Thromboelastography

SAMPLE COLLECTION AND HANDLING

Blood samples for coagulation tests should be collected carefully, with minimal tissue damage and minimal venous stasis. Patient excitement can increase the platelet count in addition to activating platelets. Increased levels of von Willebrand factor and Factors I, V, and VIII can also occur. In addition, prolonged venous stasis can activate platelets and trigger fibrinolysis. Effects occur both in vitro and in vivo.

Samples should never be collected through indwelling catheters, because small amounts of fibrinogen, fibrin, and platelets are generally found around the catheter. One of the best ways to eliminate at least some platelet activation is to use a Vacutainer or a Monovette (Fig. 15.1), rather than a syringe and needle to collect the sample. The preferred anticoagulant for most coagulation tests is sodium citrate. Citrate is supplied in liquid form, and samples collected in citrate solution are diluted by 10%. If platelet counts are done with the citrated sample, they must be corrected for this dilution. Platelet aggregates form readily in dog blood that is collected in citrate. Ethylenediaminetetraacetic acid (EDTA) is the preferred

anticoagulant for platelet counts. Citrate is also the anticoagulant that is typically used in solutions for blood collection and storage for transfusions. Samples for whole blood clotting time and activated coagulation time do not require an anticoagulant.

> **TECHNICIAN NOTE** Samples for coagulation testing are mixed with sodium citrate anticoagulant in a ratio of 1 part citrate to 9 parts whole blood.

Samples must be collected in the proper order when multiple types of samples are being drawn. Review Chapter 7 in Unit 2 of this book for the correct order of draw. The citrate tube is generally drawn first so that it is not contaminated with gel activators or anticoagulants from other tubes.

The proper ratio of citrate to blood is 1 part citrate to 9 parts whole blood. Citrate is available in 3.2% and 3.8% concentrations. These anticoagulants will provide different clotting time results. Samples should be collected with the citrate concentration used to establish laboratory reference ranges. The proper ratio of blood to anticoagulant can be achieved with

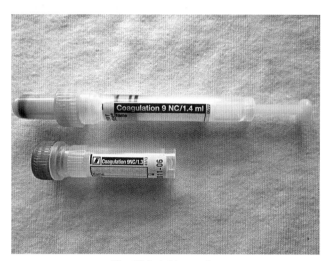

Fig. 15.1 A Monovette.

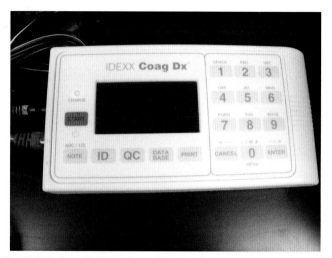

Fig. 15.2 A Coag Dx™ Analyzer. (Idexx Laboratories, Inc., Westbrook, ME.)

a Vacutainer tube, provided that the tube is at least 90% full and that the patient is not anemic, polycythemic, or dehydrated. The volume of citrate to use is based on the expected plasma volume. Consequently, if blood is added in the 1:9 ratio, anemic samples will be undercitrated, which will result in shortened clot times, and polycythemic samples will be overcitrated, which will result in prolonged clot times. Citrate volume should be adjusted accordingly for patients with significant abnormalities of the red cell mass. The volume of citrate required can be calculated with the following equation:

$$\text{Volume of citrate required} = 0.00185 \times \text{Blood volume to be collected} \times (100 - \text{Hematocrit [\%]})$$

After the sample has been collected, it should be labeled and transported rapidly to the laboratory. Tubes should be held at room temperature, remain tightly capped, and be kept upright. Vibrational trauma should be avoided. Most tests should be performed within 2 hours of sample collection. Alternatively, the sample may be centrifuged at 2500 g for 15 minutes. The plasma is then withdrawn without disturbing the platelet layer with the use of a noncontact pipette. Plasma may then be frozen in plastic tubes. Samples need to be shipped on dry ice so that they arrive frozen and can be thawed immediately before testing.

COAGULATION INSTRUMENTATION

Automated analyzers for coagulation testing are available, and some are relatively inexpensive. Automated analyzers are preferred over manual methods for the performance of these tests. The analyzers are designed to evaluate specific parts of the coagulation process. Some perform multiple analyses of the chemical phase of hemostasis, and others are designed specifically to evaluate platelet function.

Analyzers that have been designed to evaluate chemical hemostasis have mechanisms that reverse the anticoagulant in

which the sample was collected. Some make use of liquid reagents that are added to the sample. Others contain reagents in cartridges to which the sample is added. The analyzers then monitor for clot formation with either mechanical or optical systems.

Coag Dx™ Analyzer

The Coag Dx™ Analyzer (Idexx Laboratories, Inc., Westbrook, ME) is capable of performing a variety of coagulation tests that involve the use of fresh whole blood or citrate-anticoagulated blood (Fig. 15.2). The analyzer uses cartridges that contain the required reagents for the tests. Available tests include prothrombin time and activated partial thromboplastin time. Different versions of the test cartridges are used for citrated samples than for whole blood samples.

Sample is added to the cartridge, and the analyzer passes the sample back and forth through an internal channel. Light-emitting diode optical detectors are used to evaluate the rate of blood flow, which will decrease when a clot forms. The analyzer has been validated for use with canine and feline samples, and the prothrombin time test has been validated for equine samples.

> **TECHNICIAN NOTE** The Coag Dx™ Analyzer is a commonly available automated analyzer that is used to perform coagulation tests.

Fibrometer

Although no longer in widespread use, a fibrometer may still be encountered in some veterinary referral practices and laboratories. The unit is a semiautomated analyzer that can be used to perform a number of coagulation studies. The citrated patient sample is placed in a sample cup. The appropriate test reagent is drawn into the pipette that is attached to the unit. When the reagent is dispensed from the pipette, the timer is

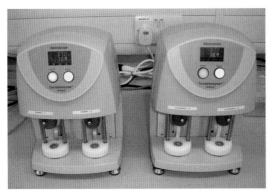

Fig. 15.3 Thromboelastography machines. (Haemonetics Corp., Braintree, MA). (From Ettinger S: *Textbook of veterinary internal medicine,* ed 7, St Louis, 2010, Saunders.)

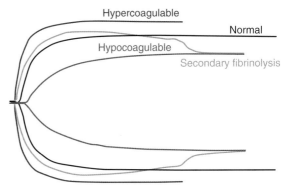

Fig. 15.4 Thromboelastograph tracings of normocoagulable, hypocoagulable, hypercoagulable, and secondary fibrinolytic states. (Redrawn from Kol A, Borjesson DL: Application of thromboelastography/thromboelastometry to veterinary medicine. *Vet Clin Pathol* 39:405, 2010. In Harvey J: *Veterinary hematology,* St Louis, 2012, Saunders.)

triggered, and the unit drops a pair of small wires into the sample cup. The wires move back and forth through the sample cup until a clot is detected.

Thromboelastograph

A variety of automated analyzers are available to perform thromboelastography (Fig. 15.3). They may vary considerably in design and the specific reagents needed. Some make use of fresh whole blood, and others involve the use of citrated samples. In general, the analyzers contain the sample in a cup to which reagent is added. The analyzer then evaluates the entire clotting process, from the formation of the initial clot through fibrinolysis. Test results are then recorded that provide a measure of the time required for clot formation, the evaluation of the strength of the clot, and the time required for the breakdown of the clot. The results are usually provided graphically and used to identify whether a patient is hypercoagulable or hypocoagulable (Fig. 15.4). There is not widespread agreement among veterinary practitioners regarding the usefulness of this analysis. Thrombocytopenia and decreased microhematocrit may demonstrate hypercoaguability. Current research has not provided definitive evidence regarding whether this is an in vitro or in vivo state. Heparin used either for anticoagulation or as a patient treatment may interfere with test results. Variations in test results may also be evident when samples are not immediately analyzed. Specific protocols for veterinary samples are not well described. Each laboratory

should develop its own protocol and expected normal ranges based on the sample collection procedure and elapsed time to perform testing.

Platelet Function Analyzers

Several analyzers are available for the assessment of platelet adhesion and aggregation. The PFA-100 analyzer (Siemens USA, Palo Alto, CA) has been validated for use with canine samples. The analyzer makes use of a disposable cartridge that contains a collagen-coated membrane with a small aperture. Blood is drawn through the aperture, and platelets adhere to the membrane. When a sufficient number of platelets have adhered and aggregated, blood can no longer flow through the aperture. The time required is then recorded.

Other analyzers are used to evaluate platelet aggregation and the secretion of platelet factors. There are a wide variety of test principles used, although few have been validated with veterinary species.

Point-of-Care Analyzers

Several additional small handheld analyzers are available for coagulation testing, but these have not been validated for use in veterinary species. They are frequently used in human emergency departments and physician offices. Some are also available for human patients who are receiving anticoagulant therapy to monitor their coagulation status.

◾ KEY POINTS

- Blood for coagulation testing must be collected carefully and with minimal trauma to avoid triggering the clotting mechanisms.
- Patient excitement and excessive venous stasis can alter coagulation test results.
- Most coagulation tests involve the use of sodium-citrate–anticoagulated plasma.

- EDTA-anticoagulated samples are preferred for the evaluation of platelet numbers.
- For coagulation testing, the proper ratio of citrate to blood is 1 part citrate to 9 parts whole blood.
- A variety of automated analyzers are available to monitor for clot formation with either mechanical or optical systems.

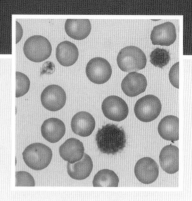

16

Platelet Evaluation

Platelets are small cytoplasmic fragments that are shed from megakaryocytes in the bone marrow. Methods for platelet evaluation include the platelet count, platelet indices, and platelet function testing. The majority of platelet evaluations are completed with automated analyzers. Thrombocytopenia is a decrease in the circulating platelet mass. Thrombocytosis is an increase in the circulating platelet mass. Thrombopathia refers to abnormal platelet function.

PLATELET COUNT

Platelets counts are performed with automated hematology analyzers. Some automated counts can be highly inaccurate as a result of platelet clumping and platelet/red blood cell overlap. A freshly collected ethylenediaminetetraacetic acid (EDTA)–anticoagulated blood sample should be used when performing platelet counts. Results from automated analyzers must be verified by viewing the peripheral blood cell film. The previously used manual counting system from Becton—Dickinson (i.e., the Unopette system) is no longer manufactured, but several alternative similar products are available. These make use of a chamber or tube that contains a premeasured volume of diluent to which the sample is added. Platelets are then counted with a hemocytometer in a manner similar to that described for the Leukopet (see Chapter 13). Morphologic changes in platelets include aggregation and giant platelets (Fig. 16.1). These abnormalities will not be evident with automated analyzers and must therefore be detected using the differential blood film.

Platelet Estimates

Indirect measurements of platelet numbers (i.e., estimates) are performed with the use of the differential blood film as described in Chapter 16. Platelet numbers should be evaluated in a monolayer area of the blood film. The numbers of platelets in a minimum of 10 microscopic fields should be counted. Generally, 8 to 10 platelets per oil-immersion field are seen in normal patients. However, this number can vary greatly depending on the field of view of the microscope used. Multiplying the estimated platelet number (as averaged over 10 fields) by 15,000 or 20,000 is also used as an indirect measure of the platelet count.

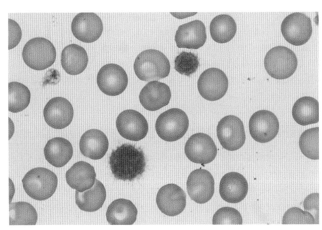

Fig. 16.1 A giant and a slightly enlarged platelet in a canine patient. (From Valenciano AC, Cowell RL: *Cowell and Tyler's diagnostic cytology and hematology of the dog and cat*, ed 4, St Louis, 2014, Mosby.)

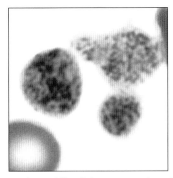

Fig. 16.2 The intense basophilia of these macrothrombocytes suggests that they may be reticulated platelets. (From Harvey J: *Veterinary hematology*, St Louis, 2012, Saunders.)

> **TECHNICIAN NOTE** Platelet estimates are performed with the use of the blood smear used for the differential blood cell count.

Platelet Morphology

Patients with thrombocytopenia may have larger than normal platelets (megaplatelets). However, normal cats and dogs are routinely found to have megaplatelets when the sample is viewed on the blood smear used for the differential blood cell count. These are often counted as erythrocytes by automated analyzers. All blood smears should be evaluated for the presence of platelet clumps. Reticulated platelets represent newly released platelets, and they contain high levels of RNA (Fig. 16.2). They are analogous to reticulocytes in that they demonstrate bone marrow responsiveness. Specialized staining is used to identify these, and they are then enumerated with flow cytometry.

PLATELET INDICES

Some automated analyzers provide an evaluation of platelet mass, individual platelet size, and platelet distribution width

(PDW). The methods differ depending on the type of analyzer. In addition to the PDW, platelet indices include a measurement of plateletcrit (PCT) and the mean platelet volume (MPV). Some analyzers may also provide the platelet–large cell ratio (P-LCR). Depending on the analyzer, these may be direct measurements, or they may be calculated from other reported values. Note that although many analyzers report these parameters, their clinical usefulness has not been well documented for veterinary species.

> **TECHNICIAN NOTE** Many analyzers provide platelet indices, including MPV, PCT, and PDW.

Mean Platelet Volume

The MPV, which is measured in femtoliters, is the mathematical average of the size of the individual platelets counted by the analyzer. An increased MPV may be expected in situations in which the increased loss, destruction, or consumption of platelets is accompanied by megakaryocytic hyperplasia. Accelerated thrombopoiesis tends to result in the release of larger platelets; however, healthy cats tend to have larger platelets, so the value may not be useful for feline patients. Certain canine breeds, such as Cavalier King Charles Spaniels, have larger platelets than other breeds. Some automated analyzers may count larger platelets as white blood cells.

A high MPV in dogs indicates an adequate bone marrow response. However, a normal or low MPV in thrombocytopenic dogs does not predict an inadequate bone marrow response. Different results may also occur depending on the anticoagulant and specific analyzer used. Exposure to EDTA has been demonstrated to cause platelets to swell. Some studies have demonstrated as much as a 30% increase in volume during the first hour after the sample is collected. However, not all studies have been in agreement. Similar results have been seen with citrated samples. Studies of MPV with impedance methods have demonstrated that the MPV increases with time, whereas laser flow cytometry methods have been shown to record decreased MPV with time. When performing serial evaluations, test samples at the same elapsed time after venipuncture.

Plateletcrit

The plateletcrit, which is also referred to as thrombocrit, is a measure of the percentage of the total blood volume that is comprised of platelets. It is comparable to the packed cell volume that is recorded for red blood cells. This value is generally determined by multiplying the total platelet count by the MPV. For most mammals, the value is typically less than 1%.

Platelet Distribution Width

PDW assesses variations in the size of the platelets. Many automated analyzers provide a histogram that provides a visual evaluation of PDW (Fig. 16.3). Larger platelets may be seen in patients with thrombocytopenia. Platelet width may be altered

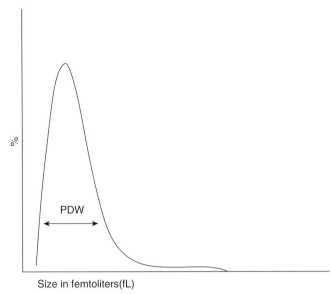

Fig. 16.3 Platelet histogram.

depending on how recently the platelet was released from the bone marrow. Platelet width is also increased when platelets are activated. However, variations in platelet size can occur in normal patients, and PDW has not been well correlated with bone marrow responsiveness or hypercoagulable states. Similarly, some analyzers report a value for the platelet–large cell ratio, which is a measure of the percentage of platelets that are larger than normal.

PLATELET FUNCTION TESTS

Thrombopathia, or an alteration in platelet function, can be assessed in a variety of ways. Automated analyzers (see Chapter 13) provide an evaluation of the ability of the platelets to aggregate and secrete platelet factors. Other measures of platelet function are indirect (see Chapter 16).

ADDITIONAL EVALUATIONS

Veterinary reference and referral laboratories offer a variety of platelet evaluations that are generally not practical for performance in the practice laboratory. These include the antiplatelet antibody assays. Antiplatelet antibody assays are immunoassays designed to identify antibodies that have adhered to the surface of platelets.

KEY POINTS

- Platelet evaluation includes a platelet count, platelet indices, and tests of platelet function.
- Platelet estimates can be performed in a variety of ways using the blood smear from the differential blood cell count.
- Specialized tests for reticulated platelets and antiplatelet antibodies are performed at reference laboratories.
- Platelet indices include plateletcrit, platelet distribution width, and mean platelet volume.

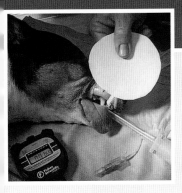

17

Coagulation Testing

LEARNING OBJECTIVES

After studying this chapter, you will be able to:

- List the commonly performed tests of blood coagulation.
- Describe the procedure for performing the buccal mucosa bleeding time test.
- Describe the procedure for performing the activated clotting time test.
- Describe the principles of the activated partial thromboplastin time test and the prothrombin time test.
- Describe the procedure for performing the heat precipitation fibrinogen test.

OUTLINE

KEY TERMS

Activated clotting time
Activated partial thromboplastin time

Buccal mucosa bleeding time
Clot retraction
D-Dimer

PIVKA
Prothrombin time tests

Tests of the blood coagulation mechanisms are designed to evaluate specific phases of the coagulation process (Fig. 17.1). Some require specialized instrumentation, whereas others are performed manually. The manual methods are less preferable as a result of variability in their performance. When these methods are used, it is vital that a consistent approach be used. Reference ranges should be established within the veterinary laboratory with the use of the specific supplies and procedures used. Many of the tests will be altered when platelet numbers are low. A platelet count should be performed to identify the presence of thrombocytopenia, which could invalidate some test results.

> **TECHNICIAN NOTE** Tests of coagulation are designed to evaluate specific parts of the coagulation pathways.

BUCCAL MUCOSA BLEEDING TIME

The buccal mucosa bleeding time (BMBT) is a primary assay for the detection of abnormalities in platelet function. The test requires a spring-loaded lancet (e.g., Surgicutt, SimPlate), blotting paper or filter paper, a stopwatch, and a tourniquet (Procedure 17.1). Always use the same device when performing the test, because the devices differ with regard to the width, depth, and number of incisions made. The patient should be sedated or anesthetized and placed in lateral recumbency. A strip of gauze is used to tie the upper lip back to expose the mucosal surface. An incision is made with the lancet, and standard blotting paper or filter paper is used to blot the incision site (Fig. 17.2). This is done by lightly touching the paper to the drop of blood and allowing the blood to be absorbed without touching the incision. The blood will be wicked away from the incision. Blotting is repeated every 5 seconds until the bleeding has stopped. The normal bleeding time for domestic animals is 1 to 5 minutes. A prolonged bleeding time occurs with most platelet dysfunction syndromes as well as with deficiencies in von Willebrand factor. It will also be prolonged in patients with thrombocytopenia, so a platelet count must be performed. Some patients will tolerate this test when they are not anesthetized. However, the patient must not

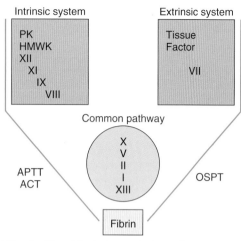

Fig. 17.1 The traditional intrinsic, extrinsic, and common coagulation pathways. (From Couto N: *Small animal internal medicine*, ed 4, St Louis, 2009, Mosby.)

PROCEDURE 17.1 Buccal Mucosa Bleeding Time Test

1. Anesthetize the patient, and place the patient in lateral recumbency.
2. Fold back the patient's lip, and secure it with gauze.
3. Place the lancet device against the mucosal surface at the level of the premolars.
4. Depress the trigger on the device without pressing against the mucosa, and simultaneously start the timer.
5. After 5 seconds, wick the blood away from the incision site with filter paper.
6. Continue the removal of the blood drop every 5 seconds until the filter paper comes up clean.
7. Record the time.

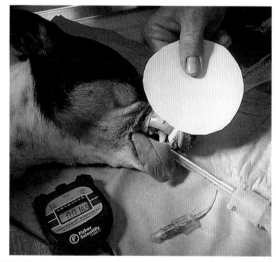

Fig. 17.2 The buccal mucosa bleeding time test. (Courtesy B. Miztner, DVM.)

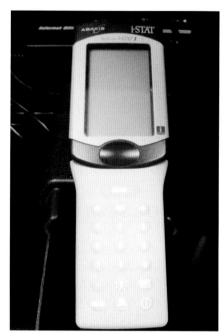

Fig. 17.3 The i-STAT analyzer has cartridges that are used for the performance of coagulation tests.

be allowed to disturb the incision with the tongue, so sedation is usually required.

ACTIVATED CLOTTING TIME

The activated clotting time (ACT) test can evaluate every clinically significant clotting factor except Factor VII. The manual method for performing the test requires a Vacutainer tube that contains an additive such as diatomaceous earth or kaolin that triggers the activation of the coagulation pathways. The tube must be prewarmed with a 37° C (98.6° F) water bath or heat block. Venipuncture is performed, and 2 mL of blood is collected directly into the tube. A timer is started as soon as the blood enters the tube. The tube is mixed once by gentle inversion and placed in a 37° C incubator or water bath. The tube is observed at 60 seconds and then at 5-second intervals for the presence of a clot. Normal values are approximately 60 to 90 seconds. Severe thrombocytopenia (i.e., <10,000 platelets/mL) and abnormalities associated with the intrinsic coagulation cascade prolong the activated clotting time. Automated analyzers are also available for the performance of ACT testing (Fig. 17.3).

WHOLE BLOOD CLOTTING TIME

The whole blood clotting time test, which is performed via the Lee–White method, is an older test of the intrinsic clotting mechanism. Whole blood clotting time tests are not commonly performed, because the ACT is more sensitive. The test is performed by collecting 3 mL of blood in a plastic syringe, noting the time that the blood first appears in the syringe by using a stopwatch. Immediately, 1 mL of blood is placed in each of three 10- × 75-mm tubes that have been rinsed with saline. The tubes are then placed in a 37° C (98.6° F) water bath. The first and then the second tubes are tilted at 30-second intervals until coagulation occurs. The third tube is tilted in a similar manner. The time elapsed between the appearance of blood in the syringe and clot formation in the third tube is the clotting time. The normal whole blood clotting time for dogs is 2 to 10 minutes; for horses, it is 4 to 15 minutes; and for cattle it is 10 to 15 minutes.

ACTIVATED PARTIAL THROMBOPLASTIN TIME

The activated partial thromboplastin time (APTT) evaluates the intrinsic and common clotting mechanisms. Depending on the specific analyzer use, some methods require multiple reagents. The Coag Dx™ analyzer (see Fig. 15.2) is a handheld analyzer that performs both the prothrombin time test and the APTT test. Citrated plasma is incubated with an activator of Factor XII, platelet substitute (i.e., cephaloplastin). After the addition of calcium, the time that it takes to form fibrin is determined. A variety of acquired and hereditary disorders, in addition to the administration of heparin, can reduce one or more factors that are necessary for the normal intrinsic coagulation cascade.

> **TECHNICIAN NOTE** Many coagulation assays are performed with automated analyzers.

PROTHROMBIN TIME TEST

Prothrombin time (PT) tests, which are also referred to as one-stage prothrombin time tests (OSPT), are usually performed by automated analyzers. This test evaluates the extrinsic and common coagulation pathways. The manual test involves the use of a citrated plasma sample to which tissue thromboplastin reagent is added. A reagent that has been designed to recalcify the sample is then added. Under normal conditions, a clot should form within 6 to 20 seconds. The normal range for dogs is 7 to 10 seconds. A prolonged prothrombin time may be associated with severe liver disease, disseminated intravascular coagulation (DIC), or hereditary or acquired deficiencies of any factors of the extrinsic coagulation cascade. The test is sensitive to vitamin K deficiency or antagonism such as warfarin toxicity.

CLOT RETRACTION TEST

The clot retraction procedure is an older test that allows for the evaluation of platelet number and function and of intrinsic and extrinsic pathways. One method involves drawing blood into a plain sterile tube and incubating the tube at 37° C. The tube is examined at 60 minutes and then reexamined periodically over a 24-hour period. A clot should be evident in 60 minutes, retracted in approximately 4 hours, and markedly compact at 24 hours. Abnormalities in the test result do not provide information regarding the cause or source of the coagulopathy.

FIBRINOGEN DETERMINATION

Automated methods for fibrinogen determination that involve photometric analysis are not commonly performed in veterinary practice. Automated electrochemical methods are available for the veterinary practice laboratory (Fig. 17.4). One manual method that may be used for fibrinogen estimation involves the use of two hematocrit tubes. The tubes are centrifuged as they would be for the determination of the packed cell volume, and the total solids of one tube are determined, usually with a refractometer. The second tube is then incubated at 58° C for 3 minutes. The second tube is recentrifuged, and the total solids are measured. The total solids in grams per deciliter are multiplied by 1000 to obtain the concentration in milligrams per deciliter. The fibrinogen estimate is then calculated with the use of the following equation, with all values given in milligrams per deciliter:

$$\text{Total solids}_{(\text{nonincubated})} - \text{Total solids}_{(\text{incubated})}$$
$$= \text{Fibrinogen mg/dL}$$

PIVKA

The acronym PIVKA refers to proteins that are induced (invoked) by the absence of vitamin K. Vitamin K is required to activate coagulation Factors II, VII, IX, and X. When vitamin K is deficient, precursor proteins of Factors II, VII, IX, and X build up and can be detected by PIVKA testing or

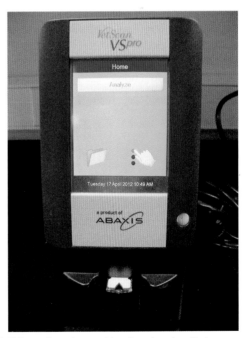

Fig. 17.4 This analyzer is capable of performing fibrinogen assays as well as other coagulation tests, chemical analyses, and electrolyte evaluations.

by the Thrombotest (Axis-Shield PoC, Oslo, Norway). The test may help to differentiate rodenticide toxicity from primary hemophilia when activated clotting time is prolonged. It is a slightly more sensitive test than the prothrombin test when the vitamin K—dependent factors are depleted. PIVKA testing may become prolonged within 6 hours of the ingestion of antico-agulant rodenticides, whereas prothrombin time is prolonged within 24 hours, and activated partial thromboplastin time is prolonged within 48 hours. Some controversy exists regarding the usefulness of this test, and many practitioners prefer the prothrombin time test. If the PT is prolonged, the PIVKA provides no additional information to the clinician. If initial treatment of the patient involves any administration of vitamin K, the PIVKA test must be performed prior to initi-ation of treatment.

D-DIMER AND FIBRIN DEGRADATION PRODUCTS

Both the D-dimer and fibrin degradation product tests are used to evaluate tertiary hemostasis (i.e., fibrinolysis). D-Dimers and fibrin degradation products (or fibrin split products) are formed as a clot is degraded. These tests are therefore useful aids in identifying the presence of DIC and to provide diag-nostic information in cases of liver failure, trauma, and hemangiosarcoma. A canine in-house test is available for D-dimer analysis. Fibrin degradation products and D-dimer tests are immune assays. Several types are available, but most involve the use of latex agglutination methods (see Unit 9, Chapter 50). The D-dimer test is considered more specific and sensitive for the evaluation of fibrinolysis, because fibrin degradation products can be produced before a clot forms.

> **TECHNICIAN NOTE** D-Dimer and fibrin degradation product tests are used to evaluate fibrinolysis.

VON WILLEBRAND FACTOR

von Willebrand factor (vWF) is required for platelet adhesion. When platelet function defects are evident, a vWF assay is generally performed. There are several types of immunoassays available in reference laboratories that can be used to quantify vWF. Additional tests are available for the evaluation of vWF function.

COAGULATION FACTOR ASSAYS

Deficiencies in clotting factors occur with a variety of heredi-tary and acquired conditions and may alter a variety of coag-ulation test results. Assays that can be used to identify specific factor deficiencies are performed in reference laboratories, and they are generally performed to identify specific hereditary factor deficiencies. The majority of these assays involve the use of photometric principles.

KEY POINTS

- Coagulation tests evaluate specific parts of the coagulation pathways.
- Most coagulation assays are performed with automated analyzers.
- Buccal mucosa bleeding time provides an evaluation of platelet number and function.

- Coagulation factor assays are performed in reference labora-tories when a specific factor deficiency must be identified.
- vWF evaluations are performed in reference laboratories via immunologic methods.

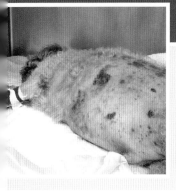

18

Disorders of Hemostasis

LEARNING OBJECTIVES

After studying this chapter, you will be able to:

- Describe the types of hemostatic disorders seen in veterinary species.
- Differentiate between hereditary and acquired defects of hemostasis.
- List and describe the common clinical signs of hemostatic disorders.

- List the common inherited disorders of coagulation and the species and breeds usually affected.
- Describe the mechanisms involved in disseminated intravascular coagulation.

OUTLINE

KEY TERMS

Disseminated intravascular coagulation

Hemophilia

von Willebrand disease

HEMOSTATIC DEFECTS

Bleeding disorders may be caused by congenital or acquired defects in coagulation proteins, platelets, or the vasculature. Most bleeding disorders found in veterinary species are secondary to some other disease process. Primary coagulation disorders are rare, and they are usually the result of an inherited defect in the production of coagulation factors. Signs of congenital or acquired deficiencies in coagulation proteins usually involve delayed deep-tissue hemorrhage and hematoma formation. Clinical signs associated with congenital or acquired defects or deficiencies of platelets include superficial petechial and ecchymotic hemorrhages (Fig. 18.1), epistaxis (Fig. 18.2), melena, and prolonged bleeding at injection and incision sites. With functional defects or deficiencies in the concentration of coagulation proteins, clinical signs usually appear before the animal reaches 6 months of age. The majority of congenital coagulation factor disorders in veterinary species involve a deficiency or abnormality of a single factor.

TECHNICIAN NOTE Clinical signs associated with defects or deficiencies of platelets include superficial petechial and ecchymotic hemorrhages, epistaxis, melena, and prolonged bleeding at injection and incision sites.

HEREDITARY COAGULATION DISORDERS

Coagulopathies that are inherited include a variety of factor deficiencies. Some common inherited coagulation factor disorders of veterinary species are listed in Table 18.1. Although the diagnosis of a specific factor deficiency or defect requires testing completed at a reference laboratory, a number of coagulation tests can be performed in the veterinary practice laboratory to aid in diagnosis. Factors XII, XI, IX, and VIII are components of the intrinsic coagulation pathway. Tests designed to evaluate the intrinsic pathway (e.g., activated clotting time, activated partial thromboplastin time) will likely

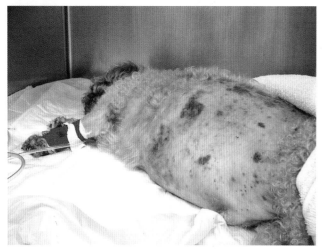

Fig. 18.1 Petechiae may signify a coagulation abnormality. (From Sirois M: *Principles and practice of veterinary technology,* ed 3, St Louis, 2011, Mosby.)

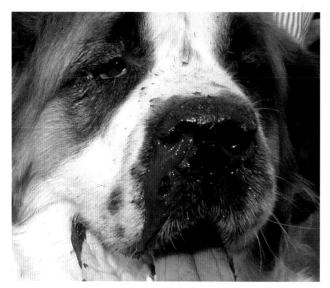

Fig. 18.2 Epistaxis in a Saint Bernard. (From Green CE: *Infectious diseases of the dog and cat,* ed 3, St Louis, 2006, Saunders.)

TABLE 18.1 Common Inherited Coagulation Disorders of Dogs	
Disorder	**Breeds Affected**
Prothrombin deficiency	Cocker spaniel, beagle
Factor VII deficiency	Beagle, malamute
Factor VIII deficiency	Many breeds (hemophilia A)
Factor IX deficiency	Many breeds (hemophilia B)
Factor X deficiency	Cocker spaniel
Factor XI deficiency	Great Pyrenees, English Springer spaniel
Factor XII deficiency	Poodle, Shar Pei

demonstrate abnormal results. Hemophilia A is the most common inherited coagulation factor deficiency in dogs, and it is caused by Factor VIII deficiency. Hemophilia B, which is also called Christmas disease, results from Factor IX deficiency. Both Hemophilia A and B involve X-linked recessive traits.

Von Willebrand Disease

The most common inherited coagulation disorder of domestic animals is von Willebrand disease (vWD). The disease results from the decreased or deficient production of von Willebrand factor. von Willebrand factor (vWF) is a large glycoprotein that circulates with Factor VIII and functions to assist with platelet aggregation at the initiation of the coagulation pathways. The disease occurs with relative frequency in Dobermans, and it has been reported in dozens of other canine breeds as well as in rabbits and swine. Several distinct forms of the disease have been identified on the basis of their patterns of inheritance (Table 18.2). Type 1 vWD shows an autosomal-dominant inheritance pattern with incomplete penetrance, and it is characterized by low levels of circulating vWF with normal structure. Animals affected by type 2 vWD have low circulating levels of vWF, and their vWF is abnormal in both structure and function. Type 3 vWD is characterized by the near absence of any vWF. Type 2 is inherited as a dominant trait; type 3 is inherited as autosomal-recessive traits. Dogs with Types 2 and 3 vWD tend to experience the most severe bleeding. Prolonged bleeding during estrus, after venipuncture, and after surgery are common findings, and the buccal mucosa bleeding time is prolonged. Specific genetic tests are available for both type 1 and type 3 von Willebrand disease. Affected animals should not be used for breeding.

> **TECHNICIAN NOTE** The most common inherited coagulation disorder of domestic animals is vWD.

ACQUIRED COAGULATION DISORDERS

Coagulation disorders can result from the decreased production or the increased destruction of platelets as well as from nutritional deficiencies, liver disease, and the ingestion of certain medications or toxic substances. The liver is the primary site for the production of coagulation factors. Any disease that alters liver function can result in coagulopathy.

Thrombocytopenia

Thrombocytopenia refers to a decreased number of platelets, and it is the most common coagulation disorder seen in small animal veterinary practice. The causes of platelet deficiencies are often unknown. However, infection with certain bacterial, viral, and parasitic agents can result in thrombocytopenia (Table 18.3). Thrombocytopenia can also occur as a result of bone marrow depression that reduces the production of platelets, or it may result from autoimmune disease that increases the rate of platelet destruction. A variety of medications have also been implicated in thrombocytopenia (Box 18.1). Aspirin and acetaminophen are common toxins encountered in small animal patients. These medications may destroy or

TABLE 18.2 Canine von Willebrand Disease

Type	Plasma Von Willebrand Factor	Examples of Breeds With Known Mutations
1	Variably reduced levels; all multimer sizes proportionately reduced; most common and recognized in >70 breeds; hemorrhage tendency variable, often with surgery or trauma	Doberman pinscher, German shepherd, golden retriever, rottweiler, Manchester terrier, Cairn terrier, Pembroke Welsh corgi, Bernese mountain dog, Kerry blue terrier, poodle, papillon
2	Disproportionately low activity; deficiency of high molecular weight multimers; larger and more effective multimers absent; bleeding can be severe	German shorthair pointer, German wirehair pointer
3	Complete deficiency (<1% plasma von Willebrand factor); most severe in that all multimers absent	Scottish terrier, Shetland sheepdog, Chesapeake Bay retriever, Kooiker

Enzyme-linked immunosorbent assay results: normal = >70%; borderline = 50% to 69%; and affected = 0% to 49%.
From Battaglia A: *Small animal emergency and critical care for veterinary technicians*, ed 2, St Louis, 2007, Saunders.

TABLE 18.3 Infectious Causes of Thrombocytopenia in Dogs and Cats

Disease	Species	Mechanism	Diagnostic Tests*	Therapy
Viral				
Canine distemper	C	U	Ag detection, PCR, serology	Supportive
Canine herpes virus	C	V	Ag detection, serology, VI	Supportive
Canine parvovirus infection: canine parvovirus 2	C	P, U	Ag detection, EM feces, PCR, serology	Supportive
Infectious canine hepatitis: canine adenovirus 1	C	U, V	Serology, PCR, VI	Supportive
Feline immunodeficiency virus	F	P	Serology, PCR	Supportive
Feline infectious peritonitis: feline corona virus	F	U, V	Ag detection, histopathology, PCR, serology	Supportive
Feline leukemia virus	F	P	Ag detection, PCR, serology	Supportive
Feline panleukopenia/feline parvovirus	F	P, U	Ag detection, EM, fecal VI, PCR, serology	Supportive
Rickettsial, Neorickettsial, Anaplasmal, and Mycoplasmal				
Canine granulocytotropic anaplasmosis: *Anaplasma phagocytophilum*	C	D, U	Blood smear, PCR, serology	Doxycycline (10 mg/kg PO q24h for 21 days)
Canine granulocytotropic ehrlichiosis: *Ehrlichia ewingii*	C	D, U	Blood smear, PCR, serology	Doxycycline (10 mg/kg PO q24h for 21 days)
Canine monocytotropic ehrlichiosis: *Ehrlichia canis, Ehrlichia chaffeensis*	C	D, P, U	Blood smear, PCR, serology	Doxycycline (10 mg/kg PO q24h for 21 days)
Feline granulocytotropic anaplasmosis: *A. phagocytophilum*	F	D?	PCR, serology	Doxycycline (10 mg/kg PO q24h for 21 days)
Feline mononuclear ehrlichiosis: *E. canis, Neorickettsia risticii?*	F	D?	PCR, serology	Doxycycline (10 mg/kg PO q24h for 21 days)
Hemotropic mycoplasmosis: *Mycoplasma haemofelis, Mycoplasma haemominutum, Mycoplasma haemocanis*	C, F	D, S	Ag detection, blood smear, PCR	Doxycycline (10 mg/kg PO q24h for 21 days), Enrofloxacin (5 mg/kg PO q24h for 14 days)
Rocky Mountain spotted fever: *Rickettsia rickettsii*	C	D, V	Ag detection (skin), PCR, serology	Doxycycline (10 mg/kg PO q24h for 21 days)
Salmon poisoning disease: *Neorickettsia helminthoeca*	C	D, U	Cytology, fecal examination	Doxycycline (10 mg/kg PO q24h for 21 days)
Thrombocytotropic ehrlichiosis: *Anaplasma platys*	C	D, U	Ag detection, blood smear, PCR, serology	Doxycycline (10 mg/kg PO q24h for 21 days)

Continued

TABLE 18.3			Infectious Causes of Thrombocytopenia in Dogs and Cats—cont'd	
Disease	**Species**	**Mechanism**	**Diagnostic Tests***	**Therapy**
Bacterial				
Bacteremia/septicemia	C, F	D, U, V	Blood, urine, body fluid culture	Ampicillin sulbactam (30 mg/kg IV q8h) and Enrofloxacin (10 mg/kg IV q24h)
Bartonellosis: *Bartonella vinsonii*	C	D, V	Culture, PCR, serology	Optimal treatment is unknown. Azithromycin (5 mg/kg PO q24h for 5 days, then EOD for 45 days) has been recommended.
Endotoxemia: most often *Escherichia, Klebsiella, Enterobacter, Proteus, Pseudomonas*	C, F	S	Blood, urine, wound culture, often presumptive	Ampicillin sulbactam (30 mg/kg IV q8h) and Enrofloxacin (10 mg/kg IV q24h)
Leptospirosis	C	D, U, V	Ag detection, histopathology, PCR, serology, urine dark-field microscopy, urine or blood culture	Ampicillin (22 mg/kg IV q8h for 2 weeks) followed by Doxycycline (5 mg/kg PO q12h for 3 weeks). Some recommend Doxycycline for initial therapy.
Plague: *Yersinia pestis*	F	S, U	Ag detection, culture, PCR, serology	Doxycycline (10 mg/kg PO q24h for 21 days), Enrofloxacin (5 mg/kg PO q24h for 14 days)
Salmonellosis	C, F	D, S, U, V	Culture, PCR	Enrofloxacin (5—10 mg/kg IV q24h) reserved for patients with septicemia
Tularemia: *Francisella tularensis*	C, F	D, U, V	Ag detection, culture, PCR, serology	Doxycycline (5 mg/kg PO q12h)
Protozoal				
Babesiosis: *Babesia canis, Babesia gibsoni*	C	U, S	Blood smear, PCR, serology	Imidocarb dipropionate (6.6 mg/kg IM twice, 2 weeks apart) for *B. canis*, Atovaquone (13.5 mg/kg PO q8h for 10 days) and azithromycin 10 mg/kg PO q24h for 10 days) for *B. gibsoni*
Cytauxzoonosis: *Cytauxzoon felis*	F	U, S	Blood smear, cytology, PCR[†]	Imidocarb dipropionate (2—3 mg/kg IM twice, 1 week apart) or Atovaquone (15 mg/kg PO q8h for 10 days) and azithromycin (10 mg/kg PO q24h for 10 days)
Leishmaniasis	C	U	Ag detection, cytology, PCR, serology, western blot analysis	Meglumine antimonite (100 mg/kg SQ q24h) and allopurinol (15 mg/kg PO q12h) for 3—4 months, allopurinol indefinitely
Toxoplasmosis: *Toxoplasma gondii*	C, F	U	Fecal (cats), serology, cytology	Clindamycin (12.5—25 mg/kg PO q12h)
Nematodal				
Heartworm disease: *Dirofilaria immitis*	C	D, U, V	Ag detection, blood smear, Knott's test, serology	Melarsomine (2.5 mg/kg IM)
Fungal				
Disseminated candidiasis	C, F	U	Culture, cytology	Itraconazole (5—10 mg/kg PO q12h)
Histoplasmosis: *Histoplasma capsulatum*	C, F	U	Ag detection, culture, cytology, serology	Itraconazole (5—10 mg/kg PO q12h)

*Refer to Greene CE: *Infectious diseases of the dog and cat,* ed 3, for more information on diagnostic tests, available test kits, specimens, and commercial diagnostic laboratories.
[†]Available at the North Carolina State University, Tick-Borne Disease Laboratory, Raleigh, NC.
[?]Uncertain.
Ag, Antigen; *C,* canine; *D,* destruction; *EM,* electron microscopy; *F,* feline; *PCR,* polymerase chain reaction; *S,* sequestration; *U,* utilization; *V,* vasculitis; *VI,* virus isolation.
From Bonagura J: *Kirk's current veterinary therapy XIV,* ed 14, St Louis, 2009, Saunders.

BOX 18.1 Drugs Associated With Thrombocytopenia in Dogs and Cats

Acetaminophen
Antiarrhythmics
Anticonvulsants
Anti-inflammatory drugs (nonsteroidal)
Barbiturates
Benzocaine
Cephalosporins
Chemotherapeutic agents
Chloramphenicol
Cimetidine
Estrogen
Gold salts
Griseofulvin
Immunosuppressive agents
Levamisole
Methimazole
Methionine
Methylene blue
Metronidazole
Penicillins
Phenobarbital
Phenothiazines
Phenylbutazone
Propylene glycol
Propylthiouracil
Sulfa derivatives
Sulfamethoxazole/trimethoprim
Zinc

BOX 18.2 Conditions That May Result in Disseminated Intravascular Coagulation

Septicemia (various gram-negative and gram-positive bacteria)
Viremia (infectious canine hepatitis, feline infectious peritonitis, African swine fever, hog cholera, African horse sickness)
Protozoal parasites (babesiosis, trypanosomiasis, sarcocystosis, leishmaniasis, cytauxzoonosis)
Metazoal parasites (heartworms, lungworms)
Marked tissue injury (heatstroke, trauma, surgical procedures)
Intravascular hemolysis
Obstetric complications
Malignancy (hemangiosarcoma, disseminated carcinomas, leukemia, lymphoma)
Traumatic shock
Liver disease
Pancreatitis
Gastric dilatation-volvulus and abomasal displacement
Toxins (snake and insect venoms, aflatoxin, insecticides)

From Harvey J: *Veterinary hematology*, St Louis, 2012, Saunders.

permanently inhibit the circulating platelets, so clinical signs may not resolve until undamaged platelets begin to be released from the bone marrow.

Vitamin K Deficiency

Vitamin K is required for the synthesis and activation of some coagulation factors. The vitamin-K–dependent factors include Factors II, VII, IX, and X. Vitamin K deficiency can occur as a result of dietary insufficiency or bile duct obstruction. Any disease that alters vitamin K activity can lead to bleeding disorders. The ingestion of toxic substances (e.g., warfarin, moldy sweet clover) can also create bleeding disorders. Anticoagulant rodenticide toxicity is a significant cause of secondary hemostasis in small animal veterinary practice. Warfarin is one of several compounds that are found in rodenticides that have anticoagulant properties. Clinical signs may not appear for several days after ingestion and include lethargy, anorexia, and dyspnea as a result of bleeding into the thoracic cavity. Ecchymosis, petechiae, and hemarthroses may also occur. Bleeding into the brain or spinal cord may result in neurologic signs. The prothrombin time is generally the first coagulation test to increase, followed by activated partial thromboplastin time and activated clotting time. The PIVKA test has also been suggested as a diagnostic aid. Patients are usually decontaminated when ingestion is known to be recent. Vitamin K therapy

is sometimes initiated and may require several weeks for successful treatment.

> **TECHNICIAN NOTE** Anticoagulant rodenticides result in vitamin K deficiency.

DISSEMINATED INTRAVASCULAR COAGULATION

Although it is not a disease entity on its own, disseminated intravascular coagulation (DIC) is associated with many pathologic conditions. DIC is often seen in trauma cases as well as with many infectious diseases. A large number of events can trigger DIC. Box 18.2 contains a summary of some common conditions associated with DIC. The resulting hemostatic disorder may manifest as systemic hemorrhage or microvascular thrombosis. Microthrombi can result in tissue hypoxia, and the formation of thrombi consumes platelets and coagulation factors, which leads to an increased tendency for hemorrhage. Fibrinolysis of the microthrombi leads to the formation of excess fibrin degradation products and D-dimers. Shock can also occur.

> **TECHNICIAN NOTE** DIC is a consumptive coagulopathy that occurs secondary to other disease conditions.

Because the triggering event and the resulting disorder are diverse, the laboratory findings are highly variable. There is no single test that can be used for diagnosis, and not all tests exhibit abnormal results in all patients. Most patients with DIC have a prolonged activated partial thromboplastin time and prothrombin time as well as significant thrombocytopenia.

TABLE 18.4   Expected Laboratory Test Results for Common Bleeding Disorders

Disorder	BMBT	ACT	PT	APTT	Platelets	Fibrinogen	FDPs	D-Dimers
Thrombocytopenia	↑	N	N	N	↓	N	N	N
Thrombopathia	↑	N	N	N	N	N	N	N
von Willebrand disease	↑	↑/N	N	D/N	N	N	N	N
Hemophilias	N	↑	N	↑	N	N	N	N
Warfarin toxicity	N	↑	↑	↑	N/↓	N/↓	N/↑	N
Disseminated intravascular coagulopathy	↑	↑	↑	↑	↓	N/↓	↑	↑

ACT, Activated clotting time; *APTT,* activated partial thromboplastin time; *BMBT,* buccal mucosa bleeding time; *FDP,* fibrin degradation products; *N,* normal; *PT,* prothrombin time.
From Ford RB, Mazzaferro E: *Kirk & Bistner's handbook of veterinary procedures and emergency treatment,* ed 9, St Louis, 2012, Saunders.

Schistocytes are often present on the blood film. Fibrinogen may be normal or decreased. Buccal mucosal bleeding time is prolonged, and fibrin degradation products and D-dimers are generally all increased. Table 18.4 contains a summary of the laboratory data seen with DIC as well as with other common hemostatic disorders.

▌ KEY POINTS

- Bleeding disorders may be caused by congenital or acquired defects in coagulation proteins, platelets, or the vasculature.
- Clinical signs of bleeding disorders include delayed deep-tissue hemorrhage, hematoma formation, superficial petechial and ecchymotic hemorrhages, epistaxis, melena, and prolonged bleeding at injection and incision sites.
- The most common inherited coagulation disorder of domestic animals is vWD.
- Thrombocytopenia refers to a decreased number of platelets, and it is the most common coagulation disorder seen in small animal veterinary practice.

- Vitamin-K–dependent factors include Factors II, VII, IX, and X.
- Thrombocytopenia can be the result of a wide variety of conditions, including infection with certain bacterial, viral, and parasitic agents. It may also be caused by bone marrow depression or autoimmune disease.
- DIC is a consumptive coagulopathy that occurs secondary to other disease conditions.
- Clinical signs and laboratory results are highly variable for patients with DIC.

UNIT 4

Clinical Chemistry

Unit Outline

Unit Objectives

List and describe the types of clinical chemistry analyzers available for the veterinary practice laboratory.
Describe proper sample collection and handling for clinical chemistry assays.
List the commonly performed clinical chemistry evaluations and the significance of abnormal test results.
Describe electrolyte and acid—base analyses and the significance of abnormal test results.

In both human and veterinary medical practice, current trends indicate a move toward greater point-of-care capabilities. This translates into better customer service, and it enhances the practice of veterinary medicine. Determinations of levels of the various chemical constituents in blood can be an important aid in the formulation of an accurate diagnosis, the prescription of proper therapy, and the documentation of the response to treatment. The chemicals being assayed are generally associated with particular organ functions. They may be enzymes associated with particular organ functions or metabolites and metabolic by-products that are processed by certain organs. Analysis of these components usually requires a carefully collected blood serum sample. Plasma may be used in some cases.

Many veterinary practices own or lease chemistry analyzers to perform routine chemical assays. This focus on in-house laboratory work makes veterinary technicians' laboratory skills perhaps their biggest asset to the practice. As the person most likely to be in charge of the laboratory, the veterinary technician must become familiar with the types of analytic instruments available, the variety of testing procedures used, and the rationales underlying the analyses. The most important contribution that the technician can make to the practice laboratory is providing accurate and reliable test results. In vitro results must reflect, as closely as possible, the actual in vivo levels of blood constituents.

There are literally hundreds of biochemical tests that can be performed on serum samples. The average veterinary practice laboratory probably performs a few dozen of these. The more common ones are included in this unit. Additional tests that are commonly performed at veterinary reference laboratories are also discussed. Although the tests are categorized primarily by the organs involved, it should be noted that some tests may be affected by the function of more than one organ or system. For example, amylase has multiple organ sources, and protein levels can be affected by many factors, including liver and kidney damage, metabolic status, and dehydration.

19

Sample Collection and Handling for Clinical Chemistry

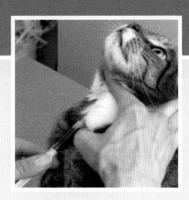

LEARNING OBJECTIVES

After studying this chapter, you will be able to:
- Describe proper sample processing for serum samples.
- Describe proper sample processing for plasma samples.
- Discuss the effects of sample quality on test results.
- List common causes of sample compromise and mechanisms to minimize those causes.

OUTLINE

KEY TERMS

Hemolysis
Icterus

Lipemia
Plasma

Reference range
Serum

Most chemical analyses require the collection and preparation of serum samples. Whole blood or blood plasma may be used for some test methods or with specific types of equipment. The instructions that accompany the chemistry analyzers should be consulted for the type of sample required. The collection of a high-quality sample on which to perform an assay has a direct effect on the quality of test results. Most adverse influences on sample quality can be avoided with careful consideration of sample collection and handling.

Chemical measurements should be completed within 1 hour after blood collection. If testing will be delayed, freezing of the sample will preserve the integrity of most of the constituents. Freezing may interfere with some test methods, however. Once thawed, the sample must not be re-frozen. Certain anticoagulants may also interfere with particular chemical analyses. Many factors other than disease influence the results of chemistry tests. These factors may be preanalytical, analytical, or postanalytical (see Chapter 5).

> **TECHNICIAN NOTE** Samples should be analyzed within 1 hour after collection.

Specific blood collection protocols vary depending on the patient species, the volume of blood needed, the method of restraint, and the types of samples needed. Blood samples for chemical testing should always be collected before treatment is initiated. The administration of certain medications and treatments may affect the results of biochemical testing. Preprandial samples (samples from an animal that has not eaten for 12 hours) are preferred. Postprandial samples (samples collected after an animal has eaten) may produce erroneous results. Samples taken after the patient has eaten can produce false values for a number of blood components, including glucose, urea, and lipase. Regardless of the method of blood collection, the sample must be labeled immediately after it has been collected. The tube should be labeled with the date and time of collection, the owner's name, the patient's name, and the patient's clinic identification number. If the sample will be submitted to a laboratory, include a request form that contains all necessary sample identification and a clear indication of which tests are requested. Additional specific information regarding general blood collection protocols and the order in which to draw the various sample types is presented in Chapter 7.

> **TECHNICIAN NOTE** Preprandial samples taken before the initiation of treatment are preferred.

PLASMA

Plasma is the fluid portion of whole blood in which the cells are suspended. It is composed of approximately 90% water and 10% dissolved constituents, such as proteins, carbohydrates, vitamins, hormones, enzymes, lipids, salts, waste materials, antibodies, and other ions and molecules. Procedure 19.1 describes the method for obtaining a plasma sample. The sample must not be contaminated with any cells from the bottom of the tube after centrifugation. If the sample cannot be centrifuged within 1 hour, it must be refrigerated. If heparinized plasma has been stored overnight after separation or has been frozen, the sample should be centrifuged again to remove any fibrin strands that may have formed. Freezing may affect certain test results; the test instructions should be consulted for all of the tests that must be run before a plasma sample is frozen.

> **TECHNICIAN NOTE** Always check the information provided by the analyzer manufacturer to determine whether serum or plasma samples are required.

SERUM

Serum is plasma from which fibrinogen (a plasma protein) has been removed. During the clotting process, the soluble fibrinogen in plasma is converted to an insoluble fibrin clot matrix. When blood clots, the fluid that is squeezed out around the cellular clot is serum. The steps for obtaining a serum sample is described in Procedure 19.2. Centrifuging at speeds of more than 2000 to 3000 rpm or for a prolonged time may result in hemolysis. Serum separator tubes (SSTs) contain a gel that forms a physical barrier between serum or plasma and blood cells during centrifugation. The inside walls of the tube also contain silica particles that assist with clot activation. Blood collected into an SST should be mixed by inverting the tube several times and then allowing the sample to clot for 30 minutes before centrifugation. Serum separator transport tubes are also available. These contain approximately double the amount of gel found in a standard SST. The additional gel barrier helps to minimize any interaction between the serum and the cells after centrifugation so that test results are not likely to be affected if tests are delayed. Any prolonged delays in

testing require that the serum be removed from the SST and placed in a sterile tube. The tube can then be refrigerated or frozen. Freezing may affect some test results; therefore, the test instructions should be consulted for all tests that must be run before a serum sample is frozen.

FACTORS THAT INFLUENCE RESULTS

Many factors other than disease influence the results of chemistry tests. Hemolysis, lipemia, icterus, certain medications, and inappropriate sample handling can all lead to inaccurate results. Effects of sample compromise are summarized in Table 19.1.

Hemolysis

Hemolysis may be produced as an artifact when a blood sample is drawn into a moist syringe, mixed too vigorously after sample collection, forced through a needle when being transferred to a tube, or frozen as a whole blood sample. A syringe must be completely dry before it is used, because water in the syringe may cause hemolysis. The needle from a syringe should be removed before blood is transferred to a tube. Forcing blood through a small needle opening may rupture cells. When

---

PROCEDURE 19.2 Serum Sample Preparation

1. Collect a whole blood sample in a container that contains no anticoagulant.
2. Allow the blood to clot in its original container at room temperature for 20 to 30 minutes.
3. Gently separate the clot from the container by running a wooden applicator stick around the wall of the container between the clot and the wall.
4. Cover the sample and centrifuge it at 2000 to 3000 rpm for 10 minutes.
5. With a capillary pipette, remove the serum from the clot.
6. Transfer the serum to a container that has been labeled with the date, the time of collection, the patient's name, and the case or clinic number.
7. Refrigerate or freeze the sample, as appropriate.

PROCEDURE 19.1 Plasma Sample Preparation

1. Collect a blood sample in a container with the appropriate anticoagulant.
2. Mix the blood-filled container with a gentle rocking motion 12 times.
3. Make sure that the container is covered to prevent evaporation during centrifugation.
4. Centrifuge (within 1 hour of collection) at 2000 to 3000 rpm for 10 minutes.
5. With a capillary pipette, carefully remove the fluid plasma layer from the bottom layer of cells.
6. Transfer the plasma to a container that has been labeled with the date, the time of collection, the patient's name, and the case or clinic number.
7. Process the sample immediately, or refrigerate or freeze it, as appropriate.

TABLE 19.1 Effects of Sample Compromise

Sample Characteristic	Effect	Result
Lipemia	Light scattering	↑
	Volume displacement	↓
	Hemolysis*	↑↓
Hemolysis/blood substitutes	Release of analytes	↑
	Release of enzymes*	↑↓
	Reaction inhibition	↓
	Increased optical density (absorbance)	↑
	Release of water	↓
Icterus	Spectral interference	↑
	Chemical interaction	↑
Hyperproteinemia	Hyperviscosity	↓
	Analyte binding*	↑↓
	Volume displacement	
Medications	Reaction interference*	↑↓

*Variable effect, depending on the analyte and test method used.

transferring a blood sample to a tube, the veterinary technician should expel the blood slowly from the syringe without causing bubbles to form. Hemolysis can also result when excess alcohol is used to clean the skin and not allowed to dry before beginning the blood collection procedure.

Hemolysis, regardless of cause, can greatly alter the makeup of a serum or plasma sample. For example, fluid from ruptured blood cells can dilute the sample, thereby resulting in falsely lower concentrations of constituents than are actually present in the animal. Certain constituents that are normally not found in high concentrations in serum or plasma escape from ruptured blood cells, thus causing falsely elevated concentrations in the sample. Hemolysis may elevate levels of potassium, organic phosphorus, and certain enzymes in the blood. Hemolysis also interferes with lipase activity and bilirubin determinations. Plasma or serum are frequently the preferred sample types over whole blood, and serum is frequently preferred over plasma.

> **TECHNICIAN NOTE** Hemolysis, lipemia, and icterus are commonly encountered conditions that compromise sample quality.

Chemical Contamination

Sterile tubes are not necessary for the collection of blood samples for routine chemical assays. However, the tubes must be chemically pure. Detergents must be completely rinsed from reusable tubes so that the detergents do not interfere with test results.

Improper Labeling

Serious errors may result if a tube that contains a sample is not labeled immediately after the sample is collected. The tube should be labeled with the date, the time of collection, and the patient's identifying number or name. The veterinary technician should double check the sample identification with the request form, if one is used, as the sample is prepared and the test is run.

Improper Sample Handling

Ideally, all chemical measurements should be completed within 1 hour of sample collection, but this is not always feasible. In this case, samples must be properly handled and stored so that the levels of their chemical constituents approximate those in the patient's body at the time of collection. Samples must not be allowed to become too warm. Heat may be detrimental to a sample, and it may destroy some chemicals and activate others

(e.g., enzymes). If a serum or plasma sample has been frozen, it must be thoroughly mixed by gentle inversion after thawing to avoid concentration gradients.

Patient Influences

If practical, a sample should be obtained from a fasting animal. The blood glucose level can be elevated, and the inorganic phosphorus level decreased, immediately after a meal. In addition, postprandial lipemia results in turbid or cloudy plasma or serum. Kidney assays are also affected as a result of the transient increase in the glomerular filtration rate after eating. Water intake need not be restricted before obtaining a blood sample.

REFERENCE RANGES

Reference ranges are also known as normal values. The reference range for a particular blood constituent is a range of values that has been derived when a laboratory has repeatedly assayed samples from a significant number of clinically normal animals of a given species via specific test methods. Therefore, reference ranges may differ depending on the specific test method and analyzer used. Numerous medicine and clinical pathology books list the reference ranges of blood constituents for domestic species. Alternatively, reference ranges may be formulated by local diagnostic laboratories or in individual practice laboratories. Appendix B contains reference ranges for common biochemical constituents.

> **TECHNICIAN NOTE** Reference ranges are specific to the test method and analyzer used.

Establishing reference range values for any laboratory is time consuming and expensive. To establish a list of reference values for the laboratory, the veterinary technician would have to assay samples from a significant number of clinically normal animals. Some investigators recommend the analysis of at least 20 animals, and others recommend the analysis of more than 100 animals with similar characteristics. Other considerations include the variety of breeds and species most often seen in the veterinary practice; the gender and reproductive status (e.g., intact, neutered) of the tested animals; and the environment, including husbandry and nutrition, of these animals. Climate is also a consideration, because drastic seasonal changes may affect assay results.

KEY POINTS

- Clinical chemistry testing usually requires either a serum or plasma sample.
- Consult the manufacturer of the test kit used in the practice for the proper sample type.
- Samples must be analyzed within 1 hour to avoid changes to the sample that can affect test results.
- The ideal sample is collected from a preprandial patient before the initiation of therapy.

- Common sample interferences include hemolysis, lipemia, and icterus.
- Samples that are hemolyzed, icteric, or lipemic may provide inaccurate results.
- Reference ranges may vary with different test methods and analyzers.

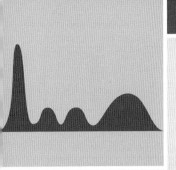

20

Protein Assays and Hepatobiliary Function Tests

LEARNING OBJECTIVES

After studying this chapter, you will be able to:

- List potential causes of alterations in serum proteins.
- Describe commonly performed tests to measure total protein and albumin.
- Describe the common method for determining globulin concentration.
- List the commonly performed tests for the evaluation of the hepatobiliary system.
- Describe the metabolism of bilirubin.
- Differentiate between conjugated and unconjugated bilirubin.
- List the leakage enzymes, and explain the significance of altered enzyme activity.
- Describe the circulation of bile acids and the significance of altered bile acid activity.

OUTLINE

KEY TERMS

Acute-phase proteins
Alanine transaminase
Albumin
Alkaline phosphatase
Aspartate transaminase
Bile acids
Bilirubin

Cholesterol
Conjugated bilirubin
Gamma glutamyltransferase
Globulins
Glutamate dehydrogenase
Hepatoencephalopathy
Hyperlipoproteinemia

Hyperproteinemia
Hypoalbuminemia
Hypoglycemia
Hypoproteinemia
Iditol dehydrogenase
Jaundice
Protein

PROTEIN ASSAYS

Although protein assays are not specifically considered liver function tests, the majority of plasma proteins are produced by the liver. Additional plasma proteins are produced by the immune system (i.e., reticuloendothelial tissues, lymphoid tissues, and plasma cells). Proteins have many functions in the body, and alterations in plasma protein concentrations occur in a variety of disease conditions, especially disease of the liver and kidneys. More than 200 plasma proteins exist. Some plasma protein concentrations change markedly during certain diseases and can be used as diagnostic aids. Other protein concentrations change little during disease. Age-related changes in plasma protein concentrations are also seen.

Major plasma protein functions are summarized in Box 20.1. The plasma protein chemical assays that are commonly performed in veterinary medicine include total protein, albumin, and fibrinogen.

Total Protein

- Elevated in
  - Dehydration
  - Hyperglobulinemia
  - Hemolysis
  - Lipemia
- Decreased in
  - Hemorrhage
  - Hypoalbuminemia

BOX 20.1 Plasma Protein Functions

- Help form the structural matrix of all cells, organs, and tissues
- Maintain osmotic pressure
- Serve as enzymes for biochemical reactions
- Act as buffers in acid–base balance
- Serve as hormones
- Function in blood coagulation
- Defend the body against pathogenic microorganisms
- Serve as transport/carrier molecules for most constituents of plasma

- Liver failure
- External plasma loss
- GI fluid loss
- Malassimilation
- Starvation
- Overhydration
- Glomerular loss
- Cancer cachexia

Total plasma protein measurements include fibrinogen values, whereas total serum protein determinations measure all of the protein fractions except fibrinogen, which is removed during the clotting process. The total protein concentration may be affected by altered hepatic synthesis, altered protein distribution, and altered protein breakdown or excretion, as well as by dehydration and overhydration.

Total protein concentrations are especially valuable for determining an animal's state of hydration. A dehydrated animal usually has a relatively elevated total protein concentration (hyperproteinemia), whereas an overhydrated animal usually has a relatively decreased total protein concentration (hypoproteinemia). Total protein concentrations are also useful as initial screening tests for patients with edema, ascites, diarrhea, weight loss, hepatic and renal disease, and blood clotting problems.

Two methods are commonly used for the determination of total protein levels: the refractometric method and the biuret photometric method. The refractometric method measures the refractive index of serum or plasma with a refractometer (see Procedure 2.1). The refractive index of the sample is a function of the concentration of solid particles in the sample. In plasma, the primary solids are the proteins. This method is a good screening test, because it is fast, inexpensive, and accurate. The biuret method measures the number of molecules that contain more than three peptide bonds in serum or plasma. This method is commonly used by analytic instruments in the laboratory. It is a simple method that yields accurate results. Other chemical tests to measure protein include dye-binding methods and precipitation methods. These tests are not commonly performed in veterinary practice. They are usually used to measure a small amount of protein in urine and cerebrospinal fluid. Specialized tests to separate the various protein populations are performed in some reference laboratories and research facilities. These methods include salt fractionation, chromatography, and gel electrophoresis (Fig. 20.1). These tests

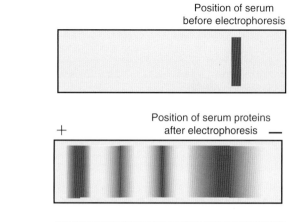

Position of serum before electrophoresis

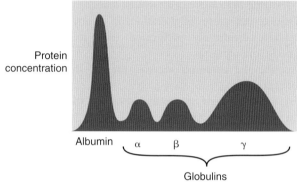

Position of serum proteins after electrophoresis

Protein concentration

Albumin   α   β   γ

Globulins

Fig. 20.1 Schematic diagram showing the results of the electrophoresis of whole serum. Four major peaks develop consistently: the albumin and three globulin peaks. (From Tizard I: *Veterinary immunology,* ed 9, St Louis, 2013, Saunders.)

can be performed on samples other than serum and plasma (e.g., urine, cerebrospinal fluid). Other tests that are also used to test a variety of body fluids include the sulfosalicylic acid test and the Pandy test. The sulfosalicylic acid test is described in Unit 5, Chapter 29.

> **TECHNICIAN NOTE** Total protein is estimated with a refractometer or measured chemically with the biuret method.

Albumin

- Elevated in
  - Dehydration
  - Hemolysis
  - Lipemia
  - Laboratory error
- Decreased in
  - Protein-losing nephropathy
  - Gastroenteropathy
  - Liver failure
  - Malnutrition
  - Exudative skin disease
  - Neonates
  - External blood loss
  - Chronic effusions

- Hyperglobulinemia
- Multiple myeloma

Albumin is one of the most important proteins in plasma or serum. It makes up 35% to 50% of the total plasma protein in most animals, and any significant state of hypoproteinemia is most likely caused by albumin loss. Hepatocytes synthesize albumin, and any diffuse liver disease may result in decreased albumin synthesis. Renal disease, dietary intake, and intestinal protein absorption may also influence the plasma albumin level. Albumin is the major binding and transport protein in the blood, and it is responsible for maintaining the osmotic pressure of the plasma. The primary photometric test for albumin in veterinary patients is the bromocresol green dye-binding method.

Box 20.2 summarizes diseases and conditions that are associated with alterations in serum proteins.

Globulins

- Elevated in
  - Dehydration
  - Infection
  - Immune-mediated diseases
  - Neoplasia
- Decreased in
  - Unremarkable

The globulins are a complex group of proteins. Alpha globulins are synthesized in the liver and primarily transport and bind proteins. Two important proteins in this fraction are high-density lipoproteins and very-low-density lipoproteins. Beta globulins include complement (C3, C4), transferrin, and ferritin. They are responsible for iron transport, heme binding, and fibrin formation and lysis. Gamma globulins (immunoglobulins) are synthesized by plasma cells, and they are responsible for antibody production (immunity). The immunoglobulins (Ig) that have been identified in animals are IgG, IgD, IgE, IgA, and IgM.

Direct chemical measurements of globulin are rarely performed. Globulin concentration is normally estimated by determining the difference between the total protein and albumin concentrations.

BOX 20.2 Conditions Associated With Altered Serum Protein

- Hyperproteinemia and/or hyperalbuminemia
- Hemoconcentration (dehydration)
- Inflammatory disease
- Plasmacytoma
- Lymphoma
- Hypoproteinemia and/or hypoalbuminemia
- Hemodilution (overhydration)
- Blood loss
- Glomerulonephritis
- Hepatic insufficiency
- Malabsorption
- Malnutrition

Albumin/Globulin Ratio

- High total protein with a normal A/G ratio
  - Dehydration
- High total protein with low A/G ratio
  - Hyperglobulinemia
- A/G ratio of 1
  - Hemorrhage

An alteration in the normal ratio of albumin to globulin (A/G) is frequently the first indication of a protein abnormality. The ratio is analyzed in conjunction with a protein profile. The A/G can be used to detect increased or decreased albumin and globulin concentrations. Many pathologic conditions alter the A/G. However, if the albumin and globulin concentrations are reduced in equal proportions, such as with hemorrhage, no alteration in A/G will be present.

The A/G is determined by dividing the albumin concentration by the globulin concentration. In dogs, horses, sheep, and goats, the albumin concentration is usually greater than the globulin concentration (i.e., the A/G is more than 1.00). In cattle, pigs, and cats, the albumin concentration is usually equal to or less than the globulin concentration (i.e., the A/G is less than 1.00).

TECHNICIAN NOTE Globulin concentration is estimated by calculating the difference between the total protein and albumin concentrations.

Fibrinogen

- Elevated in
  - Acute inflammatory disease
- Decreased in
  - DIC
  - Severe liver disease

Fibrinogen is synthesized by hepatocytes. It is the precursor of fibrin, which is the insoluble protein that forms the matrix of blood clots, and it is one of the factors necessary for clot formation. If fibrinogen levels are decreased, blood does not form a stable clot or does not clot at all. Fibrinogen makes up 3% to 6% of the total plasma protein content. Because it is removed from plasma by the clotting process, no fibrinogen is found in serum. Fibrinogen assays are performed as part of a coagulation profile but may be a useful tool as part of the chemistry profile. Acute inflammation or tissue damage may elevate plasma fibrinogen levels and has been used to detect subclinical inflammation in horses. One method of fibrinogen evaluation is the heat precipitation test described in Unit 3, Chapter 17. The fibrinogen value is calculated by subtracting the total plasma protein value of the heated tubes from that of the unheated tubes. This protein measurement of the heated tubes should be lower because fibrinogen has been removed from the plasma. Some automated analyzers may also provide fibrinogen values.

Acute-Phase Proteins

- Elevated in
  - Inflammation prior to an inflammatory leukogram
- Decreased in
  - Responses to treatment

Acute-phase proteins are primarily produced by hepatocytes immediately following injury or inflammation. There are about 30 recognized acute-phase proteins, and different species produce different ones at different levels. In addition to serum amyloid A (SAA), significant acute-phase proteins of domestic animals include C-reactive protein (CRP), fibrinogen, haptoglobin (HP), ceruloplasmin, α_1-acid glycoprotein (AGP), and major acute-phase protein (MAP) (Fig. 20.2). Albumin and transferrin are referred to as negative acute-phase proteins because their plasma concentration decreases following injury or inflammation. Although serum electrophoresis can aid in identifying increased levels of acute-phase proteins, measurements of specific acute-phase proteins is more useful. Most of the acute-phase proteins of significance in domestic animals are measured with immunoassays, although a chemical test is available for measurement of haptoglobin. A handheld portable analyzer is available for measurement of SAA in horses.

SAA is a major acute-phase protein of many species of mammals and is of particular importance in cats, cattle, and horses. Serum amyloid levels rise within hours following injury or inflammation. The magnitude of the increase can aid in determining the presence of specific disease states. For example, in healthy cats, SAA is generally below 20 mg/L. Increases in SAA are correlated to specific disease states in cats (Table 20.1). SAA values are used to differentiate infectious disease from noninfectious disease in horses and to track response to therapy.

CRP is a biomarker for inflammation produced in the liver. Levels of CRP rise dramatically in a variety of disease states, including cardiac disease, sepsis, and neoplasia. The response occurs within 6 hours after the inflammatory event or trauma and peaks in 24 to 48 hours. The levels of CRP drop rapidly as the triggering event is treated.

HEPATOBILIARY ASSAYS

The liver is the largest internal organ. It is complex in structure, function, and pathologic characteristics. It has many functions, including the metabolism of amino acids, carbohydrates, and

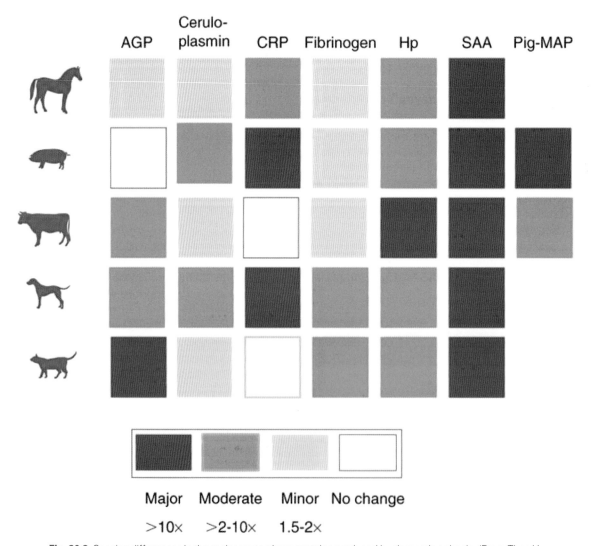

Fig. 20.2 Species differences in the major acute-phase proteins produced by domestic animals. (From Tizard I: *Veterinary immunology*, ed 9, St Louis, 2013, Elsevier.)

TABLE 20.1 SAA Values for Specific Disease States in Cats

Disease	Expected SAA Value (mg/L)
Acute pancreatitis	56.9
Feline infectious peritonitis (FIP)	29.4
Hyperthyroidism	16.5
Diabetes mellitus	14.9
Lymphoma	13.7
Chronic renal failure	8.7

BOX 20.3 Major Hepatobiliary Assays

Enzymes Released From Damaged Hepatocytes
- Alanine transaminase
- Aspartate transaminase
- Iditol dehydrogenase
- Glutamate dehydrogenase

Enzymes Associated With Cholestasis
- Alkaline phosphatase
- Gamma glutamyltransferase

Hepatocyte Function Tests
- Bilirubin
- Bile acids

lipids; the synthesis of albumin, cholesterol, plasma proteins, and clotting factors; the digestion and absorption of nutrients related to bile formation; the secretion of bilirubin and bile; and elimination, such as the detoxification of toxins and the catabolism of certain drugs. These functions are controlled by enzymatic reactions. The gallbladder is closely associated with the liver, both anatomically and functionally. Its primary function is as a storage site for bile. Malfunctions in the liver or gallbladder result in predictable clinical signs of jaundice, hypoalbuminemia, problems with hemostasis, hypoglycemia, hyperlipoproteinemia, and hepatoencephalopathy.

Hepatic cells exhibit extreme diversity of function and are capable of regeneration if damaged. As a result, more than 100 different types of tests are available to evaluate liver function. Usually liver disease has progressed significantly before clinical signs appear. Some liver function tests are designed to measure substances that are produced by the liver, modified by the liver, or released when hepatocytes are damaged. Other liver function tests measure those enzymes that have altered serum concentrations as a result of cholestasis. Liver cells also compartmentalize the work so that damage to one zone of the liver may not affect all liver functions. Liver function tests are usually performed with serial determinations and several different types of liver tests completed to assist with verifying the functional status of the organ. No single test is superior to any other for detecting hepatobiliary disease. New tests are being developed to allow for the detection of hepatic disease before the liver is severely damaged. The primary tests used in veterinary medicine for the evaluation of the liver and gallbladder are summarized in Box 20.3.

Hepatocyte Function Tests

Many substances are taken up, modified, produced, and secreted by the liver. Alteration in the ability to perform these specific functions provides an overview of liver function. Tests of hepatocyte function that are performed in veterinary practice include bilirubin and bile acids. Other substances produced by hepatocytes are less-sensitive indicators of liver function, because test results may not show abnormalities until two thirds to three fourths of liver tissue is damaged. These less-sensitive tests include albumin and cholesterol.

Bilirubin
- Elevated in
  - Prehepatic conditions
  - Hemolytic anemia
  - Cholestasis
  - Intrahepatic conditions
  - Duodenal perforation
  - Ruptured gallbladder
- Decreased in
  - Unremarkable

Bilirubin is an insoluble molecule derived from the breakdown of hemoglobin by macrophages in the spleen. The molecule is bound to albumin and transported to the liver. The hepatic cells metabolize and conjugate the bilirubin to the molecule bilirubin glucuronide. This molecule is then secreted from the hepatocytes, and it becomes a component of bile. Bacteria within the gastrointestinal system act on the bilirubin glucuronide and produce a group of compounds collectively referred to as urobilinogen. Urobilinogen is broken down into urobilin before being excreted in the feces. Bilirubin glucuronide and urobilinogen may also be absorbed directly into the blood and excreted by the kidneys (Fig. 20.3). Bilirubin can also be broken down with exposure to light. It is important that samples be protected from light to ensure accurate results.

Measurements of the circulating levels of these various populations of bilirubin can help to pinpoint the cause of jaundice. Differences in the relative solubility of each of these molecules allow them to be individually quantified. In most animals, the prehepatic (bound to albumin) bilirubin comprises approximately two thirds of the total bilirubin in serum. Increases in this population indicate problems with uptake (hepatic damage). Increases in conjugated bilirubin indicate bile duct obstruction.

TECHNICIAN NOTE Increases in the unconjugated bilirubin population indicate problems with uptake (hepatic damage). Increases in conjugated bilirubin indicate bile duct obstruction.

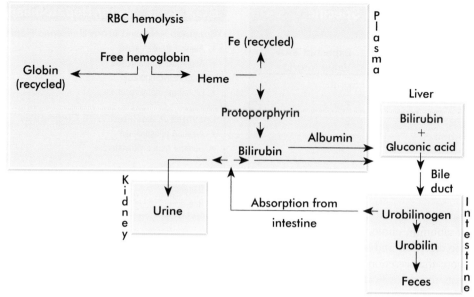

Fig. 20.3 Bilirubin metabolism.

Assays can directly measure total bilirubin (conjugated bilirubin plus unconjugated bilirubin) and conjugated bilirubin. Conjugated bilirubin is sometimes referred to as direct bilirubin, because test methods directly measure the amount of conjugated bilirubin in the sample. Unconjugated bilirubin is sometimes referred to as indirect bilirubin, because its concentration is indirectly calculated by subtracting the conjugated bilirubin concentration from the total bilirubin concentration of the sample.

Bilirubin is assayed to determine the cause of jaundice, to evaluate liver function, and to check the patency of bile ducts. Blood levels of conjugated (direct) bilirubin are elevated with hepatocellular damage or with bile duct injury or obstruction. Blood levels of unconjugated (indirect) bilirubin are elevated with excessive erythrocyte destruction or defects in the transport mechanism that allow bilirubin to enter hepatocytes for conjugation.

Bile Acids

- Elevated in
  - Hepatocellular disease
  - Cholestatic disease
  - Portosystemic shunt
- Decreased in
  - Delayed gastric emptying
  - Malabsorptive disorders
  - Rapid intestinal transport
  - Ileal resection

Bile acids serve many functions. They aid in fat absorption by enabling the formation of micelles in the gastrointestinal system and modulate cholesterol levels via bile acid synthesis. Bile acids are synthesized by hepatocytes from cholesterol, and they are conjugated with glycine or taurine. Conjugated bile acids are secreted across the canalicular membrane, and they reach the duodenum by way of the biliary system. The

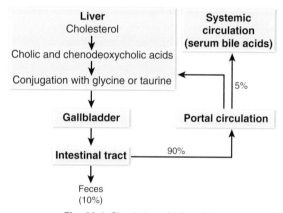

Fig. 20.4 Circulation of bile acids.

gallbladder stores bile acids (except in the horse) until contraction associated with feeding. When bile acids reach the ileum, they are transported to the portal circulation and travel back to the liver. Approximately 90% to 95% of the bile acids are actively resorbed in the ileum, and the remaining 5% to 10% are excreted in the feces. The reabsorbed bile acids are carried to the liver, where they are reconjugated and excreted as part of the enterohepatic circulation of bile acids (Fig. 20.4).

Spillover bile acids that escape from the enterohepatic circulation may be detected in normal animals; serum concentrations of bile acids correlate with portal concentrations. As a result, postprandial serum bile acid (SBA) concentrations are higher than fasting concentrations. Any process that impairs the hepatocellular, biliary, or portal enterohepatic circulation of bile acids results in elevated SBA levels. The great advantages of SBA determinations as liver function tests are that they evaluate the major anatomic components of the hepatobiliary system and that they are stable in vitro.

The SBA level is normally elevated after a meal, because the gallbladder has contracted and released increased amounts of bile into the duodenum. Paired serum samples performed after 12 hours of fasting and 2 hours postprandial are needed to perform the test. The difference in the bile acid concentration of the samples is reported. In horses, a single sample is tested. Inadequate fasting or spontaneous gallbladder contraction can increase fasting bile acid levels. Exposing the patient to even the aroma of food can result in spontaneous gallbladder contraction. Prolonged fasting and diarrhea can decrease bile acids.

Elevated SBA levels usually indicate liver diseases such as congenital portosystemic shunts, chronic hepatitis, hepatic cirrhosis, cholestasis, or neoplasms. Bile acid levels are unspecific with regard to the type of liver problem that exists and are therefore used as a screening test for liver disease. Bile acid levels may detect liver problems before an animal becomes icteric. They may also be used to follow the progress of liver disease during treatment. Increased bile acid concentrations can also result from extrahepatic diseases that secondarily affect the liver. A decreased bile acid concentration may be seen with intestinal malabsorptive diseases. In horses, increased bile acid concentrations can be the result of hepatobiliary disease or decreased feed intake. The reference ranges for bile acids in cows are widely variable. Bile acid testing is not a sensitive indicator of disease in cows.

Bile acids may be determined by several methods, and the most commonly used is an enzymatic method. The 3-hydroxy bile acids react with 3-hydroxisteroid dehydrogenase and then with diformazan. Color generation is measured by end point spectrophotometry. Lipemic postprandial samples must be cleared by centrifugation to avoid interference with spectrophotometry. A bile acid test that uses immunologic methods (e.g., enzyme-linked immunosorbent assay) is now available for use in the veterinary clinic.

Cholesterol

- Elevated in
  - Postprandial
  - Primary hyperlipidemia
  - Endocrine disorders
  - Cholestasis
  - High cholesterol diets
  - Nephrotic syndrome
  - Protein losing nephropathy
  - Idiopathic
- Decreased in
  - Liver failure
  - Malabsorption
  - Maldigestion
  - Protein losing enteropathy
  - Portosystemic shunt
  - Lymphangiectasia
  - Starvation
  - Hypoadrenocorticism
  - Neoplasia

BOX 20.4 Causes of Secondary Hyperlipidemia
- Cholestasis
- Diabetes mellitus
- Hepatic lipidosis
- Hypothyroidism
- Hyperadrenocorticism
- Acute necrotizing pancreatitis
- Nephrotic syndrome
- Corticosteroid administration

Cholesterol is a plasma lipoprotein that is produced primarily in the liver, and it is also ingested in food. Cholestasis causes an increase in serum cholesterol in some species. However, large differences exist in the lipoprotein profiles of different species, and the clearance of lipoproteins is not well characterized in most veterinary species. A number of automated analyzers are available that provide cholesterol and other lipoprotein values. Hyperlipidemia is often secondary to other conditions (Box 20.4). Primary hyperlipidemia is rare, and it is associated with inherited conditions in some breeds.

A cholesterol assay is sometimes used as a screening test for hypothyroidism. Thyroid hormone controls the synthesis and destruction of cholesterol in the body. Insufficient thyroid hormone (hypothyroidism) results in hypercholesterolemia, because the rate of cholesterol destruction is relatively slower than the rate of synthesis. Other diseases associated with hypercholesterolemia include hyperadrenocorticism, diabetes mellitus, and nephrotic syndrome. Dietary causes of hypercholesterolemia are rare but may include high-fat diets and postprandial lipemia.

Cholesterol by itself does not cause the grossly lipemic plasma that is seen after eating; triglycerides are also usually present. The administration of corticosteroids may also cause an elevated blood cholesterol concentration. Fluoride and oxalate anticoagulants may elevate enzymatic method results.

Enzymes Released From Damaged Hepatocytes

When hepatocytes are damaged and enzymes leak into the blood, a detectable rise in the blood levels of enzymes associated with liver cells occurs. These components, which are commonly referred to as the "leakage enzymes," include the transferase enzymes alanine transaminase (alanine aminotransferase) (ALT) and aspartate transaminase (aspartate aminotransferase) (AST), as well as the dehydrogenase enzymes iditol dehydrogenase (sorbitol dehydrogenase) (ID) and glutamate dehydrogenase (GLDH). Transaminases catalyze the reactions that transfer amine groups from amino acids to keto acids during the production of new amino acids. The enzymes are therefore found in tissues that have high rates of protein catabolism. Although other transaminases are present in hepatocytes, the only readily available tests are for ALT and AST. Dehydrogenases catalyze the transfer of hydrogen groups, primarily during glycolysis. Transaminases and dehydrogenases are found either free in the cytoplasm of hepatocytes or bound to the cell membrane. The serum levels of these enzymes vary in different species, and most also have nonhepatic sources.

> **TECHNICIAN NOTE** The common enzyme tests of liver function that are performed in small animal veterinary practices are AST and ALT.

Alanine Transaminase

- Elevated in
  - Liver inflammation
  - Liver infection
  - Toxins
  - Neoplasia
  - Drugs
  - Endocrine
  - Liver trauma
  - Hypoxia
  - Feline hepatic lipidosis
  - Copper storage diseases
  - Liver lobe torsion
  - Hepatocellular regeneration
  - Cirrhosis
- Decreased in
  - End-stage liver disease
  - Unremarkable

In dogs, cats, and primates, the major source of ALT is the hepatocyte, where the enzyme is found free in the cytoplasm. ALT is considered a liver-specific enzyme in these species. Horses, ruminants, pigs, and birds do not have enough ALT in the hepatocytes for this enzyme to be considered liver specific. Other sources of ALT are renal cells, cardiac muscle, skeletal muscle, and the pancreas. Damage to these tissues may also result in increased serum ALT levels. The administration of corticosteroids or anticonvulsant medications may also lead to increases in serum ALT. ALT is used as a screening test for liver disease, because it is not precise enough to identify specific liver diseases. No correlation exists between the blood levels of the enzyme and the severity of hepatic damage. Increases in ALT are usually seen within 12 hours of hepatocyte damage, and peak levels are seen at 24 to 48 hours. The serum levels will return to reference ranges within a few weeks unless a chronic liver insult is present.

Aspartate Transaminase

- Elevated in
  - See ALT
- Decreased in
  - See ALT

> **TECHNICIAN NOTE** AST is not considered clinically significant in the dog or cat. It is very sensitive but not very specific; significant amounts can be found in the muscle.

AST is present in hepatocytes, which are found free in the cytoplasm as well as bound to the mitochondrial membrane.

More severe liver damage is required to release the membrane-bound AST. AST levels tend to rise more slowly than do ALT levels, and they return to normal levels within a day provided chronic liver insult is not present. AST is found in significant amounts in many other tissues, including erythrocytes, cardiac muscle, skeletal muscle, the kidneys, and the pancreas. An increased blood level of AST may indicate nonspecific liver damage, or it may be caused by strenuous exercise or intramuscular injection. The most common causes of increased blood levels of AST are hepatic disease, muscle inflammation or necrosis, and spontaneous or artifactual hemolysis. If the AST level is elevated, the serum or plasma sample should be examined for hemolysis. Creatine kinase activity should also be assessed to rule out muscle damage before attributing an AST increase to liver damage.

Iditol Dehydrogenase (Sorbitol Dehydrogenase)

- Elevated in
  - Artifact
  - Hepatic injury
- Decreased in
  - Unremarkable

The primary source of ID is the hepatocyte. Smaller amounts of the enzyme are found in the kidney, the small intestine, skeletal muscle, and erythrocytes. ID is present in the hepatocytes of all common domestic species, but it is especially useful for evaluating liver damage in large animals such as sheep, goats, swine, horses, and cattle. Large animal hepatocytes do not contain diagnostic levels of ALT, so ID offers a liver-specific diagnostic test. The plasma level of ID rises quickly with hepatocellular damage or necrosis. ID assay can be used in all species to detect hepatocellular damage or necrosis, thereby eliminating the need for other tests (e.g., the ALT assay). The disadvantage of ID analysis is that ID is unstable in serum, so its activity declines within a few hours. If testing is delayed, samples should be frozen. ID tests are not readily available to the average veterinary laboratory. Samples to be sent to outside laboratories should be packed in ice for transport.

Glutamate Dehydrogenase

- Elevated in
  - Liver injury
- Decreased in
  - Unremarkable

GLDH is a mitochondrial-bound enzyme found in high concentrations in the hepatocytes of cattle, sheep, and goats. An increase in this enzyme is indicative of hepatocyte damage or necrosis in cattle and sheep. GLDH could be the enzyme of choice for evaluating ruminant and avian liver function, but no standardized test method has been developed for use in a veterinary practice laboratory.

Enzymes Associated With Cholestasis

Blood levels of certain enzymes become elevated with cholestasis (bile duct obstruction), metabolic defects in liver cells, the administration of certain medications, and as a result of the action of certain hormones, especially those of the thyroid. These enzymes are primarily membrane bound. The exact mechanism that induces increased levels of these enzymes when cholestasis is present is not well documented.

Alkaline Phosphatase

- Elevated in
  - Liver conditions
  - Gall bladder condition
  - Steroids
  - Growth
- Decreased in
  - Unremarkable

Alkaline phosphatase (AP) is present as isoenzymes in many tissues, particularly osteoblasts in bone, chondroblasts in cartilage, the intestine, the placenta, and cells of the hepatobiliary system in the liver. The isoenzymes of AP tend to remain in circulation for approximately 2 to 3 days, with the exception of the intestinal isoenzyme, which circulates for just a few hours. A corticosteroid isoenzyme of AP has been identified in dogs with exposure to increased endogenous or exogenous glucocorticoids. Because AP occurs as isoenzymes in these various tissues, the source of an isoenzyme or the location of the damaged tissue may be determined by electrophoresis and other tests that are performed in commercial or research laboratories.

In young animals, most AP comes from osteoblasts and chondroblasts as a result of active bone development. In older animals, nearly all circulating AP comes from the liver as bone development stabilizes. The assays that are used for AP in a practice laboratory determine the total blood AP concentration. AP concentrations are most often used to detect cholestasis in adult dogs and cats. Because of wide fluctuations in normal blood AP levels in cattle and sheep, this test is not as useful for detecting cholestasis in these species.

> **TECHNICIAN NOTE** Alkaline phosphatase can be used to evaluate cholestasis in small animals.

Gamma Glutamyltransferase

- Elevated in
  - Cholestasis
  - Drugs
  - Hepatocellular disease
- Decreased in
  - Laboratory error
  - Lipemia
  - Hemolysis

Gamma glutamyltransferase (GGT or gGT) is sometimes referred to as gamma-glutamyl transpeptidase. GGT is found in many tissues, including renal epithelium, mammary epithelium (particularly during lactation), and biliary epithelium, but its primary source is the liver. Cattle, horses, sheep, goats, and birds have higher blood GGT activity than dogs and cats. Other sources of GGT include the kidneys, the pancreas, the intestine, and the muscle cells. The blood GGT level is elevated in patients with liver disease, especially in those with obstructive liver disease.

Other Tests of Liver Function

A large number of additional tests may help the veterinarian to develop a diagnosis and a prognosis. Many of these tests are biochemical tests that are associated with other organs as well, and thus they are not specific for liver disease. For example, blood glucose is generally associated with pancreatic function. However, the liver aids in the modulation of glucose values, and liver disease often results in hyperglycemia or hypoglycemia. Additional tests to assess liver function (e.g., dye excretion, caffeine clearance) are primarily performed only in research settings.

▮ KEY POINTS

- Total plasma protein measurements include fibrinogen values, whereas total serum protein determinations measure all of the protein fractions except fibrinogen.
- Total protein concentrations are especially valuable for determining an animal's state of hydration.
- Albumin comprises 35% to 50% of the total plasma protein in most animals.
- Serum amyloid is an acute-phase protein that is correlated to specific diseases in some species.
- Some liver function tests are designed to measure substances that are produced by the liver, modified by the liver, or released when hepatocytes are damaged. Other liver function tests measure those enzymes that have altered serum concentrations as a result of cholestasis.

- In most animals, unconjugated bilirubin comprises approximately two thirds of the total bilirubin in the serum.
- Bile acids aid in fat absorption and modulate cholesterol levels via bile acid synthesis.
- Elevated SBA levels usually indicate liver disease, such as congenital portosystemic shunts, chronic hepatitis, hepatic cirrhosis, cholestasis, or neoplasms.
- The "leakage enzymes" include alanine transaminase, aspartate transaminase, iditol dehydrogenase, and glutamate dehydrogenase.
- ALT and AST are the most commonly performed liver function tests for small animals.
- Alkaline phosphatases are derived from many organs.

21

Kidney Function Tests

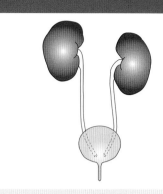

The kidneys play a major role in maintaining homeostasis in animals. Their primary functions are to conserve water and electrolytes in times of a negative balance and to increase water and electrolyte elimination in times of a positive balance, to excrete or conserve hydrogen ions to maintain blood pH within normal limits, to conserve nutrients (e.g., glucose, proteins), and to remove the end products of nitrogen metabolism (e.g., urea, creatinine, allantoin) so that blood levels of these end products remain low. Additional functions include the production of renin (an enzyme involved in the control of blood pressure), erythropoietin (a hormone necessary for erythrocyte production), and prostaglandins (fatty acids used to stimulate the contractility of uterine and other smooth muscle). The kidneys also function to lower blood pressure, to regulate acid secretion in the stomach, to regulate body temperature and platelet aggregation, to control inflammation, and to aid in vitamin D activation.

The kidneys receive blood from the renal arteries. The blood enters the glomerulus of the nephrons, where nearly all water and small dissolved solutes pass into the collecting tubules. Each nephron contains sections that function to reabsorb or secrete specific solutes. The resorption of glucose occurs in the proximal convoluted tubule. The secretion and reabsorption of mineral salts occur in the ascending limb of the loop of Henle and the distal convoluted tubule. The nephron has a specific resorptive capability for each substance, which is called the renal threshold. Most water is reabsorbed as well. As a result of water reabsorption, the volume excreted is less than 1% of the volume that originally entered the kidney. Blood returns from the kidneys to the rest of the body through the renal veins, which connect to the caudal vena cava. Urine and blood may be analyzed to evaluate kidney function. Unit 5 details urinalysis procedures. The primary serum chemistry tests for kidney function are urea nitrogen and creatinine. Other tests include various assays that have been designed to evaluate the rate and efficiency of glomerular filtration. It should be noted that serum chemistry tests along with the urinalysis are commonly utilized together to get a better idea of kidney function.

BLOOD UREA NITROGEN

- Elevated in
  - Prerenal azotemia
  - Renal conditions
  - Postrenal azotemia
  - Bladder conditions
- Decreased in
  - Diuresis
  - Diabetes insipidus
  - Liver failure
  - Low protein diets
  - Malnutrition
  - Neonates

Some references use the term serum urea nitrogen (SUN) rather than blood urea nitrogen (BUN). Urea is the principal end product of amino acid breakdown in mammals. BUN levels are used to evaluate kidney function on the basis of the ability of the kidney to remove nitrogenous waste (urea) from blood. Under normal conditions, all urea passes through the glomerulus and enters the renal tubules. Approximately half of the urea is reabsorbed in the tubules, and the remainder is excreted in the urine. If the kidney is not functioning properly, sufficient urea is not removed from the plasma, thereby leading to increased BUN levels.

Contamination of the blood sample with urease-producing bacteria (e.g., *Staphylococcus aureus*, *Proteus* spp., *Klebsiella* spp.) may result in the decomposition of urea and subsequently in decreased BUN levels. To prevent this, analysis should be completed within several hours of collection, or the sample should be refrigerated. A variety of photometric tests are available for the measurement of urea nitrogen. All of these have an acceptable level of accuracy and precision. Chromatographic dipstick tests are also available and provide a semiquantitative serum urea nitrogen result (Fig. 21.1). These methods tend to be less accurate and should be used only as quick screening tests.

Urea is an insoluble molecule, and it must be excreted in a high volume of water. Dehydration results in the increased retention of urea in the blood. High-protein diets and strenuous exercise may cause an elevated BUN level as a result of increased amino acid breakdown rather than decreased glomerular filtration. Differences in the rate of protein catabolism in male versus female animals as well as in young versus older animals will also affect BUN levels.

SERUM CREATININE

- Elevated in
  - Azotemia

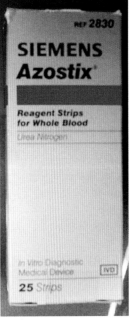

Fig. 21.1 A dipstick test for blood urea nitrogen.

- Decreased in
  - Decreased muscle mass

Creatinine is formed from creatine, which is found in skeletal muscle, as part of muscle metabolism. Creatinine diffuses out of the muscle cell and into most body fluids, including the blood. If physical activity remains constant, the amount of creatine metabolized into creatinine remains constant, and the blood level of creatinine remains constant. The total amount of creatinine is a function of the animal's total muscle mass. Under normal conditions, all serum creatinine is filtered through the glomeruli and eliminated in urine. Any condition that alters the glomerular filtration rate (GFR) will alter the serum creatinine levels. Creatinine may also be found in sweat, feces, and vomitus, and it may be decomposed by bacteria.

Blood creatinine levels are used to evaluate renal function on the basis of the ability of the glomeruli to filter creatinine from the blood and eliminate it in urine. Like BUN, creatinine is not an accurate indicator of kidney function, because nearly 75% of the kidney tissue must be nonfunctional before blood creatinine levels rise. Commonly used test methods for serum creatinine include the Jaffe method as well as several enzymatic methods. Postprandial decreases in creatinine occur in response to the transient increase in the GFR after a meal.

BLOOD UREA NITROGEN/CREATININE RATIO

Because BUN and creatinine both have a wide range of reference intervals, their use as indicators of renal function is limited. The GFR may be decreased as much as four times below normal before changes are seen in the BUN or serum creatinine levels. In addition, healthy animals often have values that are below the reference ranges. In patients with renal disease, hyperplasia of the renal tissue may mask early signs of renal failure. The ratio of BUN to creatinine is used in human medicine for the diagnosis of renal disease. Although this is not yet well established for veterinary species, it can be used to assess the patient's status during treatment.

BUN and creatinine have an inverse logarithmic relationship. The reciprocal of creatinine tracked over time can be used to track the progress of disease and the effectiveness of treatment. A disproportionate increase in BUN can indicate dehydration, dietary treatment failure, or owner noncompliance with treatment regimens.

URINE PROTEIN/CREATININE RATIO

- P/C Ratio Between 1 and 5
  - Prerenal
- P/C Ratio Greater than 5
  - Renal

The quantitative assessment of renal proteinuria is of diagnostic significance for renal disease. In the absence of inflammatory cells in the urine, proteinuria indicates glomerular disease. For the accurate determination of proteinuria, a 24-hour urinary protein value should be determined. This is a tedious task, and errors are common. A mathematical method that compares the urine protein level with the urine creatinine levels in a single urine sample is more accurate and comprehensive. This urine protein-to-creatinine (P/C) ratio is based on the concept that the tubular concentration of urine increases both the urinary protein and creatinine concentrations equally.

This method has been validated for the canine species. Usually 5 to 10 mL of urine are collected between 10 AM and 2 PM, preferably by cystocentesis. The urine sample should be kept at 4° C or stored at 20° C. The sample is centrifuged, and the supernatant is used. The protein and creatinine concentrations for each sample can be determined by a variety of photometric methods. The urine P/C ratio for healthy dogs should be less than 1. A urine P/C ratio of between 1 and 5 may have a prerenal origin (e.g., hyperglobulinemia, hemoglobinemia, myoglobinemia) or a functional origin (e.g., exercise, fever, hypertension), whereas a urine P/C ratio of greater than 5 is caused by renal disease.

URIC ACID

- Elevated in
  - Renal failure in birds
  - Postprandial in carnivorous birds
  - Fecal contamination

Uric acid is a metabolic by-product of nitrogen catabolism, and it is found mainly in the liver. Uric acid is usually transported to the kidneys while bound to albumin. In most mammals, the compound passes through the glomerulus, and it is largely reabsorbed by the tubule cells. It is then converted to allantoin and excreted in the urine. In Dalmatian dogs, a defect in uric acid uptake into the hepatocytes results in decreased conversion to allantoin. Therefore, this breed excretes uric acid (rather than allantoin) in the urine.

Uric acid is the major end product of nitrogen metabolism in avian species. It constitutes approximately 60% to 80% of the total nitrogen excreted in avian urine, and it is actively secreted by the renal tubules. The measurement of plasma or serum uric acid is used as an index of renal function in birds. Uric acid can also be increased artifactually in samples from toenail clippings because of fecal urate contamination. Uric acid concentrations will increase after a meal in carnivorous birds. With renal disease, uric acid concentrations increase when the kidney has lost more than 70% of its functional capacity.

> **TECHNICIAN NOTE** Uric acid is the primary end product of nitrogen metabolism in birds. It is also seen in the urine of Dalmatian dogs.

SDMA (SYMMETRIC DIMETHYLARGININE) TEST

SDMA is considered a sensitive and early marker (more sensitive than serum creatinine) of declining GFR in dogs and cats.

TESTS OF GLOMERULAR FUNCTION

In patients with azotemia or in those that are symptomatic for renal disease without azotemia, several additional tests can be performed to evaluate kidney function. These clearance studies require the collection of timed, quantified urine samples along with concurrent plasma samples. Two primary types of clearance studies are performed: the effective renal plasma flow (ERPF) and GFR. The ERPF uses test substances that are eliminated by both glomerular filtration and renal secretion (typically the amide p-aminohippuric acid). The GFR involves the use of test substances that are eliminated only by glomerular filtration (typically creatinine, inulin, or urea). The test substance is administered, and urine and plasma samples collected. The ERPF and GFR are then calculated as follows:

$$\text{GFR or ERPF (mL/kg per minute) of substance} = U_x \times V/P_x$$

U_x represents the substance present in urine (in milligrams per milliliter), V represents the amount of urine collected over a defined period (in milligrams per kilogram per minute), and P_x represents the plasma concentration of the substance.

> **TECHNICIAN NOTE** The ERPF uses test substances that are eliminated by both glomerular filtration and renal secretion.

Creatinine Clearance Tests
Endogenous Creatinine Clearance

Because creatinine appears in the glomerular filtrate with negligible tubular secretion, it is a natural tracer of glomerular filtration. Fortunately, its short-term blood concentrations are stable enough to satisfy the clearance formula used for steady infusion studies of inulin and p-aminohippuric acid. The test is relatively simple (Box 21.1). A measure of blood creatinine and an accurate timed urine collection are required for this test. Precision is of the utmost importance. Sloppy bladder catheterization and sampling ruin the results, especially with the briefer methods. The bladder must be rinsed before and after the test, with the after-rinses saved with the urine for creatinine analysis. Clearance is calculated by dividing urinary creatinine excretion (Urine creatinine concentration × Urine volume) by plasma creatinine concentration. The estimate, if imprecise, provides practical information.

To avoid errors, plasma creatinine should be determined with the use of the combination creatinine PAP test instead of the Jaffe method. The combination creatinine PAP test is an enzymatic chromogenic method to determine creatinine concentration. The Jaffe method also determines noncreatinine chromogens in plasma, which do not appear in urine. Excess serum ketones, glucose, and proteins all falsely elevate GFR estimates due to chromatic interference and cross-reactivity.

Exogenous Creatinine Clearance

Exogenous creatinine clearance is an accurate method for measuring GFR in small animals. Plasma creatinine concentration increases, thereby making the plasma concentration of noncreatinine chromogens negligible. This allows for the application of the Jaffe method to determine creatinine concentrations (Box 21.2). Avoiding dehydration in the animal is critical for the performance of this test; free access to water must be ensured before any glomerular filtration test is performed.

Iohexol Clearance

Iohexol clearance can be used to estimate GFR in dogs and cats. Iohexol is a radiographic agent that is given as a single intravenous dose after a 12-hour fast during which the patient has free access to water. Serum samples are taken at 2, 3, and 4

hours after administration and sent to the reference laboratory for the evaluation of the transit of iohexol and the calculation of the GFR.

Single-Injection Inulin Clearance

Inulin is excreted entirely by glomerular filtration, without tubular secretion, reabsorption, or catabolism. As a result, inulin clearance tests that make use of a constant infusion rate and quantitative urine sampling may be considered the best method for the evaluation of GFR. Single-injection inulin clearance is a simpler method that alternatively may be used. After a 12-hour fast (free access to water is permitted during the test), inulin is injected intravenously at a dosage of 100 mg/kg or 3 g/m^2 (body surface calculation gives more accurate results); serum samples are then obtained at 20, 40, 80, and 120 minutes. Total inulin clearance is calculated from the decrease of the serum inulin concentration by using a two-compartment model. Normal dogs have a GFR of 83.5 to 144.3 mL/min/m^2 of body surface area.

Water-Deprivation Tests

Polyuria or polydipsia may lead to suspicions about the kidney, which may be erroneous. Diuresis and subsequent polydipsia may mean failing nephrons or kidney function disrupted by hyperadrenocorticism (Cushing's disease), diabetes mellitus, or nephrogenic diabetes insipidus. The kidneys may be normal, but they may not receive the signal to concentrate urine, which occurs with neurogenic diabetes insipidus. In addition, the diuresis may be a totally appropriate renal compensation for pathologic water intake (i.e., psychogenic polydipsia).

Vasopressin or antidiuretic hormone (ADH) from the neurohypophysis signals the kidneys to retain water by increasing the collecting duct's permeability to water. Water in the urine passes out of the collecting duct and into the hypertonic renal medulla, thereby concentrating the urine that remains behind in the collecting duct. If the system fails (e.g., inappropriate diuresis), either the neuroendocrine pathway that releases ADH in response to hypovolemia or plasma hyperosmolarity has been interrupted or the nephrons are unable to respond.

BOX 21.1 Overview of the Endogenous Creatinine Clearance Test

- A pretest blood sample is obtained for plasma creatinine analysis.
- The urinary bladder is catheterized and rinsed several times with saline.
- All voided urine is collected over a specified time frame (most commonly 24 hours).
- The urinary bladder is catheterized at the end of the specified time, and the remainder of the urine is collected.
- The saline bladder rinse is repeated, and the creatinine concentration of the urine rinse is determined.
- Creatinine clearance is calculated with the following equation, where Uv stands for urine volume (mL/min), Uc stands for urine creatinine concentration (mg/dL), and Pc stands for plasma creatine concentration (mg/dL):

$$\text{Creatinine clearance} = \frac{[Uv \times Uc/Pc]}{\text{Body weight (kg)}}$$

- Normal clearance in dogs is 2.8 ± 0.96 mL/min/kg.

BOX 21.2 Overview of the Exogenous Creatinine Clearance Test

- A subcutaneous injection of creatinine is administered.
- A measured volume of water is administered per os via gastric intubation.
- The urinary bladder is catheterized and rinsed with saline after a specified time period (typically 40 minutes).
- A blood sample is obtained for plasma creatinine analysis.
- All voided urine is collected for a specified time period, and a second blood sample is obtained.
- Calculate the creatinine clearance using the mean values of both samples.
- Normal values in the dog are 4.09 ± 0.52 mL/kg/min.
- A related procedure for evaluating the glomerular filtration rate involves the use of an iohexol injection and does not require the collection of urine samples.

This test involves observing the patient's response to endogenous or exogenous ADH. The basis of this test is to dehydrate the patient safely until a definite stimulus exists for endogenous ADH release (usually at approximately 5% body weight loss). That end point may vary. When denied water, patients dehydrate at different rates and must be monitored for weight loss, clinical signs of dehydration, and increased urine osmolarity or specific gravity. At the end point, the kidney should be under strictest endocrine orders to concentrate urine. Continued diuresis and dilute urine indicate a lack of endogenous ADH or unresponsive nephrons. In dogs with kidney failure, this unresponsiveness precedes azotemia.

Contraindications to this test include dehydration and azotemia. Dehydrated patients risk hypovolemia and shock. They already should have maximal ADH release; if they could concentrate urine, they would. Under those conditions, the test is useless and dangerous, especially for animals with diabetes insipidus or neurogenic diabetes insipidus. Azotemia already demonstrates kidney dysfunction. Again, the test reveals nothing new and adds a prerenal component to the azotemia.

Vasopressin Response

When patients demonstrate the previously mentioned signs or when a prior water-deprivation test has failed, a vasopressin response test is indicated. The vasopressin response test is simply a challenge with exogenous ADH; it focuses on the ability of the kidneys to respond. Urine osmolarity or specific gravity is the index of function. Normal kidneys should concentrate urine with this technique, despite the patient's free access to water. Vasopressin must be handled carefully, because it is a labile drug that settles out in oil suspensions. Test failures may result from the use of old or poorly mixed solutions. In addition, intramuscular vasopressin injection causes pain. As a result of vasopressin's vasomotor activity, its use is theoretically contraindicated during pregnancy.

In both tests, even normal kidneys may be unable to concentrate urine to normal extremes. Diuresis quickly washes solutes from the renal medulla, weakening the osmotic gradient that draws water from the collecting ducts. Gradual water deprivation over a 3- to 5-day period before use of the water deprivation test is recommended to renew renal solutes and allow an evaluation of the impact of dehydration on the animal.

The basic water deprivation and vasopressin response tests may be combined in a single protocol that may differentiate several causes of polyuria and polydipsia (Box 21.3). The modified water-deprivation test is specifically contraindicated for patients with known renal disease, with uremia that results from prerenal or primary renal disorder, or with suspected or obvious dehydration.

Fractional Clearance of Electrolytes

The fractional clearance (FC)—which is also referred to as the fractional excretion (FE)—of electrolytes is a mathematical manipulation that describes the excretion of specific electrolytes (particularly sodium, potassium, and phosphorus) relative to the GFR. The most commonly used FE test is that of sodium.

BOX 21.3 Overview of the Water Deprivation/Vasopressin Response

- Water intake is gradually reduced over a 72-hour period before the initiation of the test.
- All food and water are then withdrawn, and the urinary bladder is emptied at the start of the test.
- An accurate exact body weight is obtained at the start of the test and repeated every 30 to 60 minutes.
- Urine specific gravity, osmolality, and serum urea nitrogen are recorded, and hydration and central nervous system (CNS) status are evaluated at the start of the test, repeated every 30 to 60 minutes, and then evaluated again at the conclusion of the test.
- The test is ended when the animal is clinically dehydrated, appears ill, or has lost about 5% of its body weight.
- A final blood sample is obtained for the determination of the vasopressin concentration before the vasopressin response test.

Vasopressin Response
- Aqueous vasopressin is administered via intramuscular injection.
- At 30-minute intervals for a maximum of 2 hours, the urinary bladder is emptied. Body weight, urine specific gravity, osmolality, and serum urea nitrogen are recorded, and hydration and CNS status are evaluated.

After Testing
- Small amounts of water are provided every 30 minutes for 2 hours.
- If the patient shows no evidence of vomiting, dehydration, or CNS abnormalities 2 hours after the test, water is provided ad libitum.

Bicarbonate and chloride FE testing is rarely performed. The tests can differentiate prerenal from postrenal azotemia. Random, concurrent blood and urine samples are required. The FE_X is calculated as follows:

$$FE_X = (U_X / P_X) \times (P_{CR} / U_{CR}) \times 100$$

X is the electrolyte measurement used, which can be any of the four (sodium, potassium, phosphorus, and chloride); U_X and P_X are the urine and plasma concentrations, respectively, of that specific electrolyte; and P_{CR} and U_{CR} are the urine and plasma concentrations of creatinine, respectively. Normal results are as follows:

- Dogs: sodium, 1; potassium, 20; chloride, 1; phosphorus, 39
- Cats: sodium, 1; potassium, 24; chloride, 1.3; phosphorus, 73

TECHNICIAN NOTE The fractional excretion of electrolytes is a mathematical manipulation that describes the excretion of specific electrolytes relative to the GFR.

Inorganic Phosphorus

Serum inorganic phosphorus (Pi) is usually the reciprocal of serum calcium. Normally, serum Pi is reabsorbed in the kidney tubules. This mechanism is under the hormonal control of the parathyroid hormone, and it is affected by serum pH. Initially, renal damage that alters the GFR leads to decreased urinary Pi and increased serum Pi. Subsequent alterations in calcium and

Pi lead to increases in serum calcium and decreases in serum Pi. See the electrolyte information later in this chapter for additional information about testing for Pi.

Enzymuria

Enzymuria refers to the presence of enzymes in the urine. Many of the chemical tests performed on serum or plasma can also be performed on urine samples. Enzymes that may be present in the urine of patients with renal disease include urinary GGT and urinary N-acetyl-β-d-glucosaminidase (NAG). Urinary GGT and NAG are enzymes that are released from damaged tubule cells. A comparison of the units of GGT or NAG per milligram of creatinine can indicate the extent of renal damage. Both GGT and NAG increase rapidly with nephrotoxicity, and increases occur sooner than changes in serum creatinine, creatinine clearance, or fractional excretion of electrolytes.

KEY POINTS

- The kidneys play a major role in the maintenance of homeostasis in animals by modulating water and electrolyte concentrations, maintaining blood pH, conserving nutrients, removing waste products, and producing renin, erythropoietin, and prostaglandins.
- The primary serum chemistry tests for kidney function are urea nitrogen and creatinine.
- Urea is the principal end product of amino acid breakdown in mammals.
- Dehydration results in the increased retention of urea in the blood, because urea must be excreted in a large volume of water.
- Any condition that alters the GFR will alter the serum creatinine levels.
- In Dalmatian dogs, a defect in uric acid uptake into the hepatocytes results in the excretion of uric acid in the urine.
- Uric acid is the major end product of nitrogen metabolism in avian species.
- Clearance studies that may be performed in azotemic patients include the ERPF and the GFR.
- The ERPF uses test substances eliminated by both glomerular filtration and renal secretion.
- The fractional excretion of electrolytes is a mathematical manipulation that describes the excretion of specific electrolytes relative to the GFR.
- Serum Pi is usually the reciprocal of serum calcium.

22

Pancreatic Function Tests

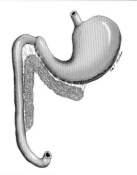

Photo from Christenson DE: *Veterinary medical terminology*, ed 2, St Louis, 2008, Saunders.

LEARNING OBJECTIVES

After studying this chapter, you will be able to:

- Differentiate between the acinar and endocrine functions of the pancreas.
- List and describe the common tests for the evaluation of the exocrine pancreas.
- Explain the relationship between insulin, glucagon, and blood glucose.
- Describe the common tests that are used to evaluate patients for hyperglycemia.
- Discuss the general concepts involved in the performance of glucose tolerance tests.

OUTLINE

KEY TERMS

Acinar
Amylase
Amyloclastic
Endocrine
Fructosamine

Glucagon
Glucose
Glucose tolerance
Glycosylated hemoglobin
Hyperglycemia

Insulin
Lipase
Pancreatic lipase immunoreactivity
Trypsin
Trypsinogen

The pancreas is actually two organs—one exocrine and the other endocrine—that are held together in one stroma. The exocrine portion, which is also referred to as the acinar pancreas, comprises the greatest portion of the organ. This portion secretes an enzyme-rich juice that contains the enzymes necessary for digestion in the small intestine. The three primary pancreatic enzymes are trypsin, amylase, and lipase. These digestive enzymes are released into the lumen of other organs through a duct system. Trauma to pancreatic tissue is often associated with pancreatic duct inflammation that results in a backup of digestive enzymes into the peripheral circulation.

> **TECHNICIAN NOTE** The pancreas has both acinar and endocrine functions.

Interspersed within the exocrine pancreatic tissue are arrangements of cells that, in a histologic section, take on the appearance of "islands" of lighter-staining tissue. These are called the islets of Langerhans. Four types of islet cells are present, but they cannot be distinguished on the basis of their morphologic characteristics. The four cell types are designated as α, β, δ, and pancreatic polypeptide (PP) cells. The δ and PP cells comprise less than 1% of the islet cells, and they secrete somatostatin and pancreatic polypeptide, respectively. β-Cells comprise approximately 80% of the islet, and they secrete insulin. The remaining nearly 20% of the islet consists of α-cells that secrete glucagon and somatostatin. The pancreas has little regenerative ability. When pancreatic islets are damaged or destroyed, pancreatic tissue becomes firm and nodular, with areas of hemorrhage and necrosis. These islets are no longer able to function. Diseases of the pancreas may result in inflammation and cellular damage that causes the leakage of digestive enzymes or the insufficient production or secretion of enzymes.

EXOCRINE PANCREAS TESTS

The tests that are commonly performed to evaluate the acinar functions of the pancreas include amylase and lipase. Trypsinlike immunoreactivity and serum pancreatic lipase immunoreactivity are also available as tests for pancreatic function. In cats, serum amylase and lipase activities have been shown to have limited clinical significance for the diagnosis of pancreatitis. In experimentally induced pancreatitis in cats, serum amylase actually decreases. The serum activities of both enzymes are frequently normal in cats with pancreatitis. Several immunoassays are available that provide either quantitative or semi-quantitative evaluation of the specific lipase of dogs and cats to rapidly differentiate pancreatitis from other disease states.

Amylase

- Elevated in
  - Pancreatic conditions
  - Enteritis
  - Renal disease
- Decreased in
  - Unremarkable

The primary source of amylase is the pancreas, but amylase is also produced in the salivary glands and the small intestine. Increases in serum amylase are nearly always caused by pancreatic disease, especially when accompanied by increased lipase levels. The rise in blood amylase level is not always directly proportional to the severity of pancreatitis. Serial determinations provide the most information.

Amylase functions to break down starches and glycogen in sugars, such as maltose and residual glucose. Increased levels of amylase appear in blood during acute pancreatitis, flare-ups of chronic pancreatitis, or obstruction of the pancreatic ducts. Enteritis, intestinal obstruction, or intestinal perforation may also result in increased serum amylase from the increased absorption of intestinal amylase into the bloodstream. In addition, because amylase is excreted by the kidneys, a decrease in the glomerular filtration rate for any reason can lead to increased serum amylase. Serum amylase activity that is greater than three times the reference range usually suggests pancreatitis.

Two amylase test methods are available: the saccharogenic method and the amyloclastic method. The saccharogenic method measures the production of reducing sugars as amylase catalyzes the breakdown of starch. The amyloclastic method measures the disappearance of starch as it is broken down to reduce sugars through amylase activity. Calcium-binding anticoagulants (e.g., EDTA) should not be used, because amylase requires the presence of calcium for activity. The presence of lipemia may reduce amylase activity. The saccharogenic method is not ideal for canine samples, because maltase in canine samples may artificially elevate assay results. Normal canine and feline amylase values can be up to 10 times higher than those found in human beings. Therefore, samples may have to be diluted if tests designed for human samples are used.

Lipase

- Elevated in
  - Pancreatic conditions
  - Enteritis
  - Renal disease
  - Hepatic disease
  - Glucocorticoids
- Decreased in
  - Unremarkable

The majority of serum lipase is derived from the pancreas. The function of lipase is to break down the long-chain fatty acids of lipids. Excess lipase is normally filtered through the kidneys, so lipase levels tend to remain normal during the early stages of pancreatic disease. Gradual increases are seen as disease progresses. With chronic progressive pancreatic disease, damaged pancreatic cells are replaced with connective tissue that cannot produce enzyme. As this occurs, a gradual decrease in both amylase and lipase levels are seen.

Chemical test methods for the determination of lipase levels are usually based on the hydrolysis of an olive oil emulsion into fatty acids by the lipase present in patient serum. The quantity of sodium hydroxide required to neutralize the fatty acids is directly proportional to lipase activity in the sample. Newer tests for lipase that are capable of detecting canine and feline pancreatic lipase by using immunologic methods are available. These tests have been demonstrated to have a high degree of sensitivity for the diagnosis of pancreatitis in dogs and cats.

Lipase assay may be more sensitive for the detection of pancreatitis as compared with the amylase assay. The degree of lipase activity, like amylase activity, is not directly proportional to the severity of pancreatitis. Determinations of blood lipase and amylase activities are usually requested at the same time to evaluate the pancreas.

Increased lipase activity is also seen with renal and hepatic dysfunction, although the exact mechanisms for this are unclear. Steroid administration is correlated with increased lipase activity, with no concurrent change in amylase activity.

Amylase and Lipase in Peritoneal Fluid

The comparison of amylase and lipase activity in peritoneal fluid with serum may provide additional diagnostic information. A finding of higher amylase and lipase activity in peritoneal fluid than in serum strongly suggests pancreatitis, provided that intestinal perforation has first been ruled out.

Trypsin

- Elevated in:
  - Unremarkable
- Decreased in:
  - Pancreatic disorders

Trypsin is a proteolytic enzyme that aids digestion by catalyzing the reaction that breaks down the proteins of ingested food. Trypsin activity is more readily detectable in feces than in blood. For this reason, most trypsin analyses are performed on fecal samples. Trypsin is normally found in feces, and its absence is abnormal. A variety of fecal testing methods are available in the reference laboratory.

Serum Trypsinlike Immunoreactivity

- Elevated in
  - Pancreatitis
  - Renal disease
- Decreased in
  - Exocrine pancreatic insufficiency

Serum trypsinlike immunoreactivity (TLI) is a radioimmunoassay that uses antibodies to trypsin. The test can detect both trypsinogen and trypsin. The antibodies are species specific. Trypsin and trypsinogen are both produced only in the pancreas. With pancreatic injury, trypsinogen is released into the extracellular space and converted to trypsin, which diffuses into the bloodstream. The test is available only for the dog and the cat.

TLI provides a sensitive and specific test for the diagnosis of exocrine pancreatic insufficiency (EPI) in dogs. Dogs with EPI have a serum TLI of less than 2.5 mg/L. Normal dogs have a range of 5 to 35 mg/L. Dogs with other causes of malassimilation may have normal serum TLI levels. Dogs with chronic pancreatitis may have normal TLI values or values of between 2.5 and 5 mg/L. Normal cats have TLI rates of 14 to 82 mg/L, whereas cats with EPI have rates of less than 8.5 mg/L. Assays for folate and cobalamin (vitamin B_{12}) are usually performed in conjunction with TLI to evaluate the extent of gastrointestinal disorders.

Serum TLI decreases in parallel with functional pancreatic mass. The inflammation associated with acute and probably chronic pancreatitis may enhance the leakage of trypsinogen and trypsin from the pancreas and increase TLI. In addition, a decreased glomerular filtration rate increases TLI (trypsinogen is a small molecule that easily passes into the glomerular filter). Serum TLI is an important indicator of functional pancreatic mass. It is most informative if it is coupled with N-benzoyl-l-tyrosyl-p-aminobenzoic acid and fecal fat results to characterize and diagnose malassimilation.

Serum TLI increases after eating (especially proteins), but values remain within reference intervals. In addition, pancreatic enzyme (exogenous) supplementation does not alter TLI. Therefore, food should be withheld for at least 3 hours (and preferably 12 hours) before a blood sample is taken. The blood is coagulated at room temperature and the serum stored at 20° C until the assay takes place.

Serum Pancreatic Lipase Immunoreactivity

- Positive
  - Pancreatitis
- Negative
  - Unremarkable

Serum feline pancreatic lipase immunoreactivity (fPLI) and canine pancreatic lipase immunoreactivity (cPLI) are specific for pancreatitis, and their use is now recommended instead of the previously validated serum TLI test as a serum test to diagnose patients with symptoms of pancreatitis. More information regarding immunoassays can be found in Unit 4. Snap cPL and fPL tests are also available for in house use. These test are canine and feline pancreas-specific lipase tests.

Table 22.1 describes the advantages and disadvantages of various tests used for the diagnosis of acute and chronic pancreatitis in dogs and cats.

ENDOCRINE PANCREAS TESTS

A variety of tests are available to evaluate the endocrine functions of the pancreas. In addition to the traditional blood glucose tests, other tests that are available include fructosamine, β-hydroxybutyrate, and glycosylated hemoglobin. Urinalysis, serum cholesterol, and triglyceride tests also provide information about the function of the pancreas.

TECHNICIAN NOTE Tests of the endocrine functions of the pancreas include glucose, fructosamine, and glycosylated hemoglobin.

Glucose

- Elevated in
  - Diabetes mellitus (fasting blood glucose elevations)
  - Stress
  - Hyperadrenocorticism
  - Pancreatitis
  - Drugs
  - Parenteral nutrition
  - Dextrose-containing fluids
  - Postprandial
  - Acromegaly
  - Diestrus
  - Neoplasia
  - Renal failure
  - Head trauma
- Decreased in
  - Fasting
  - Sepsis
  - Hepatic insufficiency
  - Prolonged sample storage
  - Iatrogenic
  - Neoplasia

TABLE 22.1 Advantages and Disadvantages of Various Tests Used in the Diagnosis of Acute and Chronic Pancreatitis in Dogs and Cats

Assay	Advantages	Disadvantages
Catalytic Assays		
(dogs only—of no use in cats)		Either may be normal in severe ± chronic pancreatitis due to enzyme depletion ± loss of tissue; degree of elevation of no prognostic value, except where stated; both renally excreted and elevated 2 or 3 times in azotemia
Amylase	Widely available on in-house analyzers. Steroids do *not* elevate it so can help diagnose pancreatitis in dogs with hyperadrenocorticism	Low sensitivity and specificity because of high background level from other sources, including small intestine
Lipase	Widely available on practice analyzers; more sensitive than amylase; degree of elevation may have prognostic significance	Extrapancreatic sources so high background level; steroids elevate up to 5×
Immunoassays		
Canine TLI	Elevations high specificity for pancreatitis	Low sensitivity for diagnosis of pancreatitis (but high sensitivity for EPI); said to rise and fall more quickly than lipase or amylase; renally excreted: elevated 2 or 3 times in azotemia. May be inappropriately low in severe ± chronic cases due to pancreatic depletion ± loss of tissue mass; no clear prognostic significance
Feline TLI	One of only two assays available for cats	Lower sensitivity and specificity than canine TLI—better used for diagnosis of EPI; renally excreted so elevated in azotemia
Canine PLI	Early indications most sensitive and specific test for canine pancreatitis; organ specific, so no interference from extrapancreatic sources. Now available as in-house test	Increased in renal disease but may not be significantly so? (Unclear yet if affected by steroids)
Feline PLI	Very new test but appears most sensitive and specific test available for feline pancreatitis	Very little published data available on its use

EPI, Exocrine pancreatic insufficiency; *PLI,* pancreatic lipase immunoreactivity; *TLI,* trypsinlike immunoreactivity.
From Nelson R, Couto C: *Small animal internal medicine,* ed 4, St Louis, 2009, Mosby.

- Hypoadrenocorticism
- Hypopituitarism
- Idiopathic
- Renal failure
- Glycogen storage disease
- Severe polycythemia
- Prolonged starvation
- Laboratory error

The regulation of the blood glucose levels is complex. Glucagon, thyroxine, growth hormone, epinephrine, and glucocorticoids are all agents that favor hyperglycemia. They boost blood glucose levels by encouraging glycogenolysis, gluconeogenesis, and lipolysis while discouraging glucose entry into cells. Insulin is the hypoglycemic hormone. By promoting glucose flux into its target cells, it also triggers anabolism, which is a process that converts glucose into other substances. This regulatory effect prevents the blood glucose concentration from exceeding the renal threshold and the spilling of glucose into the urine.

The pancreatic islets respond directly to blood glucose concentrations, and they release insulin (from the β cells) or glucagon (from the α cells) as needed. Glucagon release also directly stimulates insulin release. Epinephrine is under direct sympathetic neural control; hyperglycemia is one aspect of the classic "fight or flight" state. The other hormones mentioned respond to hypothalamic/pituitary command. At any point in time, most of these agents are acting to shift the blood glucose concentration up or down.

Because only insulin lowers blood glucose levels, aberrations of insulin action have the most obvious clinical effects. Hypofunction (diabetes mellitus) or hyperfunction (hyperinsulinism) can occur.

The blood glucose level is used as an indicator of carbohydrate metabolism in the body, and it may also be used as a measure of endocrine function of the pancreas. The blood glucose level reflects the net balance between glucose production (e.g., dietary intake, conversion from other carbohydrates) and glucose utilization, which involves expended energy and conversion into other products. It also may reflect the balance between blood insulin and glucagon levels. Glucose levels can fluctuate significantly due to a variety of factors, including nutritional status and stress. An individual blood glucose measurement reflects the level present at the time the sample was collected.

Glucose utilization depends on the amount of insulin and glucagon produced by the pancreas. As the insulin level increases, so does the rate of glucose use, thereby resulting in decreased blood glucose levels. Glucagon acts as a stabilizer to prevent blood glucose levels from becoming too low. As the insulin level decreases (e.g., with diabetes mellitus), so does glucose use, thereby resulting in increased blood glucose concentration.

Many tests are available for blood glucose. Some of these react only with glucose, whereas others may quantitate all sugars in the blood. End point and kinetic assays are available. The kinetic enzymatic assays tend to be the most accurate and precise. Samples must be taken from a properly fasted animal. Serum and plasma for glucose testing must be separated from the erythrocytes immediately after blood collection. Glucose levels may drop 10% per hour if the sample of plasma is left in contact with erythrocytes at room temperature. Even the use of a serum separator tube may not be adequate to prevent this. Mature erythrocytes use glucose for energy, and, in a blood sample, they may decrease the glucose level enough to give false-normal results if the original sample had an elevated glucose level. If the sample originally had a normal glucose level, erythrocytes may use enough glucose to decrease the level to below normal or to zero. If the plasma cannot be removed immediately, the anticoagulant of choice is sodium fluoride at 6 to 10 mg/mL of blood. Sodium fluoride may be used as a glucose preservative with EDTA at 2.5 mg/mL of blood. Refrigeration slows glucose use by erythrocytes.

> **TECHNICIAN NOTE** Glucose levels may drop 10% per hour if the sample of plasma is left in contact with erythrocytes at room temperature.

Blood Glucose Curves

A blood glucose curve (BGC) involves performing serial measurements of blood glucose during the duration of action of insulin. Glucose curves have the advantage of enabling veterinarians to establish onset of action, glucose nadir, and duration of action of the insulin. These curves then allow veterinarians to make the proper adjustments, if any are needed to a patients insulin dosages, times or meals. It is important to remember that blood glucose curves are important, but the clinical signs of a patient should dictate any changes. When the patient has no clinical signs and the body weight is steady or increasing, DM is likely controlled. When starting a blood glucose curve. Blood glucose curves serve two very useful purposes that other monitoring parameters do not. They identify clinically undetectable hypoglycemia. More importantly, although other techniques and clinical signs may suggest control is lacking, multiple reasons for poor control exist, including too low and too high an insulin dose. The only way to know how to appropriately change an insulin dose is to perform a BGC.

A BGC should be performed:
1. After the first dose of a new kind of insulin;
2. At 7 to 14 days after an insulin dose change;
3. At least q 3 mo even in well-controlled diabetics;

4. At any time clinical signs recur in a controlled patient; and
5. When hypoglycemia is suspected.

A normal insulin treatment and feeding schedule must be maintained as much as possible during the BGC. Patients should eat their amount and type of food; otherwise a BGC should probably not be performed. It is ideal if the feeding and insulin injection are done in the hospital so the injection can be observed. However, this may not be possible if normal feeding time occurs before a hospital opens or if a dog or cat will not eat in the hospital. If an owner's technique is suspect, the injection time can be changed to occur in front of the veterinarian. Clearly, cooperation between client and veterinarian is necessary to optimize the information obtained with minimal disturbance to routine.

Obtaining a fasting blood sample for BG measurement prior to insulin injection can also aid in appraisal of glycemic control. To perform a BGC the blood glucose is measured every 2 hours for a period of 12 hours. If the blood glucose falls below 150 mg/dl at any point in the curve, start monitoring the blood glucose hourly. The AlphaTrak 2 glucometer may be the most accurate BG meter for veterinary patients because it has been calibrated in dogs and cats.

The goal of the BGC is to establish the duration of the insulin effect and what the lowest BG is. The lowest BG is known as the nadir. The ideal nadir is a BG of 80 to 150mg/dl.

The first aim in regulating a diabetic is to achieve an acceptable nadir. If an acceptable nadir is not achieved, the insulin dosage should be adjusted. An acceptable nadir with good clinical control may not be obtained if the insulin used has a short duration of activity. Hypoglycemia must always be avoided. No matter what other BG concentrations are during the day, if BG is ever <80 mg/dL, the insulin dose must be reduced.

Once an acceptable nadir is achieved, duration of action, roughly defined as the amount of time BG is controlled, can be determined. Duration cannot be evaluated until the nadir is optimized. The BG should be controlled for as close to 24 hr per day as possible.

The Somogyi effect, also called hypoglycemia-induced hyperglycemia, refers to hypoglycemia followed by marked hyperglycemia. It results from a physiological response when an insulin dose causes BG to be <60 mg/dL or when BG concentration decreases quickly. For this reason, it is extremely important to get a glucose every 1 to 2 hours on time during the BGC. As we are often trying to rule this effect out. Technicians often get busy and miss testing times, which results in having to repeat the BGC.

Blood glucose curves can be performed by clients at home as well with proper instruction for veterinary technicians, and with the invention of the Free Style Libre 2 this can be achieved with much more success. Completing blood glucose curves at home is strongly recommended for both dogs and cats because it takes the stress hyperglycemia of being in the clinic out of the equation.

Commonly used sites of blood collection are the ear, gums, non—weight bearing or accessory foot pads, or elbow callus. A hypodermic needle can also be used, especially if the marginal ear vein is the site of blood collection.

Not all owners are suited to the task of obtaining a home BGC, something that takes time and patience to master. The most frequent problems encountered by owners are the need for more than one puncture to obtain a blood drop, obtaining a sufficient volume of blood, the need for assistance in restraining a pet, and the pet's resistance to obtaining a blood sample. Curves can vary from day to day even when done at home and must always be interpreted in light of clinical signs.

Fructosamine

- Elevated in
  - Persistent hyperglycemia
- Decreased in
  - Persistent hypoglycemia

Glucose can bind a variety of structures, including proteins. Fructosamine represents the irreversible reaction of glucose bound to protein, particularly albumin. When glucose concentrations are persistently elevated in blood, as occurs in patients with diabetes mellitus, the increased binding of glucose to serum proteins occurs. The finding of increased fructosamine indicates a persistent hyperglycemia. Because the half-life of albumin in dogs and cats is 1 to 2 weeks, fructosamine provides an indication of the average serum glucose over that period. Fructosamine levels respond more rapidly to alterations in serum glucose than does glycosylated hemoglobin. However, serum fructosamine may be artifactually reduced in patients with hypoproteinemia.

> **TECHNICIAN NOTE** Increased fructosamine indicates a persistent hyperglycemia.

Glycosylated Hemoglobin (Hemoglobin A1C)

- Values between 4% and 6% are associated with adequate glycemic control.

Glycosylated hemoglobin is also referred to as hemoglobin A1C (HgbA1C) and represents the irreversible reaction of hemoglobin bound to glucose. When hyperglycemia is present, there is increased binding of hemoglobin and glucose and thus increased glycosylated hemoglobin. The finding of increased glycosylated hemoglobin indicates a persistent hyperglycemia. The test result is a reflection of the average glucose concentration over the life span of an erythrocyte, which is 3 to 4 months in dogs and 2 to 3 months in cats. Therefore, HgbA1C indicates blood glucose concentration over a longer period of time than either fructosamine or a single blood glucose measurement. HgbA1C is a more specific diagnostic indicator of diabetes mellitus and more sensitive in monitoring control of diabetes. With older test methods, patients that were anemic often had artifactually reduced levels of glycosylated hemoglobin. Newer test methods that are immunoassays are not subject to errors from reduced hemoglobin.

β-Hydroxybutyrate

Ketone bodies can also be detected in plasma. The ketone produced in greatest abundance in ketoacidotic patients is β-hydroxybutyrate. However, many tests for serum ketones only detect acetone. Tests for β-hydroxybutyrate that use enzymatic, colorimetric methods are now becoming available for use in the veterinary clinic.

Glucose Tolerance

Glucose tolerance tests directly challenge the pancreas with a glucose load and measure insulin's effect by evaluating blood or urine glucose concentrations. If adequate insulin is released and its target cells have healthy receptors, then the artificially elevated blood glucose level peaks 30 minutes after ingestion and begins to drop, reaching normal value within 2 hours, and no glucose appears in the urine. A normal glucose blood level at 2 hours postprandial may rule out diabetes mellitus. Prolonged hyperglycemia and glucosuria are consistent with diabetes mellitus. Profound hypoglycemia after challenge may indicate a glucose-responsive, hyperactive β-cell tumor of the pancreas. This test may be simplified by determining a single 2-hour postprandial glucose.

> **TECHNICIAN NOTE** Prolonged hyperglycemia and glucosuria after the glucose tolerance test are consistent with diabetes mellitus.

Oral glucose tolerance is affected by abnormal intestinal function (e.g., enteritis, hypermotility) and excitement (e.g., from gastric intubation); an intravenous glucose tolerance test is preferred. The intravenous test is the only practical option for ruminants. With the intravenous glucose tolerance test (Procedure 22.1), a challenge glucose load is injected after a 12- to 16-hour fast (except in ruminants). Blood glucose is subsequently checked, and its progress is mapped as a tolerance curve. Results are standardized as disappearance half-lives or glucose turnover rates expressed as percent per minute:

$$\text{Turnover rate} = (0.693/\text{Half} - \text{life}) \times 100$$

Decreased glucose tolerance (i.e., increased half-life, decreased turnover rate) occurs with diabetes mellitus and less consistently with hyperthyroidism, hyperadrenocorticism, hyperpituitarism, and severe liver disease. Increased glucose tolerance (i.e., decreased half-life, increased turnover rate) is observed with hypothyroidism, hypoadrenocorticism, hypopituitarism, and hyperinsulinism. However, results may be erroneous. Normal animals that are consuming low-carbohydrate diets may manifest "diabetic curves." The effect of this can be minimized by providing the animal with 2 to 3 days of high-carbohydrate meals before testing. The intravenous glucose tolerance test results are so variable in normal horses, depending on diet and fasting, that they are not useful.

Glucose tolerance tests are usually unnecessary to obtain a diagnosis of diabetes mellitus. Persistent hyperglycemia and glucosuria—frequently with a history of polyuria, polydipsia,

PROCEDURE 22.1   Intravenous Glucose Tolerance Test

1. Evaluate the animal's diet. Patients that are consuming low-carbohydrate diets should be fed a high-carbohydrate diet (e.g., 100 to 200 g/day for dogs) for 3 days before the test.
2. Fast the animal for 12 to 16 hours to lower the blood glucose level to 70 mg/dL in patients with suspected hyperinsulinism (do not fast ruminants or dogs with insulinoma).
3. Obtain a preinjection blood sample in a sodium fluoride tube for a baseline blood glucose determination.
4. Begin timing the trial at the start of the intravenous infusion of glucose solution at 1.0 g/kg administered over a 30-second period.
5. Obtain blood samples at 5, 15, 25, 35, 45, and 60 minutes after glucose infusion with the use of sodium fluoride as an anticoagulant, and submit all blood samples for glucose assay. An additional blood sample is collected after 120 minutes for feline patients.
6. Plot the glucose values on semilogarithmic graph paper, and determine the time required for glucose levels to decrease by 50% (i.e., the glucose half-life).
7. Results: The postinfusion blood glucose level should fall to approximately 160 mg/dL in 30 to 60 minutes and return to baseline values after 120 to 180 minutes.

polyphagia, and weight loss—are sufficient for the diagnosis of diabetes mellitus. The test may be of value for detecting hyperinsulinism, because most β-cell tumors of the pancreas are not rapidly responsive to glucose. They may even cause diabetic glucose tolerance curves, because insulin-antagonist hormones are released as a result of the initial hypoglycemia. Patient stress and chemical restraint also affect glucose tolerance test results. Serum glucose measurements themselves may be erroneously low if blood samples are not subjected to anticoagulants and are allowed to sit at room temperature. However, the test is still used.

The best use for the glucose tolerance test is in animals with borderline hyperglycemia without persistent glucosuria. However, this test is not cost-effective for the owner, and it may not result in significant therapeutic change. This dilemma is most often seen in cats in which high renal thresholds for glucose and stress-induced hyperglycemia are common and misleading. Extra information may be obtained from the intravenous glucose tolerance test if immunoreactive insulin concentrations are followed simultaneously. This protocol may differentiate diabetes mellitus that results from an absolute lack of insulin (type 1) from that caused by target-cell insensitivity (type 2) or inappropriate slow insulin release (type 3).

Insulin Tolerance

The insulin tolerance test also probes the causes of diabetes mellitus. Specifically, it checks the responsiveness of target cells to challenge with regular crystalline (short-acting) insulin 0.1 IU/kg subcutaneously or intramuscularly. Serum glucose levels are measured in blood samples that have been obtained before insulin injection (i.e., fasting blood glucose) and every 30 minutes after injection for 3 hours. If the serum glucose level fails

to drop to 50% of the fasting concentration within 30 minutes of insulin injection (i.e., insulin resistance), then the insulin receptors are unresponsive or insulin action is being severely antagonized. The latter may occur with hyperadrenocorticism and acromegaly. Insulin resistance profoundly influences prognostic and therapeutic decisions. If the insulin-induced hypoglycemia persists for 2 hours (i.e., hypoglycemia unresponsiveness), hyperinsulinism, hypopituitarism, or hypoadrenocorticism should be suspected. The test may cause hypoglycemia, and the patient may suffer from weakness and convulsions. A glucose solution should always be on hand for rapid intravenous administration.

Glucagon Tolerance

The main indications for the glucagon tolerance test are repeated normal or borderline results with the amended insulin/glucose ratio test (discussed later in this chapter) or the lack of an insulin assay. The glucagon tolerance test provides another assessment of hyperinsulinism. Glucagon stimulates the pancreatic β cells both directly and indirectly to increase the blood insulin level. In normal animals, glucagon injection (0.03 mg/kg intravenously up to a total of 1.0 mg in dogs and 0.5 mg in cats) transiently elevates the blood glucose level to greater than 135 mg/dL. In normal animals, this concentration level is greater than 135 mg/dL. In normal animals, this concentration returns to fasting concentrations. In normal cats, the peak insulin level occurs at 15 minutes and declines to a basal concentration at 60 minutes. Type 1 diabetic cats present a flat insulin response. If the animal has a pancreatic β-cell tumor, the serum glucose level peak is lower than normal. It is followed within 1 hour by hypoglycemia (i.e., the serum glucose level is less than 60 mg/dL), because excessive insulin is secreted by the stimulated neoplasm.

To perform the test, the patient is fasted until the serum glucose level dips below 90 mg/dL (usually less than 10 hours). Glucagon is injected, and sodium fluoride anticoagulated blood samples are obtained before glucagon injection and 1, 3, 5, 15, 30, 45, 60, and 120 minutes after injection to monitor the glucose response. Unfortunately, the test is insensitive, and it may cause hypoglycemia convulsions up to 4 hours later. Patients must be fed immediately after the test and then observed for hours.

Insulin/Glucose Ratio

The cause of hyperinsulinism may be assessed by taking simultaneous measurements of serum glucose and insulin levels in a fasting animal. Hypoglycemia normally inhibits insulin secretion. Pancreatic β-cell tumors that are hyperactive and unresponsive to glucose secrete an abundance of insulin that is inappropriate for the prevailing blood glucose concentration. Although fasting serum insulin concentrations are often normal in patients with hyperinsulinism, ratios of insulin-to-glucose concentrations are usually aberrant.

The absolute ratio of insulin to glucose can be amended to increase diagnostic accuracy. The amended insulin/glucose ratio subtracts 30 from the serum glucose concentration. At a serum glucose level of 30 mg/dL or less, insulin is normally undetectable, so this discriminant puts the zero of both the glucose and insulin scale at the same physiologic place. Because abnormally high insulin concentrations are more obvious at low serum glucose concentrations, the amended insulin/glucose ratio is most valuable in animals with a confirmed hypoglycemia of less than 60 mg/dL. Insulin and glucose have to be measured from the same serum sample, at which point serial determinations may be performed to select an insulin concentration in hypoglycemia. However, the test is not totally dependable. If the results are unconvincing, then the procedure should be repeated or other tests tried. Specifically, diagnostic imaging and insulinlike growth factor

tests should be tried to rule out or confirm paraneoplastic hypoglycemia.

Miscellaneous Tests of Insulin Release

When the results of a glucagon response test or an amended insulin/glucose ratio are equivocal, glucose, epinephrine, leucine, tolbutamide, or calcium challenges may be attempted. These substances, like glucagon, may provoke a hyper-insulinemic response from pancreatic islet cell tumors, thereby resulting in decreased serum glucose levels. However, tumors vary with regard to their sensitivity to these agents, and false-negative results (i.e., no response) can occur. These tests are also dangerous, because they can precipitate severe and prolonged hypoglycemia.

KEY POINTS

- The pancreas has both acinar and endocrine functions.
- The tests that are commonly performed to evaluate the acinar functions of the pancreas include amylase and lipase.
- Immunologic tests are available for the detection of pancreatitis.
- Tests of the endocrine functions of the pancreas include glucose, fructosamine, and glycosylated hemoglobin.
- Glucose use depends on the amount of insulin and glucagon produced by the pancreas.
- Glucose tolerance tests challenge the pancreas with a glucose load and measure insulin's effect via the evaluation of blood or urine glucose concentrations.
- Serum and plasma for glucose testing must be separated from the erythrocytes immediately after blood collection.
- Increased fructosamine indicates a persistent hyperglycemia of 1 to 2 weeks' duration in dogs and cats.
- Increased glycosylated hemoglobin indicates a persistent hyperglycemia of 3 to 4 months' duration in dogs and 2 to 3 months' duration in cats.
- The ketone produced in greatest abundance in ketoacidotic patients is β-hydroxybutyrate.
- Prolonged hyperglycemia and glucosuria after the glucose tolerance test are consistent with diabetes mellitus.

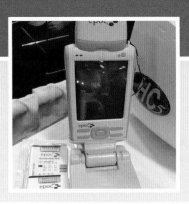

23

Electrolytes and Acid–Base Status

LEARNING OBJECTIVES

After studying this chapter, you will be able to:

- Describe the blood buffer systems and their role in maintenance of the acid–base balance.
- Explain the effect of respiratory rate on the acid–base balance.
- Define respiratory acidosis, respiratory alkalosis, metabolic acidosis, and metabolic alkalosis.
- List the major cations and anions in plasma, and describe their roles.
- List common conditions related to altered serum electrolyte levels.
- Describe the anion gap evaluation, and explain how it is calculated.

OUTLINE

KEY TERMS

Acid–base balance
Acidosis
Alkalosis
Anion
Anion gap
Base excess
Bicarbonate
Buffers
Calcium

Cation
Chloride
Electrolytes
Hypercalcemia
Hypercapnia
Hyperkalemia
Hypernatremia
Hyperphosphatemia
Hypocalcemia

Hypocapnia
Hypokalemia
Hyponatremia
Hypophosphatemia
Inorganic phosphorus
Magnesium
Potassium
Sodium

Electrolytes are the negative ions (anions) and positive ions (cations) of elements that are found in all body fluids of all organisms. Some of the functions of electrolytes include the maintenance of water balance, fluid osmotic pressure, and normal muscular and nervous functions. Electrolytes also function in the maintenance and activation of several enzyme systems and in acid–base regulation. Acid–base status depends on electrolytes, so these two things should be interpreted together.

ACID–BASE BALANCE

Acid–base balance refers to the steady state of the pH of the body. pH is used to describe the hydrogen ion concentration (Fig. 23.1). Every change on the pH scale of one number indicates a power-of-10 difference in the hydrogen ion concentration. Normal pH has a fairly narrow range of approximately 7.35 to 7.45. Should pH values begin to fall outside of the ideal range, the functioning of many of the body's

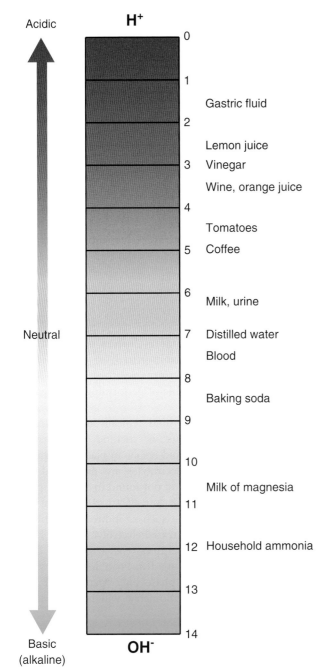

Fig. 23.1 The pH Scale. Many common chemicals are either acidic or basic. As the concentration of H⁺ increases, the solution becomes more acidic, and the pH value decreases. As the OH⁻ concentration increases, the solution becomes more basic or alkaline, and the pH value increases. (From Bassert J, Colville T: *Clinical anatomy and physiology for veterinary technicians*, ed 2, St Louis, 2008, Mosby.)

proteins is diminished or destroyed. When the pH value of body fluids is less than 7.3, the condition is called acidosis, which is characterized by excess hydrogen ions. When the pH value is more than 7.4, the condition is called alkalosis, and it is characterized by a low hydrogen ion concentration.

Normal metabolic processes continually generate acids, and other processes work to counteract the effect of those acids.

Buffer systems are responsible for counteracting those effects. Buffers are substances that can alter the hydrogen ion concentration. Buffers are located both intracellularly and extracellularly, and multiple buffering systems are present in the body. Some of the components of the buffer systems can move freely between the intracellular and extracellular compartments, and they are capable of either binding or releasing hydrogen ions in response to blood pH. Both the respiratory and renal systems work to regulate pH in the presence of acid—base imbalance. The respiratory system works in a matter of minutes whereas the renal system continues to function for days to restore the pH level within normal limits.

> **TECHNICIAN NOTE** Acid—base balance refers to the steady state of the pH of the body.

Bicarbonate Buffer

Should the blood pH become acidic, bicarbonate (HCO_3) binds to excess free hydrogen ions to form carbonic acid (H_2CO_3). Carbonic acid is then broken down to water and carbon dioxide in a reaction that is mediated by carbonic anhydrase. Carbon dioxide is removed from the body through normal respirations. The kidneys play a major role in regulating the concentration of bicarbonate by actively secreting or resorbing it from the filtrate in response to the blood pH. Under normal conditions, the bicarbonate—carbonic acid buffer maintains the blood pH in equilibrium as shown in the chemical equation in Fig. 23.2. Note that the reactions are reversible.

Potassium Buffer

Changes in the concentration of potassium in the plasma and the extracellular fluid (ECF) affect the plasma concentration of hydrogen ions. Potassium and hydrogen ions are both positively charged ions that freely move between the intracellular fluid (ICF) and the ECF. Decreases in the concentration of plasma potassium cause potassium to move from the cells to the ECF and hydrogen ions to move from the ECF into the cells. Conversely, increased plasma potassium levels result in potassium moving into the cells and hydrogen ions moving into the ECF. Therefore, plasma potassium affects acid—base balance, and acid—base balance affects the plasma potassium concentration.

Protein Buffer

Numerous proteins are also capable of binding and releasing hydrogen ions. The hemoglobin molecule serves as a blood buffer as a result of its ability to bind carbon dioxide and hydrogen. The carbon dioxide is then transported to the lungs, released, and eliminated through respiration.

> **TECHNICIAN NOTE** The primary blood buffer system is the bicarbonate—carbonic acid buffer.

$$2\,H_2O + CO_2 \longleftrightarrow H_2CO_3 + H_2O \longleftrightarrow H_3O^+ + HCO_3^-$$

| Water + Carbon Dioxide $\longleftrightarrow$ | Carbonic acid + water $\longleftrightarrow$ | Bicarbonate + hydronium (hydrogen ions in solution) |

Fig. 23.2 Reactions of the bicarbonate–carbonic acid buffer system.

ACIDOSIS AND ALKALOSIS

Acidosis and alkalosis are categorized by the cause of the condition. Respiratory acidosis or respiratory alkalosis results from abnormalities of the respiratory system. Metabolic acidosis or metabolic alkalosis results from all causes other than abnormal respiratory functions. It is important to note that these conditions are interrelated and that they can also occur simultaneously. As acidosis or alkalosis develops, the respiratory and renal systems will both attempt to work to correct the imbalance. For example, as metabolic acidosis or alkalosis develops, the respiratory system will react by increasing or decreasing the respiratory rate as appropriate.

Respiratory Acidosis and Alkalosis

If the respiratory rate decreases, the rate at which carbon dioxide is eliminated decreases. The excess carbon dioxide reacts with water to form carbonic acid. Carbonic acid then dissociates into water and hydrogen ions. This will be evidenced in part by an increased partial pressure of carbon dioxide (PCO_2) in the blood (hypercapnia). Abnormalities in the respiratory system that cause an increase in respiratory rate (hyperventilation) result in a decrease in the concentration of carbon dioxide in the blood and a subsequent decrease in PCO_2 in the blood (hypocapnia).

Metabolic Acidosis and Alkalosis

Any metabolic condition that results in the buildup of acids in the body creates the condition of metabolic acidosis. For example, excess ketones that are produced when glucose metabolism is abnormal (e.g., diabetes mellitus) can overwhelm the buffer systems. The result is generally a decrease in the blood bicarbonate levels. Disorders that alter electrolyte levels (e.g., vomiting) can cause metabolic alkalosis and a subsequent increase in the blood bicarbonate levels.

Base Excess

Base excess is the amount of strong acid or base that is required to titrate 1 L of blood to a pH of 7.4 at 37° C while the PCO_2 is held constant at 40 mm Hg. This value is generally calculated from pH, PCO_2, and hematocrit measurements. Base excess may be used to evaluate the degree of metabolic acid–base disturbances. A negative value indicates metabolic acidosis, and a positive value indicates metabolic alkalosis.

ELECTROLYTE ASSAYS

The major electrolytes in plasma are calcium, inorganicphosphorus, magnesium, sodium, potassium, chloride, and bicarbonate (Table 23.1). Changes in electrolyte concentration

TABLE 23.1	Major Electrolytes in Plasma
Cations	**Anions**
Na^+	Cl^-
K^+	HCO_3^-
Ca^{++}	PO_4
Mg^{++}	
H^+	

can result from increased or decreased intake, shifts of electrolytes between the ECF and the ICF, and increased renal retention of electrolytes or increased loss of electrolytes via the kidneys, the gastrointestinal tract, or the respiratory system.

Automated analyzers for the evaluation of electrolytes are readily available and reasonably priced, so many veterinary practices have the ability to perform electrolyte testing. Many of these analyzers are also capable of performing blood gas analysis (Fig. 23.3).

Volume displacement by lipid typically affects electrolyte measurement, although this is method dependent. An increased concentration of lipid results in plasma volume with decreased water content. Electrolytes are distributed in the aqueous portion of plasma and not found in the lipid portion. Therefore, procedures that measure electrolytes in total plasma volume (per unit of plasma), such as indirect potentiometry, will result in artifactually decreased electrolyte values. This will occur only in very lipemic samples (e.g., triglyceride concentrations of more than 1500 mg/dL). Procedures that measure electrolytes in the aqueous phase only (per unit of plasma water), such as direct potentiometry, will result in accurate electrolyte concentrations.

Arterial samples are ideal for the analysis of electrolytes and blood gases. Venous samples have significantly different normal reference ranges. Samples must be analyzed immediately after collection. Exposure to room air results in alterations in the concentration of dissolved gases in the sample and affects sample pH.

> **TECHNICIAN NOTE** Arterial samples are preferred for the analysis of electrolytes and blood gases.

Sodium

- Elevated in
  - Dehydration
  - Renal failure
  - Fluid loss

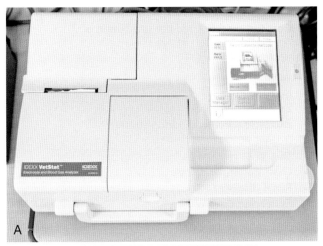

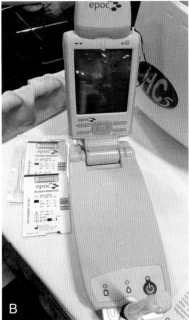

Fig. 23.3 **A** and **B**, These analyzers are capable of performing multiple electrolyte and blood gas analyses on whole blood, plasma, or serum samples.

- Hyperaldosteronemia
- Evaporation of serum sample
- Decreased in
  - Hypoadrenocorticism
  - Fluid loss
  - Severe liver disease
  - Hookworms
  - Renal disease
  - Diuretics
  - Hypotonic fluids
  - Diabetes mellitus
  - Diet
  - Hyperlipidemia
  - Marked hyperproteinemia

Sodium is the major cation of plasma and ECF. It plays an important role in water distribution and body fluid osmotic pressure maintenance. In the kidney, sodium is filtered through the glomeruli and resorbed back into the body as needed through the tubules in exchange for hydrogen ions. In this manner, sodium plays a vital role in the pH regulation of urine and acid—base balance. Hypernatremia refers to an elevated blood level of sodium. Hyponatremia is a decreased blood level of sodium. The sodium salt of heparin should not be used as an anticoagulant, because it can falsely elevate the results. Hemolysis does not significantly alter results, but it may dilute the sample with erythrocyte fluid and cause falsely lower results.

> **TECHNICIAN NOTE** Sodium is the major cation of plasma and ECF.

Potassium

- Elevated in
  - Renal failure
  - Postrenal conditions
  - Hypoadrenocorticism
  - Acidosis
  - Gastrointestinal conditions
  - Massive muscle trauma
  - Dehydration
  - Drugs
  - Hypoaldosteronism
  - Thrombocytosis
  - Hyperkalemic periodic paralysis
- Decreased in
  - Alkalosis
  - Dietary deficiency
  - Potassium free fluids
  - Bicarbonate administration
  - Drugs
  - Gastrointestinal fluid loss
  - Hyperadrenocorticism
  - Hyperaldosteronism
  - Insulin therapy
  - Diuresis
  - Diabetic ketoacidosis
  - Renal conditions
  - Total parenteral nutrition
  - Hypokalemic periodic paralysis

Potassium is the major intracellular cation. It is important for normal muscular function, respiration, cardiac function, nerve impulse transmission, and carbohydrate metabolism. In acidotic animals, potassium ions leave the ICF as they are replaced by hydrogen ions, thereby resulting in elevated plasma potassium levels, or hyperkalemia. The plasma potassium level may also be elevated in the presence of cellular damage or necrosis, which causes the release of potassium ions into the blood. Decreased plasma potassium levels, or hypokalemia, may be associated with inadequate potassium intake, alkalosis, or fluid loss as a result of vomiting or diarrhea.

Plasma is the preferred sample, because platelets may release potassium during the clotting process and cause artificially elevated potassium levels. Hemolysis should be avoided, because the concentration of potassium within erythrocytes is higher than the concentration in plasma. Hemolysis releases potassium into the plasma and results in artificially elevated potassium levels. The sample should not be refrigerated until the plasma has been separated from the cells, because cooler temperatures promote the loss of potassium from the cells without evidence of hemolysis. Samples should not be frozen without first separating the blood cells, because the resulting hemolysis makes the sample unsuitable for testing.

Chloride

> **TECHNICIAN NOTE** Proportional to sodium, look for the change in sodium.

Chloride is the predominant extracellular anion. It plays an important role in the maintenance of water distribution, osmotic pressure, and the normal anion/cation ratio. Chloride is usually included in electrolyte profiles because of its close relationship to sodium and bicarbonate levels. Hyperchloremia is an elevated blood chloride level, and hypochloremia is a decreased blood chloride level. Hemolysis may affect test results by diluting the sample with erythrocyte fluid. Prolonged storage without first separating out the blood cells may cause slightly low results.

> **TECHNICIAN NOTE** Potassium is the major intracellular cation. Chloride is the predominant extracellular anion.

Bicarbonate

- If Acidemic
  - Elevated in: Metabolic alkalosis with compensatory acidosis
  - Decreased in: Metabolic acidosis
- If Alkalotic
  - Elevated in: Metabolic alkalosis
  - Decreased in: Metabolic acidosis with compensatory alkalosis

Bicarbonate is the second most common anion of plasma. The kidneys help to regulate bicarbonate levels in the body by excreting excesses after resorbing all that is needed. Bicarbonate levels are frequently estimated from blood carbon dioxide levels. The bicarbonate level is approximately 95% of the total carbon dioxide measured. Arterial blood is the sample of choice for bicarbonate determinations. If plasma is used, lithium heparin is the anticoagulant of choice. The sample should be chilled in ice water to prevent glycolysis from altering the

acid–base composition. Freezing the sample results in hemolysis. Most test methods require incubation at 37° C.

Magnesium

- Elevated in
  - Renal failure
  - Excessive oral intake
  - Excessive parenteral administration
- Decreased in
  - Diet
  - Gastrointestinal disease
  - Renal diseases
  - Endocrine diseases
  - Sepsis
  - Blood transfusions
  - Parenteral nutrition
  - Hypothermia
  - Dialysis
  - Drugs

Magnesium is the fourth most common cation in the body and the second most common intracellular cation. Magnesium is found in all body tissues. More than 50% of the magnesium in the body is found in bones, and it is closely related to calcium and phosphorus. Magnesium activates enzyme systems and is involved in the production and decomposition of acetylcholine. Imbalance of the magnesium/calcium ratio can result in muscular tetany as a result of the release of acetylcholine. Cattle and sheep are the only domestic animals that show clinical signs related to magnesium deficiencies. Hypermagnesemia refers to an elevated blood magnesium level. Hypomagnesemia is a decreased blood magnesium level. Anticoagulants other than heparin may artificially decrease the results. Hemolysis may elevate the results through the liberation of magnesium from erythrocytes.

Calcium

- Elevated in
  - Primary hyperparathyroidism
  - Renal failure
  - Hypoadrenocorticism
  - Neoplasia
  - Hypervitaminosis D
  - Dehydration
  - Granulomatous disease
  - Skeletal disorders
  - Iatrogenic situations
  - Serum lipemia
  - Postprandial
  - Young animals
  - Laboratory error
  - Idiopathic
- Decreased in
  - Renal failure
  - Acute pancreatitis
  - Intestinal malabsorption

- Primary hypoparathyroidism
- Eclampsia
- Ethylene glycol toxicity
- Hypoproteinemia
- Hypomagnesemia
- Nutrition
- Neoplasia
- Phosphate-containing enemas
- Anticonvulsant medications
- Hypovitaminosis D
- Rhabdomyolysis
- Sodium bicarbonate administration
- Laboratory error

More than 99% of the calcium in the body is found in the bones. The remaining 1% or less has major functions in the body, which include the maintenance of neuromuscular excitability and tone (decreased calcium can result in muscular tetany), the maintenance of activity of many enzymes, the facilitation of blood coagulation, and the maintenance of inorganic ion transfer across cell membranes. Calcium in whole blood is found almost entirely in plasma or serum. Erythrocytes contain little calcium.

Calcium concentrations are usually inversely related to inorganic phosphorus concentrations. As a general rule, if the calcium concentration rises, the inorganic phosphorus concentration falls. Hypercalcemia is an elevated blood calcium concentration. Hypocalcemia is a decreased blood calcium concentration.

Samples for calcium testing should not be collected using EDTA or oxalate or citrate anticoagulants, because these substances bind with calcium and make it unavailable for assay. Hemolysis results in a slight decrease in calcium concentration in samples as the fluid from the ruptured erythrocytes dilutes the plasma.

> **TECHNICIAN NOTE** Calcium concentrations are inversely related to inorganic phosphorus concentrations.

Inorganic Phosphorus

- Elevated in
  - Young animals
  - Decreased glomerular filtration rate
  - Postrenal conditions
  - Primary hypoparathyroidism
  - Nutrition
  - Hyperthyroidism
  - Acromegaly
  - Hemolysis
  - Toxicity
  - Hypoparathyroidism
  - Diet
  - Metabolic acidosis
  - Iatrogenic

- Osteolysis
- Rhabdomyolysis
- Neoplasia
- Sample hemolysis
- Delayed serum separation
- Decreased in
  - Primary hyperparathyroidism
  - Nutrition
  - Renal tubular acidosis
  - Vomiting/diarrhea
  - Neoplasia
  - Insulin therapy
  - Diabetic ketoacidosis
  - Fanconi syndrome
  - Decreased intestinal absorption
  - Eclampsia
  - Hyperadrenocorticism
  - Vitamin D deficiency
  - Hyperaldosteronism
  - Aggressive fluid therapy
  - Bicarbonate administration
  - Respiratory or metabolic acidosis

More than 80% of the phosphorus in the body is found in bones. The remaining 20% or less has major functions, such as energy storage, release, and transfer; involvement in carbohydrate metabolism; and the composition of many physiologically important substances, such as nucleic acids and phospholipids.

Most of the phosphorus in whole blood is found within the erythrocytes as organic phosphorus. The phosphorus in plasma and serum is inorganic phosphorus, and this is the phosphorus that is assayed in the laboratory. Inorganic phosphorus levels in plasma and serum provide a good indication of the total phosphorus in an animal. Plasma or serum phosphorus and calcium concentrations are inversely related. As phosphorus concentrations decrease, calcium concentrations increase.

> **TECHNICIAN NOTE** The phosphorus in plasma and serum is inorganic phosphorus. Phosphorus within the erythrocytes is organic phosphorus.

Hyperphosphatemia is an increased serum or plasma phosphorus concentration. Hypophosphatemia is a decreased serum or plasma phosphorous concentration. Hemolyzed samples should not be used. The organic phosphorus that is liberated from the ruptured erythrocytes may be hydrolyzed to inorganic phosphorus, which results in a falsely elevated inorganic phosphorus concentration. The serum or plasma should be separated from the blood cells as soon as possible after blood collection and before the sample is stored.

Anion Gap

- Elevated in
  - Lactic acidosis
  - Uremia

- Ketoacidosis
- Ethylene glycol toxicosis
- Decreased in
  - Hypoalbuminemia
  - IgG multiple myeloma

Under normal circumstances, the total number of positive charges (cations) equals the total number of negative charges (anions). This electrical neutrality is maintained through the buffer systems. Any difference between the total positive charges and the total negative charges is an anion gap. This value is calculated from the measured electrolyte values, and it is primarily used to identify metabolic acidosis. In general, only the commonly measured electrolytes are used in the calculation.

The anion gap is calculated as follows:

$$\left(Na^+ + K^+\right) - \left(Cl^- + HCO_3^-\right) = \text{Anion gap}$$

The normal anion gap measurement is approximately 12 to 24 mEq/L in dogs and 13 to 27 mEq/L in cats. Increases are usually seen with lactic acidosis, renal failure, and diabetic ketoacidosis. Hypoalbuminemia is a common cause of a decreased anion gap.

KEY POINTS

- Electrolyte assays performed in the veterinary practice laboratory include sodium, potassium, and chloride.
- Some electrolyte analyzers can also evaluate calcium, phosphorus, magnesium, bicarbonate, and blood gases.
- The major electrolytes in plasma are calcium, inorganic phosphorus, magnesium, sodium, potassium, chloride, and bicarbonate.
- Changes in the electrolyte concentration can result from increased or decreased intake, shifts of electrolytes between the ECF and ICF, and increased renal retention of electrolytes or increased loss of electrolytes via the kidneys, the gastrointestinal tract, or the respiratory system.
- Arterial and venous blood samples have different normal values (reference ranges) for electrolytes and blood gases.
- Sodium is the major cation of the plasma and ECF, whereas chloride is the predominant extracellular anion.
- Potassium is the major intracellular cation.
- Calcium concentrations are usually inversely related to inorganic phosphorus concentrations.
- The phosphorus in plasma and serum is inorganic phosphorus. Phosphorus within the erythrocytes is organic phosphorus.

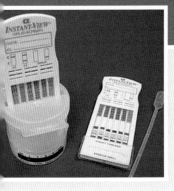

24

Miscellaneous Tests in Clinical Chemistry

LEARNING OBJECTIVES

After studying this chapter, you will be able to:

- Describe the relevance of creatine kinase testing for the diagnosis of liver or skeletal muscle damage.
- Describe the uses of lactate evaluation for critical patients.
- Discuss the indications for adrenocorticotropic hormone stimulation and dexamethasone suppression tests.
- Discuss the production and action of thyroxine.
- Describe the chemical tests of gastrointestinal function.
- Describe the handling of samples for toxicology testing.
- Describe common toxicology testing.

OUTLINE

KEY TERMS

ACTH stimulation test
Addison's disease
Adrenocorticotropic hormone
Cortisol
Creatine kinase
Cushing's disease

Dexamethasone suppression test
Ethylene glycol
Hematochezia
Hyperadrenocorticism
Hyperthyroidism
Hypoadrenocorticism

Lactate
Melena
Mucin clot test
Plumbism
Thyroid-stimulating hormone
Thyroxine

A variety of other assays may be performed in veterinary practice. These include assays designed to detect abnormalities in the endocrine systems as well as other biochemical tests that are not specific to any organ or system but can still provide diagnostic and prognostic information (e.g., blood lactate measurements). Other than blood lactate measurements, which can easily be performed in the veterinary practice laboratory, many of these tests are not performed in-house but rather are sent out to reference or referral practice laboratories. Some are available as immunoassays that can be performed in-house.

CREATINE KINASE

- Elevated in
  - Trauma
  - Myositis

- Infectious
- Surgery
- Nutritional
- Taurine deficiency
- Prolonged recumbency
- IM injections
- Pyrexia
- Hypothermia
- Cardiomyopathy
- DIC
- Seizures
- Decreased in
  - Unremarkable

Creatine kinase (CK) is found in a wide variety of tissues. Small amounts are present in the bladder, gastrointestinal tract, thyroid, kidney, lung, spleen, and pancreas. The majority of CK activity is in skeletal and cardiac muscle and in the brain. When skeletal muscle, including cardiac muscle, is damaged or destroyed, CK leaks out of the cells and produces an elevated blood CK level. CK is frequently assayed if an animal has an elevated blood aspartate aminotransferase (AST) level but shows no clinical signs of liver disease (Fig. 24.1). CK is also evaluated in the cerebrospinal fluid (CSF), because its measurement in CSF has been suggested as an ancillary diagnostic test for nonspecific damage to neural tissue (e.g., neural hypoxia, trauma, inflammation, compression by a space-occupying lesion such as a tumor). The CSF CK value may therefore be a useful guide for prognosis in canine neurologic cases and in premature foals. Increased values may also be observed after seizures.

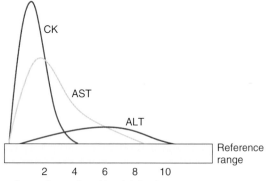

Dog and Cat
↑ ALT greater than ↑ AST; no ↑ CK → liver injury
↑ AST greater than ↑ ALT; ↑ CK → skeletal muscle injury

Horse and Ruminant
↑ AST; no ↑ CK → liver injury
↑ AST and ↑ CK → skeletal muscle injury or concomitant skeletal muscle injury and liver injury

CK

AST

ALT

Reference range

2   4   6   8   10

Approximate time (days) following severe skeletal muscle injury with resolution

Fig. 24.1 The approximated magnitude and duration of increases in creatinine kinase, aspartate transaminase, and alanine transaminase levels in the circulation after severe injury to the skeletal muscle may help to differentiate between predominantly liver or skeletal muscle injury. (From Meyer D, Harvey JW: *Veterinary laboratory medicine: interpretation and diagnosis*, ed 3, St Louis, 2004, Saunders.)

Although anything that damages the muscle cell membrane can cause an increased blood CK level, fractionation of the isoenzymes of CK can isolate the source of the CK and aid in diagnosis. CK exists as three primary isoenzymes: CK-BB (brain type), CK-MB (cardiac type), and CK-MM (skeletal muscle type). Increases in CK-MB indicate cardiac muscle damage while increases in CK-MM indicate other muscle damage or trauma.

Muscle damage that leads to increased CK may stem from intramuscular injections, persistent recumbency, surgery, vigorous exercise, electric shock, laceration, bruising, and hypothermia. Myositis and other myopathies also cause elevated blood CK levels. CK levels in samples may be artificially increased by oxidizing agents such as bleach, ethylenediaminetetraacetic acid (EDTA), citrate, fluoride, exposure to sunlight, or a delay in the performance of the assay.

TROPONIN AND BRAIN NATRIURETIC PEPTIDE

- Elevated in
  - Cardiac muscle damage
  - Heart failure

Cardiac muscle damage can also be evaluated with the troponin assay. Cardiac troponins (CTns) are proteins involved in regulating the initiation of skeletal muscle contraction. Increases in CTn levels indicate cardiac muscle damage, and the level of increase can aid in determining the degree of damage and elapsed time since the damage occurred. Brain natriuretic peptide (BNP) is a hormone secreted by myocytes that function in maintenance of blood pressure. Elevated levels occur with increased ventricular filling pressure and may aid in the diagnosis of heart failure. Both CTn and BNP are immunoassays. Results are interpreted in conjunction with other diagnostic tests and clinical signs.

LACTATE

- Elevated in
  - Hypoxia
  - Hypoperfusion

Lactate (lactic acid) is produced by anaerobic cellular metabolism. Its presence does not indicate any specific disease. However, increased lactate levels indicate hypoxia or hypoperfusion. Lactate levels may be measured in plasma, peritoneal fluid, and CSF. Hypoxia of a section of bowel wall results in increased lactate production, much of which diffuses into the peritoneal cavity before it enters the circulation and is removed by the liver. The use of paired blood and peritoneal fluid lactate measurements has been advocated as a diagnostic aid in equine colic cases. The blood lactate concentration of normal horses is always greater than that of peritoneal fluid. Horses with gastrointestinal disorders generally have peritoneal fluid lactate concentrations that are greater than the corresponding blood values. Less severe gastrointestinal disorders (e.g., impactions) tend to cause a smaller difference between peritoneal fluid and blood lactate concentrations as compared with more serious

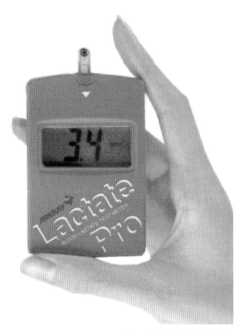

Fig. 24.2 Handheld lactate meter. (From Sirois M: *Principles and practice of veterinary technology*, ed 3, St Louis, 2011, Mosby.)

conditions (e.g., intestinal torsion [a twisted section of bowel]). Peritonitis also increases peritoneal fluid lactate values.

> **TECHNICIAN NOTE** Increased lactate levels generally indicate hypoxia or hypoperfusion.

The sample used for lactate measurement (i.e., blood or peritoneal fluid) should be collected in a fluoride oxalate or lithium heparin anticoagulant tube. The fluoride stops cellular metabolism of glucose and the consequent production of lactate, and the oxalate prevents sample clotting. Handheld lactate meters that have been validated for veterinary species are also available (Fig. 24.2).

Lactate Dehydrogenase

Lactate dehydrogenase (LD) is a serum enzyme that catalyzes the conversion of lactate into pyruvate. Like CK, LD has many isoenzymes. Different amounts of isoenzymes are present in different tissues. Almost all tissues have LD, although the liver, muscle, and erythrocytes are the major sources of increased blood LD levels. As compared with CK, the magnitude of LD rise is less dramatic after muscle injury. LD values are frequently included in biochemistry profiles. This enzyme is not considered organ-specific, because it has many sources and because the concentrations in each tissue are not high enough to result in significant elevations.

ENDOCRINE SYSTEM ASSAYS

In addition to the pancreas, a variety of organs and tissues release hormones that function in the endocrine system. The primary organs of the endocrine system are the adrenal glands, the thyroid and parathyroid glands, and the pituitary gland. These glands produce and secrete hormones directly into capillaries, and they have a variety of target organs and effects.

Adrenocortical Function Tests

Adrenocortical function tests are commonly performed. Adrenal dysfunction is increasingly common and often the result of misuse of corticosteroids. The adrenal axis starts with the hypothalamus. Stimuli that originate in the brain (e.g., as a result of stress) cause the hypothalamus to secrete corticotropin-releasing factor. Under the influence of corticotropin-releasing factor, the adenohypophysis secretes adrenocorticotropic hormone (ACTH), which is a hormone that stimulates adrenocortical growth and secretion, particularly of glucocorticoid-synthesizing tissue. Cortisol is the major hormone that is released in domestic mammals. It, in turn, feeds back to inhibit both corticotropin-releasing factor and ACTH release, thereby completing a balanced system.

True or mimicked hyperfunction of the system is a common complaint. Brain or pituitary tumors that lead to secondary bilateral adrenal hyperplasia, idiopathic adrenal hyperplasia, or neoplasia of one or both glands may cause excessive cortisol release and hyperadrenocorticism. Overenthusiastic glucocorticoid therapy is the most common cause of cortisol excess. Because exogenous (like endogenous) glucocorticoids inhibit adrenotropic hormones, iatrogenic hyperadrenocorticism is accompanied by the paradox of atrophied adrenal glands. The sudden withdrawal of exogenous glucocorticoids leads to adrenal hypofunction. However, hypoadrenocorticism (Addison's disease), by definition, includes mineralocorticoid deficiency, which does not occur with iatrogenic disease caused by the rapid withdrawal of glucocorticoids. Addison's disease may also result from the overuse of mitotane (Lysodren; for adrenal hyperplasia) or from idiopathic causes.

> **TECHNICIAN NOTE** Overenthusiastic glucocorticoid therapy is the most common cause of cortisol excess.

Screening tests for hyperadrenocorticism must be carefully interpreted, because many dogs with nonadrenal disease (e.g., diabetes mellitus), liver disease, or renal disease may have false-positive results. Thereafter, the final diagnosis of hyperadrenocorticism is made on the basis of clinical signs in conjunction with several of the various laboratory tests. Conversely, if negative laboratory testing occurs with consistent clinical evidence, the animal should be retested 1 to 2 months later if clinical signs persist.

ACTH and cortisol concentrations may be helpful diagnostic aids for the differentiation of primary (adrenal-dependent) hypoadrenocorticism from secondary (pituitary-dependent) hypoadrenocorticism. However, a single measurement has limited usefulness, because levels can fluctuate on a diurnal cycle. More often, these measurements are taken as baseline data and compared with data obtained from challenge to the adrenal gland with ACTH or dexamethasone. Animals with functioning adrenocortical tumors have low concentrations as a result of the negative feedback effect. Animals with pituitary-dependent hypoadrenocorticism should have higher concentrations. Low to undetectable ACTH concentrations occur with secondary Addison's disease, whereas normal (or increased) concentrations are expected with primary Addison's disease. ACTH is a labile protein, and special handling of the plasma sample is needed. Aprotinin (protease inhibitor) within the EDTA tube or immediate freezing of the plasma may be required. Tests for cortisol and ACTH are immunoassays, and some are available to the veterinary practice laboratory. Some tests are performed on serum, while others can be performed only on plasma samples. A few tests can also be performed on urine samples. Urine cortisol/creatinine ratios have also been used as screening tests for adrenal function.

Adrenocorticotropic Hormone Stimulation Test

Animals with suspected hypoadrenocorticism (Addison's disease) or hyperadrenocorticism (Cushing's disease) may be evaluated with an ACTH response test. In addition, the test is indicated to distinguish among iatrogenic and spontaneous hyperadrenocorticism (Procedure 24.1). It also may test the efficacy of mitotane, ketoconazole, or metyrapone therapy. The ACTH stimulation test evaluates the degree of adrenal gland response to the administration of exogenous ACTH. The degree of response to stimulation by glucocorticoid should be in proportion to the glands' size and development. Hyperplastic adrenal glands have exaggerated responses, whereas hypoplastic adrenal glands show diminished responses. The test can detect these abnormalities but not reveal their ultimate cause. The ACTH response test is a screening test. Adrenal glands that are hyperactive from neoplasia may be insensitive to ACTH. Nonetheless, current figures indicate that the test is more than 80% accurate for the diagnosis of adrenocortical hyperfunction in the dog and more than 50% accurate for the cat.

> **TECHNICIAN NOTE** The ACTH response test may help to distinguish between iatrogenic and spontaneous hyperadrenocorticism.

Dexamethasone Suppression

Dexamethasone suppression tests evaluate the adrenal glands differently by using the adrenal feedback loops. The low-dosage test confirms or replaces the ACTH response test for hyperadrenocorticism (Cushing's disease). The high-dosage test goes further and is used to differentiate pituitary causes of hyperadrenocorticism from adrenal causes (Procedure 24.2). In cats, only a high-dose dexamethasone suppression test is suitable.

PROCEDURE 24.1 Adrenocorticotropic Hormone Stimulation Test

1. Collect a plasma sample for the determination of a baseline plasma cortisol concentration.
2. Administer synthetic adrenocorticotropic hormone (ACTH; cosyntropin) via intravenous injection.
   a. Dosage varies by species: 125 mg for cats; 250 mg for dogs; and 1 mg for horses.
3. Collect a second plasma sample for cortisol determination at 30 minutes after ACTH administration in dogs and cats and at 2 hours after ACTH administration in horses.
4. Collect a third plasma sample for cortisol determination 1 hour after ACTH administration in dogs and cats and 4 hours after ACTH administration in horses.
5. Results:
   a. Normal pretest cortisol concentration:
      Dog: 0.5 to 4 mg/dL or 14 to 110 nmol/L
      Cat: 0.3 to 5 mg/dL or 8.3 to 138 nmol/L
   a. Normal post-ACTH cortisol concentration:
      Dog: 8 to 20 mg/dL or 220 to 552 nmol/L
      Cat: 5 to 15 mg/dL or 138 to 414 nmol/L
6. Interpretation:
   a. An exaggerated post-ACTH cortisol concentration is observed in most dogs (80%) and 51% of cats (borderline increased in 16%) with hyperadrenocorticism. Cats may have an increased level of only one of the post-ACTH cortisol determinations.
   b. A reduced post-ACTH cortisol concentration is observed, consistently, with both Addison's disease and iatrogenic Cushing's disease as well as with mitotane, ketoconazole, or metyrapone therapy.
   c. A normal post-ACTH cortisol concentration does not rule out Cushing's disease, because it occurs in 50% of dogs with adrenal-dependent Cushing's disease.

PROCEDURE 24.2 Dexamethasone Suppression Tests

Low Dosage
1. Obtain a blood sample for a baseline plasma cortisol determination at 8 AM. (Some clinicians also do a 2- or 3-hour test as well.)
2. Immediately administer intravenous dexamethasone at 0.01 mg/kg for dogs and 0.1 mg/kg for cats.
3. Obtain a second plasma sample for cortisol determination 8 hours after dexamethasone injection.
4. Results:

Adrenal Condition	Pretest Cortisol Level	Posttest Cortisol Level
Normal	1.1–8.0 mg/dL	0.1–0.9 mg/dL (<1.4)
Hyperadrenal	2.5–10.8 mg/dL	1.8–5.2 mg/dL (>1.4)

High Dosage
1. Use the same protocol as described previously, except increase the dexamethasone dosage to 0.1 mg/kg for dogs and 1.0 mg/kg for cats.
2. Results:
   a. Pituitary-dependent hyperadrenocorticism: Normal values as shown previously
   b. Adrenal-dependent hyperadrenocorticism: As for hyperadrenal values shown previously
   Note: Successful suppression is defined as a 50% decrease in the plasma cortisol concentration from the baseline value. In 15% of dogs with pituitary-dependent hyperadrenocorticism, the plasma cortisol level is not suppressed by 50%. About 20% of dogs with adrenal-dependent hyperadrenocorticism have suppression of the plasma cortisol level by less than 50%, but all values that remain above these are considered adequate for suppression (i.e., greater than 1.5 mg/dL).

Dexamethasone, which is a potent glucocorticoid, suppresses ACTH release from the normal pituitary gland and results in a drop in the plasma cortisol concentration. Hyperadrenocorticism of any etiology is usually resistant to suppression from small dexamethasone doses, because a diseased pituitary gland is abnormally insensitive to the drug and continues to elaborate excessive ACTH, although 35% of dogs with pituitary-dependent hyperadrenocorticism have a 4-hour post-dexamethasone cortisol level of less than 1 mg/dL or 50% of the baseline concentration. Neoplastic adrenal glands are autonomously secreting cortisol independent of endogenous ACTH control. The excessive cortisol production suppresses the secretion of ACTH by the normal pituitary gland through negative feedback inhibition. Small doses of dexamethasone do not affect plasma cortisol measurements. However, such doses may complicate test results and may differentiate only normal animals from those with hyperadrenocorticism.

With larger dexamethasone doses, more differences appear. The sensitivity of a diseased pituitary gland to dexamethasone is incomplete; large dexamethasone doses overcome it, and the abnormally high plasma ACTH and cortisol concentrations fall. However, abnormal adrenal glands continue to secrete cortisol autonomously. Thus, plasma cortisol concentrations that are unresponsive to all dexamethasone doses are probably caused by primary adrenal gland disease. Suppression by large (but not small) doses suggests pituitary gland disease. The test has 73% accuracy for differentiating pituitary from adrenal causes in dogs and 75% sensitivity for diagnosing hyperadrenocorticism in cats.

A dual high-dosage dexamethasone test and ACTH response test are described in Procedure 24.3. Although the combined protocol is a step saver, possibly ambiguous results necessitate more tests and expense. The ACTH response segment of the test is particularly prone to error. Because dexamethasone alters adrenal responsiveness to ACTH (it enhances or inhibits such responsiveness, depending on the duration of activity), the timing of the test is crucial. Normal standards must be newly established for any changes in protocol.

Corticotropin-Releasing Hormone Stimulation

This test may be indicated to differentiate between pituitary-dependent hyperadrenocorticism and primary hyperadrenocorticism. Plasma cortisol concentration and ACTH should not be elevated after corticotropin-releasing hormone stimulation in dogs with adrenal-dependent Cushing's disease.

The protocol of this test consists of obtaining a pretest sample to determine the cortisol and ACTH levels, administering 1 mg/kg of corticotropin-releasing hormone, and obtaining blood samples again 15 and 30 minutes later to evaluate the cortisol and ACTH levels.

Thyroid Assays

Thyroid hormones have pervasive effects, and they influence the metabolic rate, growth, and differentiation of all body cells.

PROCEDURE 24.3 Protocol for Combined Dexamethasone Suppression and Adrenocorticotropic Hormone Corticotropin Stimulation Test

1. Collect a plasma sample for cortisol determination.
2. Administer dexamethasone (0.1 mg/kg intravenously).
3. Collect a plasma sample for cortisol determination 4 hours after injection.
4. Immediately administer synthetic adrenocorticotropic hormone (ACTH) intravenously at a dose of 125 mg for cats and 250 mg for dogs.
5. Collect a third plasma sample for cortisol determination at 30 minutes after ACTH administration in dogs and cats and at 2 hours after ACTH administration in horses.
6. Collect a fourth plasma sample for cortisol determination 1 hour after ACTH administration in dogs and cats and 4 hours after ACTH administration in horses.
7. Results:
   a. Normal pretest cortisol concentration:
      Dog: 0.5 to 4 mg/dL or 14 to 110 nmol/L
      Cat: 0.3 to 5 mg/dL or 8.3 to 138 nmol/L
   b. Normal post-dexamethasone cortisol concentration:
      1 to 1.4 mg/dL or 28 to 39 nmol/L
   c. Normal post-ACTH cortisol concentration:
      Dog: 8 to 20 mg/dL or 220 to 552 nmol/L
      Cat: 5 to 15 mg/dL or 138 to 414 nmol/L
8. Interpretation:
   a. Elevated post-dexamethasone and elevated post-ACTH cortisol concentrations indicate hyperadrenocorticism.
   b. Elevated post-dexamethasone and normal post-ACTH cortisol concentrations indicate hyperadrenocorticism.
   c. Normal post-dexamethasone and exaggerated post-ACTH cortisol concentrations indicate pituitary-dependent hyperadrenocorticism.

Because the clinical signs of thyroid malfunction are numerous and confusing, function tests are valuable. The thyroid glands are governed like the adrenal cortices. Thyrotropin-releasing factor (TRF) from the hypothalamus encourages the anterior pituitary to release thyrotropin or thyroid-stimulating hormone (TSH). TSH enhances thyroid growth, function, and thyroxine release. Thyroxine is really composed of two varieties of hormones, triiodothyronine (T_3) and thyroxine (T_4), which vary in their extent of iodination. T_4 is also converted to the more active T_3 in tissues. Thyroxine completes the regulatory cycle by inhibiting TRF and TSH release.

Thyroid disease is manifested primarily as hypofunction in dogs, horses, ruminants, and swine and as hyperfunction in cats. The cause may be dietary iodine deficiency or excess or goitrogens, which are most common in large animals. Primary glandular disease (e.g., neoplasia, autoimmune disease, idiopathic atrophy) comprises most cases, whereas pituitary disease (secondary thyroid disease) comprises 5% of cases of hypothyroid dogs. In food animals, the diagnosis is based on clinical signs (e.g., abortion, stillbirths, alopecia, goiter in fetuses and neonates), serum T_4 concentrations, serum protein-bound iodine concentrations, and pasture iodine analyses. Feeds may be examined for goitrogenic plants (i.e., *Brassica* spp.) or for excess calcium, which decreases iodine uptake.

> **TECHNICIAN NOTE** In-house thyroid testing is generally performed with immunologic methods.

Baseline thyroxine concentrations are used diagnostically, but normal values vary dramatically. Immunologic tests are available for the measurement of T_4 concentrations. Some drugs (e.g., insulin, estrogens) may increase T_4 concentrations; others (e.g., glucocorticoids, anticonvulsants, antithyroid drugs, penicillins, trimethoprim sulfamides, diazepam, androgens, sulfonylureas) may decrease T_4 concentrations. In addition, total T_4 (TT_4) may be increased in hypothyroid dogs as a result of the presence of anti-T_4 antibodies. The specific determination of the active form of thyroxine non–protein-bound or free T_4 (FT_4) is a more accurate approach to thyroid function.

Thyroid-Stimulating Hormone Response

The thyroid-stimulating hormone response test is used on small animals (except cats with hyperthyroidism) and horses, and it provides a reliable diagnostic separation of patients with normal versus abnormal thyroid function (Box 24.1). Exogenous TSH challenge may sort out borderline cases and separate real hypothyroid patients from those with other illness or drug-depressed thyroxine concentrations, and it may also pinpoint the site of the lesions.

The test is usually used to explore canine hypothyroidism. After TSH is injected, thyroid response (usually serum T_4 levels, which provide the most reliable index) is followed. An increase in the serum T_4 level occurs in normal animals. Primarily exhausted or insensitive thyroids do not respond to exogenous TSH. Indeed, endogenous TSH concentrations are already high from failing T_4 inhibition. Therefore, the serum T_4 level is not increased in these animals. With pituitary or brain disease, however, the thyroid glands remain responsive. Such lesions result in too little endogenous thyrotropin. Although an increase in the serum T_4 level is expected in animals with pituitary lesions, 2 to 3 days of TSH challenge may be necessary before increased serum T_4 levels are seen. The extra TSH is required to overcome chronic glandular atrophy, a method that is comparable to "priming the pump."

BOX 24.1 Overview of the Thyroid-Stimulating Hormone Response Test

- A pretest blood sample is collected for baseline serum T_4 determination.
- Thyroid-stimulating hormone is administered, and T_4 determination is made with the use of a second blood sample that is collected 4 to 6 hours after injection.
- Results: The T_4 level after thyroid-stimulating hormone administration in normal dogs should be approximately twice the baseline value, or it should exceed 2.0 mg/dL or 25 nmol/L.

Glucocorticoids seem to inhibit both TSH and T_4 secretion, so euthyroidism with low serum T_3 levels only often accompanies Cushing's disease or vigorous glucocorticoid therapy. Fortunately, the TSH and ACTH response tests may be performed simultaneously. In such animals, the glands remain responsive to TSH, but the absolute values of prechallenge and postchallenge serum T_4 are low or low resting with normal post-TSH values. Feline hyperthyroidism is usually caused by functional thyroid adenomas. Oddly, with exogenous TSH challenge, little or no increase occurs in the serum T_4 level, as in canine primary hypothyroidism. This phenomenon suggests that the neoplasm either functions independently of the trophic hormone or that it is already manufacturing and leaking T_4 at maximum capacity. A lack of TSH responsiveness, appropriate clinical manifestations, and high baseline plasma T_4 concentrations all attest to feline hyperthyroidism.

In horses, iodine-deficiency hypothyroidism is rare, because iodized salt is usually offered freely or in feeds. Overzealous iodine supplementation with kelp meal or vitamin and mineral mixes can provoke hypothyroidism and goiter. The excessive use of iodine inhibits thyroid function. The normal serum T_4 values in horses are 1 to 3 mg/dL, which is lower than what is found in other species. Hypothyroidism should be suspected only with serum T_4 concentrations of less than 0.5 mg/dL.

Rare tumors of the pars intermedia of the pituitary, which compress the anterior pituitary, may cause secondary hypothyroidism in older horses. Because pituitary damage induces a plethora of signs, the TSH response test may be especially helpful.

Thyrotropin-Releasing Hormone Response

The thyrotropin-releasing hormone (TRH) response test is used on small animals, and it provides a reliable diagnostic separation of patients with normal versus abnormal thyroid function. FT_4 is the fraction of thyroxine that is not bound to protein. FT_4 levels are less influenced by nonthyroidal diseases or drugs than total T_4 concentrations. Exogenous TRH challenge may sort out borderline cases and separate real hypothyroid and hyperthyroid patients from those with other illness or drug-depressed thyroxine concentrations. The test is usually used to explore canine hypothyroidism when TSH is not available. Baseline serum TT_4 and FT_4 concentrations are determined. Four hours after 0.1 mg/kg or 0.2 mg (total dose) of TRH are injected intravenously, thyroid response (serum TT_4 and FT_4 levels) is followed. An increase in the serum TT_4 concentration of 50% and in the FT_4 concentration of 1.9 times as compared with baseline concentrations occurs in normal animals. The evaluation of FT_4 levels allows for a clearer distinction between euthyroid and hypothyroid dogs when TT_4 results are equivocal. The TRH response test may be used to diagnose mild to moderate feline hyperthyroidism. Baseline serum TT_4 and FT_4 concentrations are determined. Approximately 4 hours after 0.1 mg/kg of TRH are injected intravenously, serum TT_4 and FT_4 levels are determined. An increase of the serum TT_4 of less than 50% as compared with baseline concentrations occurs in hyperthyroid cats. Increases of between 50% and 60% are borderline, and increases of more than 60% rule out hyperthyroidism.

> **TECHNICIAN NOTE** Free T_4 is the fraction of thyroxine that is not bound to protein.

Triiodothyronine Suppression Test

Hyperthyroidism is common in middle-age to old cats in the United States and Great Britain. Diagnosis may be based on resting thyroid hormone concentrations. The determination of both TT_4 and FT_4 may help to distinguish a nonthyroidal disease. The combination of a high FT_4 value with a low TT_4 level is indicative of nonthyroidal illness, whereas a high FT_4 concentration and a high-normal TT_4 concentration indicate hyperthyroidism. However, some cases may require a functional test to confirm or rule out the disease.

Thyroid suppression testing is based on the expected negative feedback regulation of TSH, which is induced by high concentrations of circulating thyroid hormone. Hyperthyroid cats should not have a normal pituitary–thyroid regulation. As a result, the administration of exogenous T_3 must induce a decrease in endogenous T_4, unless feedback TSH regulation is altered.

To perform the test, a basal T_3 and T_4 determination is required. Seven T_3 doses of 25 mg given orally every 8 hours are administered at home. Approximately 2 to 4 hours after the seventh dose, a blood sample is obtained for T_3 and T_4 determination. Cats with hyperthyroidism have serum T_4 concentrations of more than 1.5 mg/dL or 20 nmol/L, whereas nonhyperthyroid cats have lower values. Low posttest T_3 concentrations indicate an invalid test as a result of a failure of exogenous T_3 administration.

Pituitary Function Tests

The diagnosis of canine acromegaly may be based on the documentation of an elevated growth hormone (GH) level. Serial GH determinations (i.e., from three to five samples taken at 10-minute intervals) are performed because affected dogs have constant levels of GH rather than fluctuating GH concentrations. In addition, affected dogs do not respond to stimulation with GH-releasing hormone. This test requires the intravenous administration of 1 mg/kg of GH-releasing hormone or 10 mg of clonidine. In normal dogs, the posttest plasma GH level increases 5 to 15 mg/L, and the posttest plasma clonidine level increases 13 to 25 mg/L.

CHEMICAL TESTS OF GASTROINTESTINAL FUNCTION

The principal functions of the gastrointestinal (GI) tract are the assimilation of nutrients (via digestion and absorption) and the excretion of waste products. Most nutrients are ingested in a form that is either too complex or insoluble for absorption. Within the GI tract, these substances are solubilized and degraded enzymatically to simple molecules that may be absorbed across the mucosal epithelium.

GI diseases are common in veterinary practice. Specific diagnosis is essential, especially when the disease is chronic. In cases of malabsorption, intestinal biopsy tends to be required to obtain a definitive diagnosis. Function tests are performed to rule out other diseases and to confirm the need for more invasive diagnostic procedures.

Malassimilation may be classified by pathophysiologic process into maldigestive and malabsorptive forms. Maldigestion results from altered gastric secretion and a lack of or decreased amounts of digestive enzymes, which are usually secreted by the pancreas and, less often, by the intestinal mucosa. Malabsorption is most often caused by an acquired disease of the small intestinal wall or by bacterial overgrowth syndromes. Before clinical signs of maldigestion are seen, approximately 90% of the pancreas must be either nonfunctional or destroyed. The small intestine of a dog can function well with up to 85% loss, but a loss of more than 50% may result in "short bowel syndrome," which cannot be compensated for by adaptive mechanisms.

Laboratory tests may evaluate gastric hydrochloric acid secretion, but most of them are directed to detect malassimilation and its origin. Gastric acid secretion may also be indirectly estimated by determining gastric juice pH; normal dogs have a fasting gastric pH of between 0.9 and 2.5. Gastric juice pH may be continuously monitored via a radiotelemetric technique.

Malassimilation tests are based on the examination of feces for fecal dietary nutrients and fecal enzyme activities as well as serum for concentrations of orally administered substrates or metabolites and specific tests for endogenous substances.

Fecal Occult Blood

Blood loss into the gut is another cause of protein-losing gastroenteropathy. Dramatic bleeding is evident as black feces (melena) or frank fecal blood (hematochezia). Less-obvious subtle bleeding is a significant sign of GI ulcers, neoplasia, or parasitism. Chronic low-level bleeding may lead to iron-deficiency anemia.

The reagent that is used to detect occult bleeding is guaiac. Impregnated strips or tablets are oxidized to a colored product by hemoglobin peroxidase activity in the feces. The reagent responds to dietary hemoglobin and myoglobin; therefore, the patient's diet must be meat-free for 3 days before the test. This precaution is less pertinent to herbivores, but the technician must check that the diet has not been supplemented with meat or bone meal. Another fecal occult blood test is available that uses immunochromatographic methods, but it has not been validated with veterinary species.

Monosaccharide Absorption Tests

These tests more specifically probe intestinal function. Again, the agent is given orally; blood concentrations are the measure of absorption.

d-Xylose Absorption

d-Xylose is a five-carbon sugar that is absorbed passively in the jejunum and excreted rapidly by the kidneys. Because xylose absorption is simple and the agent is not metabolized, its fate is readily traced. Xylose absorption is inefficient and often affected by some intestinal diseases. Nonetheless, the test is relatively insensitive, because control values are variable.

The test is primarily performed in horses, and it can be performed in dogs as well, as described in Box 24.2. Interference from rumen flora precludes the use of the oral test in cattle and sheep; the alternative injection of monosaccharides into the abomasum is difficult enough to make its use rare.

Abnormal xylose absorption indicates intestinal malassimilation and, specifically, malabsorption. However, only slight differences separate normal and abnormal ranges; diseased animals may have normal results. Animals with lymphangiectasia still may have normal results, because the lymphatics do not participate in xylose absorption. The rate of xylose absorption depends only on the amount given, the size of the absorptive area, the intestinal blood circulation, and gastric emptying. The latter may be delayed by cold or hypertonic solutions, pain, apprehension, or feeding. Fasting or radiographs to confirm an empty stomach are required. Vomiting, however, falsely lowers blood values, as does ascites (xylose enters pooled fluids). Bacteria have the ability to metabolize xylose; therefore, bacterial overgrowth may be monitored by this test. If bacterial overgrowth is suspected (e.g., in cases of intestinal stasis or pancreatic enzyme deficiency), the test should be repeated after 24 hours' use of oral tetracycline. Finally, renal disease falsely elevates blood xylose concentrations.

The fate of xylose has also been followed in dogs by collecting a 5-hour urine sample after a 25-g oral dose and

determining the total xylose excreted. This method is more laborious, but it requires only one xylose assay.

Cats were thought to have plasma concentrations and kinetics that were similar to dogs. Other studies found xylose uptake to be variable in cats; the plasma concentration did not increase to the levels found in dogs. Peak plasma concentrations of xylose in normal cats ranged between 12 and 42 mg/dL when a dosage of 500 mg/kg body weight was used.

False-negative results may be caused by delayed gastric emptying, abnormal intestinal motility, reduced intestinal blood flow, bacterial overgrowth, and the sequestration of xylose in the ascitic fluid. False-positive results may be caused by decreased glomerular filtration rate; therefore, ensuring that the patient is fully hydrated and not azotemic at the time of testing is important.

Of the oral dose of xylose, 18% is excreted through the kidneys within 5 hours. This test has been improved by performing a d-xylose and 3-O-methyl-d-glucose absorption test that compares the differential absorption of two sugars to eliminate the nonmucosal effects of d-xylose absorption.

Serum Folate and Cobalamin

Serum concentrations of folate and cobalamin may be assessed by immunoassay. Both concentrations tend to be decreased with malabsorption. Folate is absorbed in the proximal intestine, whereas cobalamin is absorbed in the ileum. Bacterial overgrowth may also alter these concentrations; folate synthesis is increased with bacterial overgrowth, whereas some bacteria may decrease the cobalamin availability. Assays for folate and cobalamin (vitamin B_{12}) are usually performed in conjunction with TLI to evaluate the extent of gastrointestinal disorders.

Mucin Clot Test

Synovial fluid mucin forms a clot when it is added to acetic acid. The nature of the resultant clot reflects the quality and concentration of hyaluronic acid. One method used to perform the test involves adding 1 mL of non-anticoagulated synovial fluid to a 7-N glacial acetic acid that has been diluted 0.1 : 4. The synovial fluid/acetic acid solution is gently mixed and allowed to stand at room temperature for 1 hour before it is evaluated for the presence of a clot. The mucin clot is generally graded as good (a large, compact, ropy clot in a clear solution), fair (a soft clot in a slightly turbid solution), fair-poor (a friable clot in a cloudy solution), or poor (no actual clot, but some large flecks present in a turbid solution). Clot assessment is enhanced by gently shaking the tube. Good clots remain ropy, whereas poor clots fragment. If only a few drops of synovial fluid are obtained with arthrocentesis, an abbreviated mucin clot test may be performed. If available after the preparation of a cytologic smear (and possibly after a total nucleated cell count), a drop of non–EDTA-preserved fluid is placed on a clean microscope slide. Three drops of diluted acetic acid are added and mixed. The resultant clot is graded after approximately 1 minute. Assessment may be easier against a dark background.

BOX 24.2   Overview of Monosaccharide Absorption Test in Dogs and Horses

Oral Xylose Absorption in Dogs
- The patient is fasted, and the baseline xylose measurement determined.
- Xylose solution is administered via a stomach tube, and xylose measurements are obtained from post-administration blood samples that are collected 30, 60, 90, 120, 180, and 240 minutes after xylose administration.
- Blood xylose concentrations are graphed over time.
- A peak of less than 45 mg/dL between 30 and 90 minutes is abnormal. Peak values of 45 to 50 mg/dL are possibly abnormal. A peak of more than 50 mg/dL is probably normal.

Glucose and Xylose Absorption in Horses
- Glucose and xylose tests are performed separately with the same general protocol.
- The patient is fasted for 12 to 18 hours, and water is then withheld.
- Baseline xylose (or glucose) concentrations are obtained.
- The xylose (or glucose) solution is administered via a stomach tube, and blood samples are collected at 30-minute intervals for 4 to 5 hours.
- The maximum blood xylose level of 20.6 ± 4.8 mg/dL is expected at 60 minutes. The preadministration blood glucose concentration should be doubled by 120 minutes.

TOXICOLOGY

Numerous agents may be involved in common poisonings of dogs, cats, horses, and food animals. These agents include herbicides, fungicides, insecticides, rodenticides, heavy metals (especially lead), household products (including phenols), automotive products (especially ethylene glycol), drugs (including medications), and various poisonous plants and animals. Often a presumptive diagnosis may be attained from an accurate history (including environmental factors) and a thorough clinical examination followed by response to therapy or by necropsy. However, the establishment of a specific etiologic diagnosis may be difficult in some cases.

A few simple tests may be performed in the veterinary practice laboratory. In such situations, personnel must be familiar and competent with the test procedure, reagents must not be outdated, and special equipment may be required. These requirements, together with a sporadic demand for such tests, frequently dictate that practitioners send all toxicologic specimens to a specially equipped laboratory for analysis.

Toxicologic Specimens

Suggestions for appropriate specimens and preferred methods of handling, packaging, and transport can be obtained by consultation with the toxicology laboratory. Such contact also ensures that the laboratory offers the procedures requested. Submitted specimens should be free from contamination by extraneous environmental compounds or debris. Specimens should not be washed, because this may remove toxic residues. Samples of different fluids, tissues, and feeds must be submitted in separate, clean, leak-proof (airtight) plastic or glass containers. All containers should be individually identified by the owner's and veterinarian's names, the animal's name or identification number, and the nature of the specimen before it is packaged into a large container for submission to the laboratory.

Samples of whole blood (at least 10 mL, usually heparinized), serum (at least 10 mL), vomitus, gastric lavage fluid, feces, and urine (approximately 50 mL) may be submitted from live animals. Samples of feed (portions of at least 200 g), water, and suspected baits may also be helpful in some cases. In cases of fatal poisoning, samples collected during a thorough necropsy should include whole blood or serum; urine; gut (especially stomach) contents (at least 200 g, noting the site of collection); and organ or tissue samples, especially liver and kidney but sometimes also brain, bone, spleen, or fat (generally, where practical, at least 100 g of each tissue). Sending too large a sample is always better than not sending enough, because excess can be discarded.

In general, serum or blood samples are best submitted refrigerated, whereas gut contents and tissues are best frozen. Preservatives are usually not required. An exception would be tissue samples that are submitted for histopathologic examination, which require fixation in 10% formalin and must not be frozen. If a preservative is used on a specimen that is submitted for chemical analysis, it is probably worthwhile to also submit an aliquot of preservative for reference analysis. Frozen samples should be insulated from other specimens and should arrive at the laboratory while they are still frozen. Dispatch to the laboratory by courier is recommended.

Because litigation may result from poisoning cases, accurate and detailed records should be kept from the outset of the case. The establishment of a good working relationship with the toxicology laboratory, including the provision of a good case history (and necropsy findings in cases of fatal poisoning) when samples are submitted, helps to ensure the best results.

The main advantage of the following tests is that they can be performed reasonably quickly in the practice laboratory. Results are therefore available more rapidly than if the sample were sent to a toxicology laboratory. However, they are best viewed as screening procedures that can be used to suggest appropriate avenues of investigation and treatment. The verification of findings (especially positive ones) by a reputable toxicology laboratory is advisable, especially if subsequent legal action by the client is a possibility.

Lead Poisoning

Lead is a fairly common environmental pollutant that can be found in the air of cities as well as in old lead-based paints, lead shot (ammunition), linoleum, car batteries, solder, roofing materials, and petroleum products. Lead poisoning (plumbism) can occur in all species. Clinical signs vary with the species, and they are chiefly related to the GI tract and the nervous system (Fig. 24.3). Hematologic examination of blood from an animal with lead poisoning may reveal basophilic stippling of some erythrocytes and increased numbers of circulating nucleated red blood cells (metarubricytosis). Such findings in an animal that is not anemic and that has clinical signs that are consistent with lead poisoning strongly suggest plumbism.

No simple, reliable in-house tests exist to detect lead in blood, feces, urine, milk, or tissues. Blood lead levels can be determined readily at a toxicology laboratory from whole blood that has been collected in EDTA, heparin, or citrate blood

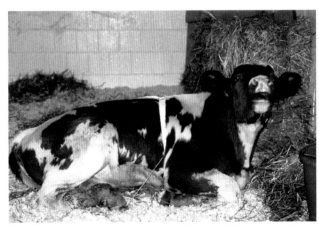

Fig. 24.3 Lead poisoning causing recumbency, blindness, and bellowing. There also were uncontrolled jerking actions in this 16-month-old heifer. (From Drivers T, Peek S: *Rebhun's diseases of dairy cattle*, ed 2, St Louis, 2008, Saunders.)

tubes. Tissue samples (especially liver and kidney) and feces may also be tested. Histopathologic examination of liver, kidney, or bone stained with the Ziehl-Neelsen technique may reveal characteristic eosinophilic, acid-fast intranuclear inclusion bodies in hepatocytes, renal tubular cells, and osteoclasts, respectively.

Nitrate or Nitrite Poisoning

Nitrate or nitrite poisoning may occur in ruminants, pigs, and horses that ingest feeds with high concentrations of these compounds. Such may be the case in cereals, grasses, and root crops that have been heavily fertilized with nitrogenous compounds. Water, especially from deep wells that are filled with seepage from heavily fertilized ground, may contain large quantities of nitrate. Nitrates are converted to nitrites in the feed or in the intestinal tract. Nitrites absorbed from the gut decrease the oxygen-carrying capacity of the blood by degrading hemoglobin to methemoglobin in erythrocytes. Consequently, the animal's blood becomes dark-red to brown. The severity of clinical signs is related to the quantity ingested. Death can be acute, and many animals can be affected.

A rapid and fairly specific semiqualitative test uses diphenylamine, which is converted into quinoidal compounds with an intensely blue color by nitrates and nitrites. Diphenylamine (0.5 g) is dissolved in 20 mL of distilled water and the solution made up to 100 mL with concentrated sulfuric acid. This stock solution may be used undiluted or diluted 1:1 with 80% sulfuric acid. The solution is applied to the inner portion of the plant's stem. An intense blue color within 10 seconds of application of the undiluted solution suggests that more than 1% nitrate is present (and thus that the feed is potentially toxic). False-positive results may occur with numerous substances, the most significant of which is iron. Such iron is generally on the outside of the stalk; therefore, careful application circumvents this problem.

A more dilute diphenylamine solution (i.e., the previous stock solution diluted 1:7 with concentrated sulfuric acid) may be used to test for nitrates and nitrites in serum, plasma, other body fluids, and urine. Three drops of the diluted diphenylamine are added to one drop of the sample on a glass slide over a white background. Nitrate and nitrite produce an intense blue color immediately. Hemolysis may mask the color change.

Anticoagulant Rodenticides

Anticoagulant rodenticides (e.g., warfarin, diphacinone, pindone) act by inhibiting the metabolism of vitamin K in the body. The latter is required for the production of factors II, VII, IX, and X in the liver. Anticoagulant rodenticide poisoning initially prolongs the prothrombin time, because factor VII is the first to be depleted. Subsequently, the partial thromboplastin time and the activated coagulation time are prolonged as other factors also become depleted. When an animal is bleeding as a result of such poisoning, both the prothrombin time and the partial thromboplastin time (or the activated coagulation time) are usually prolonged. A diagnosis of anticoagulant rodenticide poisoning is often based on these screening tests

and the patient's response to treatment with vitamin K (see Unit 3).

Chemicals That Denature Hemoglobin

A variety of compounds, when ingested, may result in damage to (i.e., the oxidative denaturation of) hemoglobin in erythrocytes with the formation of Heinz bodies. Such substances include paracetamol and methylene blue (cats), onions (dogs), red maple leaves (horses), and onions and brassicas (ruminants). The demonstration of Heinz bodies on a blood film is diagnostic of such poisoning.

Selenium-deficient animals are more prone to such oxidative injury as a result of a deficiency of glutathione peroxidase (an enzyme in erythrocytes that helps protect against such damage).

Ethylene Glycol

Ethylene glycol is the major constituent of most antifreeze solutions. Accidental ingestion can cause serious or fatal toxicosis, usually in dogs and cats. Ethylene glycol and its metabolites (Fig. 24.4) can be detected in whole blood or serum samples by a toxicology laboratory. The presence of ethylene glycol is strongly suggested when urine sediments from poisoned dogs or cats contain masses of calcium oxalate monohydrate crystals (see Unit 5). The histopathologic examination of the kidneys of fatally affected animals reveals renal tubular nephrosis and numerous oxalate crystals.

Drugs of Abuse

Animals (especially dogs and cats) may be exposed to a variety of illegal and prescription medications. Many times, patients are not presented for treatment until after the onset of clinical signs. The diagnosis of toxic exposures to human drugs of abuse may be complicated by a lack of specific information regarding the potential of exposure. Clients may be unaware

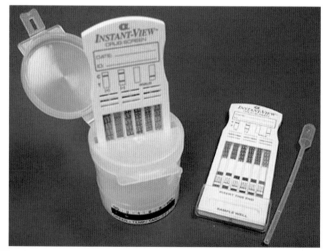

Fig. 24.4 An immunoassay to test for human drugs of abuse. (From Proctor D, Adams A: *Kinn's the medical assistant: an applied learning approach*, ed 11, St Louis, 2011, Saunders. Courtesy Alfa Scientific, Poway, CA.)

that an exposure has occurred, or they may fear prosecution by admitting to possessing drugs of abuse without a legal prescription. Clinical signs can vary considerably depending on the drug and the total amount ingested.

Few studies exist regarding the mechanisms of action of many of these medications in animals. In addition, the mode of exposure often differs from that seen with humans. Drugs that would normally be inhaled or injected by a human user usually result in exposure by ingestion in a pet animal. An additional complication of exposure relates to the potential presence of other substances mixed with the drugs that may not be identifiable or readily apparent. Studies have demonstrated that up to 50% of illicit drugs may contain none of the drug that they are supposed to, or they may contain other drugs and stimulants.

Routine biochemical analysis of blood and urine rarely demonstrates any abnormality in otherwise healthy patients after an acute exposure. A variety of rapid screening tests are available that can aid diagnosis. The vast majority of these tests utilize a competitive binding immunoassay technique contained within a lateral flow assay (Fig. 24.5). The tests are highly accurate with strict adherence to sample collection, processing, and test performance requirements. The tests are similar to the type first marketed for use as home pregnancy tests, and correlation data indicate a high degree of agreement between laboratory and field test results. The most common types of tests are urine dipstick assays. These are available in numerous configurations that test for a single analyte or for multiple analytes. A few of these tests can be used with other body fluids as well. Some manufacturers allow for the purchase of very small quantities of such tests.

The accuracy of the tests depends somewhat on the dose consumed and the time elapsed since exposure. The tests make use of standardized minimum concentration levels established by international regulatory authorities, specifically the National Institute on Drug Abuse, the World Health Organization, and the Substance Abuse and Mental Health Services Administration of the U.S. Department of Health and Human Services. Detailed published studies of the validity of these tests for use in veterinary species are not available.

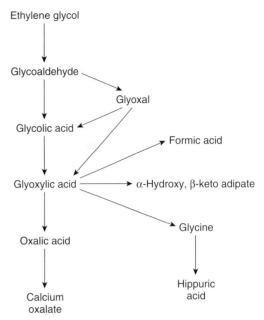

Fig. 24.5 Pathways of ethylene glycol metabolism. The pathway by which the toxicologically significant metabolites are generated is shown vertically. (From Plumlee K: *Clinical veterinary toxicology*, St Louis, 2004, Mosby.)

KEY POINTS

- Creatine kinase can be used to differentiate liver disease from skeletal muscle damage.
- Increased lactate levels generally indicate hypoxia or hypoperfusion.
- ACTH and cortisol concentrations may be helpful diagnostic aids for the differentiation of primary from secondary hypoadrenocorticism.
- Thyroxine is composed of two varieties of hormones: triiodothyronine (T_3) and thyroxine (T_4).
- Free T_4 is the fraction of thyroxine that is not bound to protein.
- In-house thyroid testing is generally performed with immunologic methods.
- Ethylene glycol ingestion can cause serious or fatal toxicosis.
- Immunochromatographic tests are available to evaluate patients for potential poisoning with human drugs of abuse.

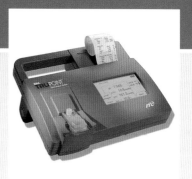

25

Automated Analyzers

LEARNING OBJECTIVES

After studying this chapter, you will be able to:
- Describe the principle of refractometry.
- Describe the principle of photometry.
- Differentiate between kinetic and end point assays.
- List the features and benefits of common analyzers.

OUTLINE

KEY TERMS

A variety of different chemistry analyzers are available for use in the veterinary practice laboratory. Veterinarians are better able to diagnose disease and monitor patient therapy when results are available immediately. Most chemistry analyzers used in the veterinary practice use the principles of photometry to quantify the constituents found in the blood. Analyzers that use electrochemical methods are also available for in-house use.

PHOTOMETRY

Several types of photometers are used in in-house diagnostic equipment (Fig. 25.1). Spectrophotometers are designed to measure the amount of light transmitted through a solution. The basic components of spectrophotometers are the same regardless of the specific manufacturer of the equipment. All spectrophotometers contain a light source, a prism, a wavelength selector, a photodetector, and a readout device (Fig. 25.2). The light source is typically a tungsten or halogen lamp. The prism functions to fragment the light into its component wavelength segments. The majority of spectrophotometric tests use wavelengths that are in the visible portion of the electromagnetic spectrum. A few tests are also available that use wavelengths in the near-infrared and ultraviolet portions of the spectrum. The wavelength selector is usually a cam that only allows one specific wavelength of light to pass into the

sample. The photodetector receives whatever light is not absorbed by the sample. The photodetector signal is then transmitted to the readout device. Depending on the model of the instrument, the readout units may be in percent transmittance, percent absorbance, optical density, or concentration units. Some automated analyzers use variations of the basic photometric procedure. The type of photometer that uses a filter to select the wavelength is referred to as a colorimeter. Another type detects light that is reflected off of a test substance rather than transmitted light. This type is referred to as a reflectometer (Fig. 25.3), and the tests are referred to as reflectance assays.

The wavelength that is used for the measurement of a specific blood constituent is chosen on the basis of the absorbance properties of the constituent being measured. The wavelength of light chosen for a given measurement is the one that results in the greatest light absorbance (i.e., the least amount of light transmission) through the sample. For example, if a solution appears blue-green, it will transmit the greatest amount of blue-green light, whereas light in the red portion of the spectrum will be absorbed. Therefore, a wavelength in the red portion of the spectrum provides maximal absorbance and would be used for the measurement of the component. For a solution to be measured with spectrophotometry, the solution must adhere to the principle of Beer's law, which is also known as Beer—Lambert's law. This principle states that a direct linear relationship exists between the concentration of an analyte and light absorption when monochromatic light (i.e., light of a single wavelength) is passed through the sample. The law also states that the transmission of monochromatic light through a sample and the concentration of an analyte in the sample have an inverse exponential relationship. The degree of color change is proportional to the solution's concentration.

END POINT VERSUS KINETIC ASSAYS

Most photometric analysis procedures are end point assays. In other words, the reaction that occurs between the sample and the reagent reaches a stable end. The analyzer then uses either a one-point calibration or an internal standard curve to calculate the patient results. Either method requires the use of a standard. A standard is a nonbiologic solution of the analyte, usually in distilled water, with a known concentration. For a one-point calibration, the standard is analyzed concurrently and in the same manner as the patient sample, and the reaction

characteristics are mathematically compared with the patient sample. The specific type of calculation varies, depending on the analyzer. In general, however, the ratio of the optical density (OD) of the reacted standard is compared with the OD of the patient sample. OD is a logarithmic function that describes the degree to which light is transmitted through a medium. An example of this type of calculation is as follows:

$$\text{Patient sample concentration} = \frac{\text{Patient sample OD} \times \text{Concentration of standard}}{\text{OD of standard}}$$

The internal standard curve is created when the analyzer is calibrated. To perform a standard curve, serial dilutions of the standard solution are created, and each is analyzed to determine its absorbance or transmittance of light. The results from each dilution are plotted on a graph as a straight line. The concentrations of subsequent patient samples are determined by locating the intersection of the absorbance of the reacted patient sample with the line on the graph. Analyzers that use standard curve methods must be recalibrated each time a new reagent is purchased.

Some analyzers use kinetic methods rather than end point methods. These are primarily used for enzyme assays or when the reagent is enzyme based. Enzymes induce chemical changes in other substances (called substrates), but they are not

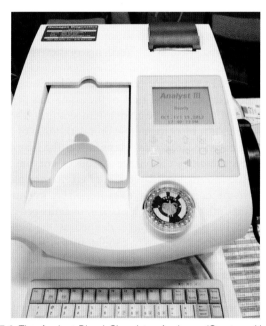

Fig. 25.1 The Analyst Blood Chemistry Analyzer. (Courtesy Hemagen Diagnostics, Columbia, MD.)

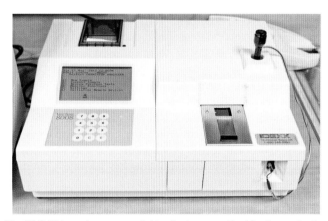

Fig. 25.3 This analyzer uses a light reflectance method for the evaluation of chemical components in the sample.

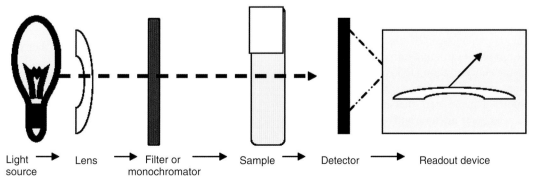

Light source → Lens → Filter or monochromator → Sample → Detector → Readout device

Fig. 25.2 Principles of spectrophotometry.

inherently changed. An enzyme may increase the rate of a biochemical reaction by acting as a catalyst to the reaction. Most enzymes are formed and function intracellularly, so they are found in their highest concentrations within cells. For this reason, the blood level of most enzymes is low in a healthy animal. The blood level of an enzyme may be elevated if the enzyme has leaked out of damaged cells or if the cells have increased production of the enzyme and the excess amount has leaked out of the cells into the blood. Each specific enzyme catalyzes the reaction of one specific substrate. Each enzymatic reaction produces a specific product from the interaction of the substrate and the enzyme. The reaction forms a product, but there is no change in the enzyme.

Because blood levels of enzymes are so low, directly measuring enzyme concentrations is difficult. The tests performed to determine enzyme concentrations in the blood indirectly measure the enzyme concentration that is present by directly measuring the rate of the formation of the product of the enzymatic reaction or the rate of reduction in the substrate. Kinetic assays do not reach a stable end point. The reaction results are recorded at a specific time after the initiation of the reaction even though the reaction continues beyond that time. Measurements that are not made at the correct time are usually not accurate. One-point calibrations are not generally performed for kinetic measurements. However, several points can be evaluated, and the change in absorbance for both the standard and the patient sample can be used to calculate patient results. When standard curves are created for kinetic methods, the graph is created by choosing the reaction time during which the graphed rates of absorbance form as close to a straight line as possible. The specific time after the initiation of the reaction when the reaction is closest to linear is different for each analyte.

Enzymes are most active when the substrate concentration is high and the product concentration is zero. If the enzyme concentration in the patient sample exceeds the substrate available in the test reagents, then the enzyme activity is no longer proportional to the product formed, and the assay is invalid. (The substrate concentration has become a limiting factor for the enzymatic reaction.)

Substrate concentrations must be kept high enough so that they do not invalidate the measurement. Enzymatic/kinetic test kits are manufactured so that a large amount of substrate is initially present to avoid this problem. If the amount of enzyme present in the patient sample is doubled, then the rate of the reaction is doubled and the amount of product formed is doubled, as long as the time is constant. If the amount of enzyme present in the patient sample is the same but the time is doubled, then the amount of product doubles. Therefore, if the time and the enzyme concentration are kept constant, then the rate of the reaction may be determined.

The most important parameters that influence the proper measurement of any enzyme are time and temperature. Enzyme activity continues as long as substrate is available. It is vital that the measurement be recorded at the appropriate time in the reaction. Enzyme activity may be inhibited by low temperatures and accelerated by high temperatures. Other factors that interfere with enzyme activity include ultraviolet light and the presence of salts of heavy metals (e.g., copper, mercury). Enzymes are proteins, and they may be denatured by temperature and pH extremes or by organic solvents. Even a small change in an enzyme's polypeptide chain structure may cause it to lose activity, so samples for enzyme assays must be handled with care.

Each enzyme has an optimal temperature at which it works most efficiently. This temperature is typically listed in the instructions that accompany the test kit or analyzer. Most assays are performed at temperatures of between 30° C and 37° C (86° F to 98.6° F). For every 10° C (18° F) above the optimal temperature, the enzyme activity doubles. Close monitoring of the incubator or water bath temperature used in enzyme assays is important.

UNITS OF MEASUREMENT

Enzyme concentrations are measured as units of activity. These units of measurement may be confusing. For example, enzyme activity is proportional to the enzyme concentration only under certain conditions. Each investigator who developed an enzymatic analytic method assigned his or her own unit of measurement to the results, and these often reflected the developer's name. Examples include the Bodansky, Somogyi, and Sigma-Frankel units. Because each of the assays was performed under different conditions (e.g., pH, temperature), the correlation of the results reported in one unit with those of another unit became difficult. To avoid this confusion, the International Union of Biochemistry established a unit of enzyme activity known as the International Unit (U or IU). According to this system, enzyme concentration is expressed as milliunits per milliliter (mU/mL), units per liter (U/L), or units per milliliter (U/mL). An International Unit is defined as the amount of enzyme that, under given assay conditions (particularly temperature and pH), will catalyze the conversion of 1 micromole of substrate per minute. Box 25.1 shows how to convert various units into International Units. Some laboratories have replaced the International Unit system with one better related to the Système International d'Unités (SI) set of basic units, which is based on the metric system. In this system, the katal is the basic unit of enzyme activity, and it reflects the amount of activity that converts 1 mole of substrate per second.

Enzymes are usually named for the substrate on which they act or the biochemical reaction in which they participate. Most enzyme names end with the -ase suffix. For example, lipase is an enzyme that catalyzes biochemical reactions that result in the hydrolysis of lipids (fats) to fatty acids, and lactate dehydrogenase participates in a reaction that involves the oxidation or dehydrogenation of lactate to pyruvate.

Some enzymes that are found in different tissues occur as isoenzymes. An isoenzyme is one of a group of enzymes with similar catalytic activities but different physical properties. The

---

BOX 25.1 Factors for Converting Various Enzyme Units Into International Units

Alkaline Phosphatase
Bodansky units × 5.37 = IU/L
Shinowara-Jones-Reinhart units × 5.37 = IU/L
King-Armstrong units × 7.1 = IU/L
Bessey-Lowry-Brock units × 16.67 = IU/L
Babson units × 1.0 = IU/L
Bowers-McComb units × 1.0 = IU/L

Amylase
Somogyi (saccharogenic) units × 1.85 = IU/L
Somogyi (37° C; 5 mg starch/15 min/100 mL) × 20.6 = IU/L

Lipase
Roe-Byler units × 16.7 = IU/L

Transaminases
Reitman-Frankel units × 0.482 = IU/L
Karmen units × 0.482 = IU/L
Sigma-Frankel units × 0.482 = IU/L
Wroblewski-LaDue units × 0.482 = IU/L

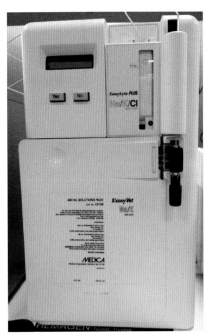

Fig. 25.4 This electrolyte analyzer utilizes ion-selective electrode technology.

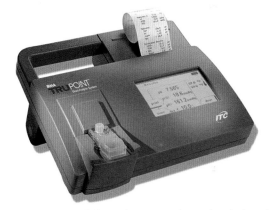

Fig. 25.5 The IRMA TruPoint analyzer uses electrochemical methods to measure blood gases and electrolytes. (Courtesy International Technidyne, Edison, NJ.)

serum concentration of an enzyme that occurs as isoenzymes is the total of the concentrations of all of the isoenzymes present from various tissues. The identification of which isoenzyme is present in the sample also allows for the identification of the source of that particular isoenzyme. For example, serum alkaline phosphatase is found in many tissues, particularly osteoblasts and hepatocytes. If the total serum alkaline phosphatase level is elevated, ascertaining whether the increase is from damaged bone cells or damaged liver cells is impossible. However, if the respective levels of the various isoenzymes of alkaline phosphatase are assayed, levels of the isoenzyme from the damaged tissue are elevated, thereby identifying the damaged tissue. The alkaline phosphatase assay performed in the practice laboratory is for total serum alkaline phosphatase, because individual isoenzyme assay methods have not yet been developed for the practice laboratory. Another clinically significant isoenzyme is creatine kinase (CK). The isoenzymes are widely distributed in many tissues, with the highest activity in brain, cardiac, and skeletal muscle. Fractionation of CK into the three primary isoenzymes, CK-BB (brain type), CK-MB (hybrid type), and CK-MM (muscle type) is a more sensitive indicator of specific pathological conditions.

ION-SELECTIVE ELECTRODE AND ELECTROCHEMICAL METHODS

Some analyzers use the related principles of electrochemistry or ion-selective electrode (ISE) technology to determine analyte concentrations. A few analyzers combine electrochemical and photometric methods within self-contained cartridges. Electrochemical and ISE methods are most often used for the evaluation of electrolytes and other ionic components. These types of tests vary considerably in configuration, but they function in a similar manner (Fig. 25.4). ISE analyzers, which are sometimes referred to as potentiometers, are designed with specific electrodes that are configured to allow for interaction with just one ion. For each ion being evaluated, the analyzer contains an electrode that is specific for that ion with a known concentration of the ion. This is referred to as the reference electrode. The sample interacts with the second ion-specific electrode and creates an electrical potential or voltage difference. The difference in electrical potential between the two electrodes is proportional to the concentration of ions in the sample. Electrochemical analyzers incorporate electrodes within biosensor reagent strips or cartridges. The sample interacts with reagents that are impregnated in the biosensor device and creates a measurable current that corresponds to the ion concentration (Fig. 25.5).

FEATURES AND BENEFITS OF COMMON CHEMISTRY ANALYZER TYPES

Most automated analyzers use liquid reagents, dry reagents, or slides that contain dry reagents. Liquid reagents may be purchased in bulk or in unitized disposable cuvettes. Dry reagents are available in unitized form. Bulk liquid reagents are the least expensive, but they require additional handling and storage space. Some reagents are flammable and toxic. The purchase of unitized reagents eliminates the hazards that are associated with handling these reagents. Dry slide reagents pose little or no handling or storage concerns but tend to be more expensive.

Analyzers that use dry systems include those with reagent-impregnated slides, pads, or cartridges. Most of these use reflectance assays. Dry systems tend to have comparatively higher costs associated with them than other analyzer types. Many are not configured for veterinary species and have fairly high incidences of sample rejection, particularly with samples that are lipemic or hemolyzed or that come from large animals. However, they do have the benefit of not requiring reagent handling, and the performance of single tests is relatively simple. Running profiles (i.e., large numbers of tests on a single patient sample) on some of these types of systems tends to be a bit more time-consuming as compared with most other analyzer types. A few dry slide type analyzers allow for the loading of large numbers of slides at once, thereby minimizing the time required to prepare the analyzer to evaluate a profile (Fig. 25.6). Some dry systems use reagent strips similar to those that are used for urine chemical testing.

Liquid systems include those that make use of a lyophilized reagent or an already prepared liquid reagent. The most common type of lyophilized reagent system for veterinary clinical practice uses rotor technology. The rotors consist of individual cuvettes to which diluted samples are added (Fig. 25.7). Cuvettes are optical-quality reservoirs used in the photometer, and they may be plastic or glass. Rotor-based systems tend to be quite accurate, although some are not configured for veterinary species. They are usually cost-effective for profiles, but they are not configured to run single tests. Other liquid systems in common use include those with unitized reagent cuvettes or bulk reagent. The unitized systems have the advantage of not requiring reagent handling, but they tend to be the most expensive of all of the liquid reagent systems. In addition, running profiles with these systems is somewhat time-consuming, but single testing is simple. Bulk reagent systems may supply reagent in either concentrated form, which must be diluted, or working strength. Working-strength reagent systems do not usually require any special reagent handling. These analyzers are the most versatile in that they can perform either profiling or single testing with relative ease (Fig. 25.8). Most require little preparation time. However, a few have extensive maintenance time, particularly with the calibration of test parameters. Some systems that use bulk reagent may have a flow cell instead of a cuvette. Sample and reagent can be aspirated directly through the analyzer without the need for the transfer

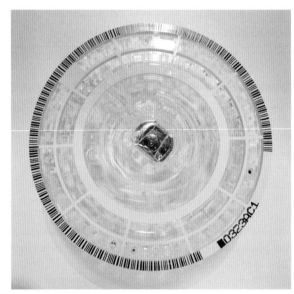

Fig. 25.7 Reagent rotor for use in some liquid chemistry systems.

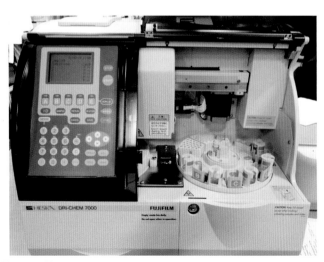

Fig. 25.6 This analyzer utilizes dry-slide technologies. Multiple slides can be loaded into the analyzer at one time.

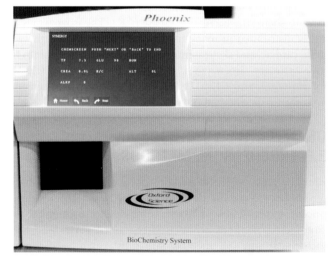

Fig. 25.8 This chemistry analyzer involves the use of working-strength reagents. It can perform single tests and profiles for multiple patients at the same time.

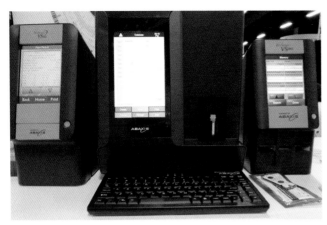

Fig. 25.9 Most analyzer manufacturers allow for the integration of multiple analyzers with programs to record results in patient records.

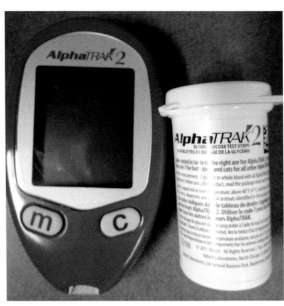

Fig. 25.10 This dedicated glucose-measuring instrument is available over the counter in many pharmacies.

of the reactants into cuvettes. Regardless of the test methods or the tests available for a specific analyzer, nearly all major manufacturers provide the ability to integrate all analyzer types (i.e., hematology, chemistry, blood coagulation, and electrolytes) into a software system that enables results to be recorded automatically and integrated with patient records (Fig. 25.9).

Dedicated-use analyzers are available for certain tests. Many of these utilize electrochemical technology and sample for only one substance, such as blood glucose (Fig. 25.10). Dedicated analyzers can be used if only a single test is requested or in emergency situations.

INSTRUMENT CARE AND MAINTENANCE

Chemistry analyzers are sensitive instruments that must be carefully maintained. Veterinary technicians should follow the manufacturer's operating instructions. Instruments generally have a warm-up period to allow the light source, photodetector, and incubator, if present, to reach equilibrium before they are used. Ideally, laboratory personnel should turn on the instrument in the morning and leave it on all day. The instrument is therefore ready to use at any time during the day, especially during emergency situations.

Following the manufacturer's maintenance schedule prolongs the life of the chemistry analyzer. A schedule sheet should be established for each instrument in the laboratory to allow for the quick and easy review of the maintenance history of any instrument. Most manufacturers have a toll-free number to call if problems arise.

KEY POINTS

- Most clinical chemistry analyzers use spectrophotometric methods and test principles that are based on Beer's law.
- Analyzers that use reflectance methods are also widely available.
- Chemistry assays may use end point or kinetic methods.
- Electrochemical analyzers are primarily used for electrolyte assays.
- Chemistry analyzers have different advantages, benefits, and limitations.

UNIT 5

Urinalysis

Unit Outline

Unit Objectives

Describe the formation of urine.
List and describe a variety of urine sample collection methods.
List and describe physical and chemical evaluations performed with urine samples.
Describe the formed elements that may be encountered in urine samples.
Describe the procedure for preparing urine for microscopic examination.
Describe the procedure for evaluating the formed elements in a urine sample.

Urinalysis is a relatively simple, rapid, and inexpensive laboratory procedure. It evaluates the physical and chemical properties of urine as well as the urine sediment. A urinalysis provides information to the veterinarian about the status of the urinary system, the metabolic and endocrine systems, and the electrolyte and hydration status. Therefore, the veterinarian may request that the owner bring a urine sample for initial testing. Samples may also be collected in-house using a variety of techniques.

Abnormalities in the urine may reflect a variety of disease processes involving several different organs. The basic equipment needed to perform a urinalysis is minimal and readily available in most veterinary clinics.

Quality assurance begins with proper specimen identification and handling. All samples should be labeled immediately after collection, and urinalysis should be performed as soon as possible. Reagent strips and tablets must be kept in tightly sealed bottles, and outdated reagents must be replaced with fresh reagents. Reactions for most constituents in the urine may be checked against available controls (e.g., Chek-Stix, Bayer Corporation, Leverkusen, Germany; Uritrol, YD Diagnostics, Seoul, Korea; Liquid Urine Control, Kenlor Industries, Inc., Santa Ana, CA). In addition, urine samples with distinct reactions for certain constituents sometimes may be preserved and used as positive controls. The results obtained from control samples and made-up controls should be plotted to determine whether observer drift or reagent decomposition is occurring. The urinalysis laboratory report should include patient information, collection technique, date and time collected, method of preservation (if used), and complete urinalysis results, including the results of microscopic examination results. A standard protocol for reporting results must be followed. Precision and accuracy need to be maintained by the veterinary technician for the proper interpretation of results.

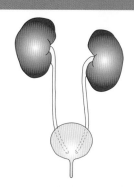

26

Anatomy and Physiology of the Urinary System

LEARNING OBJECTIVES

After studying this chapter, you will be able to:
- List and describe the components of the urinary system.
- Explain the formation of urine.
- Describe the structure of the nephron.
- Name the hormones involved in the regulation of urine volume.

OUTLINE

KEY TERMS

Anuria
Glomerulus

Nephron
Oliguria

Polyuria
Renal threshold

The many metabolic reactions that take place in the body's cells generate a variety of chemical by-products. Some of these substances are still useful to the body and are recycled, but others would be harmful if they were allowed to accumulate in the body. These harmful waste products must be eliminated. The urinary system is the primary means by which waste products are removed from the blood. It consists of two kidneys, two ureters, the urinary bladder, and the urethra (Fig. 26.1). The left and right kidneys are located in the dorsal part of the abdominal cavity, just ventral to the most cranial lumbar vertebrae. Most animals have smooth, bean-shaped kidneys. However, the right kidney of the horse is heart-shaped, and bovine kidneys have a lobulated appearance.

Blood and lymph vessels, nerves, and the ureter enter and leave the kidney through the indented area called the hilus. A rough-appearing outer cortex is wrapped around a smooth-appearing inner medulla. The area deep to the hilus region is the renal pelvis, which is the funnel-like beginning of the ureter. The work of the kidneys is done within the nephrons. Depending on the animal's size, each kidney may contain from several hundred thousand to several million nephrons. Each nephron is a tube composed of epithelial cells with several bends. Each portion of the nephron is characterized by a different type of epithelial cell. A small number of these epithelial cells are regularly sloughed off. Increased numbers of specific types of epithelial cells can aid in determining the cause of renal damage or dysfunction.

The nephron has the following parts; see Fig. 26.2:
- Renal corpuscle
- Proximal convoluted tubule
- Loop of Henle
- Distal convoluted tubule
- Collecting tubule

Each renal corpuscle is composed of a glomerulus surrounded by a Bowman's capsule. The glomerulus is a tuft of capillaries between the arterioles that enter and leave the renal corpuscle.

> **TECHNICIAN NOTE** The urinary system consists of two kidneys, two ureters, the urinary bladder, and the urethra.

FORMATION OF URINE

When blood enters the renal corpuscles, a portion of the plasma, along with its wastes, is filtered through the glomerulus into the proximal convoluted tubule. Large proteins and cells do not enter the tubule unless there is damage to the glomerulus. The filtered fluid passes slowly through the rest of the

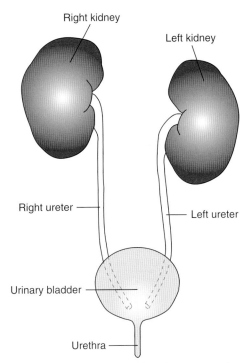

Fig. 26.1 Parts of the urinary system. The urinary system is made up of two kidneys, two ureters, one urinary bladder, and one urethra. (From Colville TP: *Clinical anatomy and physiology for veterinary technicians*, ed 2, St Louis, 2008, Mosby.)

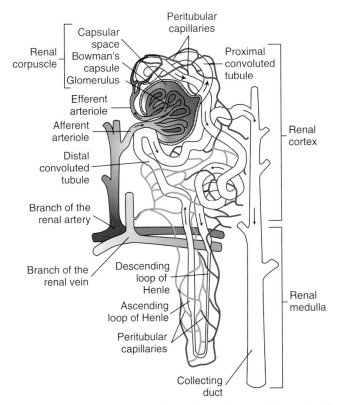

Fig. 26.2 Microscopic anatomy of a nephron. *Arrows* indicate the direction of fluid flow through the nephron. (From Colville TP: *Clinical anatomy and physiology for veterinary technicians*, ed 2, St Louis, 2008, Mosby.)

nephron and is modified as it moves along. Substances such as water and glucose are resorbed back into the blood of the capillary network. The nephron has a specific limit for the resorption of specific substances known as the renal threshold. Should the filtrate contain extremely high concentrations of any of those substances, the excess is not resorbed and is instead excreted in the urine. By the time the fluid in the nephron reaches the collecting tubules, it has become urine. Collecting tubules of all nephrons drain urine into the renal pelvis to the opening of the ureter (Fig. 26.3).

> **TECHNICIAN NOTE** The term *renal threshold* refers to the maximum absorptive capabilities of the nephron for specific substances.

Ureters

From each renal pelvis, urine is transported to the urinary bladder by the ureters, which are muscular tubes that conduct the urine via smooth-muscle contractions. The ureters enter the bladder at oblique angles, which form valvelike openings that prevent the backflow of urine into the ureters as the bladder fills.

Urinary Bladder

The urinary bladder is a muscular sac lined with transitional epithelial cells that stores urine and releases it periodically to the outside during a process called urination. The kidneys constantly produce urine. As urine accumulates in the urinary bladder, the bladder enlarges, and stretch receptors in the bladder wall are activated when the volume reaches a certain point. A spinal reflex then initiates the contraction of the smooth muscle in the bladder wall. A voluntarily controlled sphincter muscle around the neck of the urinary bladder enables the conscious control of urination.

Urethra

The urethra is the tube that carries urine from the urinary bladder to the outside of the body. In females, it is relatively short, straight, and wide, and it has a strictly urinary function. In males, it is relatively long, curved, and narrow, and it serves both urinary and reproductive functions. A small amount of normal flora (bacteria) are commonly found in the distal urethra along with a small number of white blood cells.

URINE VOLUME REGULATION

The regulation of the volume of urine produced is controlled by two hormones: antidiuretic hormone, which is released from the posterior pituitary gland, and aldosterone, which is secreted by the adrenal cortex. Antidiuretic hormone acts on the collecting ducts to promote the reabsorption of water. Alterations in water volume may involve decreased production (oliguria), increased production (polyuria), or the absence of urine (anuria).

A

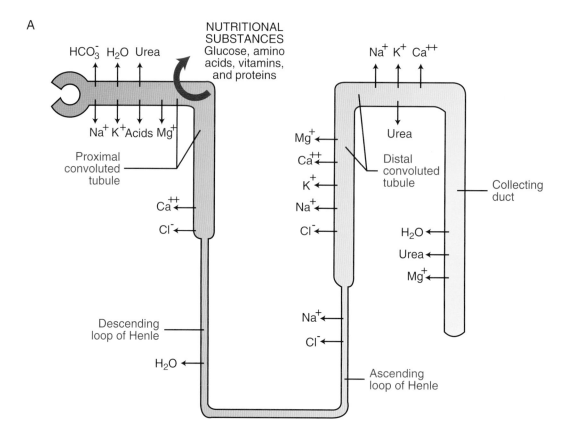

B

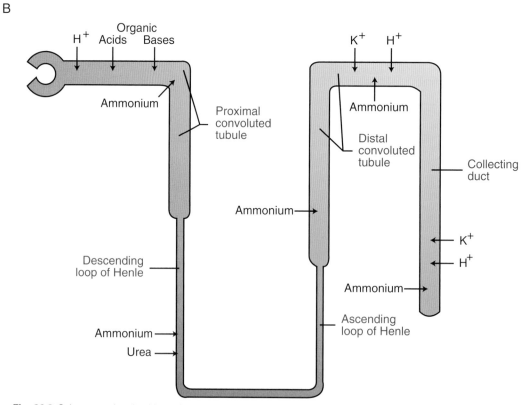

Fig. 26.3 Substances involved in reabsorption and secretion. **A,** Substances that are recovered from tubular filtrate through reabsorption into peritubular capillaries. **B,** Substances that are eliminated from the body as necessary through secretion into tubular filtrate from peritubular capillaries. (From Bassert J, Colville T: *Clinical anatomy and physiology for veterinary technicians,* ed 2, St Louis, 2008, Mosby.)

KEY POINTS

- The urinary system consists of two kidneys, two ureters, the urinary bladder, and the urethra.
- The functional unit of the kidney is the nephron.
- Parts of the nephron include the renal corpuscle (i.e., the glomerulus and Bowman's capsule), the proximal convoluted tubule, the loop of Henle, the distal convoluted tubule, and the collecting tubule.
- The term *renal threshold* refers to the maximum absorptive capabilities of the nephron for specific substances.
- Antidiuretic hormone and aldosterone are involved in the regulation of urine volume.

27

Sample Collection and Handling of Urine

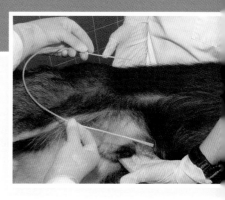

LEARNING OBJECTIVES

After studying this chapter, you will be able to:

- List the methods used to obtain samples for urinalysis.
- Discuss aspects of sample collection by free catch.
- State the equipment needed for catheterization and cystocentesis.

- State the procedures for the collection of urine samples via catheterization and cystocentesis.
- Describe the proper handling of urine samples.

OUTLINE

KEY TERMS

Bladder expression
Catheterization

Cystocentesis
Free catch

Micturition
Tom Cat catheter

The first step in performing a urinalysis is the proper collection of a urine sample, which must be carefully obtained to ensure accurate results. The analysis of urine samples should be performed only on samples taken before the administration of therapeutic agents. Urine specimens may be obtained via

1. the natural voiding of urine
2. bladder expression
3. catheterization or
4. cystocentesis.

The two preferred methods are cystocentesis and catheterization. These methods provide optimal samples for all aspects of urinalysis due to avoiding contamination from the distal genital tract and external areas. Collecting samples by voiding or the expression of the bladder may be easier, but urine collected in these ways may be of limited diagnostic value. Except for cytologic examination, performing a urinalysis on preprandial morning samples is best, although not always practical, in veterinary patients. Morning samples tend to be the most concentrated and least affected by dietary factors, thereby increasing the chances of finding formed elements.

VOIDED OR FREE-CATCH SAMPLES

The easiest sample to obtain is the voided (i.e., free-catch) sample, which is collected as the animal urinates. A sample

collected in this manner is not satisfactory for bacteriologic examination, because it is often contaminated during urination. Often voided samples contain increased white blood cell counts as a result of contamination from normal flora or inflammatory lesions of the distal genital tract. Results of other evaluations are usually unaffected.

> **TECHNICIAN NOTE** Voided samples often contain increased white blood cell counts.

A voided sample is collected in a clean and dry (although not necessarily sterile) container. If possible, the vulva or prepuce should be washed to decrease contamination of the sample before collection. Animals' owners may be asked to collect a sample when the animal spontaneously urinates. Furthermore, the cleansed tissue in the external orifice area does not remain clean for long. A mid-urination (midstream) sample is best because it is less likely to be contaminated. However, the initially voided urine is sometimes collected as a precaution against not being able to collect sufficient volume with a mid-urination sample.

Dogs may begin to urinate and then stop when collection is attempted. Chances of successfully obtaining urine may be increased by attaching a paper cup to a long pole and collecting the sample without disturbing the animal. A voided sample from a cat is difficult to obtain. Occasionally cats will urinate in an empty litter box, but veterinarians may prefer to give cat owners nonabsorbent granules to use in the litter box. Cows may be stimulated to urinate by rubbing a hand or a dry hay ventral on the vulva in a circular fashion. Sheep may be stimulated to urinate by occluding their nostrils. Horses may be stimulated to urinate by rubbing a warm, wet cloth on their ventral abdomen or by placing them in a clean stall with fresh hay.

BLADDER EXPRESSION

Urine may be collected from small animals via manual compression of the bladder. However, samples obtained in this manner are also unsatisfactory for bacteriologic culturing. As with the collection of a voided sample, the external genitalia should be cleansed before bladder expression. With the animal standing or in lateral recumbency, the bladder is palpated in the caudal abdomen, and gentle, steady pressure is applied. Care must be taken not to exert too much pressure, which could injure or rupture the bladder. Relaxation of the bladder sphincters often takes a few minutes. Occasionally an increase in red blood cells (RBCs) will be found as a result of pressure applied to the bladder, and an increase in white blood cells may result from contamination that originates in the distal genital tract. If bacteria are in the urine, the kidneys may become infected by these bacteria. This method should never be used on animals with urethras that may be obstructed or with bladder walls that may be fragile, because excessive pressure can cause the bladder to rupture. In large animals, urination may be stimulated by maintaining pressure on the bladder through the rectal wall while performing rectal palpation.

CATHETERIZATION

Catheterization is the insertion of a polypropylene or rubber catheter into the bladder by way of the urethra. A variety of catheters exist for different species and genders (Fig. 27.1). As with the previous two methods of collection, the external genitalia should be cleansed before the procedure, and sedation is sometimes required. Sterile catheters should always be used, and sterile gloves must be worn. Care must be taken to maintain sterility and to prevent trauma to the urinary tract.

This method may be used for culture and sensitivity if a cystocentesis cannot be performed. For female animals, a speculum improves visualization of the urethral orifice and thus facilitates the catheterization (Fig. 27.2). The catheter should pass easily through the urethra. A small amount of sterile water-soluble lubricating jelly, such as K-Y Jelly (Johnson & Johnson, Arlington, TX), should be placed on the tip of the catheter (Fig. 27.3). Care must be taken to avoid trauma to the sensitive urethral mucosa. The distal end of many catheters is designed for attachment to a syringe so that urine can be collected with gentle aspiration. Collection into a sterile syringe is especially advantageous if bacteriologic culture is anticipated. Often the first portion of the sample obtained is discarded because possible contamination may occur as the catheter is advanced through the distal urethra. Occasionally an increase in RBCs and epithelial cells may be seen in the sample as a result of urethral mucosa damage from the catheter. Procedures 27.1, 27.2, and 27.3 summarize catheterization procedures for male and female dogs and male cats.

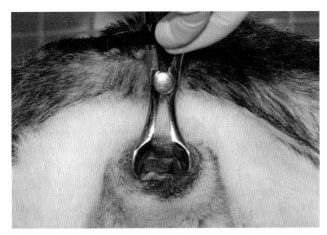

Fig. 27.2 A vaginal speculum is used to facilitate visualization of the urethral orifice in female patients. (From Taylor S: *Small animal clinical techniques*, St Louis, 2010, Saunders.)

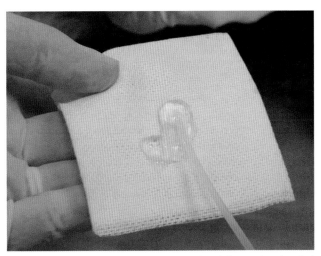

Fig. 27.3 Use sterile water-soluble lubricating jelly on the tip of the catheter. (From Taylor S: *Small animal clinical techniques*, St Louis, 2010, Saunders.)

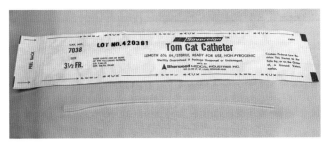

Fig. 27.1 Tom Cat Catheter. This is a 3.5-Fr polypropylene catheter used to obtain urine samples from male cats. (From Sonsthagen T: *Veterinary instruments and equipment*, ed 2, St Louis, 2011, Mosby.)

PROCEDURE 27.1   Urinary Catheterization: Male Cat

Materials
- Sedation drugs
- Sterile gloves
- Sterile water-soluble lubricating jelly
- Antiseptic solution
- Saline
- Urinary catheter
- Syringe

Procedure
1. Sedate the cat, if necessary.
2. Place the cat in lateral or dorsal recumbency.
3. Extrude the penis by pushing the penis caudally and pulling the prepuce forward.
4. Gently wash the end of the penis with antiseptic solution and then rinse it with saline.
5. Lubricate the tip of the catheter with sterile water-soluble lubricating jelly.
6. Gently insert the tip of the catheter into the external urethral orifice, and advance it into the lumen of the bladder.

TECHNICIAN NOTE A 4- to 10-Fr polypropylene catheter is usually used to collect urine samples by catheterization from dogs.

CYSTOCENTESIS

Cystocentesis is often used to collect sterile urine samples from dogs and cats, but only when the bladder is sufficiently distended so that it can be easily isolated. This procedure should be performed only on calm, easily restrained patients (Fig. 27.4). An ultrasound-guided cystocentesis may also be performed. The bladder must be palpated before the procedure to avoid damage to other internal organs. When performing a cystocentesis, a 22- or 20-gauge needle that is 1 to 1.5 inches long and a 10-mL syringe should be used. Once the needle is through the skin, it should never be redirected because of the potential for damage to other internal organs. With the animal in lateral or ventral recumbency or standing, the bladder is gently palpated and immobilized, and the needle is inserted into the caudal abdomen and directed dorsocaudally (Fig. 27.5). For male dogs, insert the needle caudal to the umbilicus and to the side of the sheath. For female dogs and for cats, insert the needle on the ventral midline caudal to the umbilicus. Gently aspirate urine into the syringe, and properly label the syringe with the patient information. If transferring the sample from the syringe into a collection tube, remove the needle from the syringe before transferring the sample. Ideally, the sample will be transferred directly into a sterile tube. Alternately, a larger-bore needle can be placed on the syringe and the sample then transferred by puncturing the stopper of the collection tube. A sample collected by cystocentesis can also be used for culture and sensitivity testing. Occasionally, samples contain an increase in RBCs as a result of bladder trauma. The

PROCEDURE 27.2   Urinary Catheterization: Male Dog

Materials
- Sterile gloves
- Sterile water-soluble lubricating jelly
- Antiseptic solution
- Saline
- Urinary catheter
- Syringe

Procedure
1. Place the dog in lateral or dorsal recumbency.
2. Estimate the length of the catheter to be inserted by holding the catheter next to the dog.

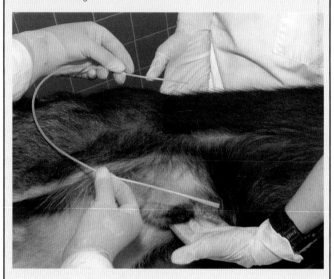

3. Extrude the penis by pushing the penis cranially from the base while pushing the prepuce caudally off of the penis.
4. Gently wash the end of the penis with antiseptic solution and then rinse it with saline.
5. Lubricate the tip of the catheter with sterile water-soluble lubricating jelly.
6. Gently insert the tip of the catheter into the external urethral orifice, and advance it into the lumen of the bladder, being careful not to advance it too far.
7. Collect and discard the first few milliliters of urine, and then collect a sample for urinalysis and culture.

Figure from Taylor S: *Small animal clinical techniques,* St Louis, 2010, Saunders.

urine S-Monovette system (Sarstedt AG & Co., Nümbrecht, Germany) is a commercially available urine-collection device that consists of a sterile, individually wrapped syringe with a disposable tube (Fig. 27.6). This system can simplify cystocentesis collection, and it minimizes the potential for contamination when samples are transferred between a syringe and a collection tube, because the sample is drawn directly into the tube. The tube can also be centrifuged for urine sediment examination. A special tip is also included to collect catheter specimens. The technique for cystocentesis is summarized in Procedure 27.4. Smaller patients can be placed in lateral recumbency to avoid puncturing the descending aorta on midline.

PROCEDURE 27.3 **Urinary Catheterization: Female Dog**

Materials
- Sedation drugs
- Sterile gloves
- Sterile water-soluble lubricating jelly
- Antiseptic solution
- Saline
- Vaginal speculum
- Urinary catheter
- Syringe

Procedure
1. Restrain the dog standing or in sternal recumbency with the feet off the end of the table.
2. Cleanse the external genitalia with antiseptic solution and rinse it with saline.
3. Flush the vagina and vestibule with sterile saline injected through a syringe.
4. Insert a vaginal speculum directed dorsally, and spread the wings of the speculum to visualize the urethral orifice on the ventral floor of the vagina.
5. Lubricate the tip of the catheter with sterile water-soluble lubricating jelly.
6. Gently insert the tip of the catheter into the external urethral orifice, and advance it into the lumen of the bladder, being careful not to advance it too far.

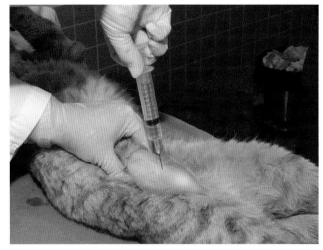

Fig. 27.5 Direct the needle dorsocaudally for cystocentesis. (From Taylor S: *Small animal clinical techniques*, St Louis, 2010, Saunders.)

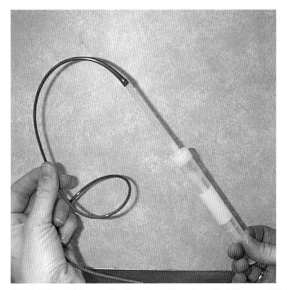

Fig. 27.6 Urine S-Monovette System. (Courtesy B. Mitzner, DVM.)

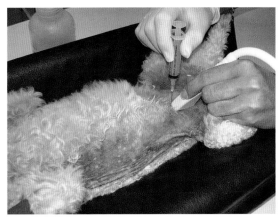

Fig. 27.4 Collection of a urine sample through ultrasound-guided cystocentesis.

> **TECHNICIAN NOTE** Cystocentesis is preferred for sample collection when culture and sensitivity testing is needed.

SPECIMEN STORAGE AND HANDLING

> **TECHNICIAN NOTE** Ideally samples should be analyzed within 30 minutes to 1 hour of collection to avoid postcollection artifacts and degenerative changes. If immediate analysis is not possible, refrigeration preserves most urine constituents for an additional 6 to 12 hours.

All of the aforementioned methods of collection are satisfactory for qualitative analysis. However, for quantitative analysis, a 24-hour sample must be collected. Ratios of certain urine constituents (e.g., protein/creatinine) have been used to obtain data that may be interpreted in a similar manner to 24-hour urinary excretions (Table 27.1).

Refrigeration may have an impact on urine specific gravity, so this test should be done before refrigeration. If a urine sample is going to be refrigerated, it should have a tight-fitting lid to prevent evaporation and contamination. Crystals may form when the urine cools. Decreased glucose and bilirubin concentrations, increased pH as a result of the bacterial

PROCEDURE 27.4   Urine Collection by Cystocentesis

Materials
- Alcohol
- 22- × 1½-in needle
- Syringe or S-Monovette system

Procedure
1. Place the patient in dorsal recumbency.
2. Palpate the bladder to assess its size and location, and clean the skin surface with alcohol.
3. Localize and immobilize the urinary bladder, if possible. Do not apply excessive digital pressure before, during, or after cystocentesis.
4. Attach the needle to the syringe, or use the S-Monovette system.
5. Advance the needle through the ventral abdominal wall to the bladder.
   a. Insert the needle through the bladder wall at an oblique angle directed dorsocaudally so that, as the bladder shrinks, the needle tip remains within the bladder lumen.
   b. Apply suction.
   c. Release all suction after the sample has been obtained to minimize the chance of sample contamination.
6. Withdraw the needle from the abdomen.

breakdown of urea into ammonia, crystal formation with increased sample turbidity, the breakdown of casts and RBCs (especially in dilute or alkaline urine), and bacterial proliferation may occur in samples that are allowed to stand for long periods at room temperature. Many crystals may form in refrigerated samples. Refrigerated urine should be warmed to room temperature before evaluation, but crystals that formed during cooling may not dissolve when the sample is brought to room temperature. The urine sample should be mixed by gentle inversion before evaluation so that formed elements are evenly distributed. Cells tend to break down rapidly in urine, so if cytologic evaluation is to be performed, the urine should be centrifuged soon after collection, and 1 to 2 drops of the patient's serum or bovine albumin should be added to the sediment to preserve cell morphologic characteristics.

TECHNICIAN NOTE Urine samples should be analyzed within 30 minutes to 1 hour of collection.

Samples to be transported to an outside laboratory or held for more than 6 to 12 hours may be preserved by adding one of the following: 1 drop of 40% formalin to 1 oz of urine; toluene sufficient to form a layer on top of the sample; a single thymol crystal; or one part 5% phenol to nine parts urine. If formalin is used as a preservative, chemical tests should be performed before the addition of formalin, because formalin interferes with some chemical analyses (especially that for glucose). However, formalin is the best preservative for formed elements in urine.

FEAR-FREE COLLECTION

The goal of fear-free collection is to alleviate fear, anxiety, and stress (FAS) in our patients. Although not always possible to achieve the best diagnostic results, free-catch methods can be the least stressful way to collect urine samples. With cats, utilize non-absorbent litter substrates. However, the need for catheterization or cystocentesis cannot be avoided in all patients and when restraint is required there are some key concepts to remember. Use gentle control. This means use the least amount of restraint needed. In general, it is beneficial to use treats before, during, and after procedures. Constant communication between team members is critical to ensure that our touches with the patient and treats are timed correctly.

Touch gradient is another fear-free tool. It is a term used to describe how to touch our canine and feline patients to minimize FAS during veterinary procedures. Touch gradient encompasses both gentle control and considerate approach.

Touch gradient has two components:
- It begins by maintaining continual physical hands-on contact throughout the entire procedure or examination whenever possible.

TABLE 27.1   Pros and Cons of Urine Collection Methods

	Pros	Cons
Voided	No risk to the animal Fear free Avoids iatrogenic hematuria	May contain debris from lower urinary and genital tract Quantitative urine culture required
Manual Expression		May induce trauma to urinary tract, resulting in hematuria May be stressful for animal, especially if bladder is painful May contain debris from lower urinary and genital tract Quantitative urine culture required
Catheterization	Provides method to obtain urine sample when other methods of collection have failed	Potential for trauma to urinary tract, especially urethra More invasive than other methods Sedation may be required Risk of introducing bladder infection. Quantitative urine culture required
Cystocentesis	Preferred method of collection for urine culture Avoids contamination of sample from lower urinary tract	Potential risk of trauma if performed incorrectly or animal moves during procedure Potential for iatrogenic hematuria More invasive than spontaneous micturition Potential for bacterial contamination of sample if needle penetrates colon during procedure

- It includes acclimating a patient to an increasing level of touch intensity, while continuously measuring the patient's acceptance and comfort.

Remember to go slow. Let them acclimate to their environment and help them acclimate to the tools and new smells you will be introducing during the procedures.

KEY POINTS

- The best samples for urinalysis are morning samples or samples collected after several hours of water deprivation.
- Preferred methods of urine collection are cystocentesis and catheterization.
- All samples should be labeled immediately after collection.
- Urine samples should be analyzed within 30 minutes to 1 hour of collection.
- Always note the method of urine sample collection on the urinalysis report.
- If the sample cannot be examined within 1 hour of collection, it should be refrigerated or preserved.
- A refrigerated sample should be allowed to warm to room temperature before evaluation.

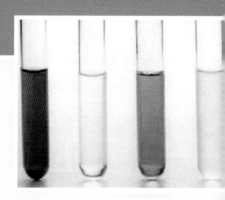

28

Physical Examination of Urine

LEARNING OBJECTIVES

After studying this chapter, you will be able to:
- List the physical evaluations completed on urine samples.
- Describe the significance of variation in urine color.
- Describe possible causes of turbid urine.
- Describe possible causes for urine odor variations.
- List and describe methods for evaluating urine specific gravity.

OUTLINE

Urine Volume, 180
Color, 181
Clarity/Transparency, 182
Odor, 182

Specific Gravity, 182
    Refractometer, 183
    Causes of Altered Urine Specific Gravity, 183
    Osmolality, 184

KEY TERMS

Anuria
Flocculent
Hematuria
Hemoglobinuria
Hypersthenuria
Hyposthenuria

Isosthenuria
Ketones
Myoglobinuria
Oliguria
Pollakiuria
Polydipsia

Polyuria
Specific gravity
Urease
Urinometer
Urochromes

Physical properties of urine include all of the observations that may be made without the aid of a microscope or chemical reagents.
- Volume
- Color
- Odor
- Transparency
- Specific gravity

Chemical analysis and sediment analysis are the other two steps needed to complete the urinalysis and will be covered in the next two chapters. Procedure 28.1 describes the procedure for a routine urinalysis.

URINE VOLUME

The animal's owner often provides information concerning the amount of urine passed. However, owners may mistake frequent urination (pollakiuria) for increased urine production (polyuria). Therefore, obtaining an estimate of the amount of urine that an animal is producing is important.

Many factors unrelated to disease influence the amount of urine produced. Some of these factors include fluid intake, external losses (especially through the respiratory system and the intestinal tract), environmental temperature and humidity, amount and type of food, level of physical activity, and size and species of the animal. Observing a single urination is not sufficient for estimating the urine output of an animal. Ideally, the 24-hour urine volume should be determined, although this is often impractical. Observing an animal in its cage or outdoors may provide a rough estimate of the volume of urine being produced. Table 28.1 lists the approximate daily urine production of common domestic species. The amount of urine produced per day is variable. Normal urine output for adult dogs and cats is approximately 20 to 40 mL/kg body weight per day.

> **TECHNICIAN NOTE** Owners often confuse pollakiuria and polyuria.

An increase in daily urine output or production is termed polyuria, and it is usually accompanied by polydipsia.

PROCEDURE 28.1 Routine Urinalysis

1. Prepare a laboratory sheet with the patient's information and the date, time, and method of urine collection.
2. If the sample was refrigerated, make note on the record and allow the sample to warm to room temperature.
3. Properly mix the sample by gentle inversion.
4. Record the physical characteristics: color, clarity, volume, and odor of sample.
5. Calibrate the refractometer with distilled water to 1.000.
6. Determine and record the specific gravity of the sample.
7. Dip a reagent test strip into the urine sample and then remove it promptly, making sure to lightly tap the edge of the strip onto a paper towel to remove excess urine.
8. Read the pad's color at the appropriate time intervals as stated by the manufacturer's directions, and record the results.
9. Properly label a 15-mL conical centrifuge tube.
10. Pour approximately 5 to 10 mL of the urine sample into the centrifuge tube.
11. Centrifuge the sample for 5 to 6 minutes at 1000 to 2000 rpm.
12. Make note of the amount of sediment.
13. Pour off the supernatant, leaving approximately 0.5 to 1 mL in the tube.
14. Resuspend the sediment by gently mixing it with a pipette or flicking the tube with the fingers.
15. Transfer a drop of reconstituted sediment to a microscope slide with a transfer pipette, and place a coverslip over it.
16. Subdue the light of the microscope by partially closing the iris diaphragm.
17. Examine the entire specimen under the coverslip with the high-power (40×) objective to identify cells, casts, crystals, and bacteria.
18. To help with the detection of these elements, the fine adjustment knob should be continuously focused.
19. Record the results.

TABLE 28.1 Normal Daily Urine Production for Domestic Species

Species	Daily Urine Output (mL/kg)
Dogs	20—40
Cats	20—40
Cattle	17—45
Horses	3—18
Sheep and goats	10—40

Polydipsia is defined as an increase in water consumption. With polyuria, the urine is usually pale or light yellow in color, with a low specific gravity.

Polyuria occurs with many diseases, including:
- nephritis
- diabetes mellitus
- diabetes insipidus
- pyometra in dogs and cats
- and liver disease.

It also occurs with administration of diuretics, corticosteroids, or fluids.

Oliguria, which is a decrease in daily urine output, may occur when an animal has restricted access to water. It can be severe when the environmental temperature increases and causes excess water loss through the respiratory system. With oliguria, the urine is usually concentrated and has a high specific gravity.

Oliguria also occurs with many disease and can be seen with:
- acute nephritis
- fever
- shock
- heart disease
- and dehydration.

Anuria, which is the absence of urine production, may be seen with:
- complete urethral obstruction
- urinary bladder rupture
- and renal shutdown.

COLOR

Normal urine color is light yellow to amber as a result of the presence of pigments called urochromes. The magnitude of yellow color in urine varies with the degree of urine concentration or dilution (Table 28.2). Colorless urine usually has a low specific gravity, and it is often associated with polyuria. Dark yellow to yellow-brown urine generally has a high specific gravity, and it may be associated with oliguria. Yellow-brown or green urine that produces a greenish-yellow foam when shaken is likely to contain bile pigments. Red or red-brown urine indicates the presence of red blood cells (RBCs; hematuria) or hemoglobin (hemoglobinuria). Urine that is brown when voided may contain myoglobin (myoglobinuria). Myoglobin is excreted when conditions that cause muscle cell lysis are present, such as rhabdomyolysis in horses. Some drugs may alter the color of urine; red, green, or blue urine may be observed. When observing urine, it should be in a clear plastic or glass

TABLE 28.2 Significance of Urine Colors

Color	Significance
Colorless or pale yellow	Dilute, low specific gravity, poorly concentrated urine
Dark yellow to orange	Concentrated urine (dark yellow) Bilirubinuria (orange to orange-brown)
Yellow-green	Photo-oxidation of bilirubin to bilirubinuria Biliverdin
Yellow-brown to brown	Bilirubinuria
Red	Hematuria Hemoglobinuria Myoglobinuria Methemoglobin
Brown to black	Methemoglobin Oxyglobin administration Metronidazole administration
Deep red to port wine	Porphyrins

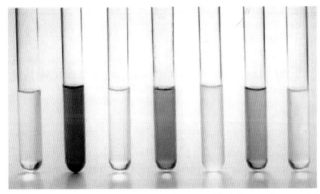

Fig. 28.1 Urine color is best assessed in good lighting against a white background. (From Little S: *The cat*, St Louis, 2012, Saunders.)

TABLE 28.3   Correlation to Urine Clarity

Urine Transparency	Description	Possible Clinical Correlation
Clear	No turbidity No visible particles Newsprint visible through the specimen	Normal Inadequately concentrated urine
Hazy, cloudy, turbid	No visible particles, although clarity is increasing obscured	Mucus Cellular elements Crystalluria
Milky	White, turbid specimen	Pyuria Lipiduria Chyluria
Flocculent	Many large particles observed	Precipitation of crystals Fecal contamination

container against a white background to be properly evaluated for color (Fig. 28.1).

> **TECHNICIAN NOTE** Evaluate the color and clarity of urine by placing it in a clear container and holding it against a white background.

CLARITY/TRANSPARENCY

In most species, freshly voided urine is transparent or clear. Normal equine urine is cloudy as a result of the high concentration of calcium carbonate crystals and mucus secreted by glands in the renal pelvis. Normal rabbit urine also has high concentrations of calcium carbonate crystals, and it appears milky. When observing urine for the degree of transparency, it should be placed against a letter-print background. Transparency is noted as clear, slightly cloudy, cloudy, or turbid (flocculent), depending on how well the letters can be read through the sample. Clear samples usually do not have much sediment on centrifugation. Cloudy samples usually contain large particles and often yield a significant amount of sediment on centrifugation. Urine may become cloudy while standing as a result of bacterial multiplication or crystal formation. Substances that cause urine to be cloudy include RBCs, white blood cells (WBCs), epithelial cells, casts, crystals, mucus, fat, and bacteria. Other causes of turbidity can include contaminants from the collection container or surface and contamination with feces. Flocculent samples contain suspended particles that are sometimes large enough to be seen with the naked eye. Table 28.3 helps correlate descriptions of transparency with possible clinical correlations.

ODOR

The odor of urine is not highly diagnostic, but it may sometimes be helpful. Normal urine has a distinctive odor that varies among species. The urine of male cats, goats, and pigs has a strong odor. An ammonia odor may occur with cystitis caused by bacteria that produce urease (*Proteus* spp. or *Staphylococcus* spp.) and that have metabolized urea to ammonia. Samples left

standing at room temperature may occasionally develop an ammonia odor as a result of bacterial growth. A characteristic sweet or fruity odor of the urine indicates ketones and is most commonly found with diabetes mellitus, ketosis in cows, and pregnancy disease in ewes. Medications can also alter the odors associated with urines.

> **TECHNICIAN NOTE** Samples left standing at room temperature may develop an ammonia odor as a result of bacterial growth.

SPECIFIC GRAVITY

Specific gravity is defined as the weight (density) of a quantity of liquid as compared with that of an equal amount of distilled water. The number and molecular weight of dissolved solutes determine the specific gravity of urine. The normal composition of urine is that it contains 5% solutes and 95% water. Specific gravity may be determined before or after centrifugation, because the particles that settle during centrifugation have little or no effect on specific gravity. Whichever method is used to perform the evaluation of specific gravity in a specific clinic and whether this evaluation occurs before or after centrifugation, the same method must be consistently performed by all clinic personnel. If the urine is turbid, the sample should be centrifuged and the supernatant used to determine the specific gravity. The specific gravity of urine from polyuric patients tends to be low, and urine from oliguric patients tends to be high. The specific gravity of normal urine depends on eating and drinking habits, the environmental temperature, and when the sample was collected. An early morning mid-urination sample tends to be the most concentrated. The interpretation of urine specific gravity (USG) yields information about the patient's hydration status and the ability of the patient's kidneys to concentrate or dilute urine. The specific gravity of normal animals is extremely variable, and it fluctuates throughout the day. Table 28.4 lists the USG ranges for normal domestic

TABLE 28.4 Urine Specific Gravity Values for Common Domestic Species

	Dog	Cat	Horse	Cattle	Sheep
Specific gravity	1.025 (1.001–1.065)	1.030 (1.001–1.080)	1.035 (1.020–1.050)	1.015 (1.005–1.040)	1.030 (1.020–1.040)

TABLE 28.5 Changes in Urine Specific Gravity for Dogs and Cats and their Significance

USG	Significance	Referred to as
In the dog: Greater than 1.030 In the cat: Greater than 1.035	Urine is more concentrated than the glomerular ultrafiltrate. Adequate rental function Dehydration or hypoperfusion should be considered in a dehydrated patient.	Hypersthenuria
In the dog: 1.013–1.029 In the cat: 1.013–1.034	Urine is more concentrated than the glomerular ultrafiltrate. Renal function may be normal. Moderately concentrated urine If patient is dehydrated or azotemic, renal insufficiency or extra-renal impairment of concentrating ability is likely.	Hypersthenuria
1.008–1.012	Urine, plasma, and glomerular ultrafiltrate osmolality are similar. Potentially normal renal function re-evaluation is warranted. If patient is dehydrated or azotemic, renal failure is likely.	Isosthenuria
Less than 1.008	Urine is more dilute than the glomerular ultrafiltrate. Renal tubules are able to reabsorb solutes from tubular fluid. Dilute urine Consider extrarenal causes of inadequate urine concentration such as osmotic diuresis and decreased medullary concentration gradient.	Hyposthenuria

animals. In normal dogs, the USG may range from 1.001 to 1.065; in normal cats, it may range from 1.001 to 1.080. Table 28.5 shows variable values and how they can be used to interpret changes in patients.

To determine the specific gravity of urine, a refractometer, a urinometer, or reagent strips can be used. Reagent strip specific gravity is the least reliable method for determining USG in animals. USG is less frequently determined with the use of a urinometer. This instrument requires a large amount of urine (approximately 10 mL), and it generally provides less-reproducible results than a refractometer.

> **TECHNICIAN NOTE** USG should NOT be measured using a reagent strip as it is the least reliable method available.

Refractometer

Specific gravity is most commonly determined by a refractometer. More information about the principle of the refractometer is presented in Procedure 2.1, which can be found in Unit 1, Chapter 2. Urine contains substances that absorb various wavelengths of light. The light waves bend as they pass through the medium, and this bend is measured by the refractometer. The refractive index of a fluid is influenced by the same factors that determine specific gravity, and it therefore provides an estimate of USG. It is important to note that refractometers that are not calibrated for veterinary patients may not provide accurate results, especially with feline samples. Research has demonstrated that canine and feline samples with identical specific gravities have different refractive indexes. Refractometers calibrated for veterinary samples are widely available, and they provide accurate evaluations of USG. It is also common for a specific gravity reading to be higher than the range that can be read by an instrument that is not designed for veterinary species. In this case, the sample must be diluted and reevaluated by mixing equal volumes of the sample with distilled water. Use a drop of that mixture to determine the specific gravity, and then multiply the numbers after the decimal point by 2. For example, if the dilution contains equal parts distilled water and urine and the specific gravity of the dilution is 1.030, then the actual specific gravity is 1.060. See Procedure 28.2.

Students should remember that glucosuria and proteinuria can both impact USG, resulting in overestimation of the USG. Protein concentrations of 1g/dL can increase USG approximately 0.003 to 0.005. Glucose concentrations of 1000 mg/dL increase USG approximately 0.004 to 0.005.

Causes of Altered Urine Specific Gravity

Increased USG is referred to as hypersthenuria, although this term is not commonly used. It is seen with decreased water

---

PROCEDURE 28.2 Calculation for Dilution of USG

1. Add 50 µL of urine sample to 50 µL deionized water. This will make a 1:2 dilution.
2. Mix well.
3. Read the specific gravity using a refractometer.
4. Multiple the result by 2.
5. Example:
   a. Initial result before dilute was >1.050
   b. Result after a 1:2 dilution was performed was 1.035
   c. Calculation: 0.035 × 2 = 0.0700
   d. Final specific gravity result = 1.070

---

intake, increased fluid loss through sources other than urination (e.g., sweating, panting, diarrhea), and increased excretion of urine solutes. Decreased water intake in animals with normal renal function rapidly causes increased USG. Increased USG may occur with acute renal failure, dehydration, and shock.

Decreased USG is referred to as hyposthenuria. It is seen with diseases in which the kidneys cannot resorb water and with increased fluid intake, such as with polydipsia or excessive fluid administration. Pyometra, diabetes insipidus, psychogenic polydipsia, some liver diseases, certain types of renal disease, and diuretic therapy may also cause decreased USG.

Isosthenuria occurs when the USG approaches that of glomerular filtrate (1.008 to 1.012). In other words, urine with this specific gravity range has not been concentrated or diluted by the kidneys. Animals with chronic renal disease frequently produce isosthenuric urine. In animals with kidney disease, the closer the specific gravity is to isosthenuric, the greater the amount of kidney function that has been lost. When these animals are deprived of water, their USG usually remains in the isosthenuric range. Animals with decreased renal function are often slightly to moderately dehydrated and have USG that is slightly greater than isosthenuric (1.015 to 1.020).

Osmolality

Osmolality is a concentration of solutes in a solution and provides a measure of urine concentration. It is more accurate than using specific gravity. However, it is impractical for clinical practice. It is available from some referral laboratories. This specific measurement is infrequently needed in clinical cases.

■ KEY POINTS

- Physical properties of urine include volume, color, odor, transparency, and specific gravity.
- Normal urine output for adult dogs and cats is approximately 20 to 40 mL/kg body weight per day.
- Normal urine color is light yellow to amber and varies with the degree of urine concentration or dilution.

- In most species, freshly voided urine is transparent or clear.
- Substances that cause urine to be cloudy include RBCs, WBCs, epithelial cells, casts, crystals, mucus, fat, and bacteria.
- USG is a measure of the dissolved solutes in urine.
- USG is normally evaluated with a refractometer.

29

Chemical Evaluation of Urine

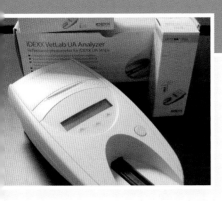

LEARNING OBJECTIVES

After studying this chapter, you will be able to:

- Describe the procedure for performing the chemical analysis of urine.
- List the chemical tests that are commonly performed on urine samples.
- Discuss the significance of proteinuria.

- Describe methods used to differentiate between hematuria and hemoglobinuria.
- Discuss the significance of glucosuria.
- List conditions that can be characterized by ketonuria.
- List conditions that can be characterized by bilirubinuria.

OUTLINE

KEY TERMS

Bence Jones protein
Bilirubinuria
Glucosuria

Hematuria
Hemoglobinuria
Ketonuria

pH
Proteinuria

Testing for various chemical constituents of urine is usually performed with reagent strips that are impregnated with appropriate chemicals or with reagent tablets. There are some automated analyzers that are used for serum chemistry that can also be used for urine testing, although modifications of the procedures may be required. Many of those tests are performed concurrent with electrolyte testing, and they are discussed further in Unit 4. The container of reagent strips must be stored at room temperature with the lid tightly closed, and the expiration date should also be noted. Some reagent strips simultaneously test for numerous constituents, whereas other strips exist for individual tests. The reagent strip should be dipped into the sample so that it is fully immersed; it should then be removed and the long edge tilted on a paper towel to allow excess urine to be wicked away. Alternatively, urine can be added to the reagent strip from a pipette, making sure that each reagent pad is fully saturated. Color changes on each reagent pad are noted at specific time intervals. The concentration of various constituents is determined by comparing the colors on the strip with the color chart on the label of the strip container (Fig. 29.1). The manufacturer's directions must be carefully followed. It is important to note that a large number of conditions (e.g., medications, dietary factors, environmental factors) can affect urinalysis test results (Table 29.1).

pH

- **Clinical Significance**
  - Result of the total body acid–base balance
- **Expected Values**
  - Dogs & Cats: 5.5–7.5
- **Acidic Urine**
  - Meat-based diet
  - Administration of acidifying agents

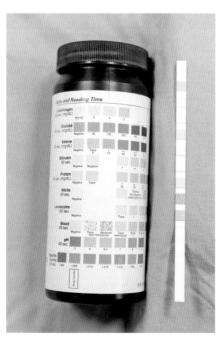

Fig. 29.1 Reagent strip test container and combination dipstick strip.

- Metabolic acidosis
- Respiratory acidosis
- Protein catabolic states
- Severe vomiting
- **Alkaline Urine**
  - Vegetable-based diet
  - Administration of alkalinizing agents
  - Urinary tract infection by urease-producing bacteria
  - Postprandial alkaline tide
  - Metabolic alkalosis
  - Respiratory alkalosis
  - Renal tubular acidosis

The pH expresses the hydrogen ion (H^+) concentration. Essentially, pH is a measure of the degree of acidity or alkalinity of urine. A pH of more than 7.0 is alkaline, whereas a pH of less than 7.0 is acidic. Proper technique must be used to obtain accurate results. The urine sample must be fresh so that accurate results can be obtained. The pH of samples left standing open at room temperature tends to increase as a result of a loss of carbon dioxide, whereas delays in reading the reaction may lead to color changes and false readings. If samples that contain urease-producing bacteria (i.e., *Proteus* spp. or *Staphylococcus* spp.) are left standing, the pH is usually increased.

The kidneys play a role in the acid–base regulation of the body. The kidneys must vary the pH of urine to compensate for the patient's diet and the products of metabolism. The pH of a healthy animal's urine depends largely on its diet. Alkaline urine is usually found in animals that consume plant-based diets, whereas high-protein cereal diets or diets of animal origin cause acidic urine. Therefore, herbivores normally have alkaline urine, carnivores have acidic urine, and omnivores have either acidic or alkaline urine, depending on what has

been ingested. Many dog foods contain substantial amounts of plant material that may cause the urine to be slightly alkaline. Nursing herbivores have acidic urine from the consumption of milk. Other factors such as stress and excitement (especially in cats) increase the urine pH and may create a transient glucosuria. Table 29.2 lists the normal urine constituents and characteristics, including pH, for common domestic species.

> **TECHNICIAN NOTE** Herbivores normally have alkaline urine, carnivores have acidic urine, and omnivores have either acidic or alkaline urine, depending on what has been ingested.

Urine pH is usually measured with reagent strips or a pH meter. Factors that may decrease the pH (acidity) include fever, starvation, a high-protein diet, acidosis, excessive muscular activity, and the administration of certain drugs. Increased pH (alkalinity) may be caused by alkalosis, high-fiber diets (plants), infection of the urinary tract with urease bacteria, the use of certain drugs, or urine retention such as that which occurs with urethral obstruction or bladder paralysis. If the pH of the urine is too acidic or too alkaline, specific crystals or uroliths can form. The pH can be manipulated with diet to help dissolve the solids or prevent them from forming.

PROTEIN

- **Clinical Significance**
  - Can indicate prerenal, overflow proteinuria, renal, post-renal, and tubular secretion diseases
- **Expected Values**
  - 0–30 mg/dL
- **Increased in**
  - Glomerular disease
  - Inflammatory disease

Protein is usually absent or present in only trace amounts in normal urine obtained by catheterization or cystocentesis. In healthy animals, plasma proteins that pass into the glomerular filtrate are resorbed in the renal tubules before the filtrate reaches the renal pelvis. However, voided samples or those obtained by expressing the bladder may contain a small amount of protein from secretions that may contaminate urine during its passage along the urinary tract. Trauma to the urinary tract that results from cystocentesis, catheterization, or bladder expression may occasionally cause sufficient bleeding that results in a trace of protein in the urine. Urine protein measurements are interpreted in the light of the collection method, the urine specific gravity, the rate of urine formation, and contributions from any hemorrhage or inflammation noted by sample analysis. Protein levels in the urine may be measured by several methods, including reagent test strips and the sulfosalicylic acid turbidity test.

Protein Determination by Reagent Test Strips

Urine dipsticks allow for the semiquantitative measurement of protein in urine via progressive color changes on the reaction pad. Reagent strip analysis is a rapid, convenient, and

TABLE 29.1 Effect of Drugs and Other Factors on the Measurement of Constituents in Urine

Drug or Variable	Specific Gravity	Urine pH	Proteinuria	Glucosuria (Dipstick)	Ketonuria	Bilirubinuria	Urobilinogen	Hemoglobinuria/ Myoglobinuria	Nitrituria	Pyuria
Acetazolamide		↑	⇑1				⇑			
Aminoglycosides			⇑2	↑						⇑1
Ascorbic acid		↓		⇓		⇓	↓	⇓	⇓	
Cephalosporins			⇑2	↑						⇑1
Chlorpromazine			⇑2			↓				
Colchicine	↓									
Corticosteroids	↓									
Dipyrone				⇓						
Diuretics	↓									
Methionine		↓			↑					
Penicillins			⇑2			⇑	⇑		⇑	
Phenazopyridine			⇑1		⇑	⇑	⇑			
Phenolphthalein					⇑					
Phenothiazines						⇑	⇑			
Procaine							⇑			
Radiographic contrast media	⇑		⇑2							
Salicylates			⇑2	⇓		⇓				
Sodium bicarbonate		↑	⇑1				↑			
Sulfobromophthalein					⇑		⇑			
Sulfonamides			⇑2				⇑			
Urinary acidifiers		↓					↓			
Acetoacetate (ketonuria)				⇓						
Alkaline urine	⇓1		⇑1⇓2						⇓3	
Bilirubinuria							⇑			
Highly concentrated urine								⇓		
Nitrituria						⇓	⇑	⇓		
Proteinuria	⇑1		⇑1	⇓						
Refrigerated urine				⇓						
Time		⇑				⇓	⇓			
Ultraviolet light										

↑, Value increased because of physiologic change; ↓, value decreased because of physiologic change; ⇑, value increased because of interference with method; ⇓, value decreased because of interference with method or collection changes; 1, dipstick; 2, sulfosalicylic acid method; 3, sediment.

From Meyer D: *Veterinary laboratory medicine: interpretation & diagnosis*, ed 3, St Louis, 2004, Saunders.

TABLE 29.2   Urine Values for Common Domestic Species

	Dog	Cat	Horse	Cattle	Sheep
Specific gravity	1.025 (1.001–1.065)	1.030 (1.001–1.080)	1.035 (1.020–1.050)	1.015 (1.005–1.040)	1.030 (1.020–1.040)
pH	6–7	6–7	7–8.5	7–8.5	6–8.5
Glucose	None	None	None	None	None
Protein	None/trace	None/trace	None	None/trace	None/trace
Bilirubin	None/trace	None/trace	None/trace	None	None/trace
Ketone	None	None	None	None	None
Occult blood	None	None	None	None	None

reasonably accurate method of determining urinary protein levels. The accuracy of these methods is variable. Reagent strips primarily detect albumin (protein soluble in water), and they are much less sensitive to globulins (proteins insoluble in water). False-positive results may occur in alkaline urine, depending on factors such as diet, urinary tract infection, and urine retention (urethral obstruction). Protein measurements that are considered excessive or pathologic should be confirmed by a sulfosalicylic acid turbidity test or specific biochemical analysis. Microalbuminuria is the presence of albumin in urine that is not detected by the reagent strip method. The reagent strip method detects urine protein concentrations that are greater than 30 mg/dL. The albumin-capture enzyme-linked immunosorbent assay (ELISA) method is used to measure albumin levels 1 to 30 mg/dL in the urine. See Unit 9 for more information about the principles of ELISA tests.

Protein Determination by Sulfosalicylic Acid Turbidity Test

Sulfosalicylic acid turbidity determines urine protein levels via acid precipitation. The resultant turbidity is proportional to the concentration of protein. Results are compared with levels in prepared standards and thus may be reported in semiquantitative units. The advantage of this method is that it is equally sensitive to albumin and globulins, and it is quite useful to confirm strip methods, especially in alkaline urine. This test also measures Bence Jones proteins, which are light chain proteins that can pass through the glomerulus. Components of extremely alkaline urine may interact with the acid and decrease the amount of protein precipitated.

Urine Protein/Creatinine Ratio

This test is used to help confirm significant amounts of protein in the urine. To determine its significance, the urine protein concentration can be compared with that of creatinine. The sample is centrifuged to separate particulate matter (cells) from dissolved substances (protein), and the creatinine and protein concentrations of the supernatant are used. The ratio is obtained by dividing the protein concentration by the creatinine concentration. The ratio is not affected by urine concentration and volume and therefore aids in the accurate assessment of urine protein loss in patients with low specific gravity.

> **TECHNICIAN NOTE** Acute and chronic renal diseases lead to proteinuria.

Interpretation of Protein in Urine

The presence of protein in the urine (proteinuria) is usually abnormal, and it is primarily attributable to disease of the urinary tract or possibly of the genital system. Occasionally a small amount of protein is found in the urine of normal animals. Transient proteinuria may result from a temporary increase in glomerular permeability that allows excessive protein to enter the filtrate. This condition is caused by increased pressure in the glomerular capillaries, and it may be found with muscle exertion, emotional stress, or convulsions. Occasionally a small amount of urine protein is found after parturition, during the first few days of life, and during estrus.

Very dilute urine may yield a false-negative result, because the protein concentration may be below the sensitivity of the testing method. A trace amount of protein in a very dilute sample may be clinically significant, because dilute urine often occurs when a large volume of urine is being produced, such as in a patient with chronic renal failure. Trace protein in very dilute samples indicates a higher degree of proteinuria than trace amounts present in a normally concentrated sample.

In most cases, proteinuria indicates disease of the urinary tract, especially of the kidneys. Both acute and chronic renal diseases lead to proteinuria. Acute nephritis is characterized by marked proteinuria with white blood cells (WBCs) and casts in the urine, whereas with chronic renal disease, the degree of proteinuria is qualitatively less. However, with chronic renal disease, urine output is usually excessive with low specific gravity; therefore the total protein excreted is actually quite significant. The ratio of urine protein to creatinine is used to determine the degree of protein loss in a patient with chronic renal disease.

Multiple myeloma, which is a cancer of plasma cells, may produce large quantities of light chain proteins (Bence Jones proteins) that may leak through the glomerulus. In patients with myeloma, proteins may be passed in the urine because they have damaged the glomerulus or because they are the "light chains" that freely pass through the glomerulus. Because these proteins do not react with the protein pads on the reagent strips, the sulfosalicylic acid method is necessary to detect and quantify them.

Mild proteinuria is seen with passive congestion of the kidneys, as occurs with congestive heart failure or any other impediment of blood flow from the kidneys. Proteinuria of renal origin may also be caused by trauma, tumors, renal infarcts, or necrosis that results from drugs and chemicals such as sulfonamides, lead, mercury, arsenic, and ether.

Inflammation of the urinary or genital tract may cause proteinuria of postrenal origin. Proteinuria also may be seen with traumatic catheterization or bladder expression.

GLUCOSE

- **Clinical Significance**
  - Glucosuria usually occurs during hyperglycemia when the plasma glucose exceeds the renal glucose threshold levels that vary by species. In dogs the threshold is 180 mg/dL; in cats the threshold is 280 mg/dL.
- **Expected Values**
  - Negative
- **When Present**
  - Diabetes mellitus
  - Stress
  - Infusion of dextrose fluids
  - Pheochromocytoma
  - Proximal renal tubular disease
  - Aminoglycoside toxicity
  - Acute renal failure
  - Fanconi syndrome
  - Primary renal glucosuria

The presence of glucose in urine is known as glucosuria or glycosuria. Glucose is filtered through the glomerulus and resorbed by the kidney tubules. The amount of glucose in the urine depends on blood glucose levels and on the rates of glomerular filtration and tubular resorption. Glucosuria usually does not occur in normal animals unless the blood glucose level exceeds the renal threshold (approximately 170 to 180 mg/dL for dogs). At this concentration, tubular resorption cannot keep up with the glomerular filtration of glucose, and glucose passes into the urine.

> **TECHNICIAN NOTE** Glucosuria often indicates diabetes mellitus.

Glucosuria occurs in patients with diabetes mellitus as a result of a deficiency of insulin or an inability of insulin to function. Insulin is necessary to transport glucose into body cells, and a deficiency causes hyperglycemia and the spilling of glucose into the urine. A high-carbohydrate meal may lead to blood glucose levels that exceed the renal threshold and thus glucosuria. Because of this, a period of fasting is recommended before the urine glucose concentration is determined. Fear, excitement, or restraint (especially in cats) often causes hyperglycemia and glucosuria as a result of epinephrine release. Glucosuria often occurs after the intravenous administration of

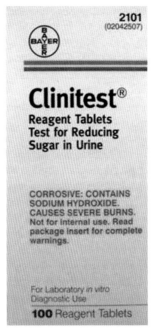

Fig. 29.2 Clinitest Reagent Tablets for the detection of sugars in the urine.

fluids that contain glucose and occasionally after general anesthesia. Rarely, glucosuria is found with hyperthyroidism, Cushing's disease, and chronic liver disease. A rare condition called renal glucosuria may occur when the blood glucose concentration is in the normal range. Renal glucosuria is caused by the reduced resorption of glucose in the renal tubules. Glucosuria may occur in some cats with chronic disease, possibly as a result of altered proximal renal tubular function.

False-positive results for glucose may be seen after the use of various drugs, including ascorbic acid (vitamin C), morphine, salicylates (e.g., aspirin), cephalosporins, and penicillin.

Various reagent test strips are available to detect glucose in urine. Clinitest Reagent Tablets (Bayer Corporation, Leverkusen, Germany) (Fig. 29.2) are also available. These tablets detect any sugar in the urine, whereas most reagent test strips detect only glucose.

KETONES

- **Clinical Significance**
  - They indicate that excess lipid mobilization is taking place.
- **Expected Values**
  - Negative
- **When Present**
  - Diabetes ketoacidosis
  - Starvation
  - Prolonged fasting
  - Glycogen storage disease
  - Low carbohydrate diets
  - Persistent fever
  - Persistent hypoglycemia

Ketones include acetone, acetoacetic acid, and β-hydroxy-butyric acid. Ketone bodies are formed during the incomplete catabolism of fatty acids. Normal animals may have small amounts of ketones in the blood. Conditions that are characterized by altered carbohydrate metabolism may result in excessive amounts of fat catabolism to provide energy. When fatty acid metabolism is not accompanied by sufficient carbohydrate metabolism, excess ketones are present in the urine, which is a condition called ketonuria.

A common cause of ketonuria is ketonemia, or ketosis, in lactating cows and pregnant ewes and cows. Ketosis usually occurs early during lactation (i.e., 3 to 6 weeks after freshening), when the energy for milk production exceeds the capacity of the cow to ingest sufficient feed to meet its energy requirements. In ewes, this condition is called pregnancy toxemia, and it is seen when the ewe is carrying twins or triplets. Ketosis is associated with hypoglycemia, and it is caused by carbohydrate intake that is insufficient to meet energy requirements. Body fat is then rapidly metabolized, which results in ketonemia and ketonuria.

Ketonuria frequently occurs in animals with diabetes mellitus. Because the animal lacks the insulin necessary for carbohydrate metabolism, fat is broken down to meet the animal's energy needs, and excess ketones are excreted in the urine. Ketones are important sources of energy, and they are normally produced during fat metabolism. However, problems develop when excessive ketones are produced. Ketones are toxic and cause central nervous system depression and acidosis. Acidosis that results from ketonemia is termed ketoacidosis.

Ketonemia with ketonuria also occurs with high-fat diets, starvation, fasting, long-term anorexia, and impaired liver function. With a high-fat diet, carbohydrates meet a relatively low percentage of energy needs, so a great amount of fat is used to meet energy needs. In the fasting, starved, or anorexic animal, body fat is used to meet energy needs, thus producing a greater-than-normal amount of ketones. With liver damage, impaired carbohydrate metabolism leads to fat serving as the main energy source, especially when the damaged liver cannot store adequate amounts of glycogen.

Measurement of Urine Ketone Content

Urinary ketones are detected by using urinary reagent strips with a ketone reagent pad. The color intensity is roughly proportional to the concentration of urine ketones. These methods are most sensitive to acetoacetic acid; they are less sensitive to acetone, and they do not detect β-hydroxybutyric acid. β-Hydroxybutyric acid is the first ketone produced by the body in any condition that causes ketosis. Urine reagent test strips may not adequately identify these patients until the ketosis has been present for some time.

BILE PIGMENTS

- **Clinical Significance**
  - It will be elevated in urine before it is elevated in the serum.

- **Expected Values**
  - Negative
  - Can be seen in trace amounts in concentrated samples and still be normal
- **When Present**
  - Hemolysis
  - Liver disease
  - Extrahepatic obstruction
  - Fever
  - Starvation

Bile pigments that are commonly detected in urine are bilirubin and urobilinogen. Only conjugated bilirubin (water soluble) is found in urine, because unconjugated bilirubin does not pass through the glomerulus into the renal filtrate; it is bound to albumin, and it is not water soluble. Normal dogs (especially males) occasionally have bilirubin in their urine (bilirubinuria) because of a low renal threshold for conjugated bilirubin and the ability of their kidneys to conjugate bilirubin. Many normal cattle also have small amounts of bilirubin in their urine. Bilirubin is usually not found in the urine of cats, pigs, sheep, or horses. In cats, the renal threshold is many times that of dogs; thus, any amount of bilirubin in cat urine is considered abnormal and suggests disease. Urobilinogen is normal in urine and indicates normal enterohepatic bilirubin circulation.

> **TECHNICIAN NOTE** Bilirubinuria is seen with a variety of conditions, including bile duct obstruction, hemolytic anemia, and liver disease.

Bilirubinuria is seen with a number of diseases, including the obstruction of bile flow from the liver to the small intestine as well as liver disease. Bilirubinuria results from the accumulation in hepatic cells of conjugated bilirubin that is released into the blood and excreted in the urine. Conditions that cause biliary obstruction include calculi in the bile duct, tumors in the area of the bile duct, acute enteritis, pancreatitis, and obstruction of the upper intestinal tract. When conjugated, bilirubin enters the bloodstream after being released from damaged liver cells and then passes into the urine.

Hemolytic anemia may also cause bilirubinuria, especially in dogs. In patients with hemolytic anemia, the liver's ability to metabolize the excess bilirubin may be exceeded, thereby resulting in the release of conjugated bilirubin into the blood and ultimately bilirubinuria. In dogs, unconjugated bilirubin from hemoglobin catabolism in the mononuclear phagocytic system can be conjugated in the kidney and passed in the urine.

Bilirubinuria is detected with the Ictotest (Bayer Corporation). A diazo compound in the reagent tablet reacts with bilirubin to produce a blue or purple color. The speed with which the color change occurs and the degree of color change indicates the amount of bilirubin present. Reagent strips are less sensitive than Ictotest tablets. Ictotest tablet tests should be performed to confirm bilirubinuria that has been detected by a dipstick test. Urine to be tested for bilirubin must not be exposed to light, because bilirubin is broken down by short-wave light.

False-negative results for bilirubin occur in urine that is exposed to sunlight or artificial light.

In the intestines, bacteria convert bilirubin into stercobilinogen and urobilinogen. The bulk of these products are excreted in the feces, but some are resorbed into the bloodstream and excreted by the liver into the intestinal tract. A small amount of resorbed urobilinogen is excreted by the kidneys into the urine. Urobilinogen in a urine sample is considered normal. The reliability of screening tests for the detection of urobilinogen is questionable as a result of the instability of urobilinogen.

BLOOD (HEMOPROTEIN)

- **Clinical Significance**
  - Doesn't differentiate between RBCs, hemoglobin, or myoglobin. Always confirm with sediment.
- **Expected Values**
  - Negative
- **Increased in**
  - Hematuria
  - Hemolysis
  - Rhabdomyolysis

Tests for blood in urine detect hematuria, which is the presence of intact red blood cells (RBCs) in urine; hemoglobinuria, which is the presence of free hemoglobin in urine; and myoglobinuria, which is the presence of myoglobin in the urine. Hematuria, hemoglobinuria, and myoglobinuria may occur simultaneously; the presence of one does not rule out the others. The urine sediment should also be examined for intact RBCs.

Hematuria

Hematuria is usually a sign of disease that is causing bleeding somewhere in the urogenital tract, whereas hemoglobinuria usually indicates intravascular hemolysis. Some systemic conditions may also cause hematuria. In very dilute or highly alkaline urine, RBCs often lyse to yield hemoglobin. Therefore, in dilute or highly alkaline urine, hemoglobinuria may not be the result of hemoglobin entering the urine through the glomerulus. Ghost cells (the shells of lysed RBCs) may be seen during the microscopic examination of sediment if the source of hemoglobin is the lysis of RBCs within the excretory pathway or in vitro.

Moderate to large amounts of blood impart a cloudy red, brown, or wine color to urine. Similar colors that have a transparent appearance that remains after centrifugation indicate hemoglobinuria. With minute amounts of blood in the urine, a visible color change is usually not evident. Occult or hidden blood occurs when the urine is not obviously discolored by blood but blood is detected by chemical analysis. More information about hematuria is found in the section on microscopic examination of urinary sediment in Chapter 30.

> **TECHNICIAN NOTE** Hematuria, hemoglobinuria, and myoglobinuria can occur simultaneously in urine samples.

Hemoglobinuria

Hemoglobinuria is usually the result of intravascular hemolysis. Hemoglobin from RBCs that are broken down intravascularly is normally bound to the plasma protein haptoglobin. When hemoglobin is bound to haptoglobin, it does not pass through the glomeruli. If intravascular hemolysis overwhelms the binding ability of haptoglobin, then hemoglobinemia leads to hemoglobinuria, because free hemoglobin filters through glomeruli. Hemoglobinuria is indicated by a positive test for hemoglobin without RBCs in the urine sediment, or the degree of the test reaction is often greater than what may be accounted for by the numbers of RBCs in the urine sediment. When hemoglobin concentration is sufficiently high in the urine to impart red discoloration, the urine remains red after centrifugation. If the discoloration is caused by intact RBCs, then the urine is clear above the pellet after centrifugation. Partial clearing after centrifugation indicates both hemoglobinuria and hematuria. The presence of hemoglobin (either as free hemoglobin or in RBCs) must be confirmed by a urine dipstick test and further evaluation by microscopic examination.

Hemoglobinuria may be seen with many conditions that cause intravascular hemolysis. Conditions that can cause intravascular hemolysis include immune-mediated hemolytic anemia, isoimmune hemolytic disease of neonates, incompatible blood transfusions, leptospirosis, babesiosis, certain heavy metals (e.g., copper), and the ingestion of certain poisonous plants. Other conditions that cause hemoglobinuria include severe hypophosphatemia, postparturient hemoglobinemia in cattle, and hemolysis that occurs when cattle drink large quantities of water after being unable to obtain water (e.g., after a long period of low temperatures has frozen their usual water source).

If the urine is dilute or very alkaline, hemoglobinuria can originate from the lysis of RBCs in the urine. This condition must be considered hematuria, because intact RBCs were initially present. Often ghost RBCs may be found when hemoglobinuria is caused by the release of hemoglobin from RBCs in vitro.

Because the test for blood in the urine detects hemoglobinuria, hematuria, and myoglobinuria, other considerations include sediment examination, history, physical examination findings, and additional laboratory procedures to determine the cause of the positive test for blood in the urine. Contamination of reagent strips or collection containers with oxidizing agents, such as bleach, can cause a false-positive test for blood in the urine.

Myoglobinuria

Myoglobin is a protein that is found in muscle. Severe muscle damage causes myoglobin to leak from muscle cells into the blood. Myoglobin passes through the glomeruli and is excreted in the urine. Urine that contains myoglobin is usually very dark brown to almost black, but at low concentrations, the urine may have a similar color to that seen in patients with hemoglobinuria. Distinguishing myoglobinuria from hemoglobinuria may be difficult. History and clinical findings that suggest muscle damage help to determine whether a positive hemoglobin test is caused by the presence of myoglobin. Myoglobinuria is frequently seen in horses with exertional rhabdomyolysis.

Several methods have been used to try to distinguish hemoglobin from myoglobin, but none of the methods are completely reliable. These conditions may sometimes be differentiated on the basis of their different molecular weights and different solubility in ammonium sulfate.

LEUKOCYTES

Presumptive evidence of leukocytes (WBCs) in urine may be obtained with the leukocyte reaction of certain reagent strips. However, many false-negative reactions occur with animal species, and microscopic evaluation is necessary to confirm a positive result. The leukocyte reagent strip test is not valid for cats because it produces false-positive results.

URINALYSIS ANALYZERS

Analyzers used for the in-house evaluation of urine samples are generally the semiautomated types that are used only for the reading and recording of test results. These analyzers use a standard urinalysis reagent dipstick to which the sample is applied by the technician. The dipstick is then loaded into the analyzer, and the results are read and recorded at the

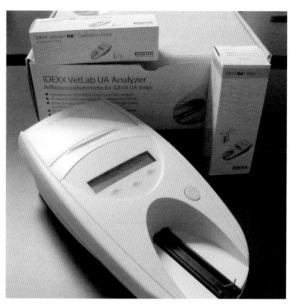

Fig. 29.3 Automated Urinalysis Analyzer.

appropriate time (Fig. 29.3). Larger reference laboratories generally have fully automated analyzers that are capable of performing a greater number of evaluations than the semiautomated analyzers. Many of these analyzers also evaluate the gross characteristics of the sample (e.g., turbidity).

KEY POINTS

- The chemical analysis of urine is performed with the use of reagent dipsticks.
- Color matching of the color changes on the reagent pads is used to determine the chemical values.
- Tablet tests are also available for the chemical analysis of urine and usually used to confirm an abnormality detected with the dipstick test.
- The pH of urine is affected by the patient's diet.

- The presence of protein in the urine is usually abnormal, and it is primarily attributable to disease of the urinary tract.
- Glucosuria and ketonuria are associated with diabetes mellitus.
- Bilirubinuria is seen with a variety of conditions, including bile duct obstruction, hemolytic anemia, and liver disease.
- Hematuria, hemoglobinuria, and myoglobinuria can occur simultaneously in urine samples.

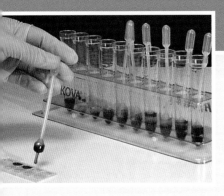

30

Urine Sediment Analysis

LEARNING OBJECTIVES

After studying this chapter, you will be able to:
- Describe the procedure for preparing urine for microscopic examination.
- Describe the procedure for performing the microscopic examination of urine sediment.
- List the cells that may be encountered in urine sediment, and explain their significance.
- List the crystals that may be encountered in urine sediment, and explain their significance.
- Describe the formation of casts, and explain their significance in a urine sample.
- List and describe parasites that may be encountered in urine sediment.
- Discuss the significance of bacteria in urine sediment.

OUTLINE

KEY TERMS

Ammonium biurate
Calcium carbonate
Calcium oxalate
Casts
Cellular casts
Crystalluria
Cystine
Fatty casts
Granular casts
Hyaline casts
Leucine
Renal epithelial cells
Struvite
Transitional epithelial cells
Tyrosine
Uric acid
Uroliths
Waxy casts

The microscopic examination of urine sediment is an important part of a complete urinalysis, especially for recognizing diseases of the urinary tract. Many abnormalities in a urine sample cannot be detected with reagent test strips or tablets, and often more specific information may be obtained by observation of the urine sediment. In addition, urine sediment examination is occasionally an aid in the diagnosis of systemic disease. In human medicine, the microscopic analysis of urine sediment is usually performed only when patients are symptomatic or when abnormalities are evident in the physical and chemical urine examinations. However, many veterinary practitioners routinely request a urine sediment examination of every urine sample.

With the exception of horse and rabbit urine, the normal urine of domestic animals does not contain a large amount of sediment. Small numbers of epithelial cells, mucus threads, red blood cells (RBCs), white blood cells (WBCs), hyaline casts, and crystals of various types can be found in the urine of normal animals. The urine of horses and rabbits usually has large amounts of calcium carbonate crystals. Urine must be collected cleanly, because bacteria and aberrant substances may be present in a urine sample that has been contaminated during collection.

The best samples for sediment examination are morning samples or samples collected after several hours of water deprivation. Because such samples are more concentrated, the chances of finding formed elements are increased. Sediment should be examined while the urine is fresh, because bacteria will multiply if the sample is allowed to stand at room temperature for a period of time. Other changes may also occur in a sample as it ages. Crystals may form as the sample cools, and casts may dissolve in alkaline urine. If a voided sample is collected, a midstream sample is preferred, because it is less likely to be contaminated by cells, bacteria, and debris from the external genital surfaces. Urine collected by cystocentesis is the best sample for microscopic examination. If the sample cannot be examined within 1 hour of collection, it should be refrigerated or preserved.

For semiquantitative measurements of the formed elements in urine, the volume of urine used and the volume of sediment obtained should be recorded. If a sufficient volume has been obtained, 5 to 10 mL of a well-mixed sample should be placed in a graduated conical centrifuge tube and centrifuged for 3 to 5 minutes at approximately 1000 to 2000 rpm, depending on the radius of the centrifuge. Excessive force compacts the sediment and may distort or disrupt formed elements. The procedure should be standardized for a particular centrifuge to yield uniform results. After centrifugation, the volume of sediment is recorded, and the supernatant is gently poured off to leave approximately 0.5 mL of urine in the bottom of the tube. The sediment is resuspended by gently flicking the bottom of the centrifuge tube with the fingers or by mixing it gently with a pipette (Procedure 30.1).

The Kova urine sediment system (Hycor Biomedical Inc., Garden Grove, CA) provides a method for the standardization of the initial sample volume, the volume of the sample used to resuspend the packed sediment, and the distribution of elements on the slide. Each specimen is processed in a specially shaped conical plastic tube with a flared opening for easy filling. When the supernatant is poured off after centrifuging, a fixed volume is retained along with the sediment. The specially designed pipette is then used to dispense a fixed volume of the resuspended sediment into a special chambered slide for microscopic examination (Fig. 30.1). This unique system provides an even distribution of microscopic elements that improves visualization.

The sediment may be examined stained or unstained. Examining the sediment unstained first allows for the better evaluation of the specimen. To examine unstained sediment, a small drop of the suspended sediment is placed on a clean glass slide, covered with a coverslip, and examined immediately. Subdued light that partially refracts the elements must be used to examine unstained urine sediment. This is achieved by partially closing the diaphragm and adjusting the condenser downward until optimal contrast is achieved. If too much light is present, some structures may be missed. The fine adjustment

PROCEDURE 30.1 Preparing Urine Sediment for Microscopic Examination

1. Pour approximately 10 mL of the urine sample into a labeled conical centrifuge tube.
2. Centrifuge the sample for 3 to 6 minutes at 1000 to 2000 rpm.
3. Pour off the supernatant to leave approximately 0.5 to 1 mL in the tube.
4. Resuspend the sediment by flicking the tube with your fingers or by gently mixing the sediment and supernatant with a pipette.
5. Transfer a drop of resuspended sediment near the end of a microscope slide with a transfer pipette, and place a coverslip over it.
6. Optional: Add 1 drop of Sedi-Stain or new methylene blue to 1 drop of urine sediment on the other end of the microscope slide, and place a coverslip over it.
7. Subdue the light of the microscope by partially closing the iris diaphragm.
8. Scan the entire unstained slide for the presence of large formed elements such as casts and clusters of cells.
9. Examine the entire specimen under the coverslip with the high-power objective lens (40×) to identify and quantify formed elements. Use the stained sediment as needed to confirm the identification of a formed element.
10. Examine a minimum of 10 microscopic fields with the high-power lens.
11. Record the results. Report cells and bacteria in numbers per high-power field and casts in numbers per low-power field. The report can list either the average number seen in 10 microscopic fields or a range that represents the lowest and highest number of each element seen in 10 microscopic fields.

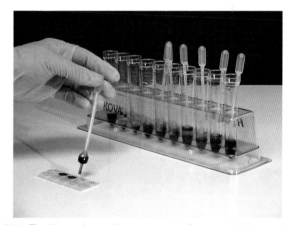

Fig. 30.1 The Kova urine sediment system. (Courtesy B. Mitzner, DVM.)

knob of the microscope should be continuously adjusted to see the depth of the object as well as other structures. The use of stain in the sediment may help to identify different cell types. However, stains often introduce artifacts into the sediment, particularly precipitate material and bacteria. Available urine sediment stains include Sternheimer-Malbin stain (Sedi-Stain, Becton, Dickinson, Franklin Lakes, NJ) (Fig. 30.2) and 0.5% new methylene blue, which contains a small amount of formalin. One drop of stain is mixed with the suspended sediment before placing a drop of sediment on a microscope slide. A coverslip is placed over the drop of stained sediment. The amount of illumination is less critical when examining a stained specimen than it is for an unstained one, although high-power lens. Epithelial cells, RBCs, and WBCs are reported as the average number observed per high-power field. Bacteria are reported as few, moderate, or many, and their morphologic characteristics (e.g., cocci, bacilli) are noted. Alternatively, elements can be reported as the range that is seen. For example, one to four cells per high-power field would indicate that nearly every microscopic field examined had at least one cell and some had as many as four. Bacteria and crystals may also be semiquantified with the use of a scale of +1 to +4.

DRY-MOUNT URINE CYTOLOGY

When cells appear abnormal with standard wet-mount preparations or when bacterial characteristics cannot be readily evaluated, a dry-mount preparation can be made from the urine sediment. The procedure is similar to that described for other fluid samples (see Chapter 38). Samples must be thoroughly air-dried so that the sample adheres to the slide. Dry-mount samples can be examined unstained or appropriate cytology stains can be added. If the sample peels off during staining, a preparation can be made by adding a small amount of normal clear serum to the sample before making the smear. The additional protein added to the sample from the serum can aid in adherence of the sample during staining of the slide.

CONSTITUENTS OF URINE SEDIMENT

Normal urine sediment in healthy animals may contain a few casts, crystals, epithelial cells, RBCs, WBCs, mucus threads, and, in males or recently bred females, spermatozoa. Fat droplets, artifacts, and contaminants may also be seen. If more than a few erythrocytes, leukocytes, hyperplastic or neoplastic epithelial cells, casts, crystals, parasite ova, bacteria, and yeast are identified in urine sediment, it is considered abnormal, and further diagnostic tests should be performed (Fig. 30.4).

Erythrocytes

Erythrocytes (RBCs) may have several different appearances, depending on the urine concentration, pH, and time elapsed between collection and examination. In a fresh sample, RBCs are small, round, usually smooth edged, somewhat refractile, and yellow or orange, but they may be colorless if their hemoglobin has diffused during standing (Figs. 30.5 and 30.6). RBCs are smaller than WBCs, and they may have a smooth, biconcave disk shape. In concentrated urine, RBCs shrink and crenate. Crenated RBCs have ruffled edges, are slightly darker, and may even appear granular as a result of membrane irregularities. In dilute or alkaline urine, RBCs swell and may lyse. Swollen RBCs have smooth edges and are pale yellow or orange. Lysed RBCs may appear as colorless rings (i.e., "shadow cells" or "ghost cells") that vary in size. However, lysed RBCs—especially when they result from marked alkalinity—often dissolve and cannot be found with microscopic examination. Normally urine sediment contains less than two to three RBCs per high-power field.

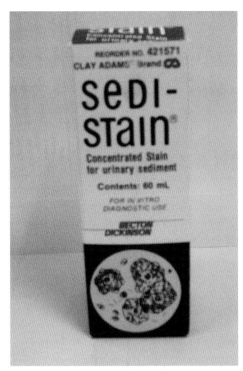

Fig. 30.2 Sedi-Stain.

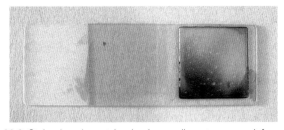

Fig. 30.3 Stained and unstained urine sediment prepared for microscopic examination.

reduced illumination also helps with the visualization of substances by providing contrast. The quantifying of elements in the sediment should never be done with a stained slide, because the stain dilutes the sample significantly. One method that may simplify the urinalysis procedure is to prepare two drops of urine sediment side by side on the same microscope slide (Fig. 30.3). The drop that has stain added to it can be used to identify cells, whereas the unstained side can be used to quantify elements in the urine.

The specimen must be initially scanned under low power (10× objective lens) to evaluate the overall quality of the preparation and to identify larger elements, such as casts or aggregates of cells. The entire area under the coverslip should be examined, because casts tend to migrate toward the edge of the coverslip. Casts and crystals are identified and reported as the number observed per low-power field. The high-power lens (40× objective lens) is necessary to identify most objects accurately, to detect bacteria, and to differentiate cell types. A minimum of 10 microscopic fields should be observed with a

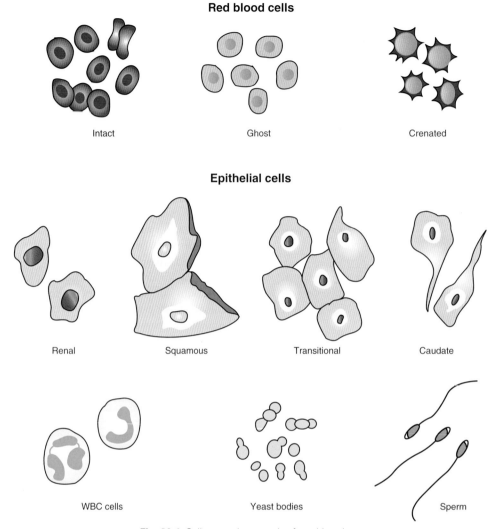

Fig. 30.4 Cell types that may be found in urine.

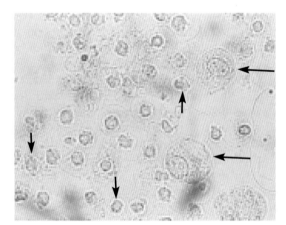

Fig. 30.5 Unstained urine showing crenated red blood cells *(short arrows)* and two epithelial cells *(long arrows)*. (From Raskin RE, Meyer DJ: *Atlas of canine and feline cytology,* St Louis, 2001, Saunders.)

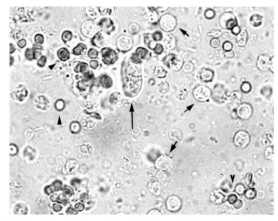

Fig. 30.6 Unstained urine sediment with a cast *(long arrow)* and several red blood cells *(arrowheads)* and white blood cells *(short arrows)*. (From Van-Steenhouse JL: Clinical pathology. In McCurnin DM, Bassert JM, editors: *Clinical textbook for veterinary technicians,* ed 7, St Louis, 2009, Saunders.)

Because mammalian RBCs contain no nucleus, they may be confused with fat globules or yeast. However, their light yellow or orange color usually allows them to be differentiated from these other elements. Furthermore, variation in RBC size is minimal, whereas fat globules vary in size. Erythrocytes in urine usually indicate bleeding somewhere in the urogenital tract or occasionally in the genital system. A voided sample from a female in proestrus or estrus or after parturition may be contaminated with RBCs. Both females and males with inflammatory conditions of the genital system may have RBCs in urine collected by free catch or expression of the bladder. Urine collected by catheterization from females with inflammatory lesions in the genital tract is usually not contaminated, but urine from males with genital tract inflammation may be contaminated. Even the slight trauma that occurs as a result of catheterization, cystocentesis, and manual expression of the bladder may slightly increase the number of RBCs in the sediment. Generally cystocentesis does not cause much increase in RBC numbers. The veterinary technician should note the method of urine collection on the laboratory report to help determine the significance of any RBCs in the urine.

Leukocytes

Leukocytes (WBCs) are larger than erythrocytes and smaller than renal epithelial cells. Leukocytes are spherical and can have a dull gray or greenish-yellow color. They are identified in urine sediment by their characteristic granules or by the lobulation of the nucleus (Fig. 30.7). Their appearance is attributable to the fact that most WBCs in urine are neutrophils, which contain a large number of granules. Few leukocytes are found in the urine of animals without urinary or genital tract disease. WBCs shrink in concentrated urine and swell in dilute urine. Leukocytes are usually in low numbers in urine (i.e., 0 to 1 per high-power field). Finding more than two to three per high-power field indicates an inflammatory process somewhere in the urinary or genital tract. The term for excessive WBCs in the urine is *pyuria*. Pyuria is indicative of an inflammatory or infectious process such as nephritis, pyelonephritis, cystitis, urethritis, or ureteritis. Urine with increased

numbers of leukocytes should be cultured for bacteria, even if organisms are not observed by microscopic examination.

Epithelial Cells

A few epithelial cells in urine are considered normal and occur as a result of the normal sloughing of old cells. A marked increase indicates inflammation. The three types of epithelial cells found in urinary sediment are squamous, transitional, and renal. The differentiation of transitional from renal epithelial cells is often difficult. In this case, reporting the cells as nonsquamous epithelial cells is acceptable.

Squamous Epithelial Cells

Squamous epithelial cells derived from the distal urethra, vagina, vulva, or prepuce are occasionally found in voided samples. Their presence usually is not considered significant. These flat, thin cells with a homogeneous appearance are the largest cells found in urine sediment. They often have straight edges and distinct corners, which sometimes curl or fold (Fig. 30.8A). They may have a small, round nucleus. Squamous epithelial cells are not normally found in samples obtained by cystocentesis or catheterization.

Transitional Epithelial Cells

Transitional epithelial cells come from the bladder, the ureters, the renal pelvis, and the proximal urethra. They are usually

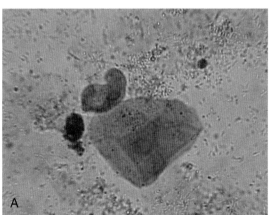
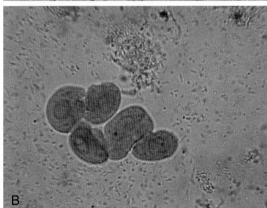

Fig. 30.8 **A,** Squamous epithelial cells in stained canine urine. **B,** Transitional epithelial cells in stained canine urine.

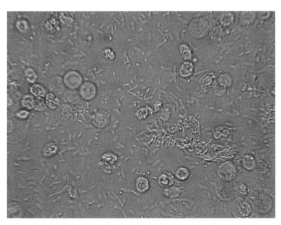

Fig. 30.7 White blood cells and bacteria in unstained canine urine.

round, but they may be pear-shaped or caudate. They are granular, have small nuclei, and are larger than WBCs (Fig. 30.8B). Low numbers of transitional cells (i.e., 0 to 1 per high-power field) may be found in urinary sediment as a result of the sloughing of old cells, but an increased number suggests cystitis or pyelonephritis. Increased numbers may also be seen if catheterization was used to obtain the sample.

Renal Epithelial Cells

Renal epithelial cells are the smallest epithelial cells observed in urine. They originate in the renal tubules, are only slightly larger than WBCs, and are often confused with WBCs. Renal epithelial cells are generally round and contain a large nucleus and nongranular or finely granular cytoplasm. They are rarely found (i.e., 0 to 1 per high-power field). Increased numbers of these cells occur with diseases of the kidney parenchyma.

Casts

Casts are formed in the lumen of the distal and collecting tubules of the kidney, where the concentration and acidity of urine are greatest. In the renal tubules, secreted protein precipitates in acidic conditions and forms casts that are shaped like the tubules in which they form. They are composed of a matrix of protein from plasma and mucoprotein secreted by the tubules. They are commonly classified on the basis of their appearance as hyaline, epithelial, cellular (i.e., epithelial cells, RBCs, WBCs, or both RBCs and WBCs), granular, waxy, fatty, or mixed casts. Which cast type is present depends in part on how quickly the filtrate is moving through the tubules and how much tubular damage is present. Faster-moving filtrate with

minor tubule damage is usually evident as a hyaline cast. Slower-moving filtrate allows time for the cells to be incorporated within the cast. If the filtrate is moving very slowly, the cells will degenerate as the cast continues through the tubules; the cast will then appear as a granular cast. Granular casts also result when cellular debris from damaged tubule cells is incorporated into the cast.

All casts are cylindrical structures with parallel sides, and their width is determined by the width of the lumen in which they are formed. Their ends may be tapered, irregular, or round. Any cells or structures in the area may also be incorporated into casts, thereby imparting the morphologic features that allow them to be specifically identified (Fig. 30.9). Casts dissolve in alkaline urine, so cast identification should be performed in fresh samples that have not become alkaline with standing. Because casts dissolve quickly in alkaline urine, they are rarely seen in the sediment of herbivores, which characteristically have alkaline urine. Casts may be disrupted with high-speed centrifugation and rough sample handling. A few hyaline casts or granular casts (i.e., 0 to 1 per high-power field) may be seen in normal urine, but larger numbers of casts indicate a lesion in the renal tubules. The number of casts observed is not a reliable indicator of the severity of the urinary disease.

Hyaline Casts

Hyaline casts are clear, colorless, and somewhat transparent structures that are composed only of protein. They are difficult to see, and they are usually identified only in dim light. Hyaline

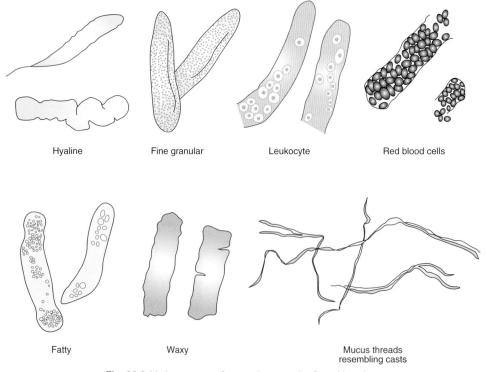

Hyaline   Fine granular   Leukocyte   Red blood cells

Fatty   Waxy   Mucus threads resembling casts

Fig. 30.9 Various types of casts that may be found in urine.

casts are cylindrical, with parallel sides and usually rounded ends (Fig. 30.10). They are easier to identify in stained sediment than in unstained sediment. Increased numbers of hyaline casts indicate the mildest form of renal irritation. Their numbers are also increased with fever, poor renal perfusion, strenuous exercise, or general anesthesia.

Granular Casts

Granular casts, which are hyaline casts that contain granules, are the most common type of cast seen in animals (Fig. 30.11). The granules come from tubular epithelial cells, RBCs, or WBCs that became incorporated in the cast and then degenerated. Cellular degeneration may occur in the tubules that produce granular casts, which may be coarse or fine in appearance. Other materials released from cells in the urinary tract may also become embedded in casts. Granular casts are seen in large numbers with acute nephritis and indicate more severe kidney damage as compared with hyaline casts.

Epithelial Casts

Epithelial casts consist of epithelial cells from the renal tubules that become embedded in a hyaline matrix (Fig. 30.12). Epithelial cells in casts are always of the renal epithelial type, because this is the only epithelial cell present at the site of cast formation. These casts are formed by epithelium sloughing in the tubules. They are seen with acute nephritis and other conditions that cause degeneration of the renal tubular epithelium.

Leukocyte Casts

Leukocyte casts contain WBCs, predominantly neutrophils. These casts can be readily identified unless cellular degeneration has occurred. The presence of WBCs and leukocyte casts indicates inflammation in the renal tubules.

Erythrocyte Casts

Erythrocyte casts are deep yellow to orange in color. The RBC membranes may or may not be visible. Erythrocyte casts contain RBCs and form when RBCs aggregate within the lumen of the tubule (Fig. 30.13). Erythrocyte casts indicate renal bleeding. Bleeding may be strictly from hemorrhage that results from trauma or bleeding disorders, or it may occur as part of an inflammatory lesion.

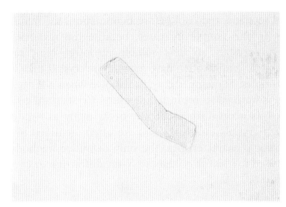

Fig. 30.10 Unstained hyaline cast. (From Cowell RL, et al: *Diagnostic cytology and hematology of the dog and cat,* ed 3, St Louis, 2008, Mosby.)

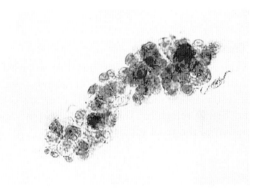

Fig. 30.12 Renal epithelial cast, stained. (From Cowell RL, et al: *Diagnostic cytology and hematology of the dog and cat,* ed 3, St Louis, 2008, Mosby.)

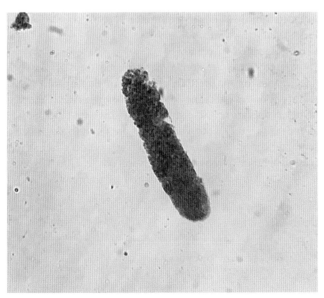

Fig. 30.11 Granular cast in stained canine urine.

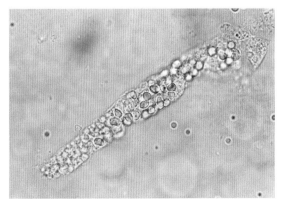

Fig. 30.13 Red blood cell cast, unstained. (From Raskin RE, Meyer DJ: *Atlas of canine and feline cytology,* St Louis, 2001, Saunders.)

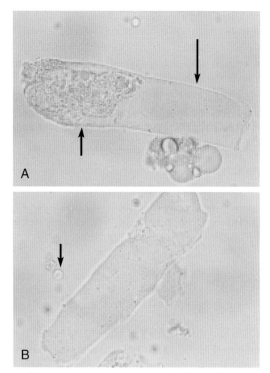

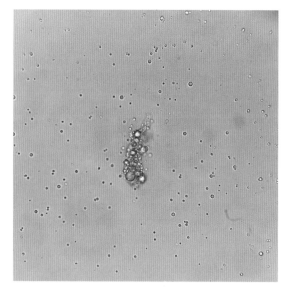

Fig. 30.15 Fatty cast in unstained urine sample.

Fig. 30.14 A, Unstained granular casts develop into waxy casts as illustrated by this cast that has the characteristics of both a waxy cast *(long arrow)* and a granular cast *(short arrow).* **B,** Unstained waxy cast *(arrow).* (From Raskin RE, Meyer DJ: *Atlas of canine and feline cytology,* St Louis, 2001, Saunders.)

Waxy Casts

Waxy casts resemble hyaline casts, but they are usually wider, with square ends rather than round ends and a dull, homogeneous, waxy appearance (Fig. 30.14). They are colorless or gray and highly refractile. They indicate chronic and severe degeneration of the renal tubules.

Fatty Casts

Fatty casts contain many small droplets of fat that appear as refractile bodies (Fig. 30.15). They are frequently seen in cats with renal disease, because cats have lipid in their renal parenchyma. They are occasionally seen in dogs with diabetes mellitus. Large numbers of fatty casts suggest the degeneration of the renal tubules.

Crystals

The presence of crystals in the urine is called crystalluria. Crystalluria may or may not be of clinical significance. Certain crystals form as a consequence of their elements being secreted into the urine by normal renal activity (Fig. 30.16). Some crystals form as a consequence of metabolic diseases. Conditions that lead to crystal formation may also cause the formation of urinary calculi. The types of crystals formed depend on the urine pH, concentration, and temperature and the

solubility of the elements (Table 30.1). If a urine sample is allowed to stand and cool before examination, the number of crystals in the sample increases, because the materials that make up crystals are less soluble at lower temperatures. Refrigerated samples often have many more crystals than warm, fresh samples. Sometimes crystals dissolve when a refrigerated sample is warmed to room temperature. Crystals are generally reported as occasional, moderate, or as many as +1 to +4. Although crystals (and uroliths) are often identified by their morphologic characteristics, the only definitive methods that can be used to identify crystals are x-ray diffraction or chemical analysis.

Struvite

- **pH**
  - Any, more often neutral to alkaline
- **Clinical Significance**
  - Often of no clinical significance
  - Urinary tract infection
  - Refrigerated specimens

Struvite crystals are sometimes referred to as triple phosphate crystals or magnesium ammonium phosphate crystals. They are found in alkaline to slightly acidic urine. Generally, struvite crystals are six- to eight-sided prisms with tapering sides and ends (Fig. 30.17). Struvite crystals are typically described as resembling coffin lids, although they may take on other shapes. Occasionally they may assume a fern-leaf shape, especially when the urine contains a high concentration of ammonia.

Calcium Oxalate

- **pH**
  - Acidic, but any pH possible

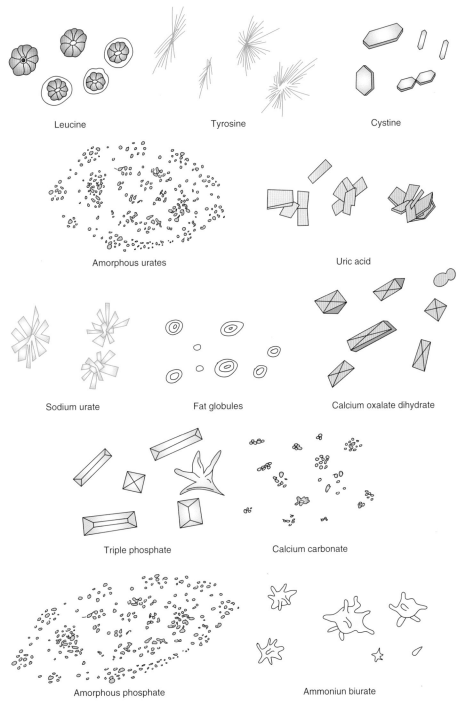

Leucine   Tyrosine   Cystine

Amorphous urates   Uric acid

Sodium urate   Fat globules   Calcium oxalate dihydrate

Triple phosphate   Calcium carbonate

Amorphous phosphate   Ammoniun biurate

Fig. 30.16 Crystals that may be found in urine.

- **Clinical Significance**
  - Can be normal finding in dogs and cats
  - Can form in urine that has been standing
  - Less often seen in ethylene glycol toxicosis

Calcium oxalate dihydrate crystals generally appear as small squares, and they contain an "X" across the crystal that resembles the back of an envelope (Fig. 30.18). Calcium oxalate monohydrate crystals may be small and dumbbell-shaped, or they may be elongated and pointed at each end (i.e., resembling a slat from a picket fence) (Fig. 30.19). Calcium dihydrate crystals are found in acidic and neutral urine, and they are commonly seen in small numbers in dogs and horses. The urine of animals that have been poisoned with ethylene glycol (antifreeze) often contains large numbers of calcium oxalate crystals, especially calcium monohydrate crystals. Animals with oxalate urolithiasis may have large numbers of calcium oxalate crystals in their urine, and large numbers of oxalate crystals may indicate a predisposition to oxalate urolithiasis.

TABLE 30.1	pH Chart for Urine Crystals
Crystal	**pH**
Ammonium biurate	Slightly acidic, neutral, alkaline
Amorphous phosphate	Neutral, alkaline
Amorphous urate	Acidic, neutral
Bilirubin	Acidic
Calcium carbonate	Neutral, alkaline
Calcium oxalate	Acidic, neutral, alkaline
Cystine	Acidic
Leucine	Acidic
Triple phosphate	Slightly acidic, neutral, alkaline
Tyrosine	Acidic
Uric acid	Acidic

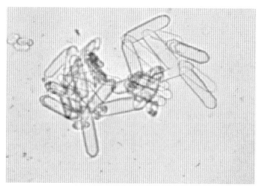

Fig. 30.19 Calcium oxalate (monohydrate form) crystals in unstained canine urine. (From VanSteenhouse JL: Clinical pathology. In McCurnin DM, Bassert JM, editors: *Clinical textbook for veterinary technicians*, ed 7, St Louis, 2009, Saunders.)

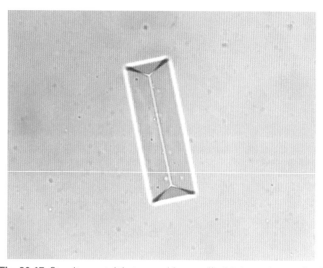

Fig. 30.17 Struvite crystal that resembles a coffin lid shown in unstained canine urine.

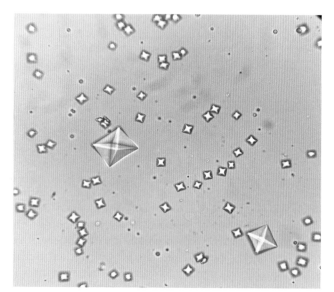

Fig. 30.18 Calcium oxalate (dihydrate form) crystals in unstained canine urine. (From VanSteenhouse JL: Clinical pathology. In McCurnin DM, Bassert JM, editors: *Clinical textbook for veterinary technicians*, ed 7, St Louis, 2009, Saunders.)

Uric Acid

- **pH**
  - Acidic
- **Clinical Significance**
  - Inherited defect in purine metabolism that can lead to hyperuricosuria
  - In Dalmatians it is a normal finding
  - Can also be normal in bulldogs and black Russian terriers
  - Patients can be at risk for uric acid uroliths
  - Liver disease
  - Acidic urine allowed to stand at room temperature

Uric acid crystals take on a variety of shapes but are usually diamond or rhomboid (Fig. 30.20B). They appear yellow or yellow-brown, and they are not commonly found in dogs and cats (except in Dalmatian dogs).

Amorphous Crystalline Material

- **pH**
  - Amorphous phosphates—alkaline
  - Amorphous urates—acidic
- **Clinical Significance**
  - No clinical significance
  - Increased formation with refrigeration

Amorphous phosphate crystals are common in alkaline urine and appear as a granular precipitate (Fig. 30.21). Amorphous urates appear as a granular precipitate similar to amorphous phosphates (see Fig. 30.20A). Amorphous urates are seen in acidic urine, whereas amorphous phosphates are found in alkaline urine.

Calcium Carbonate

- **pH**
  - Alkaline or neutral
- **Clinical Significance**
  - Normal in horses

Calcium carbonate crystals are commonly seen in the urine of horses and rabbits. They are round, with many lines

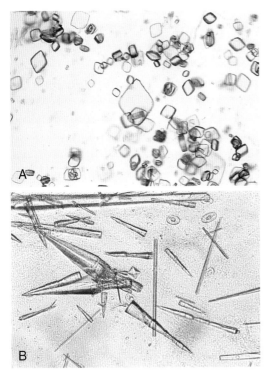

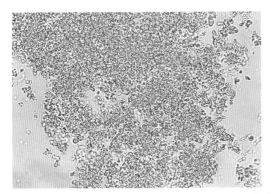

Fig. 30.20 A, Uric acid crystals, unstained. These are not commonly found in small animals, except for Dalmatian dogs. **B,** Sodium urate crystals, unstained. These may be found in association with ammonium biurate uroliths. A calcium oxalate dihydrate crystal is also present *(center).* (From Raskin RE, Meyer DJ: *Atlas of canine and feline cytology,* St Louis, 2001, Saunders.)

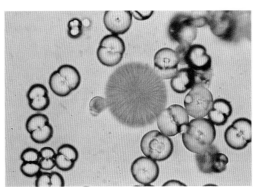

Fig. 30.22 Calcium carbonate crystals, unstained. (From Raskin RE, Meyer DJ: *Atlas of canine and feline cytology,* St Louis, 2001, Saunders.)

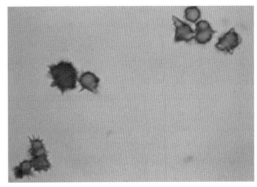

Fig. 30.23 Unstained urine sediment with ammonium biurate crystals. (From VanSteenhouse JL: Clinical pathology. In McCurnin DM, Bassert JM, editors: *Clinical textbook for veterinary technicians,* ed 7, St Louis, 2009, Saunders.)

they are round, with long, irregular spicules (i.e., they have a "thorn-apple" shape) (Fig. 30.23). Often the spicules fracture and the remaining crystal is brown, with fine radiating lines. They are most common in animals with severe liver disease (e.g., portacaval shunts).

Sulfonamide
- **pH**
  - Acidic
- **Clinical Significance**
  - Patient is being treated with sulfonamide medications

Sulfonamide crystals may be seen in animals that are being treated with sulfonamides. Sulfonamide crystals are round and usually dark, with individual crystals radiating from the center. They are less likely to be observed in alkaline urine because they are more soluble in alkaline urine. The prevention of precipitation of these crystals in the renal tubules is assisted by maintaining alkaline urine and encouraging the animal to drink.

Bilirubin
- **pH**
  - Acidic

Fig. 30.21 Amorphous phosphate crystals, unstained. (From Raskin RE, Meyer DJ: *Atlas of canine and feline cytology,* St Louis, 2001, Saunders.)

radiating from their centers, or they may appear as large granular masses (Fig. 30.22). They also may have a dumbbell shape. They are of no clinical significance.

Ammonium Biurate
- **pH**
  - Alkaline, neutral, or slightly acidic
- **Clinical Significance**
  - Hyperammonemia due to portosystemic shunt or hepatic failure

Ammonium biurate crystals are seen in slightly acidic, neutral, or alkaline urine. These crystals are brown in color, and

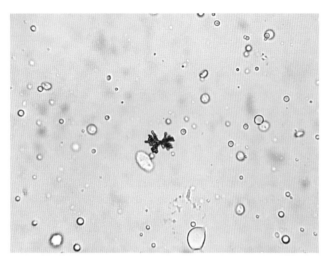

Fig. 30.24 Bilirubin crystals in unstained urine.

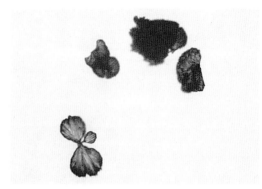

Fig. 30.25 Stained tyrosine crystals. (From Cowell RL, et al: *Diagnostic cytology and hematology of the dog and cat,* ed 3, St Louis, 2008, Mosby.)

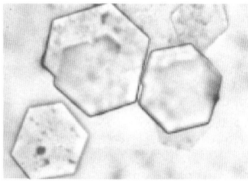

Fig. 30.26 Unstained cystine crystals. (From VanSteenhouse JL: Clinical pathology. In McCurnin DM, Bassert JM, editors: *Clinical textbook for veterinary technicians,* ed 7, St Louis, 2009, Saunders.)

- **Clinical Significance**
  - Indicate some degree of bilirubinuria
  - Can be normal in highly concentrated urine samples from dogs

Bilirubin crystals may be seen in normal acidic canine urine (Fig. 30.24). In other species, the presence of bilirubin crystals is an abnormal finding and the animal that should be investigated for an underlying disease process.

Leucine

- **pH**
  - Acidic to neutral
- **Clinical Significance**
  - Unknown possible liver disease

Leucine crystals are wheel or "pincushion" shaped and yellow or brown in color (see Fig. 30.16). Animals with liver disease may have leucine crystals in their urine.

Tyrosine

- **pH**
  - Acidic
- **Clinical Significance**
  - Severe liver disease

Tyrosine crystals are dark, with needle-like projections, and they are highly refractile (Fig. 30.25). They are often found in small clusters. Animals with liver disease may have tyrosine crystals in their urine. They are not a common finding in dogs and cats.

Cystine

- **pH**
  - Acidic
- **Clinical Significance**
  - Indicates cystinuria, an inherited defect in urinary transport

Cystine crystals appear to be flat. They are six-sided (hexagonal), colorless, and thin (Fig. 30.26). They can be associated with renal tubular dysfunction or cystine urolithiasis.

Crystals Associated With Melamine Toxicity

- **Clinical Significance**
  - Acute renal failure from ingestion of melamine and cyanuric contaminated pet food

Golden-brown round to oval crystals with radial striations may be present in animals that have been fed diets contaminated with melamine or cyanuric acid.

MICROORGANISMS

A variety of microorganisms may be found in urine sediment, including bacteria, fungi, and protozoa. Normal urine is free of bacteria, but it may be contaminated by bacteria residing on the epithelium of the vagina, vulva, or prepuce during urination. Normal urine collected by cystocentesis or catheterization does not contain bacteria and therefore is considered sterile. Because bacteria often proliferate in urine that has been left standing for some time, especially at room temperature, the urine must be immediately examined or refrigerated until it can be examined. Bacteria can be identified only under magnification. They may be round (cocci) or rod-shaped (bacilli), usually refract light, and appear to be quivering as a result of Brownian movement. They are reported as few, moderate, many, or too numerous to count (TNTC). A large number of bacteria accompanied by a large number of WBCs suggests infection and inflammation of the urinary tract (e.g., cystitis, pyelonephritis) or the genital tract (e.g., prostatitis, metritis, vaginitis). Bacteria in the urine sample are most significant when they are also identified within the cytoplasm of the WBCs. These samples should be submitted for bacterial culture (see Unit 8).

Yeasts are often confused with RBCs or lipid droplets, but they usually display characteristic budding, and they may have double refractile walls. Yeast are usually contaminants in urine samples, because yeast infections of the urinary tract are rare in domestic animals. Yeast infection of the external genitalia may cause yeast to be present in voided samples. Fungi also may be found in urine. Fungi are filamentous and usually branching. Fungal infections of the urinary tract are uncommon but quite serious when they occur.

Parasite Ova and Microfilaria

Parasite ova may be seen in the urine sediment of animals with urinary parasites, or they may result from fecal contamination at the time of collection of the urine sample. Some parasites of the urinary tract include *Pearsonema plica* (formerly *Capillaria plica*), which is a bladder worm of dogs and cats (Fig. 30.27), and *Dioctophyma renale,* which is a kidney worm of dogs. Microfilaria (e.g., *Dirofilaria immitis*) may be seen in the urine sediment of dogs with adult heartworms, and circulating microfilaria may be seen if hemorrhage into the urine occurs either from disease or as a result of trauma during collection (Fig. 30.28).

MISCELLANEOUS COMPONENTS OF URINE

Mucus Threads

Mucus threads are often confused with casts, but they do not have the well-delineated edges of casts. They resemble a twisted ribbon more than a cast. A large amount of mucus is normally present in equine urine because horses have mucus glands in the renal pelvis and ureter. In other animals, mucus indicates urethral irritation or contamination of the sample with genital secretions.

Spermatozoa

Spermatozoa are occasionally seen in the urine sediment of intact male animals. They are easily recognized and have no clinical significance. Sperm may also be present in recently bred females. Large amounts of sperm in the urine may produce false-positive results for protein.

Fat Droplets

In urine sediment, fat droplets are lightly green-tinged, highly refractile, spherical bodies of varying sizes. Because they vary in size, they can be distinguished from RBCs and yeast, which

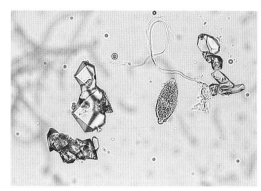

Fig. 30.27 Ova of *Pearsonema plica* in unstained urine sediment. (From Raskin RE, Meyer DJ: *Atlas of canine and feline cytology*, St. Louis, 2001, Saunders.)

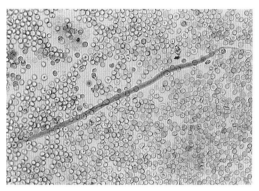

Fig. 30.28 Stained microfilaria of *Dirofilaria immitis* in a dog with hemorrhagic cystitis. (From Raskin RE, Meyer DJ: *Atlas of canine and feline cytology*, St Louis, 2001, Saunders.)

tend to be uniform in size. If a sediment smear sits for a few moments before being examined, fat droplets rise to a plane just beneath the coverslip, whereas other formed elements settle to the top of the slide. Therefore, fat droplets are often not in the plane of focus of other formed elements. Small round structures found under the coverslip are usually fat globules. Uniformly sized round structures found in a lower plane are usually RBCs. In sediment that has been stained with Sudan III stain, fat droplets appear orange or red in color. Frequently, fat droplets from catheter lubricants or from oily surfaces of collecting vials and pipettes may contaminate urine. Fat in the urine, which is called lipuria, is seen to some degree in most cats. Lipuria is also seen with obesity, diabetes mellitus, hypothyroidism, and, rarely, after a high-fat meal.

Artifacts

Many artifacts may enter the urine sample during collection, transportation, or examination. The recognition of these structures is irrelevant and not a normal part of the sediment evaluation. However, these contaminants may be a source of great confusion.

Air bubbles, oil droplets (usually as a result of lubricated catheters), starch granules (from surgical gloves), hair, fecal material, plant spores, pollen, cotton fibers, dust, glass particles or chips, bacteria, and fungi may contaminate urine. The ova of intestinal parasites may be observed as a result of fecal contamination of the urine sample.

UROLITHIASIS

Uroliths are calculi (stones) composed of various minerals that are found anywhere in the urinary tract; their occurrence is termed urolithiasis. They may cause the blockage of urine outflow from the bladder into the urethra; lodge in the urethra and cause a severe and acute inability to urinate; or remain in the bladder and cause inflammation and bleeding. Determining the composition of calculi is critical, because their prevention and the animal's prognosis depend on the identification of their composition. After the composition is determined, proper therapy may be initiated to remove the uroliths and prevent their reoccurrence. Urolithiasis may be a particular problem in castrated male ruminants. The lodging of calculi in the urethra obstructs the outflow of urine, which is a major problem in lambs and steers, particularly those that are fed high-concentrate rations. The most common calculi in these species are composed of calcium, magnesium, and ammonium carbonate or calcium, magnesium, and ammonium phosphate.

The analysis of the mineral composition of uroliths may be determined by submitting it intact to a reference laboratory for quantitative analysis. Occasionally a reasonable presumption about the composition of a urolith may be made by its gross and radiographic appearance and the crystal types found in the urine sediment. Uroliths of dogs and cats are usually struvite, and cystine and oxalate uroliths may also be observed. Urate uroliths are seen mostly in Dalmatians, because this breed excretes large amounts of uric acid.

KEY POINTS

- Subdued light must be used when examining sediment under the microscope.
- The fine adjustment knob on the microscope should be continuously adjusted so that various structures may be seen.
- To identify different cell types and bacteria accurately, the high-power objective lens (40×) is used.
- RBCs in urine sediment have several different appearances, depending on the concentration, pH, and time elapsed between collection and examination.
- WBCs are larger than RBCs, and they are identified by their characteristic granules and the lobulation of their nuclei.
- Casts are formed in the lumen of the distal and collecting tubules of the kidney.
- Casts are cylindrical structures with parallel sides that are present in acidic urine.
- Crystal formation depends on the urine pH, concentration, and temperature and the solubility of the elements.

Parasitology

Unit Outline

Unit Objectives

List the common internal parasites of domestic animals.
List the common external parasites of domestic animals.
Discuss the life cycles of common parasites of domestic animals.
Describe the treatment and control strategies for common parasites of domestic animals.
Describe the procedures that are used to diagnose parasites.

Parasitology is the study of organisms that live in (internal parasites, endoparasites) or on (external parasites, ectoparasites) another organism, the host, from which they derive their nourishment. Parasitism is a type of symbiotic relationship. Symbiosis involves two organisms living together, and there are three types: (1) Commensalism: One organism benefits, the other is unaffected; (2) Mutualism: Both organisms benefit; and (3) Parasitism: One organism benefits, the other is harmed.

The organism that the parasite lives in or on is called its host. The host may be a definitive host that shelters the sexual, adult stages of the parasite, or the host may be an intermediate host that harbors the asexual (immature) or larval stages of the parasite. There are also paratenic hosts or transport hosts for some parasites, in which the parasite survives without multiplying or developing. Parasite life cycles can be simple with direct transmission, or they may be complex and involve one or more vectors. A vector can be mechanical or biological. Mechanical vectors transmit the parasite, but the parasite does not develop in the vector. Biological vectors serve as intermediate hosts for the parasite. The term life cycle refers to the maturation of a parasite through various developmental stages in one or more hosts. For a parasite to survive, it must have a dependable means of transfer from one host to another and the ability to develop and reproduce in the host, ideally without producing serious harm to the host. This requires the following:

A mode of entry into a host (infective stage)
The availability of a susceptible host (definitive host)
An accommodating location and environment in the host for maturation and reproduction (e.g., the gastrointestinal, respiratory, circulatory, urinary, or reproductive system)
A mode of exit from the host (e.g., feces, sputum, blood, urine, smegma), with dispersal into an ecologically suitable environment for development and survival
Parasites have a wide distribution within host animals. They can have a negative impact in a number of ways, including the following:
Injury on entry (e.g., creeping eruption)
Injury by migration (e.g., sarcoptic mange)
Injury by residence (e.g., heartworms)
Chemical or physiological injury (e.g., digestive disturbances)
Injury due to host reaction (e.g., hypersensitivity, scar tissue)

Internal parasites, called endoparasites, live within an animal. These parasites derive their nutrition and protection at the expense of the infected animal, which is called the host. The various internal parasites have many different life cycles. Each parasite's life cycle is distinctive. It is composed of various developmental stages, all of which may occur within the same host or separately within sequential hosts. Endoparasites of domestic animals include unicellular protozoans, trematodes (flukes), cestodes (tapeworms, with their associated metacestode stages), nematodes (roundworms), and acanthocephalans (thorny-headed worms). A few arthropods (e.g., horse bots) are endoparasites. Ectoparasites usually live on or in skin surfaces or feed on them. Ectoparasites infest the skin or external surfaces of animals and produce an infestation on the animal.

The host that harbors the adult, mature, or sexual stages of a parasite is called the definitive host. The dog is the definitive host for *Dirofilaria immitis;* adult male and female heartworms are found in the right ventricle and pulmonary arteries of the dog's heart. The host that harbors the larval, immature, or asexual stages of a parasite is called the intermediate host. The mosquito is the intermediate host for *D. immitis;* the first, second, and third larval stages of *D. immitis* are found within the mosquito.

The life cycle of most parasites has at least one stage during which the parasite may be passed from one host to the next. Diagnostic procedures frequently detect this stage; therefore, it is referred to as the diagnostic stage. The diagnostic stage of a parasite may leave the host through excreta (e.g., feces, urine), or it may be transmitted from the bloodstream to its next host by an arthropod (e.g., a mosquito). The microfilarial stage is the diagnostic stage of *D. immitis;* the female mosquito takes in the microfilariae during a blood meal.

The diagnosis of endoparasitism is one of the most frequently performed procedures in the veterinary clinical setting. An accurate diagnosis of endoparasitism is based primarily on the veterinarian's and the technician's awareness of parasites that are prevalent in the immediate geographic area or ecosystem. However, because of the far-ranging mobility of owners and their pets in the twenty-first century, residence in or travel to another geographic region should also be considered when endoparasitism is among several differential diagnoses.

Heavily parasitized animals often show clinical signs that are suggestive of the infected organ system. Depending on the affected organ system, these signs may include diarrhea or constipation, anorexia, vomiting, blood in the stool, or fat in the stool. Parasitized animals are frequently lethargic and display an unthrifty appearance that is characterized by weight loss or stunted growth, a dull hair coat, dehydration, or anemia. The animal may also experience coughing or labored breathing.

Internal parasites of domestic animals comprise several types of organisms that live internally in animals, that feed on their tissues or body fluids, or that compete directly for their food. These organisms range in size from being too small to be seen with the naked eye (microscopic) to being more than 1 m in length. Parasites also vary with regard to their location within the host and the means by which they are transmitted from one host to another. Because of these diverse variations, no single diagnostic test can identify all endoparasites.

The time elapsed between initial infection with a parasite until the infection can be detected with the use of common diagnostic procedures is called the prepatent period. The best example of this concept is trying to diagnose hookworm disease *(Ancylostoma caninum)* in a 1-week-old puppy via the observation of eggs on fecal flotation. This attempted diagnosis is not helpful, because the minimum time from infection until adult hookworms are present in the bowel and begin to produce eggs (prepatent period) is 12 days. The astute veterinary practitioner uses fecal flotation results but also the puppy's history, clinical signs, and other laboratory tests (e.g., blood values) to arrive at a specific diagnosis of ancylostomiasis (infection with hookworms).

Classification of Parasites. Parasites of domestic animals are found in the kingdom Protista and the kingdom Animalia as well as in a large number of phyla in those kingdoms. There is some variation with regard to the classification schemes of different references, and organisms are often reclassified when new information about their biochemistry is obtained.

The majority of information in this unit is related to parasites of companion and farm animals. Lists of the major parasites of exotic species are located in Appendix L.

Zoonoses. Zoonoses are diseases that can be transmitted between animals and humans. Veterinary technicians are responsible for educating clients about preventing infection with zoonotic parasites. Parasites of zoonotic significance include protozoans, trematodes, cestodes, nematodes, and arthropods.

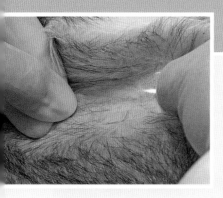

31

Sample Collection and Handling for Parasitology

LEARNING OBJECTIVES

After studying this chapter, you will be able to:
- Describe the collection of fecal samples from small animals.
- Describe the collection of fecal samples from large animals.
- Explain the procedure for the collection of samples through skin scraping.
- Explain the procedure for the collection of samples with the use of the cellophane tape preparation method.

- Describe the collection of samples for the diagnosis of blood parasites.
- Describe the collection of samples with the use of a vacuum cleaner technique.

OUTLINE

KEY TERMS

Cellophane tape preparations
Fecal loop

Pooled sample
Skin scraping

Vacuum collection

Parasites that infect the oral cavity, the esophagus, the stomach, the small and large intestines, and the other internal organs of animals are usually detected by microscopic examination of feces. Diagnosis usually involves identifying specific life-cycle stages of the parasites within the feces. These stages include eggs, oocysts, larvae, segments (tapeworms), and adult organisms. External parasites can be detected through skin scraping, cellophane tape preparations, vacuum collection, and brushing or combing the hair coat.

COLLECTION OF FECAL SAMPLES

Fecal samples that are collected for routine examination should be as fresh as possible. Specimens that cannot be examined within a few hours of excretion should be refrigerated or mixed with an equal part of 10% formalin. In older samples, the appearance of eggs, oocysts, and other life cycle stages may be altered as a result of parasite development.

Small Animal Fecal Samples

Several methods are used to collect feces from companion animals. An owner may collect a fecal sample immediately after

the animal has defecated. The feces can be stored in any type of container, such as a zippered plastic bag or a clean, small jar. Veterinary hospitals may dispense containers to their clients for this purpose. In either case, only a small amount of feces (1 g) is required for proper examination. Ideally, a small amount of sample should be collected from different areas of the defecated material. All specimens should be properly identified with the owner's name, the animal's name, and the species of the animal.

Fecal samples may also be collected directly from the animal at the veterinary hospital with the use of a gloved finger or a fecal loop (Fig. 31.1). If a glove is used, the feces may remain in the glove, with the glove turned inside out, tied, and labeled. To collect the sample with the fecal loop, apply a small amount of lubricant to the end of the loop, and then gently insert it into the animal's rectum to collect a small amount of fecal material. Samples collected with a fecal loop should be used for direct examination only, because the amount collected is relatively small.

Large Animal Fecal Samples

Fecal specimens that are collected from livestock may be obtained either directly from an individual animal's rectum or

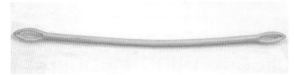

Fig. 31.1 The fecal loop is composed of a long plastic shaft with a small loop at each end. (From Sonsthagen T: *Veterinary instruments and equipment,* ed 2, St Louis, 2011, Mosby.)

from a number of animals to make up a pooled sample. Samples collected directly from an individual animal with a gloved hand can remain in the glove, with the glove turned inside out, tied, and labeled.

Pooled samples are collected from a number of animals that are housed together. The samples are then commingled in a single container. These samples are evaluated to determine the degree of infection within the group. Pooled samples can be collected in any type of container as long as it is clean and can be tightly sealed. These samples should be labeled with the species name and the pen or group number.

SKIN SCRAPING

Skin scraping is a common diagnostic procedure that is used to evaluate animals with suspected external parasites. Equipment needed to collect a skin scrape sample includes an electric clipper with a no. 40 blade, a scalpel or spatula, and mineral oil in a small dropper bottle. Typical lesions or sites that are most likely to harbor the particular parasite should be scraped (e.g., ear margins for *Sarcoptes scabiei* var. *canis*).

The scraping is performed with a no. 10 scalpel blade, with or without a handle. A 165-mm stainless steel spatula (Sargent-Welsh Scientific, Detroit, MI) may also be used. The scalpel blade should be held between the thumb and the forefinger (Fig. 31.2). Before the skin is scraped, the blade is dipped in a drop of mineral oil on the slide (Fig. 31.3), or a drop of mineral oil may be placed on the skin.

During the scraping process, the blade must be held perpendicular to the skin. Holding it at another angle may result in an accidental incision. The average area scraped should be approximately 3 cm^2 to 4 cm^2. Multiple sites should be scraped to increase the chances of collecting the parasite.

The depth of the scraping varies with the typical location of the parasite in question. When scraping for mites that live in tunnels (e.g., *Sarcoptes* species) or in hair follicles (e.g., *Demodex* species), scrape the skin until a small amount of capillary blood oozes from the scraped area (Fig. 31.4). Clipping the area with a no. 40 blade before scraping enables better visualization of the lesion and removes excess hair that impedes proper scraping and interferes with the collection of epidermal debris. Scraping at the interface between affected and unaffected sites is important. For surface-dwelling mites (e.g., *Cheyletiella, Psoroptes,* or *Chorioptes* species), the skin is scraped superficially to collect any loose scales or crusts. Clipping before scraping is not necessary when infestation with surface-dwelling mites is suspected.

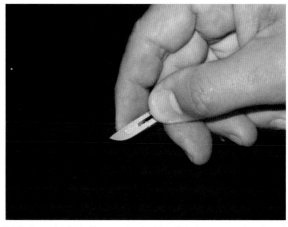

Fig. 31.2 A scalpel blade may be held safely between the thumb and forefinger for skin scrapings.

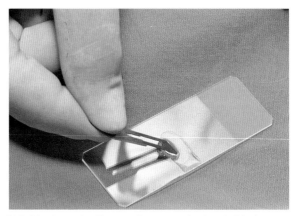

Fig. 31.3 Dip the scalpel in a small amount of mineral oil before scraping the skin. (From Taylor SM: *Small animal clinical techniques,* St Louis, 2010, Saunders.)

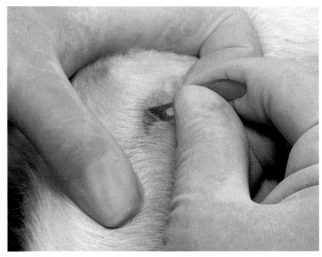

Fig. 31.4 For deep scraping, scrape the skin until a small amount of capillary blood oozes from the site. (From Taylor SM: *Small animal clinical techniques,* St Louis, 2010, Saunders.)

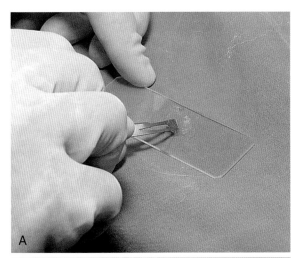

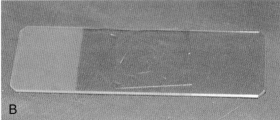

Fig. 31.5 Spread the scraped material onto the glass slide in the drop of mineral oil **(A)** and apply a coverslip **(B)**. (From Taylor SM: *Small animal clinical techniques*, St Louis, 2010, Saunders.)

All scraped debris on the forward surface of the blade is then spread in a drop of mineral oil on the glass slide (Fig. 31.5). A glass coverslip is placed on the material, and the slide is ready for microscopic examination with the use of the 4× (scanning) objective lens.

> **TECHNICIAN NOTE** When performing skin scrapes ensure you are scraping deep enough to cause bleeding.

CELLOPHANE TAPE PREPARATION

When attempting to demonstrate lice or mites that live primarily on the surface of the skin (e.g., *Cheyletiella*, *Psoroptes*, or *Chorioptes* species), a cellophane tape preparation may be used. Clear cellophane tape is applied to the skin to pick up epidermal debris (Fig. 31.6). A ribbon of mineral oil is placed on a glass slide, and the adhesive surface of the tape is then placed on the mineral oil (Fig. 31.7). Additional mineral oil and a coverslip may be placed on the tape to prevent the tape from wrinkling, but this is not necessary. The slide is then examined microscopically for parasites.

Flea collection is facilitated by spraying the pet with an insecticide. After a few minutes, dead fleas drop off of the animal. Alternatively, fleas may be collected with a fine-tooth flea comb available at any veterinary supply store or pet store.

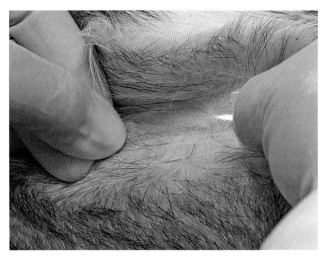

Fig. 31.6 Touch the sticky side of clear tape to the skin to collect parasites. (From Taylor SM: *Small animal clinical techniques*, St Louis, 2010, Saunders.)

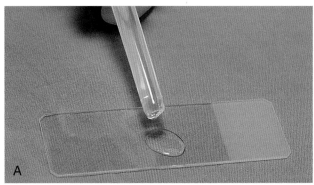

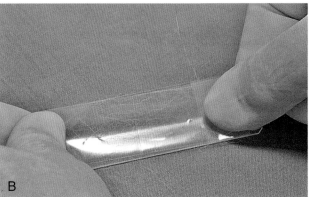

Fig. 31.7 A, Place a small amount of mineral oil on the slide. **B,** Place the sticky side of the tape down into the mineral oil. (From Taylor SM: *Small animal clinical techniques*, St Louis, 2010, Saunders.)

VACUUM COLLECTION

Parasites that are primarily present on the skin surface or on the hair can also be collected with the use of a vacuum cleaner. Gentle restraint of the patient is generally required, because the noise of the vacuum cleaner may stress some patients. To perform the procedure, place a piece of filter paper over the end

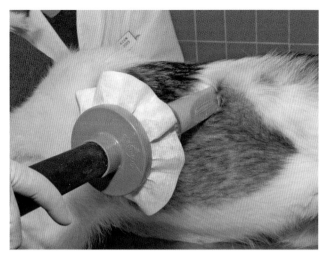

Fig. 31.8 Samples can be collected with a vacuum cleaner. Place a piece of filter paper over the end of the vacuum cleaner. (From Taylor SM: *Small animal clinical techniques*, St Louis, 2010, Saunders.)

SAMPLE COLLECTION AT NECROPSY

Necropsy (postmortem examination) is an important method of diagnosing many diseases, including parasitism. The types of lesions produced by immature parasites, any adult parasites found in the body cavity and tissues, and the histopathologic examination of infected tissues are used for diagnosis. Veterinary technicians are responsible for the samples collected and for making sure that they are properly contained, preserved, labeled, and shipped.

Two methods are used to recover parasites from the digestive tract at necropsy: the decanting method and the sieving method (Boxes 31.1 and 31.2). With either method, the veterinary technician must separate the different parts of the digestive tract and work with the contents of each section individually.

Parasites recovered from the digestive tract may be preserved in 70% alcohol or 10% neutral buffered formalin for later identification. Occasionally, bladder worms or cysticerci may be found attached to the viscera of domestic animals. These should be handled with care, because the fluid within the bladder can be allergenic and may also be zoonotic.

COLLECTION OF BLOOD SAMPLES

Sterile equipment and alcohol are required for the collection of a blood sample from an animal. Blood may be collected with the use of a syringe and needle or a Vacutainer (Becton Dickinson, Franklin Lakes, NJ). All samples should be labeled with the owner's name, the animal's name, and the date of collection. (See Chapter 7 in Unit 2 for more details regarding blood collection.)

> **BOX 31.1   Decanting Method**
> - Each section of the digestive tract is opened, and the contents are poured into a bucket.
> - The interior lining of the organ is scraped with a spatula, and the scrapings are added to the bucket or examined separately.
> - An amount of water equal to the contents of each bucket is added and thoroughly mixed.
> - The bucket is allowed to sit undisturbed for approximately 45 minutes.
> - The liquid is poured off and the sediment left in the bottom of the bucket.
> - An amount of water equal to the volume of the sediment is added and thoroughly mixed.
> - The process is repeated until the water over the sediment becomes clear.
> - The sediment is transferred to a dissecting pan and examined with a dissecting microscope or a magnifying glass.
> - Any parasites that are found are gently removed with thumb forceps and preserved.

> **BOX 31.2   Sieving Method**
> - The contents of the digestive tract, including scrapings from the interior lining, are placed in a bucket and mixed with an equal volume of water.
> - The mixture is poured through a no. 18 sieve and then through a no. 45 sieve.
> - The sieves' contents are rinsed with water.
> - The solid material in the sieves is examined with a dissecting microscope or a magnifying glass.
> - Any parasites that are found are gently removed with thumb forceps and preserved.

KEY POINTS

- The diagnosis of alimentary parasitism requires the examination of a fecal specimen for the presence of eggs (ova), oocysts, larvae, tapeworm proglottids, and adult parasites.
- Fecal samples from small animals can be collected after evacuation by the animal or with the use of a fecal loop or thermometer.
- Fecal samples from groups of large animals are often collected as pooled samples.
- Parasites that reside primarily on the surface of the skin can be collected with the cellophane tape method.
- Deep skin scraping is required to collect parasites that reside in hair follicles.

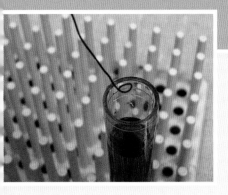

Diagnostic Techniques in Parasitology

LEARNING OBJECTIVES

After studying this chapter, you will be able to:
- Describe the gross examination of fecal samples.
- Describe the procedure for performing a fecal direct smear.
- Describe the procedure for performing fecal flotation.
- Discuss the advantages and disadvantages of various fecal flotation solutions.
- Describe the procedure for performing centrifugal flotation.
- Explain the use of the Baermann apparatus.
- Describe the procedure for performing a buffy coat smear.
- Describe the modified Knott's test.

OUTLINE

KEY TERMS

Baermann technique
Centrifugal flotation
Direct smear

Fecal sedimentation
McMaster technique
Modified Knott's test

Simple fecal flotation
Zinc sulfate

Parasites may be located in the oral cavity, the esophagus, the stomach, the small and large intestines, the internal organs, and the skin of animals. Diagnostic stages can be found in sputum, feces, blood, urine, secretions of the reproductive organs, and the epidermal layers of the skin. Samples collected for examination should be as fresh as possible and examined as soon as possible, preferably within the first 24 hours after collection. It is vital to take proper precautions when working with samples to prevent contamination of the work environment and to ensure personal health when handling agents that are transmissible to people. Wear gloves, wash your hands frequently with warm water and soap, and clean and disinfect work areas after examinations. In addition, it is important to clean equipment frequently.

TECHNICIAN NOTE Always wear gloves and proper outerwear when handling feces, because some parasites are zoonotic and can even enter the body through the skin.

The maintenance of good records is important. Label samples with the client's name, the date of collection, and the patient's name and species. Records should include identification information, the procedures performed, and the results. An adequate history that includes clinical signs, the duration of those signs, any medications given, the animal's environment, the vaccinations that the animal has received, the stocking density, and the number of animals affected for herd or flock examinations should accompany the sample.

The microscopic examination of samples is the most reliable method for the detection of parasitic infections. A binocular microscope with 10×, 40×, and 100× objective lenses is needed. A stereo microscope is also helpful for the identification of gross parasites. A calibrated ocular micrometer may be necessary to determine the sizes and specific differentiations of some parasitic stages, such as those of microfilariae (see Chapter 3 in Unit 1 of this book). Samples are generally mounted on a glass slide in a fluid medium with a coverslip on top. The sample should be thoroughly and systematically viewed with the 10× objective lens, beginning at one corner of the coverslip and ending at the opposite end. Parasite stages are usually in the same plane of focus as air bubbles or the edge of the coverslip. Any materials or objects observed can be viewed and verified with more powerful objectives. A good working knowledge of the parts of the binocular microscope and of the adjustments needed to produce Kohler illumination are essential for parasitology examinations.

EVALUATION OF FECAL SPECIMENS

Depending on clinical signs and the patient's history, it is likely that specific parasite infestations may be suspected. This information helps to guide the choice of test to be performed.

The parasitologic examination of feces begins with gross examination of the sample, noting consistency and color as well as the presence of blood, mucus, odor, adult parasites, or foreign bodies (e.g., string). Normal feces should be formed yet soft. Diarrhea or constipation can occur with parasitic infections. Most secretions are clear and moderately cellular. A yellowish discoloration with excessive mucus could signal infection. Blood in a sample can be fresh and bright red or partially digested (hemolyzed), appearing dark reddish brown to black and tarry. Excessive mucus in a sample generally indicates irritation to a mucosal membrane, with proliferation of mucus-producing cells. This is common in parasitic infections of the respiratory system and the lower digestive tract. Adult parasites such as roundworms and tapeworm proglottids can be found and identified in vomitus or feces.

> **TECHNICIAN NOTE** The gross examination of feces includes recording the consistency and color of the sample as well as the presence of blood, mucus, odor, adult parasites, or foreign bodies.

Direct Smear

Fecal direct smears are the simplest of the evaluation procedures. Feces, sputum, urine, smegma, and blood can be observed with the technique described in Procedure 32.1. This type of smear requires a minimum amount of equipment and materials, and it is a rapid scan for parasite stages. A fecal sample for a direct smear preparation may be obtained from an animal with the use of a fecal loop or a rectal thermometer (after measuring the animal's temperature). The procedure involves placing a small amount of feces on a clean glass slide and examining it microscopically for the presence of eggs and larvae. This method will also allow for the visualization of the trophozoite stages of protozoal parasites such as *Giardia*. The addition of Lugol's iodine can also help with identification of parasites.

Unfortunately, a direct smear alone is not an adequate examination for parasites. Disadvantages include the small amount of feces examined, which may not be sufficient to detect a low parasite burden, and the amount of extraneous fecal debris on the slide, which could be confused with parasitic

---

> ### PROCEDURE 32.1 Direct Smear of Feces
>
> **Materials**
> - Glass microscope slides (25 mm)
> - Glass coverslips (22 mm² [#1])
> - Wooden applicator sticks
> - Water or saline
>
> **Procedure**
> 1. Dip the applicator stick into the feces (only a small amount should adhere to the stick).
> 2. Place a drop of saline on a slide.
> 3. Mix the feces with the saline to produce a homogeneous emulsion that is clear enough to read newsprint through. (A common mistake is to make the smear too thick.)
> 4. Place the coverslip over the emulsion.
> 5. Examine the slide at 100× and 400× magnification for eggs, cysts, trophozoites, and larvae.

material. However, it should be incorporated as a routine part of any parasitology examination.

> **TECHNICIAN NOTE** The fecal direct smear technique involves the use of a small volume of sample, so parasite infections may be missed.

Fecal Flotation

Flotation methods are based on differences in the specific gravity of the life-cycle stages of parasites that are found in feces and fecal debris. Simple fecal flotation is an example of a flotation method (Procedure 32.2). Specific gravity refers to the weight of an object compared with the weight of an equal volume of distilled water, and it is a function of the total amount of dissolved material in the solution. Most parasite eggs have a specific gravity that is between 1.10 and 1.20 g/mL (Table 32.1). Flotation solutions are formulated with a specific gravity that is higher than that of common parasite ova. Therefore, the ova float to the surface of the solution. Saturated solutions of sugar and various salts are used as flotation solutions and have a specific gravity that ranges between 1.18 and 1.40. Fecal debris and eggs with a specific gravity greater than that of the flotation solution do not float. Fluke eggs are generally heavier than the specific gravity of most routinely used flotation solutions, with a few exceptions (e.g., *Paragonimus, Nanophyetus*), and they are not usually recovered with this technique. Nematode larvae can be recovered, but they are frequently distorted as a result of crenation, thereby making identification difficult. If the specific gravity of the flotation solution is too high, a plug of fecal debris floats and traps the parasite stages in it, thereby obscuring them from view.

Commonly used flotation solutions include sugar, sodium chloride, sodium nitrate, magnesium sulfate, and zinc sulfate. Each solution has advantages and disadvantages, including cost, availability, efficiency, shelf life, crystallization, corrosion of equipment, and ease of use (Table 32.2). Selection is often determined by the type of practice and the common parasites

PROCEDURE 32.2 Simple Fecal Flotation

Materials
- Glass microscope slides (25 mm)
- Glass coverslips (22 mm² [#1])
- Wooden tongue depressors
- Waxed paper cups (90–150 mL)
- Cheesecloth or gauze squares (10 cm) or a metal screen tea strainer
- Shell vial (1.25–2.0 cm or 5.0–7.5 cm) or 15-mL conical centrifuge tube
- Saturated salt or sugar flotation solution

Procedure
1. Place approximately 2 g to 5 g of feces in the paper cup.
2. Add 30 mL of flotation solution.
3. Use a tongue depressor to mix the feces and produce an evenly suspended emulsion.
4. If using cheesecloth or gauze, bend the sides of the cup to form a spout, and then cover the top with the cheesecloth squares while pouring the suspension into the shell vial. If using a metal strainer, pour the suspension through the metal strainer into another cup, and then fill the shell vial with the filtered solution.
5. Fill the shell vial to form a convex dome (meniscus) at the rim. Do not overfill the vial. Fresh solution can be used to form this dome.
6. Place a coverslip on top of the filled shell vial.
7. Allow the coverslip to remain undisturbed for 10 to 20 minutes.
8. Pick the coverslip straight up and then place it on a glass slide, with the fluid side down.
9. Systematically examine the surface under the coverslip at 100× magnification.

TABLE 32.1 Specific Gravity of Select Parasites

Species	Specific Gravity
Ancylostoma	1.06
Toxocara	1.09–1.10
Trichuris vulpis	1.15
Taenia	1.22
Cystoisospora	1.11
Toxoplasma gondii	1.11
Giardia	1.05

encountered in the area. The specific gravity of flotation solutions can be checked with the use of a hydrometer and adjusted by adding more salts or more water to the solution. Leaving extra crystals of salt on the bottom of the solution ensures that the solution is saturated.

Several companies have packaged flotation kits that include prepared solutions of sodium nitrate or zinc sulfate, disposable plastic vials, and strainers (Fig. 32.1). They are convenient, but they are also more expensive. Supplies to conduct simple flotation procedures can be acquired through suppliers of scientific equipment and chemicals. Products are also available that minimize the potential for personnel coming into contact with the fecal material (Fig. 32.2).

Centrifugal Flotation

This procedure is similar in principle to the flotation procedure except that, after the sample and solution are mixed, the specimen is strained to remove excess debris. A coverslip is added, and the specimen is centrifuged at 400 G to 650 G for 5 minutes. Centrifugal force holds the coverslips in place during spinning, provided that the tubes are balanced. A bacteriology loop is then used to remove a drop of liquid from the surface of the tube, and the drop is examined microscopically (Fig. 32.3). Centrifugal flotation is more sensitive than simple flotation. It recovers more eggs and cysts from a sample in less time (Procedure 32.3). However, it requires access to a tabletop centrifuge with a head that can accommodate rotation buckets. Fixed-angle heads do not work as well for this procedure as described, but they can be adapted for this procedure by not filling the tubes and omitting the coverslip during centrifugation.

> **TECHNICIAN NOTE** Centrifugal flotation recovers more eggs and cysts from a sample in less time than standard flotation.

Fecal Sedimentation

The fecal sedimentation procedure is used when suspected parasites produce ova that are too large to be recovered with standard flotation (e.g., fluke ova). The fecal sample is mixed in

TABLE 32.2 Commonly Used Flotation Solutions

	Specific Gravity*	Components	Comments
Magnesium sulfate (MgSO₄) (Epsom salt)	1.20	450 g of MgSO₄ 1000 mL of tap water	Corrosive; forms crystals
Zinc sulfate (ZnSO₄)	1.18–1.20	331 g of ZnSO₄ 1000 mL of warm tap water	Some trematode and pseudophyllidean tapeworm ova may not float; the use of this solution results in the least amount of distortion of common flotation solutions
Sodium nitrate solution (NaNO₃)	1.18–1.20	338 g of NaNO₃ 1000 mL of tap water	Forms crystals and distorts eggs if allowed to sit for more than 20 minutes
Modified Sheather's solution	1.27	454 g of granulated sugar 355 mL of tap water 6 mL of formaldehyde	Dissolve sugar and water in the top of a double boiler or with gentle heat; if the solution is not clear, filter it through coarse filter paper
Saturated salt (NaCl)	1.18–1.20	350 g of NaCl 1000 mL of tap water	Forms crystals and severely distorts parasite eggs; corrodes laboratory equipment

*Check the specific gravity with a hydrometer. Store solutions at room temperature.

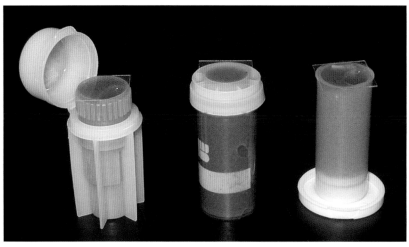

Fig. 32.1 Three commercially available fecal flotation kits: Fecalyzer *(left)*, Ovassay *(center)*, and Ovatector *(right)*. These kits are based on the principles of the simple flotation procedure. (From Hendrix CM, Robinson E: *Diagnostic parasitology for veterinary technicians*, ed 4, St Louis, 2012, Mosby.)

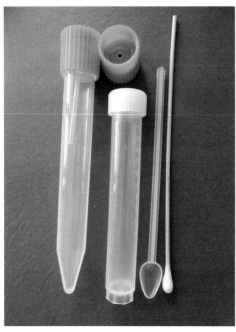

Fig. 32.2 The Fecal Parasite Concentration System replaces funnel-gauze filtration with tubes that are connected with a closed system strainer device.

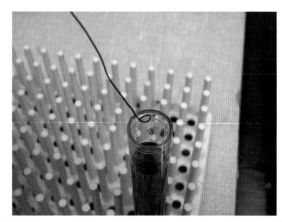

Fig. 32.3 The use of a bacteriologic loop to transfer a drop from the top of a fecal flotation emulsion after the centrifugation procedure. Note that loop is bent at a 90-degree angle to the wire handle. (From Hendrix CM, Robinson E: *Diagnostic parasitology for veterinary technicians*, ed 4, St Louis, 2012, Mosby.)

higher specific gravity, thereby making it difficult to recognize them. A few drops of liquid detergent can be added to the water as a surfactant to help remove excess fats and debris from the sample.

> **TECHNICIAN NOTE** Fecal sedimentation is used primarily when fluke infections are suspected.

CELLOPHANE TAPE PREPARATION

This method is often used to recover the ova of *Oxyuris* (pinworms). It can also help with the identification of tapeworms. A piece of cellophane tape is wrapped around a tongue depressor with the adhesive side out. The animal's tail is raised, and the tongue depressor is pressed firmly against the anus. The tape is removed, applied to a glass slide that has a small amount of water on it, and then examined microscopically (Procedure 32.5).

a small volume of water and strained into a centrifuge tube. The sample can be centrifuged at 400 G for 5 minutes or allowed to remain undisturbed for 20 to 30 minutes. The supernatant is poured off, and a pipette is used to remove a drop of the sediment. One drop from the upper, middle, and lower portions of the sediment is removed, and these three drops are then examined microscopically. Sedimentation concentrates parasite stages as well as fecal debris (Procedure 32.4). Because of the debris, parasite stages may be obscured from view. This technique is also more laborious. Sedimentation is used primarily when fluke infections are suspected. Most fluke eggs do not float, or they are distorted by flotation solutions with a

PROCEDURE 32.3 Centrifugal Flotation

Materials

- Glass microscope slides (25 mm)
- Glass coverslips (22 mm² [#1])
- Waxed paper cups
- Cheesecloth or gauze squares (10 cm) or a metal screen tea strainer
- Funnel
- Conical centrifuge tubes (15 mL)
- Test tube rack
- Flotation solution
- Centrifuge with rotating buckets*
- Wooden tongue depressors
- Balance scale

Procedure

1. Prepare a fecal emulsion using 2 g to 5 g of feces and 30 mL of the flotation solution.
2. Strain the emulsion through the cheesecloth or tea strainer into the centrifuge tube. (Suspending a funnel over the tube facilitates the filling of the tube.)
3. Fill the tube to create a positive meniscus with the flotation solution.
4. Place a coverslip on top of the tube.
5. Create a balance tube of equal weight that contains another sample or water.
6. Place the tubes in the centrifuge buckets, and weigh them on a balance. You may add water to the buckets to make them equal weights.
7. Centrifuge the tubes for 5 minutes at 400 G to 650 G (approximately 1500 rpm).
8. Remove the coverslips from the tubes by lifting straight up, and then place them on a slide.
9. Systematically examine the slides at 100× magnification.

*For centrifuges with fixed-angle heads, do not fill the tubes, and omit the coverslip during centrifugation.

PROCEDURE 32.4 Fecal Sedimentation

Materials

- Waxed paper cups (90–150 mL)
- Wooden tongue depressors
- Cheesecloth or gauze squares (10 cm) or a metal screen tea strainer
- Funnel
- Conical centrifuge tubes (50 mL)
- Disposable pipettes (2 mL)
- Glass microscope slides (25 mm)
- Glass coverslips (22 mm² [#1])

Procedure

1. Mix 2 g to 5 g of feces in a cup with 30 mL of water.
2. Strain the fecal suspension through the cheesecloth, gauze, or tea strainer into a 50-mL conical centrifuge tube. (Suspending a funnel over the tube facilitates the filling of the tube.)
3. Wash the sample with water until the tube is filled.
4. Allow the tube to sit undisturbed for 15 to 30 minutes.
5. Decant the supernatant off, and then resuspend the sediment in water.
6. Repeat Steps 4 and 5 two more times.
7. Decant the supernatant without disturbing the sediment.
8. Use a pipette to mix the sediment, and then transfer an aliquot to a slide.
9. Place a coverslip over the sediment, and systematically examine the slide with 100× magnification.
10. Repeat Steps 8 and 9 until all sediment has been examined.

PROCEDURE 32.5 Cellophane Tape Preparation

Materials

- Transparent adhesive tape
- Wooden tongue depressors
- Glass microscope slides (25 mm)

Procedure

1. Place adhesive tape in a loop around one end of the tongue depressor, with the adhesive side facing out.
2. Press the tape firmly against the skin around the anus.
3. Place a drop of water on the slide. Undo the loop of tape, and then stick the tape to the slide, allowing the water to spread out under the tape.
4. Examine the taped area of the slide microscopically for the presence of pinworm eggs.

BAERMANN TECHNIQUE

The Baermann technique is sometimes used to recover larvae from fecal samples. The procedure requires the construction of a Baermann apparatus, which consists of a large funnel supported in a ring stand. A piece of rubber tubing is attached to the end of the funnel and placed in a collection tube. The fecal sample is placed in the funnel on top of a piece of metal screen (Fig. 32.4). Warm water or warmed physiologic saline is passed

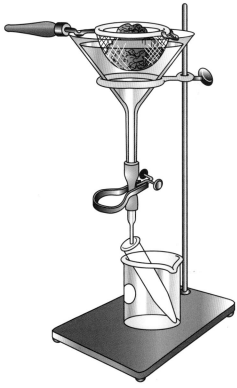

Fig. 32.4 The Baermann apparatus is used to recover the larvae of roundworms from feces, soil, or animal tissues. This apparatus is most useful for recovering the larvae of lungworms. (From Bowman D: *Georgis' parasitology for veterinarians*, ed 9, St Louis, 2009, Saunders.)

through the sample. The larvae are stimulated to move by the warm water, and they then sink to the bottom of the apparatus. A drop of the material in the collection container is examined microscopically for the presence of larvae. The Baermann technique is used to recover nematode larvae from feces, fecal cultures, soil, herbage, and animal tissues (Procedure 32.6). The warm water stimulates the larvae to migrate out of the sample and relax. They then sink to the bottom of the apparatus, where they can be collected relatively free of debris. Free-living larvae must be distinguished from parasitic ones, especially if the sample is collected off of the ground, from soil, or from herbage. This may require the expertise of an experienced helminthologist. Preserve samples by adding 5% to 10% formalin to the pellet for submission to an expert. Kill free-living larvae by adding 1% hydrochloric acid to the pellet, and examine the preparation without heat fixation. Unfortunately, the identification of motile larvae is more difficult.

The Baermann technique is performed on feces of domestic animals when lungworm infections (i.e., *Dictyocaulus, Aelurostrongylus, Filaroides, Crenosoma, Muellerius,* and *Protostrongylus*) are suspected. Ideally, samples should be fresh and collected rectally. For dogs and cats, the Baermann technique should be used when infection with *Strongyloides* species are suspected. If the sample is not fresh, a fecal culture may be needed to distinguish first-stage hookworm larvae from the first-stage larvae of *Strongyloides*. The third-stage filariform larva of *Strongyloides* is diagnostic and characterized by an esophagus that is half the length of the larva and a forked (bipartite) tail. Care should be taken when handling *Strongyloides* fecal cultures because of the zoonotic potential of this organism.

MODIFIED MCMASTER TECHNIQUE

An additional type of fecal flotation test is the modified McMaster technique. This technique provides an estimate of the number of eggs or oocysts per gram of feces, and is primarily used with livestock species and horses (Procedure 32.8). Originally it was adapted from a technique used in people infected with hookworms to estimate the worm population in the host. However, it is impossible to calculate the actual worm population in a host, especially in livestock and horses, because many factors influence egg production, and the number of eggs produced varies with the species and number of worms present.

Typically, livestock and horses are infected with several species of worms at one time, and some species are more prolific and pathogenic than others. In addition, lesions often result from damage produced by the immature stages of the parasites. In ruminants, the parasites of interest are coccidia and trichostrongyles. In horses, the parasites of interest are large and small strongyles. Both trichostrongyles and strongyles infect ruminants and horses. The eggs of trichostrongyles and strongyles cannot be readily distinguished from one another, and they are referred to collectively as strongyle eggs. Nevertheless, counts in excess of 1000 are considered indicative of heavy infections, whereas those of more than 500 indicate moderate infections. A low egg count can indicate a low level of infection or a severe infection in which the parasites are just becoming mature. Egg counts must always be interpreted in view of the clinical signs observed; the age, sex, and nutritional level of the animal; and the stocking density of the herd or flock.

Egg counts have been used in epidemiologic investigations and herd health management programs as predictors of peak pasture contamination and transmission potential for different geographic regions and individual farms. This information is applied toward prevention programs that involve the strategic use of broad-spectrum anthelmintics and pasture rotation schemes aimed at reducing the infective levels of pastures and exposure rates. When herd studies are conducted, individual samples are taken from at least 10% of the herd. Egg counts are also used to monitor the development of resistance to anthelmintics. Egg counts are done before treatment and again 3 weeks after treatment to determine the effectiveness of the anthelmintic used and the development of resistance in a given worm population.

PROCEDURE 32.6 Baermann Technique

Materials
- Baermann apparatus (i.e., ring stand, ring, funnel, rubber tubing, clamp, and wire screen)
- Cheesecloth or Kimwipes
- Disposable pipettes
- Centrifuge tubes (15 mL) or Petri dishes
- Pinch clamps

Procedure
1. Construct a Baermann apparatus by fastening the ring to the ring stand. Attach 3 to 4 inches of rubber tubing to the narrow portion of the funnel. Ensure that there is a good seal. (The tubing can be glued on.) Place the funnel in the ring. Place the wire screen in the top portion of the funnel to support the feces. Put several layers of cheesecloth or Kimwipes over the wire screen. Place the pinch clamps at the end of the rubber tubing and check, with the use of water, to ensure a tight seal. Put 30 g to 50 g of feces on top of the cheesecloth or Kimwipes, and fill the funnel with warm water (not hot) to a level above the fecal sample. (An alternative method, which is more practical in a practice setting, is to use long-stemmed plastic champagne glasses with hollow stems. The feces are wrapped in several layers of Kimwipes in a way that is similar to a teabag. The fecal pouch is then set in the glass. Fill the glass with warm water to a level above the fecal sample.)
2. Allow the apparatus to remain undisturbed for a minimum of 1 hour and up to 24 hours.
3. Collect the fluid in the rubber tubing (or the stem of the glass), and transfer it to a Petri dish or a centrifuge tube.
4. Examine the Petri dish for larvae with the use of a stereo microscope, or centrifuge the solution to pellet the larvae. Remove the supernatant from the centrifuge tube, and then place the pellet on a microscope slide.
5. Examine the slide for larvae, and identify them. The slide can be passed over the flame of a Bunsen burner several times to kill the larvae in an extended position before identification.

PROCEDURE 32.7   Fecal Culture

Materials
- Glass jar with tight-fitting lid
- Charcoal or vermiculite
- Wooden tongue depressors

Procedure
1. Moisten 50 g of charcoal or vermiculite with water. The charcoal or vermiculite should be damp but not wet.
2. Use a tongue depressor to mix an equal amount of feces with the moistened substrate.
3. Place the fecal mixture in a glass jar, and seal the jar with the lid.
4. Place the jar in indirect light at room temperature for up to 7 days.
5. Check the jar periodically to ensure that the contents remain moist. A spray bottle of water can be used to moisten the fecal mixture if it becomes too dry. Be sure not to saturate the material.
6. Perform a Baermann technique on the fecal culture at 48-hour intervals to recover developing stages. Some larvae migrate up the wall of the jar and congregate in condensation droplets. These can be collected by flushing the sides of the jar with water and then collecting the excess fluid in a centrifuge tube or Petri dish.
7. Identify the larvae that are recovered.

PROCEDURE 32.8   Modified McMaster Quantitative Egg-Counting Technique

Materials
- McMaster slides (Olympic Equine Products, Issaquah, WA)
- Waxed paper cups (90—150 mL) or beakers
- Graduated cylinder
- Balance scale
- Saturated sodium chloride solution
- Wooden tongue depressors
- Disposable pipettes
- Rotary stirrer (optional)

Procedure
1. Use the balance scale to weigh 5 g of feces, and then place the sample into a cup.
2. Add a small amount of the flotation solution to the cup.
3. Mix the feces and flotation solution together thoroughly with a tongue depressor to make an even suspension.
4. Add sufficient flotation solution to bring the total volume to 75 mL.
5. Turn the rotary stirrer on, and place the cup that contains the fecal suspension in it. If a rotary stirrer is not available, the fecal suspension can be mixed with a tongue depressor.
6. Use a pipette to withdraw a portion of the mixing suspension, and then fill the chambers of the McMaster slide.
7. Allow the slide to sit undisturbed for 10 minutes.
8. Using the 10× objective lens, focus on the grid that is etched in the McMaster slide. Count all of the eggs or oocysts seen in the six columns of the etched square, and keep a separate count for each species of parasite that is seen.
9. Multiply the numbers counted by the appropriate dilution factor (this is dependent on the number of squares counted), and record the results as eggs per gram (epg) of feces. The volume under the etched area is 0.15 mL. If 5 g per 75 mL total volume equals 1 g per 15 mL total volume, then 0.01 g is contained in 0.15 mL. Therefore, if one chamber is counted, multiply by 100. If two chambers are counted, multiply by 50 to arrive at the total epg.

NOTE: Several protocols are available; this is just one example.

MISCELLANEOUS FECAL EXAMINATIONS

Some parasites produce intestinal bleeding. This bleeding may be evident as frank blood in the fecal sample or as darkened feces. Some intestinal bleeding can only be identified with chemical testing. This is referred to as fecal occult blood testing. Several types of kits are available for this procedure, and they primarily act to identify the presence of hemoglobin in the sample.

The examination of vomitus may also aid in the diagnosis of parasitism. Some parasites (e.g., *Toxocara canis*) are often present in the vomitus of infected patients.

Fecal culture is used to differentiate parasites that have eggs or larvae that are not easily distinguished via the examination of a fresh fecal sample (Procedure 32.7). Trichostrongyle eggs in ruminant feces are indistinguishable from strongyle eggs. Small strongyle eggs found in a horse fecal sample cannot be distinguished from large strongyle eggs. First-stage hookworm larvae in a dog or cat sample and some free-living nematode larvae in soil or on grass cannot be easily distinguished from first-stage *Strongyloides* larvae. After fecal culture, the third-stage larvae of many of these parasites can be identified to the genus level. Because the life cycles, pathogenicity, and epidemiology of some species may differ, identification may be necessary for proper treatment and control. Identification may require the help of an experienced helminthologist.

STAINING PROCEDURES

Stains may also be used to recognize certain structural characteristics of trophozoites and cysts. Lugol's iodine and new methylene blue are common stains that are used with the direct smear procedure. These stains do not preserve the slide, but they do facilitate the examination of the specimen, thereby making identification easier.

If a protozoal parasite cannot be identified with a direct smear, a fecal smear that contains protozoal trophozoites can be dried; stained with Diff-Quik, Wright's, or Giemsa stain; and sent to a diagnostic laboratory.

The acid-fast staining technique is used to identify *Cryptosporidium* species in feces. Cryptosporidium is a parasite of the gastrointestinal tract of many animals, including human beings. The oocysts are 2 μm to 8 μm in diameter, and they are almost undetectable in flotation solution to the inexperienced eye. Acid-fast staining can help to detect the oocysts in a fecal smear.

Diff-Quik stain can be used to help with the identification of *Isospora* species. An intestinal mucosal scraping is stained and examined for diagnostic stages (e.g., schizonts, merozoites) of this parasite. This procedure involves scraping the mucosa of the jejunum and smearing the scrapings onto microscope slides. After the slides are air dried, they are stained with Diff-Quik and examined with the oil-immersion objective lens.

EVALUATION OF BLOOD SAMPLES

The examination of blood samples may reveal adult parasites and their various life-cycle stages, either free in the blood or intracellularly. A variety of methods can be used for this determination. Thin or thick blood smears are prepared in the same way that smears for a white blood cell differential count are prepared. (The preparation of smears for this type of count is described in Unit 2, Chapter 9.) Most parasites are carried with the laminar flow to the feathered edge of the slide. Parasites may be located between cells, on the surface of cells, or in the cytoplasm of cells. Thin blood films are most effectively used to study the morphology of protozoan and rickettsial parasites. If parasitemia is low, infections can be missed. A thick blood film or a buffy coat smear is more effective because it concentrates a larger volume of cells (Procedure 32.9).

The buffy coat smear is a concentration technique for the detection of protozoa and rickettsiae in white blood cells. A microhematocrit tube is centrifuged as is done for a packed cell volume determination. Microfilariae and some protozoa may also be found at the top of the plasma column (Fig. 32.5). The technique is quick, but it cannot be used to differentiate *Dirofilaria immitis* from *Acanthocheilonema reconditum*.

> **TECHNICIAN NOTE** The buffy coat smear is useful for the detection of protozoa and rickettsiae in white blood cells.

Direct Drop

The direct drop is the simplest of the blood evaluations, although it is also the least accurate as a result of the small sample size used. A drop of anticoagulated whole blood is examined microscopically. The movement of parasites that are extracellular can be detected with this method.

Filter Test

The filter technique is a method that is designed to concentrate microfilariae in blood (Procedure 32.10). The principles applied are similar to those of the modified Knott's test, except that the blood is passed through a Millipore filter, which collects the microfilariae. Commercial kits make use of a detergent lysing solution and a differential stain (Fig. 32.6). This

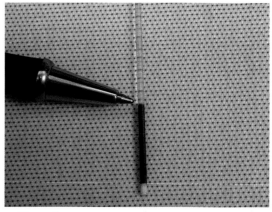

Fig. 32.5 The buffy coat in a hematocrit tube. (From Hendrix CM, Robinson E: *Diagnostic parasitology for veterinary technicians*, ed 4, St Louis, 2012, Mosby.)

PROCEDURE 32.9 Buffy Coat Smear

Materials
- Hematocrit tubes
- Sealant
- Hematocrit centrifuge
- Glass microscope slides (25 mm)
- Glass coverslips (22 mm² [#1])
- File
- Permount Mounting Medium

Procedure
1. Fill the hematocrit tube with the blood sample, and plug one end with sealant.
2. Centrifuge the sample for 5 minutes.
3. The buffy coat is located in the middle of the centrifuged sample, between the red blood cells and the plasma.
4. Use the file to etch the glass below the buffy coat. Snap the tube by applying pressure opposite the etched spot.
5. Take the end of the tube that contains the buffy coat and plasma, and tap the buffy coat onto a glass slide with a small amount of plasma. If too much plasma is released, use a clean Kimwipe to wipe away excess.
6. Apply a clean slide over the buffy coat, and rapidly pull the two slides across each other in opposite directions.
7. Allow the slides to air dry, and stain them with Romanowsky stain.
8. After staining, apply the mounting medium and a coverslip.
9. Examine the slides microscopically at 400× and 1000× magnification.

PROCEDURE 32.10 Millipore Filtration Procedure

Materials
- 5-μ Millipore filters
- Millipore filter holders
- 2.5% methylene blue stain
- 2% formalin
- Glass microscope slides (25 mm)
- Glass coverslips (22 mm² [#1])
- 12-mL disposable syringes

Procedure
1. Assemble the filter holder with a Millipore filter.
2. Place 1 mL of blood in the syringe.
3. Add 9 mL of 2% formalin to the blood in the syringe, and insert the plunger.
4. Connect the syringe to the filter apparatus, and slowly apply pressure to the syringe plunger.
5. Remove the syringe, and fill it with tap water. Allow a few milliliters of air to remain in the syringe. Flush the water through the filter apparatus.
6. Remove the filter from the filter holder, and place it topside up on a glass slide.
7. Place a drop of the methylene blue stain on the filter, and then add a coverslip.
8. Examine the slide microscopically for microfilariae at 100× magnification.

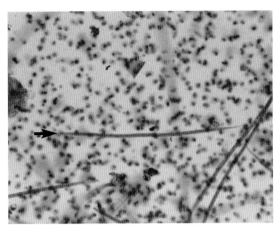

Fig. 32.6 Microfilariae of *Dirofilaria immitis* as shown by the Difil Test *(arrow).* (From Hendrix CM, Robinson E: *Diagnostic parasitology for veterinary technicians,* ed 4, St Louis, 2012, Mosby.)

TABLE 32.3 Differentiation of Microfilariae Using the Modified Knott's Technique

	Dirofilaria Immitis	*Acanthocheilonema Reconditum*
Body length	310 μm	290 μm
Mid-body width	6 μm	6 μm
Head	Tapered	Blunt
Tail	Straight	Hooked*

*Artifact of formalin fixation.

procedure is quicker and easier than the modified Knott's test, but the differential characteristics of the microfilariae are not as obvious. Identification involving the characteristics listed in Table 32.3 is not possible with commercial kits, because the characteristics of the microfilariae are based on fixation with 2% formalin.

Modified Knott's Test

The modified Knott's test is used to concentrate microfilaria, and it can help with the differentiation of *Dirofilaria* from *Acanthocheilonema (Dipetalonema).* The procedure requires a mixture of blood and formalin in a centrifuge tube. The mixture is incubated at room temperature for 1 to 2 minutes and then centrifuged for 5 minutes. The supernatant is poured off, and a drop of methylene blue is added to the sediment in the tube. A drop of this mixture is then transferred to a glass slide for microscopic evaluation (Procedure 32.11). The technique concentrates microfilariae while fixing them, and it lyses red blood cells. When preparing the 2% formalin solution, it is important to remember that 37% formaldehyde is equivalent to 100% formalin. It is also important to use water and not physiologic saline to prepare this solution, because physiologic saline does not lyse red blood cells. For the accurate differentiation of the microfilariae, the microscope must have a calibrated ocular micrometer. The most accurate differentiating characteristics are body width, body length, and the shape of

PROCEDURE 32.11 Modified Knott's Technique

Materials
- Blood collection materials
- 15-mL conical centrifuge tubes
- 2% formalin (2 mL of 37% formaldehyde/98 mL of water)
- 2.5% methylene blue (2.5 g of methylene blue/100 mL of water)
- Tabletop centrifuge
- Glass microscope slides (25 mm)
- Glass coverslips (22 mm^2 [#1])
- Pipettes

Procedure
1. Mix 1 mL of blood with 9 mL of 2% formalin in a centrifuge tube. Agitate the tube, and mix its contents well.
2. Centrifuge the tube at 1500 rpm for 5 minutes.
3. Pour off the supernatant, and then add 1 to 2 drops of methylene blue stain to the pellet at the bottom of the tube.
4. Mix the stain and the sediment using a pipette, and then transfer the mixture to a glass slide.
5. Apply a coverslip, and examine the sediment microscopically for microfilariae at 100× and 400× magnification.

the cranial end. The other characteristics are not consistent. The modified Knott's technique cannot detect occult heartworm infections.

> **TECHNICIAN NOTE** The modified Knott's test, the buffy coat smear, and the direct drop technique can help with the differentiation of the microfilaria of *Dirofilaria immitis* and *Acanthocheilonema reconditum.*

IMMUNOLOGIC AND MOLECULAR DIAGNOSTIC TESTS

A variety of tests are available to identify antigens and antibodies to specific parasites. The majority of tests are based on the enzyme-linked immunosorbent assay (ELISA) principle. The tests are highly accurate and precise, and they can detect occult infections. Canine heartworm infections and *Toxoplasma* infections are routinely diagnosed with these methods. The ELISA method involves the use of monoclonal antibodies to detect antigens of adult heartworms in the serum or plasma of dogs. These procedures are rapid and easy to perform. They are also more sensitive and specific than microfilariae detection methods. The American Heartworm Society currently recommends using antigen-detection methods for routine screening. Antigen-detection methods are preferred to microfilariae concentration methods in cats, because such aberrant hosts circulate microfilariae for only a very short time. However, antigen levels in the blood of infected cats may also be too low to detect. Other methods (e.g., radiography) may also be employed to make a diagnosis in cats.

Approximately 25% of heartworm-infected dogs have occult infections. Occult infections are characterized by a lack of circulating microfilaria. They occur if the infection is not yet patent, if the population of adult heartworms consists of only one sex, and if the immune reactions of the host to microfilariae eliminate this stage from the bloodstream. Occult infections can also occur if animals infected with adult heartworms are given heartworm-prevention medications of the ivermectin group, because these interfere with oogenesis and sterilize the worms.

The identification of specific protozoal parasites (e.g., *Cryptosporidium, Giardia*) are also performed with the use of molecular diagnostics, such as the polymerase chain reaction.

MISCELLANEOUS PARASITOLOGIC EVALUATIONS

Cellophane tape preparations, as described previously, can be used to recover external parasites that live primarily on the surface of the skin (i.e., mites, lice, and fleas). Parasites that live in hair follicles or burrows are usually diagnosed with the use of standard skin-scraping procedures.

Samples may be collected from the ear or the respiratory or genital tracts with cotton swabs. These can be examined microscopically with the use of standard preparations as for cytology samples. Transtracheal and bronchial washes can also be used to recover parasites of the respiratory system. Parasites of the urinary system are usually recovered using standard urine sediment examination techniques. Impression smears can be used for the diagnosis of intracellular parasites. They can also be useful for the diagnosis of parasitic, neoplastic, and fungal diseases antemortem and postmortem. These procedures are described in more detail in Unit 7. Frequently, protozoal organisms produce systemic disease. These organisms may be located in the reticuloendothelial cells of the lymph nodes, liver, lung, bone marrow, spleen, brain, kidneys, and muscles. In addition, the liver, lungs, lymph nodes, bone marrow, and spleen filter out damaged and abnormal cells of the blood, thereby collecting parasitized cells. Toxoplasmosis, leishmaniasis, ehrlichiosis, and babesiosis are examples of parasitic diseases that can be diagnosed with the use of cytology techniques.

Skin scrapings are used as a diagnostic tool for dermatologic conditions, especially mange in domestic animals. Because some mange mites dwell in burrows and hair follicles deep in the epidermis, superficial scrapings are not productive. Other mites live in the more superficial layers of the skin and produce crusty or scaly lesions; deep scrapings are not required to diagnose these infestations. Sometimes the thick crusts interfere with the visualization of the mites. Soaking the crust in a 10% potassium hydroxide solution helps to dissolve the keratinized skin and releases the mites. Mite infestations usually localize in specific locations (e.g., ear margin, tail head) initially, depending on the species of mite involved. Later, they may become generalized and more difficult to diagnose. *Sarcoptes* and *Cheyletiella* mites can be transmitted to people and produce pruritic reactions that require attention. The specific identification of mites can be accomplished with the aid of taxonomic keys.

Cheyletiella infestation can be diagnosed by combing the coat of infested animals over a piece of black paper and observing the paper for "moving dandruff." *Otodectes cynotis* infestations of the external ear canal can be diagnosed with otoscopic examination or by taking a swab of the dark waxy debris found in the ear and microscopically examining it in mineral oil.

Tritrichomonas foetus is a flagellated protozoan parasite of the reproductive tract of cattle that causes early-term abortions and repeat breeding. The organism can be found in fluid from the abomasum of aborted fetuses, uterine discharges, and vaginal and preputial washes. However, the numbers present are usually low, and culture of these materials facilitates diagnosis. Occasionally, intestinal flagellates can contaminate a sample. These must be differentiated from *T. foetus*, which has three cranial flagella and one caudal flagellum attached to an undulating membrane. Isolates of *T. foetus* can be propagated through several passages of culture medium, whereas intestinal flagellates usually cannot. Materials may also be collected and shipped to diagnostic facilities for culture and identification. InPouch TF (Biomed Diagnostics, White City, OR) is an excellent transport medium.

Tables 32.4 and 32.5 list the diagnostic characteristics of the internal parasites of domestic animals.

TABLE 32.4   Diagnostic Characteristics of Internal Parasites of Domestic Animals

Parasite	Prepatent Period	Diagnostic Stage	Diagnostic Test
Acanthocheilonema reconditum (formerly *Dipetalonema reconditum*)	9 weeks	Microfilaria	Modified Knott's test Millipore filtration
Aelurostrongylus abstrusus	4–6 weeks	L1 with S-shaped tail and a dorsal spine; 360 μm long; esophagus is one third of the length of the body	Baermann
Ancylostoma braziliense	3 weeks	Hookworm egg; 75–95 μm × 41–45 μm	Fecal flotation
Ancylostoma caninum	2–3 weeks	Clear, smooth, thin-walled hookworm egg; 8- to 16-celled morula zygote; 55–65 μm × 27–43 μm	Fecal flotation

TABLE 32.4	Diagnostic Characteristics of Internal Parasites of Domestic Animals—cont'd		
Parasite	**Prepatent Period**	**Diagnostic Stage**	**Diagnostic Test**
Anoplocephala spp.	1—2 months	Clear, thick-walled, square eggs with a pear-shaped (piriform) apparatus that contains a hexacanth embryo	Fecal flotation
Ascaris suum	7—9 weeks	Brownish-yellow, thick-walled, mammillated egg; single-celled zygote; 50—80 μm × 40—60 μm	Fecal flotation
Ascarops strongylina	6 weeks	Oblong, clear, smooth, thick-walled, larvated egg; 34—40 μm × 18-22 μm	Fecal flotation
Balantidium coli		Thin-walled, greenish cyst with hyaline cytoplasm, 40—60 μm; trophozoite with rows of cilia, 30—150 μm × 25—120 μm	Fecal flotation / Direct smear
Bunostomum spp.	2—3 weeks	Strongyle egg	Fecal flotation
Capillaria plica	60 days	Rough, striated, thick-walled, barrel-shaped, amber-colored egg with asymmetric bipolar plugs; single-celled zygote; 60—68 μm × 24—30 μm	Sedimentation of urine
Cryptosporidium muris	4—10 days	Clear, smooth, thin-walled oocyst that contains four sporozoites; 5 μm × 7 μm	Fecal flotation
Cryptosporidium spp.	4—10 days	Clear, thin-walled, spherical oocyst that contains four sporozoites; 5 μm × 5 μm	Fecal flotation
Cyathostoma (small strongyles)	2—3 months	Smooth, thin-walled, clear strongyle egg zygote; 8- to 16-cell morula; size varies with species	Fecal flotation
Dicrocoelium dendriticum	10—12 weeks	Dark brown, operculated egg; 36—45 μm × 22—30 μm	Sedimentation of feces
Dictyocaulus arnfieldi	2—4 months	L1 with dark, granular intestines; esophagus is one third of the length of the larva; tapered tail	Fecal flotation / Baermann
Dictyocaulus spp.	3—4 weeks	L1 with dark granular intestines; esophagus is one third of the length of the larva; straight, pointed tail; 550—580 μm long	Baermann
Dioctophyma renale	5 months	Dark brown, thick-walled, barrel-shaped egg with a pitted shell and an operculum at each pole; single-celled zygote; 71—84 μm × 46—52 μm	Sedimentation of urine
Dipylidium caninum	3 weeks	Proglottid with bilateral genital pores; eggs contain six-hooked hexacanth embryos in packets; 35—60 μm	Identification of proglottids via fecal flotation
Dirofilaria immitis	6—8 months	Microfilaria (L1) lacks an esophagus	Modified Knott's test / Millipore filtration / Enzyme-linked immunosorbent assay / Antigen test
Dracunculus insignis	309—410 days	Comma-shaped larva with an esophagus and a straight tail; 500—750 μm long	Direct smear of fluid taken from blister
Echinococcus spp.	47 days	Similar to *Taenia* eggs	Fecal flotation
Eimeria leuckarti	15—33 days	Dark brown, piriform, thick-walled oocyst 70—90 μm × 49-69 μm	Fecal flotation
Eimeria spp.	4—30 days	Smooth or rough, thin-walled, clear to yellowish-brown oocysts; single-celled zygote; size varies with species	Fecal flotation
Elaeophora schneideri	4—5 months	Microfilaria in the skin of the poll; 207 μm × 13 μm	Skin biopsy
Eucoleus aerophilus (formerly *Capillaria aerophila*)	6 weeks	Rough, granular, thick-walled, barrel-shaped, straw-colored egg with asymmetric bipolar plugs; single-celled zygote; 58—79 μm × 29—40 μm	Fecal flotation
Fasciola hepatica	10—12 weeks	Dark amber, oval, operculated egg; 130—150 μm × 63—90 μm	Sedimentation of feces
Filaroides spp.	5—10 weeks	L1 with S-shaped tail and lacking a dorsal spine; esophagus is one third of the length of the body; 230—266 μm long	Fecal flotation / Baermann
Gasterophilus spp.		2.5-cm long robust grub with rows of spines and straight spiracular slits (breathing tubes)	Identification of third instar at necropsy
Giardia spp.	7—10 days	Smooth, clear, thin-walled cyst with two to four nuclei; 4—10 μm × 8—16 μm	Fecal flotation
Giardia spp.		Piriform, bilaterally symmetric, greenish trophozoite with two nuclei and four pairs of flagella; 9—20 μm × 5—15 μm	Direct smear

Continued

TABLE 32.4   Diagnostic Characteristics of Internal Parasites of Domestic Animals—cont'd

Parasite	Prepatent Period	Diagnostic Stage	Diagnostic Test
Habronema and *Draschia* spp.	2 months	Thin-walled, larvated egg (rarely seen)	Identification of adults at necropsy
Hyostrongylus rubidus	15—21 days	Strongyle egg	Fecal flotation
Isospora spp.	4—12 days	Clear, spherical to ellipsoid, thin-walled oocyst; size varies with species	Fecal flotation
Macracanthorhynchus hirudinaceus	2—3 months	Dark brown, thick-walled egg with three membranes; zygote is an acanthor with anterior hooks; 67—110 μm × 40—65 μm	Fecal flotation
Mesocestoides spp.	16—20 days	Smooth, thin egg capsule that contains a six-hooked hexacanth embryo; 20—25 μm; globular proglottid with parauterine body	Fecal flotation Identification of proglottid
Metastrongylus spp.	24 days	Rough, clear, thick-walled, larvated egg with a corrugated surface; 45—57 μm × 38—41 μm	Fecal flotation
Moniezia spp.	6 weeks	Thick-walled, clear, triangular to square egg with a piriform apparatus that contains a hexacanth embryo	Fecal flotation
Nanophyetus salmincola	1 week	Rough, brown, operculated egg; 52—82 μm × 32—56 μm	Sedimentation of feces
Oesophagostomum spp.	32—42 days	Strongyle egg	Fecal flotation
Onchocerca spp.	1 year	Unsheathed microfilaria in the skin of the ventral midline; 200—370 μm long	Skin biopsy
Oxyuris equi	5 months	Clear, smooth, thin-walled egg with one side flattened; operculated; 90 μm × 42 μm	Cellophane tape preparation
Paragonimus kellicotti	1 month	Smooth, golden brown, urn-shaped, operculated egg; 75—118 μm × 42—67 μm	Sedimentation of urine
Paramphistomum spp.	7—10 weeks	Light greenish, oval, operculated egg; 114—176 μm × 73—100 μm	Sedimentation of feces
Parascaris equorum	10 weeks	Rough, brown, thick-walled, spherical egg; single-celled zygote; 90—100 μm	Fecal flotation
Physaloptera spp.	56—83 days	Smooth, clear, thick-walled, larvated egg; 45—53 μm × 29—42 μm	Fecal flotation
Physocephalus sexalatus	6 weeks	Clear, smooth, thick-walled, larvated egg; 31—45 μm × 12—26 μm	Fecal flotation
Platynosomum fastosum	8—12 weeks	Dark amber, oval, operculated egg that contains a miracidium; 34—50 μm × 20—35 μm	Sedimentation of feces
Protostrongylus rufescens	30—37 days	L1 with a straight, pointed tail 48 μm × μm 56 m long and without a dorsal spine; 340—400 μm × 19—20 μm	Baermann
Sarcocystis spp.	7—33 days	Thin-walled oocyst with two sporocysts that contain four sporozoites each; size varies with species	Fecal flotation
Setaria equina		Sheathed microfilaria in the blood; 190—256 μm long	Blood smear Identification of adults at necropsy
Spirocerca lupi	5—6 months	Clear, smooth, thick-walled, paper-clip—shaped, larvated egg; 30—37 μm × 11—15 μm	Flotation
Spirometra mansonoides	10—30 days	Unembryonated, thin-walled, smooth, amber-colored operculated egg; 70 μm × 45 μm	Fecal flotation
Stephanofilaria stilesi		Microfilaria in the skin along the ventral midline; 45—60 μm	Skin biopsy
Stephanurus dentatus	3—4 months	Strongyle egg	Sedimentation of urine
Strongyloides ransomi	3—7 days	Smooth, thin-walled, larvated egg with parallel sides; 45—55 μm × 26—35 μm	Fecal flotation
Strongyloides stercoralis	8—14 days	L1 with a rhabditiform esophagus and a straight pointed tail; L3 with a filariform esophagus and a bipartite tail	Baermann Fecal culture
Strongyloides westeri	8—14 days	Smooth, thin-walled, larvated egg; 40—50 μm × 32—40 μm	Fecal flotation
Taenia spp.	2 months	Dark brown, thick, radially striated eggshell; six-hooked hexacanth embryo; 32—37 μm; rectangular proglottids with unilateral genital pore	Identification of proglottid
Thelazia californiensis	3—6 weeks	Adult worm in conjunctival sac	Identification of adult

TABLE 32.4 Diagnostic Characteristics of Internal Parasites of Domestic Animals—cont'd

Parasite	Prepatent Period	Diagnostic Stage	Diagnostic Test
Thysanosoma actinoides		Thin-walled egg with hexacanth embryos; 21–45 µm	Fecal flotation
Toxascaris leonina	11 weeks	Clear, smooth, thick-walled eggshell with wavy internal membrane; single-celled zygote; does not completely fill the egg; 75 µm × 85 µm	Fecal flotation
Toxocara canis	3–5 weeks	Dark brown, thick-walled, pitted egg; single-celled zygote; 75–90 µm	Fecal flotation
Toxocara cati	8 weeks	Dark brown, thick-walled, pitted egg; single-celled zygote; 65–75 µm	Fecal flotation
Toxoplasma gondii	1–3 weeks	Clear, smooth, thin-walled spherical oocyst; single-celled zygote; 8–10 µm	Fecal flotation
Trichinella spiralis	2–6 days	L3 encysted in striated muscles; esophagus composed of stichocytes (single cells stacked on top of one another); cysts are 400–600 µm × 250 µm	Compression preparation of muscle
Trichomonads		Spindle-shaped to piriform trophozoite with three to five anterior flagella, an undulating membrane, and a posterior flagellum	Direct smear
Trichostrongyles, Haemonchus, Ostertagia, Cooperia, and Trichostrongylus spp.	15–28 days	Strongyle egg	Fecal flotation
Trichuris suis	2–3 months	Brownish-yellow, smooth, thick-walled egg with symmetric bipolar plugs; single-celled zygote; 50–56 µm × 21–25 µm	Fecal flotation
Trichuris vulpis	3 months	Smooth, amber, thick-walled, barrel-shaped egg with bipolar plugs; single-celled zygote; 72–90 µm × 32–40 µm	Fecal flotation
Uncinaria stenocephala	2 weeks	Hookworm egg; 63–93 µm × 32–55 µm	Fecal flotation

From Sirois M: *Principles and practice of veterinary technology*, ed 3, St Louis, 2011, Mosby.

TABLE 32.5 Diagnostic Characteristics of Blood Parasites of Domestic Animals

Parasite	Definitive Hosts	Location in Host	Prepatent Period	Diagnostic Stage	Diagnostic Tests
Babesia spp.	People, dogs, cattle, horses	Erythrocytes	10–21 days	Paired piriform (tear-shaped) merozoites in erythrocytes	Romanowsky-stained blood film; indirect fluorescent antibody test
Trypanosoma spp.	People, dogs, cats, cattle, sheep, horses	Blood and lymph, heart, striated muscle, reticuloendothelial muscle	Acute and chronic disease	Trypanosome form (spindle-shaped flagellate with undulating membrane, central nucleus, and kinetoplast) found in the blood	Blood smears; xenodiagnosis (a clean vector is allowed to feed on a suspect patient, and the organism is isolated from the vector); biopsy; animal inoculation; serology
				Amastigote form (intracellular spherical body with single nucleus and rod-shaped kinetoplast) found in the myocardium, striated muscle cells, and macrophages	
Leishmania donovani	People, dogs	Intracellular in the cytoplasm of macrophages of the reticuloendothelial system	Several months, up to 1 year	Amastigote form (oval body with single nucleus and a rod-shaped kinetoplast) found in clusters within the cytoplasm of macrophages	Impression smears; biopsy of skin, lymph nodes, and bone marrow

From Sirois M: *Principles and practice of veterinary technology*, ed 3, St Louis, 2011, Mosby.

KEY POINTS

- Methods for the examination of fecal specimens include both the gross and microscopic examination of feces.
- The microscopic examination of fecal samples may involve the direct examination of samples or concentration of material with fecal flotation or fecal sedimentation techniques.
- Hemoparasites (blood parasites) can be identified with microscopic examination of peripheral blood smears or by using a variety of concentration techniques (e.g., modified Knott's procedure).
- Fecal concentration methods are preferred for the identification of parasite ova, larvae, and oocysts in the feces. Larger volumes of feces are used as compared with the direct smear, thereby making it more likely the developmental stages will be seen, if present, in the feces.
- Fecal flotation solutions with a specific gravity of 1.2 to 1.25 are used to float parasite ova, cysts, and larvae while the fecal material sinks to the bottom of the container.
- The fecal solutions of choice are Sheather's sugar solution, sodium nitrate solution, and zinc sulfate solution.
- Fecal centrifugation is the method of choice for fecal flotation testing, because it floats a higher concentration of ova, cysts, and larvae as compared with simple fecal flotation.
- Fecal sedimentation is used to test for trematode eggs, which are heavier than other parasite eggs and thus do not float as well.
- A thin blood smear will reveal such blood parasites as *Babesia* and *Theileria* within the red blood cells. However, it cannot be used for the accurate differentiation of *D. immitis* and *A. reconditum*.
- The buffy coat technique and the modified Knott's technique can be used to properly differentiate between *D. immitis* and *A. reconditum*.

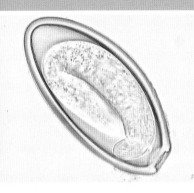

33

Nematodes

LEARNING OBJECTIVES

After studying this chapter, you will be able to:
- Describe the general characteristics of nematodes.
- Describe the generalized life cycle of nematodes.
- Differentiate between direct and indirect life cycles.
- List the common species of ascarids that affect domestic animals.
- List the common species of hookworms, lungworms, and whipworms that affect domestic animals.
- Discuss the life cycle of the canine heartworm.

OUTLINE

KEY TERMS

Ascarid
Cuticle
Definitive host
Direct life cycle

Endoparasite
Indirect life cycle
Intermediate host
Microfilaria

Nematode
Parthenogenetic
Prepatent period
Pseudocoelom

PHYLUM NEMATODA

Organisms in the phylum Nematoda are commonly called roundworms because of their cylindrical body shape. Nematodes are multicellular. They possess a body wall composed of an external, acellular, protective layer called the cuticle; a cellular layer beneath the cuticle called the hypodermis; and a layer of longitudinal somatic muscles that function in locomotion. The digestive tract and reproductive organs of roundworms are tubular, and they are suspended in the body cavity (pseudocoelom). The digestive tract is a straight tube that runs the length of the body from the mouth to the caudal end (anus). Most nematodes have separate male and female organisms. The reproductive organs are also tubular, but they are typically longer than the body and coil around the intestinal tract of the worm. Nematodes have a nervous system and an excretory system but no respiratory system.

> **TECHNICIAN NOTE** Organisms in the phylum Nematoda are commonly referred to as roundworms.

The life cycle of nematodes follows a standard pattern that consists of several developmental stages: the egg, four larval stages that are also wormlike in appearance, and sexually mature adults. The infective stage may be an egg that contains a larva, a free-living larva, or a larva within an intermediate host or transport host. A life cycle is considered a direct life cycle if no intermediate host is necessary for development to the infective stage. If an intermediate host is required for development to the infective stage, the life cycle is considered to be an indirect life cycle. Transmission to a new definitive host (i.e., the host that harbors sexually mature adults) can occur through ingestion, skin penetration of infective larvae, ingestion of an intermediate host, or deposition of infective larvae into or onto the skin by an intermediate host (Fig. 33.1).

After a nematode gains entry into a new host, development to the adult stages may occur in the area of their final location, or it may occur after extensive migration through the body of the definitive host. The diagnostic stages of parasitic nematodes are typically found in feces, blood, sputum, or urine. Most parasitic nematodes are found in the intestinal tracts of their respective definitive hosts, but some are found in the lungs, kidney, urinary bladder, or heart. Table 33.1 summarizes the nematode parasites of veterinary species.

The following 11 taxonomic superfamilies of nematodes are significant in veterinary medicine:

1. Ascaroidea
2. Strongyloidea
3. Trichostrongyloidea
4. Rhabditoidea
5. Metastrongyloidea
6. Trichuroidea
7. Oxyuroidea
8. Spiruroidea
9. Dracunculoidea
10. Dioctophymoidea
11. Filarioidea

Ascaroidea (Ascarids)
Roundworms of Dogs and Cats

Toxocara canis, *Toxocara cati*, and *Toxascaris leonina* are the ascarids of dogs and cats. These roundworms are found in the small intestine of dogs and cats in most areas of the world. All young puppies and kittens presented to a veterinary clinic should be examined for these large, robust nematodes (Fig. 33.2). Adult ascarids may vary from 3 cm to 18 cm in length. When passed, they are usually tightly coiled (Fig. 33.3). The eggs of *Toxocara* species are spherical, with a deeply pigmented center and a rough, pitted outer shell (Fig. 33.4). The eggs of *T. canis* are 75 μm to 90 μm in diameter, whereas those of *T. cati* are smaller at only 65 μm to 75 μm in diameter (Fig. 33.5). The eggs of *T. leonina* are spherical to ovoid, with dimensions of 75 μm by 85 μm. These eggs have a smooth outer shell and a hyaline or "ground-glass" central portion. Fig. 33.6 shows the characteristic ovum of *T. leonina*. The prepatent period for *T. canis* is 21 to 35 days, whereas that of *T. leonina* is 74 days.

> **TECHNICIAN NOTE** *Toxocara canis*, *Toxocara cati*, and *Toxascaris leonina* are the commonly encountered ascarids of dogs and cats.

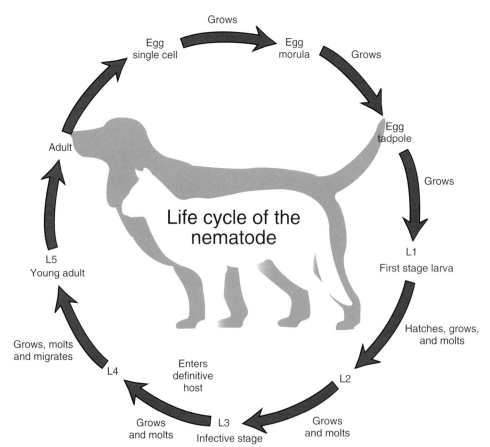

Fig. 33.1 Generalized life cycle of a nematode. (From Hendrix CM, Robinson E: *Diagnostic parasitology for veterinary technicians*, ed 4, St Louis, 2012, Mosby.)

TABLE 33.1 Selected Nematodes of Veterinary Species

Scientific Name	Common Name	Primary Location in Host
Dogs		
Acanthocheilonema reconditum (formerly Dipetalonema reconditum)	Skin filariid	Skin
Ancylostoma braziliense	Hookworm	Small intestine
Ancylostoma caninum	Hookworm	Small intestine
Pearsonema plica	Bladder worm	Urinary bladder
Dioctophyma renale	Giant kidney worm	R. kidney
Dirofilaria immitis	Canine heartworm	R. ventricle/pulmonary artery
Dracunculus insignis	Guinea worm	Skin
Eucoleus aerophilus (formerly Capillaria aerophila)		Nasal
Eucoleus böehmi		Nasal
Filaroides hirthi	Canine lungworm	Trachea/bronchi
Filaroides milksi	Canine lungworm	Nasal cavity/frontal sinus
Filaroides osleri	Canine lungworm	Lung parenchyma
Pelodera strongyloides		Skin
Physaloptera species	Stomach worm	Stomach
Spirocerca lupi	Esophageal worm	Esophagus
Strongyloides stercoralis	Threadworms	Small intestine
Strongyloides tumefaciens	Threadworms	Small intestine
Thelazia californiensis	Eyeworm	Conjunctival sac
Toxocara canis	Roundworm/ascarid	Small intestine
Trichuris vulpis	Whipworm	Large intestine
Uncinaria stenocephala	Northern canine hookworm	Small intestine
Cats		
Aelurostrongylus abstrusus	Lungworm	Bronchioles
Ancylostoma braziliense	Hookworm	Small intestine
Ancylostoma tubaeforme	Hookworm	Small intestine
Aonchotheca putorii (formerly Capillaria putorii)	Gastric capillarid of cats	Stomach
Pearsonema feliscati	Bladder worm	Urinary bladder
Eucoleus aerophilus (formerly Capillaria aerophila)		Bronchioles/alveolar ducts
Ollulanus tricuspis	Feline trichostrongyle	Lumen of small intestine
Physaloptera species	Stomach worm	Stomach
Spirocerca lupi	Esophageal worm	Esophagus
Thelazia californiensis	Eyeworm	Conjunctival sac
Toxascaris leonina	Roundworm/ascarid	Small intestine
Toxocara cati	Roundworm/ascarid	Lumen of small intestine
Trichuris campanula	Whipworm	Cecum and colon
Trichuris serrata	Whipworm	Cecum and colon
Ruminants		
Bunostomum species	Cattle hookworm	Abomasum/intestine
Chabertia species	Trichostrongyle	Abomasum/intestine
Cooperia species	Trichostrongyle	Abomasum/intestine
Dictyocaulus filaria	Lungworm of sheep/goats	Bronchi
Dictyocaulus viviparus	Lungworm of cattle	Bronchi
Elaeophora schneideri	Arterial worm of sheep	Carotid arteries
Gongylonema pulchrum	Ruminant esophageal worm	Esophagus
Haemonchus species	Bovine trichostrongyle	Abomasum/intestine
Marshallagia species	Bovine trichostrongyle	Abomasum/intestine

Continued

TABLE 33.1 Selected Nematodes of Veterinary Species—cont'd

Scientific Name	Common Name	Primary Location in Host
Muellerius capillaris	Hair lungworm or sheep/goats	Bronchioles
Nematodirus species	Bovine trichostrongyle	Abomasum/intestine
Oesophagostomum species	Bovine trichostrongyle	Abomasum/intestine
Ostertagia species	Bovine trichostrongyle	Abomasum/intestine
Protostrongylus species	Sheep and goat lungworm	Bronchioles
Setaria cervi	Abdominal worm	Peritoneal cavity
Stephanofilaria stilesi		Skin
Strongyloides papillosus	Intestinal threadworm	Intestine
Thelazia gulosa	Eyeworms	Conjunctival sac
Thelazia rhodesii	Eyeworms	Conjunctival sac
Trichostrongylus species	Trichostrongyle	Abomasum/intestine
Trichuris ovis	Whipworm	Cecum/colon
Horses		
Dictyocaulus arnfieldi	Lungworm	Bronchi/bronchioles
Draschia megastoma		Stomach mucosa
Habronema microstoma		Stomach mucosa
Habronema muscae		Stomach mucosa (adults); skin (larvae)
Onchocerca cervicalis	Filarial worm	Ligamentum nuchae
Oxyuris equi	Pinworm	Cecum/colon/rectum
Parascaris equorum	Roundworm	Small intestine
Setaria equina	Abdominal worm	Peritoneal cavity
Strongyloides westeri	Intestinal threadworm	Large intestine
Strongylus edentatus		Large intestine
Strongylus equinus		Large intestine
Strongylus vulgaris		Large intestine
Thelazia lacrymalis	Eyeworm	Conjunctival sac/lacrimal duct
Trichostrongylus axei		Stomach
Pigs		
Ascaris suum	Swine ascarid	Small intestine
Ascarops strongylina	Stomach worm	Stomach
Hyostrongylus rubidus	Red stomach worm	Stomach
Metastrongylus elongatus	Lungworm	Bronchi/bronchioles
Oesophagostomum dentatum	Nodular worm	Large intestine
Physocephalus sexalatus	Stomach worm	Stomach
Stephanurus dentatus	Kidney worm	Hepatic, renal, and perirenal tissues
Strongyloides ransomi	Intestinal threadworm	Large intestine
Trichinella spiralis	Trichina worm	Small intestine
Trichostrongylus axei		Stomach
Trichuris suis	Whipworm	Cecum/colon
Rabbits		
Obeliscoides cuniculi		Stomach
Trichostrongylus calcaratus		Small intestine
Rats		
Aspiculuris tetraptera	Pinworms	Cecum
Syphacia muris	Pinworms	Cecum
Syphacia obvelata	Pinworms	Cecum
Trichosomoides crassicauda	Bladder worm	Urinary bladder

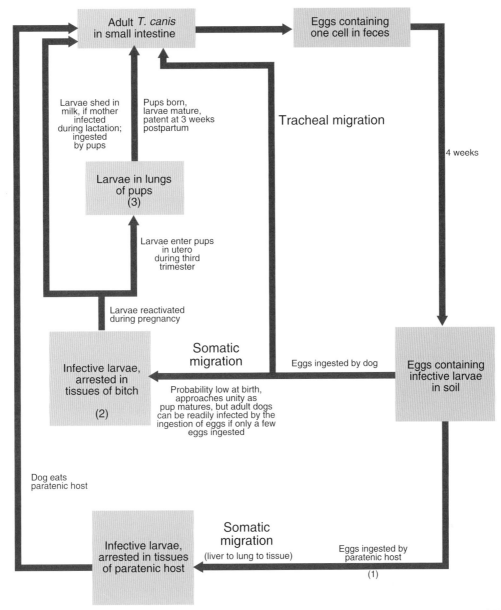

Fig. 33.2 Life cycle of *Toxocara canis*. (From Bowman D: *Georgis' parasitology for veterinarians*, ed 9, St Louis, 2009, Saunders.)

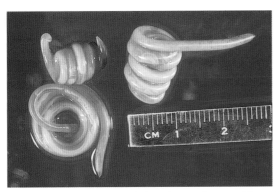

Fig. 33.3 Adult ascarids may vary in length from 3 cm to 18 cm. When passed in feces, they are usually tightly coiled. (From Hendrix CM, Robinson E: *Diagnostic parasitology for veterinary technicians*, ed 4, St Louis, 2012, Mosby.)

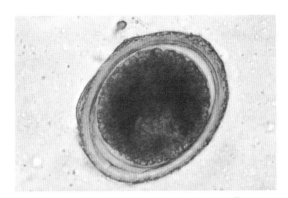

Fig. 33.4 Characteristic ovum of *Toxocara* species. These eggs are spherical, with a deeply pigmented center and a rough, pitted outer shell. Eggs of *T. canis* are 75 μm to 90 μm in diameter. (From Hendrix CM, Robinson E: *Diagnostic parasitology for veterinary technicians*, ed 3, St Louis, 2006, Mosby.)

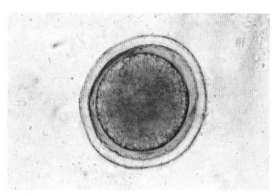

Fig. 33.5 Characteristic ovum of *Toxocara cati*. These eggs are smaller than those of *Toxocara canis*, measuring only 65 μm to 75 μm in diameter. (From Hendrix CM, Robinson E: *Diagnostic parasitology for veterinary technicians*, ed 3, St Louis, 2006, Mosby.)

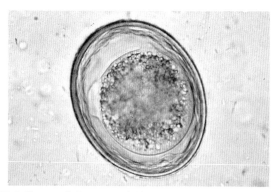

Fig. 33.6 Characteristic ovum of *Toxascaris leonina*. These eggs are spherical to ovoid, with dimensions of 75 μm by 85 μm. They have a smooth outer shell and a hyaline or "ground-glass" central portion. (From Hendrix CM, Robinson E: *Diagnostic parasitology for veterinary technicians*, ed 3, St Louis, 2006, Mosby.)

Roundworms of Horses

Parascaris equorum is often called the "equine ascarid" or "equine roundworm." It is found in the small intestine of horses, particularly young foals. The prepatent period is 75 to 80 days. Eggs recovered from the feces of young horses are oval and brown. The shell is thickened, with a finely granular surface. The eggs measure 90 μm to 100 μm in diameter. The center of the egg contains one or two cells (Fig. 33.7). Eggs may be recovered easily with standard fecal flotation.

Roundworms of Ruminants

Toxocara (Neoascaris) vitulorum is transmitted via the trans-mammary route to calves. It is a large worm, and the eggs have a thick, pitted shell.

Roundworms of Swine

Ascaris suum, the swine ascarid or the large intestinal roundworm, is the largest nematode found within the small intestine of pigs. The eggs may be recovered with standard fecal flotation.

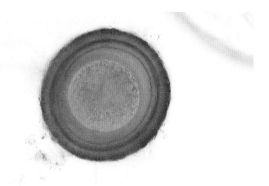

Fig. 33.7 Characteristic ovum of *Parascaris equorum*, the equine ascarid or the equine roundworm. The shell is thickened, with a finely granular surface. The eggs measure 90 μm to 100 μm in diameter. The center of the egg contains one or two cells. (From Hendrix CM, Robinson E: *Diagnostic parasitology for veterinary technicians*, ed 3, St Louis, 2006, Mosby.)

They are oval and golden brown, with a thick albuminous shell that bears prominent projections. These eggs measure 70 μm to 89 μm by 37 μm to 40 μm (Fig. 33.8).

Strongyloidea
Hookworms of Dogs and Cats

Ancylostoma caninum, a canine hookworm; *Ancylostoma tubaeforme*, a feline hookworm; *Ancylostoma braziliense*, a canine and feline hookworm; and *Uncinaria stenocephala*, a northern canine hookworm, are small intestinal nematodes. Hookworms are found throughout the world, and they are common in the tropical and subtropical areas of North America. Hookworm infection, which can produce severe anemia in young kittens and puppies, can be a serious problem in kennels and catteries. The prepatent period depends on the species of hookworm and the route of infection (Fig. 33.9). The eggs of all hookworm species are oval or ellipsoid. They have thin walls, and they contain 8 to 16 cells when they are passed in an animal's feces. Because these eggs larvate rapidly in the external environment (i.e., as early as 48 hours after feces are passed), fresh feces are needed for the diagnosis of hookworm infections. The eggs of *A. caninum* are 56 μm to 75 μm by 34 μm to 47 μm (Fig. 33.10). Those of *A. tubaeforme* are 55 μm to 75 μm by 34.4 μm to 44.7 μm. Those of *A. braziliense* are 75 μm by 45 μm, and those of *U. stenocephala* are 65 μm to 80 μm by 40 μm to 50 μm. These eggs are usually recovered with standard fecal flotation.

Hookworms of Ruminants

Bunostomum phlebotomum is the hookworm of ruminants, and it produces trichostrongyle-type eggs.

TECHNICIAN NOTE The eggs of hookworms larvate rapidly in the environment.

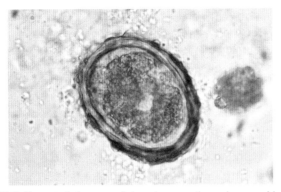

Fig. 33.8 Characteristic ovum of *Ascaris suum,* the swine ascarid or the large intestinal roundworm of pigs. The eggs are oval and golden brown, with a thick, albuminous shell that bears prominent projections. They measure 70 μm to 89 μm by 37 μm to 40 μm. (From Hendrix CM, Robinson E: *Diagnostic parasitology for veterinary technicians,* ed 3, St Louis, 2006, Mosby.)

Strongyles in Horses

Strongyles are nematodes that parasitize the large intestine of horses. They are typically divided into two types: large strongyles and small strongyles. The small strongyles comprise several genera that vary with regard to their pathogenicity. The large strongyles are included in the family *Strongyloidea,* and they are the most pathogenic of the strongyles. *Strongylus vulgaris, Strongylus edentatus,* and *Strongylus equinus* are the large strongyles (Fig. 33.11).

Regardless of whether these endoparasites are small strongyles or large strongyles, their eggs are virtually identical. Identification to the species level is accomplished with fecal culture and the identification of larvae. Strongyle eggs are most often observed in a standard fecal flotation. They contain an 8- to 16-cell morula, and they measure approximately 70 μm to 90 μm by 40 μm to 50 μm. When these characteristic eggs are

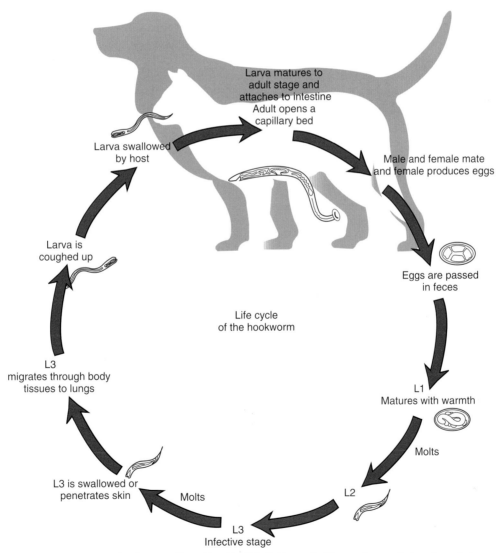

Fig. 33.9 Life cycle of the hookworm. (From Hendrix CM, Robinson E: *Diagnostic parasitology for veterinary technicians,* ed 4, St Louis, 2012, Mosby.)

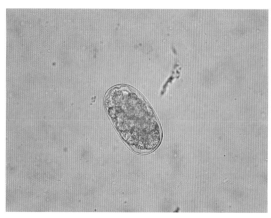

Fig. 33.10 Characteristic hookworm ovum. The eggs of *Ancylostoma caninum* are 56 µm to 75 µm by 34 µm. (From Hendrix CM, Robinson E: *Diagnostic parasitology for veterinary technicians*, ed 3, St Louis, 2006, Mosby.)

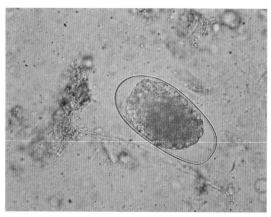

Fig. 33.11 Strongyle-type ovum of horses. These eggs contain an 8- to 16-cell morula, and they measure approximately 70 µm to 90 µm by 40 µm to 50 µm. (From Hendrix CM, Robinson E: *Diagnostic parasitology for veterinary technicians*, ed 3, St Louis, 2006, Mosby.)

found with fecal flotation, the observation is recorded as "strongyle-type ova" rather than as a particular species of strongyle.

Nodular Worm of Swine

Oesophagostomum dentatum, the "nodular worm of swine," is found in the large intestine of swine. The prepatent period is 50 days. The eggs are a trichostrongyle type; in other words, they are oval, thin-shelled eggs. They contain 4 to 16 cells, and they measure 40 µm by 70 µm. These eggs may be recovered with a standard fecal flotation. As with bovine trichostrongyles, definitive diagnosis is made only by fecal culture and larval identification.

Trichostrongyloidea
Bovine Trichostrongyles

The bovine trichostrongyles are composed of several genera of nematodes within the abomasum and the small and large

intestines of cattle and other ruminants. Genera that produce trichostrongyle-type eggs are *Bunostomum, Cooperia, Chabertia, Haemonchus, Oesophagostomum, Ostertagia,* and *Trichostrongylus.* These seven genera (and others) produce oval, thin-shelled eggs. They contain four or more cells, and they are 70 µm to 120 µm long. Some of these ova may be identified to their respective genera; however, identification is usually difficult, because mixed infections of bovine trichostrongyles are quite common.

Upon identification of the characteristic eggs, record the finding as a trichostrongyle-type egg (Fig. 33.12). These should never be recorded by individual genus names. The identification of genus and species usually can be performed only by fecal culture and larval identification.

> **TECHNICIAN NOTE** The identification of the exact species of trichostrongyle-type eggs generally requires fecal culture and larval identification.

Nematodirus species and *Marshallagia* species are also bovine trichostrongyles; however, their eggs are much larger than those of the genera mentioned previously. Their eggs are the largest in the trichostrongyle family. Fig. 33.13 shows the large eggs of *Nematodirus* species. In a standard fecal flotation, the eggs of *Nematodirus* species are large (150 µm to 230 µm by 80 µm to 100 µm), and they have tapering ends and four to eight cells. The eggs of *Marshallagia* species also are large (160 µm to 200 µm by 75 µm to 100 µm). They have parallel sides and rounded ends, and they contain 16 to 32 cells.

Bovine Lungworm

Dictyocaulus species are lungworms of cattle (*Dictyocaulus viviparus*), sheep, and goats (*Dictyocaulus filaria*). Adults are found in the bronchi of these animals. Larvae of *D. filaria* have brownish food granules in their intestinal cells, a blunt tail, and a cranial cuticular knob. They are 550 µm to 580 µm long. The larvae of *D. viviparus* also have brownish food granules in their intestinal cells, but they also have a straight tail; they lack the cranial cuticular knob. These larvae are 300 µm to 360 µm in length (Fig. 33.14).

Equine Lungworm

Dictyocaulus arnfieldi, the equine lungworm, is found in the bronchi and bronchioles of horses, mules, and donkeys. The prepatent period varies with the species, but it is approximately 28 days. The prepatent period for the equine lungworm is 42 to 56 days. Eggs are usually coughed up and swallowed. They hatch in the intestine, where they produce larvae that may be recovered in the feces.

Red Stomach Worm of Swine

Hyostrongylus rubidus is referred to as the "red stomach worm" of swine. The eggs are trichostrongyle type (i.e., they are oval,

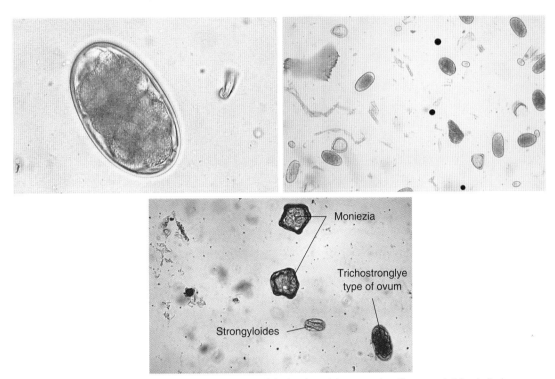

Fig. 33.12 Characteristic trichostrongyle-type ova of the bovine trichostrongyles. These oval, thin-shelled eggs contain four or more cells. They measure 70 μm to 120 μm long. Some of these ova can be identified by their respective genus; however, identification is usually difficult, because mixed infections are common. (From Hendrix CM, Robinson E: *Diagnostic parasitology for veterinary technicians*, ed 3, St Louis, 2006, Mosby.)

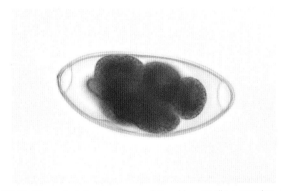

Fig. 33.13 Characteristic large ova of the *Nematodirus* species. (From Hendrix CM, Robinson E: *Diagnostic parasitology for veterinary technicians*, ed 3, St Louis, 2006, Mosby.)

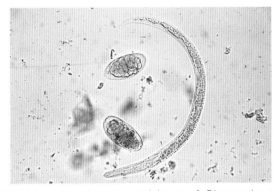

Fig. 33.14 Representative eggs and larvae of *Dictyocaulus* species (cattle lungworms). (From Hendrix CM, Robinson E: *Diagnostic parasitology for veterinary technicians*, ed 3, St Louis, 2006, Mosby.)

thin-shelled eggs). They contain four or more cells, and they measure 71 μm to 78 μm by 35 μm to 42 μm. These eggs may be recovered with fecal flotation. As with bovine trichostrongyles, definitive diagnosis can be made only with fecal culture and larval identification. The prepatent period is approximately 20 days.

Feline Trichostrongyle

Ollulanus tricuspis is the "feline trichostrongyle." This parasite is usually associated with vomiting in cats. It is most commonly identified by the examination of the cat's vomitus with a dissecting or compound microscope.

Rhabditoidea (*Strongyloides* spp.)
Strongyloides of Horses

Strongyloides stercoralis, *Strongyloides tumefaciens*, and *Strongyloides papillosus* are often referred to as "intestinal threadworms." These nematodes are unique; only a parthenogenetic female (i.e., a female that can lay eggs without copulation with a male) is parasitic in the host. Parasitic males do not exist. These females produce eggs, and, in dogs, these eggs hatch in the intestine and release first-stage larvae. Fig. 33.15 shows the parasitic adult females, eggs, and first-stage larvae of *Strongyloides* species. The larvae are 280 μm to 310 μm long. They have a rhabditiform (club-shaped) esophagus with a club-

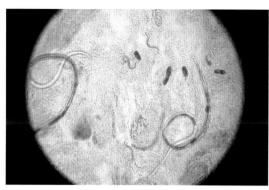

Fig. 33.15 Parasitic adult females, eggs, and first-stage larvae of *Strongyloides* species. (From Hendrix CM, Robinson E: *Diagnostic parasitology for veterinary technicians*, ed 3, St Louis, 2006, Mosby.)

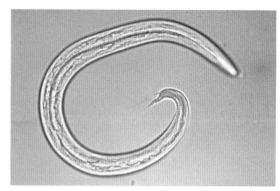

Fig. 33.16 First-stage larva of *Muellerius capillaris,* the "hair lungworm" of sheep and goats. (From Hendrix CM, Robinson E: *Diagnostic parasitology for veterinary technicians*, ed 3, St Louis, 2006, Mosby.)

shaped cranial corpus, a narrow median isthmus, and a caudal bulb. The prepatent period is 8 to 14 days. *Strongyloides westeri* is often referred to as the "intestinal threadworm" of horses. These females produce larvated eggs that measure 40 μm to 52 μm by 32 μm to 40 μm. The eggs are usually recovered with fecal flotation of fresh feces. The prepatent period is 5 to 7 days.

Strongyloides of Swine

Strongyloides ransomi, the intestinal threadworm of pigs, is found within the small intestine of pigs. These females produce larvated eggs that measure 45 μm to 55 μm by 26 μm to 35 μm. Eggs are usually recovered with fecal flotation of fresh feces. The prepatent period is 3 to 7 days.

Metastrongyloidea
Lungworm of Sheep and Goats

Muellerius capillaris is often called the "hair lungworm." Adults are found within the bronchioles, most commonly in nodules in the lung parenchyma of sheep and goats. The eggs develop in the lungs of the definitive host, and the first-stage larvae are coughed up, swallowed, and passed out with the feces. They are 230 μm to 300 μm long. The larval tail has an undulating tip and a dorsal spine (Fig. 33.16).

Adult *Protostrongylus* species occur in the small bronchioles of sheep and goats. Again, the eggs develop in the lungs of the definitive host, and the first-stage larvae are coughed up, swallowed, and passed out with the feces. These larvae are 250 μm to 320 μm long. This nematode's larval tail has an undulating tip, but it lacks a dorsal spine. The Baermann technique is used to diagnose lungworm infection in ruminants.

Lungworm of Swine

Metastrongylus apri, the swine lungworm, is found within the bronchi and bronchioles of pigs. The oval, thick-walled eggs measure 60 μm by 40 μm and contain larvae. Eggs can be recovered with fecal flotation using a flotation medium with a specific gravity of more than 1.25 or with the fecal sedimentation technique. The prepatent period is approximately 24 days.

Canine Lungworms

Filaroides (Oslerus) osleri, Filaroides hirthi, and *Filaroides milksi,* the canine "lungworms," are found in the trachea, the lung parenchyma, and the bronchioles of canids, respectively. The larva is 232 μm to 266 μm long, and it has a short, S-shaped tail. *Filaroides* species are unique among the nematodes in that their first-stage larvae are immediately infective for the canine definitive host. No period of development is required outside of the host. Diagnosis involves finding these characteristic larvae with fecal flotation or by using the Baermann technique. Fig. 33.17 shows the unique infective larvae of *F. osleri.* Nodules of *F. osleri* are usually found at the bifurcation of the trachea, where they can be observed by endoscopic examination. The prepatent period for *F. osleri* is approximately 10 weeks.

Feline Lungworm

Aelurostrongylus abstrusus is the feline lungworm. The adults live in the terminal respiratory bronchioles and the alveolar ducts, where they form small egg nests or nodules. The eggs of this parasite are forced into the lung tissue, where they hatch to form characteristic first-stage larvae that are approximately 360 μm long. Each larva has a tail with an S-shaped bend and a dorsal spine (Fig. 33.18). Characteristic larvae found with fecal flotation or the Baermann technique can determine their presence. Recovering the larvae with tracheal washing is also possible (Fig. 33.19). The prepatent period is approximately 30 days.

Trichuroidea (*Trichuris* spp., *Eucoleus* spp., and *Trichinella spiralis*)
Whipworms of Dogs and Cats

Trichuris vulpis, the canine whipworm, and *Trichuris campanula* and *Trichuris serrata,* the feline whipworms, reside in the cecum and colon of their respective hosts. Canine whipworms are common, but feline whipworms are rare in North America and

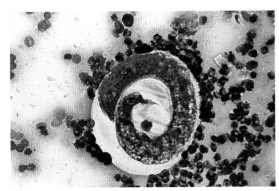

Fig. 33.17 Characteristic infective first-stage larva of *Filaroides osleri*, a canine lungworm. (From Hendrix CM, Robinson E: *Diagnostic parasitology for veterinary technicians*, ed 3, St Louis, 2006, Mosby.)

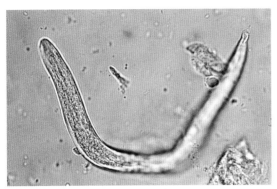

Fig. 33.18 Characteristic first-stage larva of *Aelurostrongylus abstrusus*, the feline lungworm. (From Hendrix CM, Robinson E: *Diagnostic parasitology for veterinary technicians*, ed 3, St Louis, 2006, Mosby.)

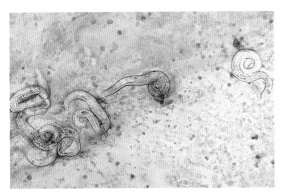

Fig. 33.19 Numerous first-stage larvae of *Aelurostrongylus abstrusus* recovered with tracheal washing. (From Hendrix CM, Robinson E: *Diagnostic parasitology for veterinary technicians*, ed 3, St Louis, 2006, Mosby.)

diagnosed only sporadically throughout the world. Whipworms derive their name from the fact that the adults have a thin, filamentous cranial end (i.e., the lash of the whip) and a thick caudal end (i.e., the handle of the whip). The egg of the whipworm is described as trichinelloid or trichuroid. It has a thick, yellow-brown, symmetric shell with polar plugs at both ends. The eggs are unembryonated (not larvated) when laid.

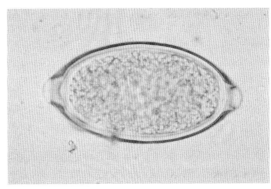

Fig. 33.20 Characteristic ovum of *Trichuris vulpis*. (From Hendrix CM, Robinson E: *Diagnostic parasitology for veterinary technicians*, ed 3, St Louis, 2006, Mosby.)

Eggs of *T. vulpis* are 70 μm to 89 μm by 37 μm to 40 μm. Fig. 33.20 shows the characteristic egg of *T. vulpis*. The prepatent period for *T. vulpis* is 70 to 90 days.

The eggs of *T. campanula* and *T. serrata* may be easily confused with those of *Aonchotheca putorii*, *Eucoleus aerophilus*, and *Personema feliscati*, which are the parasites of the feline stomach, respiratory tract, and urinary system, respectively. The eggs of *T. campanula* average 63 μm to 85 μm by 34 μm to 39 μm. When examining a cat's feces for feline trichurids, the veterinary technician should be aware of pseudoparasites; the eggs of trichurids or capillarids frequently parasitize an outdoor cat's prey via hosts such as mice, rabbits, or birds. The eggs of these trichurids or capillarids may pass unaltered through the cat's gastrointestinal system, remaining intact and unembryonated and thus appearing to infect the feline host.

Capillarids of Dogs and Cags

Aonchotheca putorii is commonly referred to as the gastric capillarid of cats. It was once known by the former name *Capillaria putorii*. This capillarid frequently parasitizes mustelids, such as mink, but it also has been reported in cats. These nematodes are rarely reported in North America. The eggs of *A. putorii* are easily confused with other trichinelloid nematodes (see the section about feline whipworms). Their eggs are 53 μm to 70 μm by 20 μm to 30 μm, and they exhibit a netlike surface similar to that of the eggs of *Eucoleus aerophilus*, an upper respiratory capillarid. The eggs of *A. putorii* are dense and less delicate than those of *E. aerophilus*, and they are organized in a longitudinal formation. They have flattened sides, and they contain a one- or two-cell embryo that fills the egg.

Eucoleus aerophilus (Capillaria aerophila) is a capillarid nematode found in the trachea and bronchi of both dogs and cats. The prepatent period is approximately 40 days. In standard fecal flotations, eggs of *Eucoleus* species are often confused with those of *Trichuris* (whipworms). Eggs of *E. aerophilus* are smaller than whipworm eggs (59 μm to 80 μm by 30 μm to 40 μm), more broadly barrel-shaped, and lighter in color. The egg also has a rough outer surface with a netted appearance. *Eucoleus böehmi* is found in the nasal cavity and frontal sinuses of dogs. Its eggs are smaller and have a smoother outer surface than those of *E. aerophilus.* Its shell has a pitted appearance. This parasite can be detected by standard fecal flotation.

Pearsonema (Capillaria) plica and *Pearsonema (Capillaria) feliscati* are nematodes of the urinary bladder of dogs and cats, respectively. Their eggs may be found in urine or in feces contaminated with urine. The eggs are clear to yellow in color, they measure 63 μm to 68 μm by 24 μm to 27 μm, and they have flattened bipolar end plugs (Fig. 33.21). Their outer surface is roughened. These eggs may be confused with those of the respiratory and gastric capillarids and with those of the whipworms.

Whipworms of Ruminants

Trichuris ovis infects the cecum and colon of ruminants. Eggs of bovine whipworms measure 50 μm to 60 μm by 21 μm to 25 μm. *Trichuris suis* is the swine whipworm. Eggs of porcine whipworms measure 50 μm to 60 μm by 21 μm to 25 μm. The prepatent period is 42 to 49 days.

> **TECHNICIAN NOTE** Eggs of *Pearsonema* species may be present in urine or in feces contaminated with urine.

Trichina Worm of Swine

Trichinella spiralis is found in many species of carnivores and omnivores, but it is often associated with raw or undercooked pork. Animals (including human beings) become infected with *T. spiralis* when they ingest infective larval stages (juveniles) in meat. The larvae mature into adults in the host's small intestine within a few weeks, and the female worms give birth to larvae. The males die after fertilizing the females, and the females die after producing larvae. The larvae enter the bloodstream of the host and eventually end up in the pig's musculature. Within the muscles, the larvae mature into infective encysted larvae. The next host becomes infected when it eats these larvae. Trichinosis is probably best known as a parasite that human beings contract from eating raw or undercooked pork. It is usually detected by proper meat inspection. Most recent outbreaks of trichinosis in the United States have been traced to pork products from pigs that have not been inspected and that have been privately slaughtered.

> **TECHNICIAN NOTE** Most animals become infected with trichinosis after the ingestion of undercooked pork.

Oxyuroidea
Pinworms of Horses

Oxyuris equi is the pinworm of horses. The adult worms are found in the animal's cecum, colon, and rectum. Adult worms are often observed protruding from the horse's anus. The adult female worms attach their eggs to the anus with a sticky, gelatinous material that produces anal pruritus in infected horses. The activity of the female worms is irritating and produces itching. Eggs also may be recovered from the feces. The eggs are 90 μm by 40 μm, with a smooth, thick shell. They are operculated and slightly flattened on one side, and they may be larvated (Fig. 33.22). The prepatent period is approximately 4 to 5 months. Diagnosis involves finding the characteristic eggs using microscopic examination of cellophane tape impressions or by scraping the surface of the anus.

Human Pinworms

Enterobius vermicularis is the human pinworm, and it does not parasitize dogs or cats. Nevertheless, the family pet is often falsely incriminated by family practitioners or pediatricians as a source of pinworm infection in young children.

Spiruroidea
Stomach Worms of Horses

Habronema species and *Draschia megastoma* are nematodes that are found in the stomachs of horses. *Habronema microstoma* and *H. muscae* occur on the stomach mucosa, just beneath a thick layer of mucus; *D. megastoma* is often associated with large, thickened, fibrous nodules within the stomach mucosa. Larvae of both may parasitize skin lesions and cause a condition

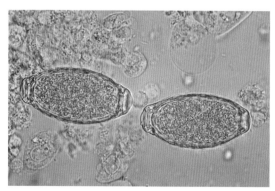

Fig. 33.21 Eggs of *Pearsonema plica,* the urinary capillarid. (From Hendrix CM, Robinson E: *Diagnostic parasitology for veterinary technicians,* ed 3, St Louis, 2006, Mosby.)

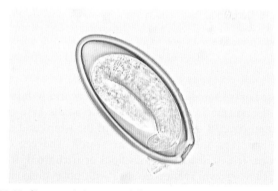

Fig. 33.22 Characteristic ovum of *Oxyuris equi,* the pinworm of horses. (From Hendrix CM, Robinson E: *Diagnostic parasitology for veterinary technicians,* ed 3, St Louis, 2006, Mosby.)

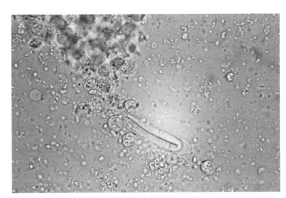

Fig. 33.23 Larvated eggs or larvae of *Habronema* and *Draschia* species may be recovered with standard fecal flotation. (From Hendrix CM, Robinson E: *Diagnostic parasitology for veterinary technicians*, ed 3, St Louis, 2006, Mosby.)

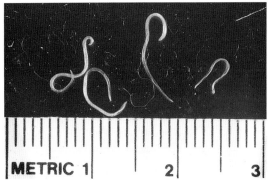

Fig. 33.24 Adult *Thelazia* species (eyeworms) from the conjunctival sac of a cow. (From Hendrix CM, Robinson E: *Diagnostic parasitology for veterinary technicians*, ed 3, St Louis, 2006, Mosby.)

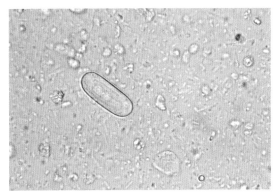

Fig. 33.25 Characteristic Ovum of *Spirocerca lupi*. (From Hendrix CM, Robinson E: *Diagnostic parasitology for veterinary technicians*, ed 3, St Louis, 2006, Mosby.)

known as "summer sores." The prepatent period is approximately 60 days. Larvated eggs or larvae may be recovered with standard fecal flotation. The eggs of both genera are elongated, with thin walls, and they measure 40 μm to 50 μm by 10 μm to 12 μm (Fig. 33.23).

Eyeworm of Dogs and Cats

Thelazia californiensis is the "eyeworm" of dogs and cats. Adult parasites can be recovered from the conjunctival sac and the lachrymal duct. Examination of the lachrymal secretions may reveal eggs or first-stage larvae. *Thelazia rhodesii* and *Thelazia gulosa* are the "eyeworms" of cattle, sheep, and goats. Fig. 33.24 shows adult *Thelazia* in the conjunctival sac of a cow.

Eyeworm of Horses

Thelazia lacrymalis is the eyeworm of horses throughout the world. Adult parasites may be recovered from the conjunctival sac and the lachrymal duct. Examination of the lachrymal secretions may reveal eggs or first-stage larvae.

Esophageal Worm of Dogs and Cats

Spirocerca lupi, the esophageal worm, is a nematode that often forms nodules (granulomas) in the esophageal wall of dogs and cats. Occasionally it may be found in nodules in the stomach of cats. Adult worms reside deep within these nodules and expel their eggs through fistulous openings in the granuloma. Eggs are passed into the lumen of the host animal's esophagus and then pass out in the feces. The thick-shelled eggs are 30 μm to 38 μm by 11 μm to 15 μm, and they contain a larva when they are laid. These eggs have a unique paper-clip shape (Fig. 33.25). Eggs are usually observed with fecal flotation, and they may be recovered when vomitus has been subjected to a standard fecal flotation procedure. Radiographic or endoscopic examination may reveal characteristic granulomas within the esophagus or within the stomach. The prepatent period is 6 months.

Stomach Worm of Dogs and Cats

Physaloptera species are stomach worms of dogs and cats. Although they occasionally are found in the lumen of the stomach or the small intestine, *Physaloptera* species are usually firmly attached to the mucosal surface of the stomach, where they suck blood. At this site, these nematodes may be viewed with an endoscope. Their diet consists of blood and tissue derived from the host's gastric mucosa. Their attachment sites continue to bleed after the parasite detaches. Vomiting, anorexia, and dark, tarry stools may be observed in affected animals.

The adults are creamy white and sometimes tightly coiled, and they are 1.3 cm to 4.8 cm long. They are often recovered in the pet's vomitus, and they may be confused with ascarids or roundworms. A quick way to differentiate these two parasites is to break open an adult specimen and, if that specimen happens to be female, examine the released eggs microscopically. The eggs of *Physaloptera* species are small, smooth, thick-shelled, and embryonated when passed in the feces. Eggs are 30 μm to 34 μm by 49 μm to 58 μm, and they contain a larva when they are laid. Fig. 33.26 shows the characteristic ovum of *Physaloptera* species. Eggs can usually be recovered with standard fecal flotation using solutions with a specific gravity of more than 1.25. The prepatent period is 56 to 83 days.

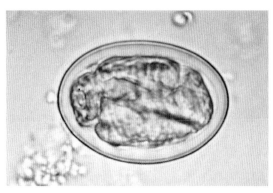

Fig. 33.26 Characteristic ovum of *Physaloptera* species. (From Hendrix CM, Robinson E: *Diagnostic parasitology for veterinary technicians*, ed 3, St Louis, 2006, Mosby.)

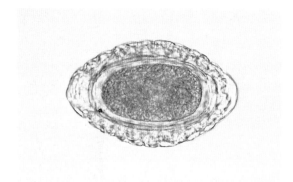

Fig. 33.27 Characteristic ovum of *Dioctophyma renale* recovered from urine sediment. (From Hendrix CM, Robinson E: *Diagnostic parasitology for veterinary technicians*, ed 3, St Louis, 2006, Mosby.)

Thick Stomach Worms of Swine

Ascarops strongylina and *Physocephalus sexalatus* are the "thick stomach worms" of the porcine stomach. Both of these nematodes produce thick-walled, larvated eggs that may be recovered with fecal flotation. The eggs of both species are similar. The eggs of *A. strongylina* are 34 μm to 39 μm by 20 μm, and they have thick shells surrounded by a thin membrane that produces an irregular outline. The eggs of *P. sexalatus* are 34 μm to 39 μm by 15 μm to 17 μm. The prepatent period for both species is approximately 42 days.

Dracunculoidea
Guinea Worm of Dogs and Cats

Dracunculus species are uncommon parasites of dogs, cats, and other carnivores. The life cycle requires a copepod intermediate host, and the definitive host becomes infected after ingestion of the copepod.

Dioctophymoidea
Giant Kidney Worm of Dogs

Dioctophyma renale is the "giant kidney worm" of dogs. This largest of parasitic nematodes frequently infects the right kidney of dogs and gradually ingests the renal parenchyma, leaving only the capsule of the kidney. Eggs may be recovered by centrifugation and examination of the urine sediment. They are characteristically barrel-shaped, bipolar, and yellow-brown. The egg's shell has a pitted appearance. Eggs measure 71 μm to 84 μm by 46 μm to 52 μm (Fig. 33.27). *D. renale* may also occur freely within the peritoneal cavity. When it is in this location, eggs are not passed to the external environment. The prepatent period is approximately 18 weeks.

Kidney Worm of Swine

Stephanurus dentatus, the swine kidney worm, is found in the kidney, ureters, and perirenal tissues of pigs. Their eggs are strongyle type (i.e., oval and thin-shelled), they contain 4 to 16

cells, and they measure 90 μm to 120 μm by 43 μm to 70 μm. Eggs may be recovered from the urine by urine sedimentation. The prepatent period is extremely long at approximately 9 to 24 months.

Filaroidea
Canine Heartworm

Dirofilaria immitis, the canine heartworm, is the most important parasite of the vascular system of domestic animals in the United States. This nematode can also parasitize cats and ferrets. Adult heartworms are found within the right ventricle, the pulmonary artery, and the fine branches of that artery. This parasite is often recovered in a variety of aberrant sites, such as the brain, the anterior chamber of the eye, and subcutaneous sites. The prepatent period in dogs is approximately 6 months and approximately 7 to 8 months in cats. The life cycle of *D. immitis* requires the mosquito intermediate host to be transmitted from animal to animal (Fig. 33.28). The adults live in the right ventricle and pulmonary artery, where they can obstruct the blood vasculature. The male and female adults mate, and the female produces microfilariae. The microfilariae are released into the host's bloodstream, where they are ingested by feeding female mosquitoes. The microfilariae grow and molt in the mosquito until they reach the infective stage. After they become infective, they enter a new host the next time the mosquito feeds. When they are in the new host, the larvae migrate and molt through various body tissues on their way to the heart. It is at this time that the larvae may grow and molt to become adults in sites other than the heart.

> **TECHNICIAN NOTE** The prepatent period for *Dirofilaria immitis* infection in dogs is approximately 6 months.

In microfilaremic dogs, a diagnosis can be made by observing microfilariae in blood samples with the use of one of several concentration techniques (e.g., modified Knott's test) or the commercially available filter techniques (Figs. 33.29 and 33.30). Microfilaremia is not commonly detected in cats. When

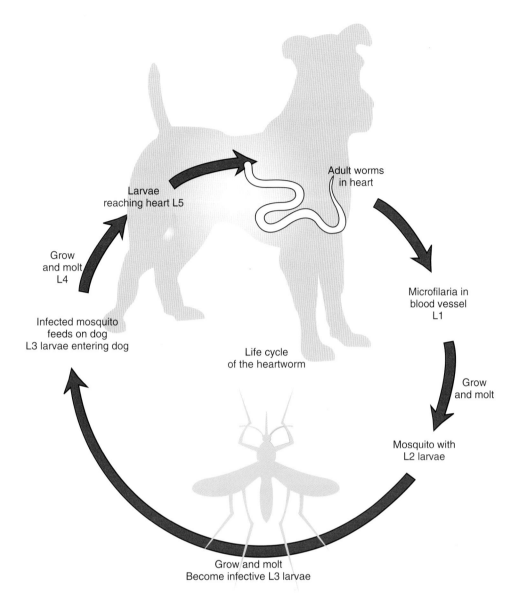

Adult worms
in heart

Larvae
reaching heart L5

Grow
and molt
L4

Infected mosquito
feeds on dog
L3 larvae entering dog

Life cycle
of the heartworm

Microfilaria in
blood vessel
L1

Grow
and molt

Mosquito with
L2 larvae

Grow and molt
Become infective L3 larvae

Fig. 33.28 Life cycle of the canine *Dirofilaria immitis*. (From Hendrix CM, Robinson E: *Diagnostic parasitology for veterinary technicians*, ed 3, St Louis, 2006, Mosby.)

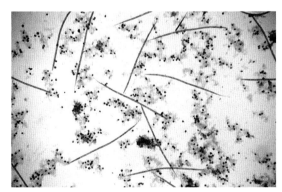

Fig. 33.29 Microfilariae of *Dirofilaria immitis* from a peripheral blood sample subjected to the modified Knott's test. (From Hendrix CM, Robinson E: *Diagnostic parasitology for veterinary technicians*, ed 3, St Louis, 2006, Mosby.)

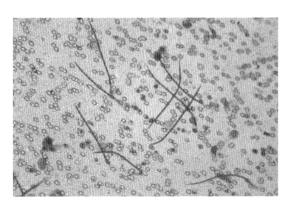

Fig. 33.30 Microfilariae of *Dirofilaria immitis* from a peripheral blood sample subjected to a commercially available filter test. (From Hendrix CM, Robinson E: *Diagnostic parasitology for veterinary technicians*, ed 3, St Louis, 2006, Mosby.)

present, the numbers of microfilaria are low and persist for only a few weeks. Infection with *Dirofilaria* is more commonly diagnosed using commercially available immunodiagnostic tests that detect the presence of antigen from adult female worms.

A subcutaneous filariid of dogs, *Acanthocheilonema (Dipetalonema) reconditum,* also produces microfilariae in the peripheral blood. The microfilariae of this nonpathogenic nematode must be differentiated from those of *D. immitis.*

Skin Worm in Horses

The unsheathed microfilariae of *Onchocerca cervicalis,* the equine filarial parasite, have been incriminated as causing recurrent dermatitis, periodic ophthalmia, and blindness in horses. Adults live in the ligamentum nuchae, and females produce microfilariae that migrate to the dermis. Biting flies of the genus *Culicoides* are the intermediate hosts.

Abdominal Worm of Cattle

Setaria cervi is the "abdominal worm" of cattle.

Abdominal Worm of Horses

Setaria equina is the abdominal worm of horses. Adults are found free within the peritoneal cavity. The sheathed microfilariae are 240 μm to 256 μm long. Diagnosis is confirmed by the demonstration of microfilariae in blood smears.

Arterial Worm of Sheep

Elaeophora schneideri, the "arterial worm," is found in the common carotid arteries of sheep in the western and southwestern United States. Microfilariae are 270 μm long and 17 μm thick, bluntly rounded cranially, and tapered caudally. They are found in the skin, usually in the capillaries of the forehead and face. Filarial dermatitis is seen on the face, the poll region, and the feet of sheep.

Diagnosis involves observation of characteristic lesions and the identification of microfilariae in the skin. The most satisfactory means of diagnosis is to macerate a piece of skin in warm saline and examine the material for microfilariae after approximately 2 hours. In sheep, microfilariae are rare, and they may not be found in the skin of infected animals. Postmortem examination may be necessary to confirm the diagnosis. The prepatent period is 18 weeks or more.

▌ KEY POINTS

- The life cycle of nematodes consists of several developmental stages: the egg, four larval stages, and sexually mature adults.
- Infective stages of nematodes may involve an egg that contains a larva, a free-living larva, or a larva within an intermediate host or a transport host.
- A life cycle is considered to be direct if no intermediate host is necessary for development to the infective stage.
- Organisms with indirect life cycles require an intermediate host for development to the infective stage.

- Transmission of a nematode parasite to a new definitive host can occur through ingestion, skin penetration of infective larvae, ingestion of an intermediate host, or deposition of infective larvae into or onto the skin by an intermediate host.
- Nematode parasites of veterinary significance are members of 11 taxonomic superfamilies.
- Common nematode parasites of dogs and cats include *Toxocara* spp., *Ancylostoma* spp., *Trichuris* spp., and *D. immitis.*

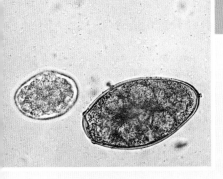

34

Cestodes, Trematodes, and Acanthocephalans

LEARNING OBJECTIVES

After studying this chapter, you will be able to:

- Differentiate between true tapeworms and pseudotapeworms.
- Describe the general characteristics of eucestodes.
- Describe the general characteristics of pseudotapeworms.
- Describe the life cycle of *Dipylidium caninum*.
- Describe the appearance of the eggs of common tapeworm species.
- Describe the zoonotic potential of cestodes.
- Describe the general characteristics of trematodes.
- Discuss the life cycle of *Fasciola hepatica*.

OUTLINE

KEY TERMS

Bothria	Metacercaria	Scolex
Cercaria	Miracidium	Sporocyst
Cestode	Proglottid	Strobila
Coracidium	Redia	Trematode
Hexacanth	Rostellum	

Phylum Platyhelminthes includes the trematodes and the cestodes. These are flatworms that lack a body cavity. The taxonomic class that includes the cestodes contains two subclasses. Members of the subclass Eucestoda are referred to as the true tapeworms, whereas members of the subclass Cotyloda are referred to as the pseudotapeworms. The phylum Acanthocephala includes the thorny-headed worms. These are not commonly encountered parasites in companion animal practice.

The life cycle of tapeworms is always indirect, and it involves one or two intermediate hosts. The intermediate hosts may be arthropods, fish, or mammals. Domestic animals can be definitive or intermediate hosts for tapeworms, or they may be both. The larval stages of some tapeworms that are found in domestic animals are called bladderworms, because they resemble fluid-filled sacks with one or multiple scoleces.

When ingested by a definitive host, the bladderworms are released from the tissue of the intermediate host and develop into adult tapeworms within the digestive tract of the definitive host. Some cestodes have larval forms that are solid bodies (i.e., procercoid, plerocercoid, and tetrathyridium). Domestic animals become infected with the larval stages of tapeworms via the ingestion of the cestode egg or procercoid.

EUCESTODES

The true tapeworms are multicellular organisms that lack a body cavity. Their organs are embedded in loose cellular tissue (parenchyma). The body of a tapeworm is long and dorsoventrally flattened, and it consists of three regions. The head (scolex) is modified into an attachment organ and bears two to four muscular suckers or acetabula. The suckers may be armed with hooks. There may also be a snout (rostellum) on the head, which can be fixed or retractable. The rostellum can also be armed with hooks (Fig. 34.1). Caudal to the head is a short neck of undifferentiated tissue, and this is followed by the body (strobila). The body is composed of segments (proglottids) in different stages of maturity. Those near the neck are immature, and these are followed by sexually mature proglottids and then by gravid segments that contain eggs. Gravid proglottids break off and pass out of the body of the definitive host in the feces (Fig. 34.2). New proglottids are continually formed from the undifferentiated tissue of the neck. Cestodes lack a digestive tract, and nutrients are absorbed directly through the body wall. The most prominent organs in cestodes are the organs of the reproductive system. Both male and female reproductive organs occur in each individual proglottid of the tapeworm. Cross-fertilization and self-fertilization both take place. Cestodes also have a nervous system and an excretory system.

> **TECHNICIAN NOTE** Tapeworms are dorsoventrally flattened and contain segments known as proglottids.

The cestode egg contains a fully developed embryo, which has six hooks in three pairs (hexacanth embryo or oncosphere) (Fig. 34.3). In most cases, the gravid proglottids are passed intact in the feces, either singly or in chains, and they then rupture and release the eggs. The eggs must then be ingested by the intermediate host, where they develop into the metacestode stage. The metacestode (larval) stage may be in the form of a cysticercus, a coenurus cyst, a hydatid cyst, or a tetrathyridium. The definitive host becomes infected after the ingestion of an intermediate host that contains the metacestode stage. The juvenile tapeworm then emerges from the metacestode stage, attaches to the lining of the small intestine, and begins to produce the strobili.

The pseudotapeworms are similar in structure to the true tapeworms except for the fact that their reproductive organs and genital pores are centrally located rather than laterally located. The organs of attachment are a pair of slitlike organs known as bothria, which are located on the lateral aspect of the scolex. The eggs of pseudotapeworms are operculated, and they are usually released from the uterus and passed in the feces. The

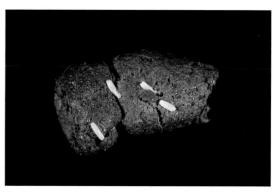

Fig. 34.2 Characteristic motile, terminal, gravid proglottids of *Dipylidium caninum* on canine feces. In the fresh state, these proglottids resemble cucumber seeds, which led to their common name, the "cucumber-seed" tapeworm.

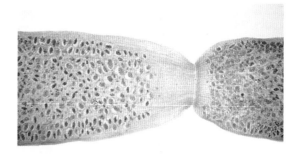

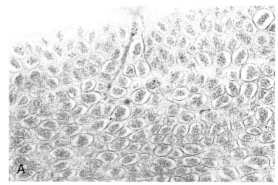

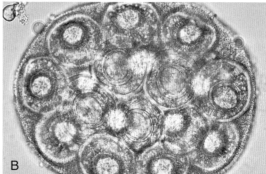

Fig. 34.3 A, Gravid proglottids of *Dipylidium caninum* are filled with thousands of egg packets. **B,** A characteristic egg packet of *D. caninum.* Each egg packet may contain up to 30 hexacanth embryos.

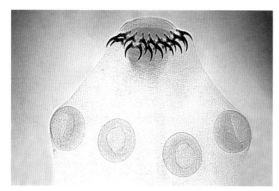

Fig. 34.1 Details of the scolex of the canine taeniid. Note the four suckers and the armed rostellum. (From Hendrix CM, Robinson E: *Diagnostic parasitology for veterinary technicians,* ed 4, St Louis, 2012, Mosby.)

egg contains an embryo referred to as a coracidium, which is released when the egg makes contact with water. The coracidium is then ingested by a microscopic aquatic crustacean, and it then develops into a stage called a procercoid. The crustacean is eventually ingested by a fish or an amphibian, and it develops into the metacestode stage (i.e., plerocercoid or sparganum) within the musculature of that host. The definitive host becomes infected after ingesting the second intermediate host.

Table 34.1 summarizes the cestode parasites of veterinary species.

TABLE 34.1 Selected Cestode Parasites of Veterinary Species

Scientific Name	Common Name	Intermediate Hosts	Prepatent Period
Dogs			
Diphyllobothrium species	Broad fish tapeworm	Copepod/fish	40 days
Dipylidium caninum	Cucumber-seed tapeworm	Flea	14—21 days
Mesocestoides species		Mites and mouse/reptile	20—30 days
Spirometra species	Zipper tapeworm	Copepod/fish/amphibians	15—30 days
Echinococcus granulosus	Hydatid disease tapeworm	Ruminants	45—60 days
Echinococcus multilocularis		Mice/rats	
Taenia multiceps		Sheep	30 days
Taenia serialis		Rabbit	30—60 days
Taenia hydatigena		Rabbit/sheep	51 days
Taenia ovis		Sheep	42—63 days
Taenia pisiformis		Rabbit/ruminant	56 days
Cats			
Echinococcus multilocularis	Hydatid disease tapeworm	Rodents	28 days
Taenia taeniaeformis or Hydatigera taeniaeformis	Feline tapeworm	Mice/rats	40 days
Diphyllobothrium species	Broad fish tapeworm	Copepod/fish	40 days
Dipylidium caninum	Cucumber-seed tapeworm	Flea	14—21 days
Mesocestoides species		Mites and mouse/reptile	
Spirometra species	Zipper tapeworm	Copepod/fish/amphibians	15—30 days
Ruminants			
Cysticercus bovis	Larval Taenia saginata		
Cysticercus cellulosae	Larval Taenia solium		
Cysticercus tenuicollis	Larval Taenia hydatigena		
Moniezia benedeni		Grain mites	40 days
Moniezia expansa		Grain mites	22—45 days
Taenia saginata or Taeniarhynchus saginata	Beef tapeworm of humans	Cattle	70—84 days
Thysanosoma actinoides	Fringed tapeworm	Psocids (lice)	Not known
Horses			
Anoplocephala magna		Oribatid mites	4—6 weeks
Anoplocephala perfoliata		Oribatid mites	4—6 weeks
Paranoplocephala mamillana	Dwarf tapeworm	Oribatid mites	4—6 weeks
Pigs			
Taenia solium		Pigs	35—84 days
Rodents			
Hymenolepis diminuta		None	
Hymenolepis nana		Fleas/grain beetles/cockroaches	

Eucestodes of Dogs and Cats

Dipylidium Caninum

Dipylidium caninum is the most common tapeworm found in the small intestine of the dog and cat. The dog or cat becomes infected by ingesting an infected flea, which is the intermediate host. Fleas often contain this parasite's infective cysticercoid stage (Fig. 34.4). This tapeworm has motile, terminal, gravid proglottids, which usually are found on the feces, on the pet's hair coat, or in the bedding of the host. If fresh proglottids of *D. caninum* are teased or broken open, they may reveal thousands of unique egg packets, each of which contains 20 to 30 hexacanth embryos (see Fig. 34.3). The proglottids of *D. caninum* often dry out in the external environment. As they lose moisture, they shrivel up and resemble uncooked grains of rice (Fig. 34.5). If reconstituted with water, the dried proglottids usually assume their former cucumber-seed appearance. The prepatent period for *D. caninum* is 14 to 21 days.

> **TECHNICIAN NOTE** *Dipylidium caninum* is the most common tapeworm of dogs and cats.

Canine Taeniid Tapeworms

Taenia pisiformis, Taenia hydatigena, and *Taenia ovis* are the canine taeniids. As with *D. caninum, Taenia* tapeworms appear as motile, terminal, gravid proglottids on the feces, on the pet's hair coat, or in the bedding of the host. In the fresh state, these

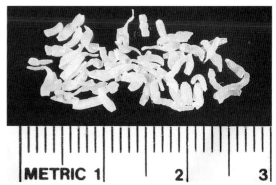

Fig. 34.5 Dried proglottids of *Dipylidium caninum* resemble uncooked grains of rice. When water is added, they assume their natural state. (From Hendrix CM, Robinson E: *Diagnostic parasitology for veterinary technicians,* ed 4, St Louis, 2006, Mosby.)

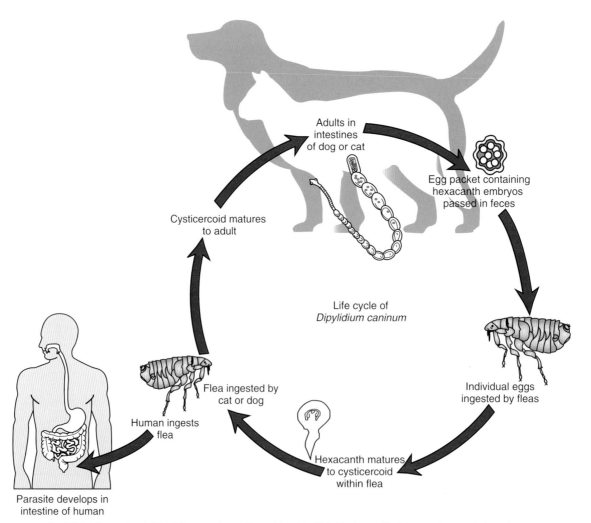

Fig. 34.4 Life cycle of *Dipylidium caninum.* (From Hendrix CM, Robinson E: *Diagnostic parasitology for veterinary technicians,* ed 4, St Louis, 2012, Mosby.)

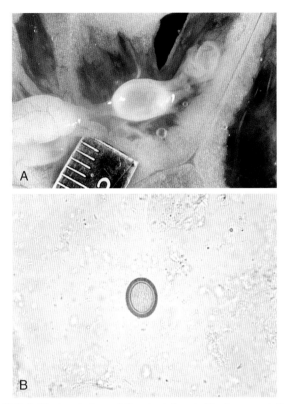

Fig. 34.6 **A,** The larval stage of *Taenia pisiformis (Cysticercus pisiformis)* is usually attached to the greater omentum or other abdominal organs of the rabbit intermediate host. **B,** Ova of *Taenia pisiformis.* (From Hendrix CM, Robinson E: *Diagnostic parasitology for veterinary technicians*, ed 4, St Louis, 2012, Mosby.)

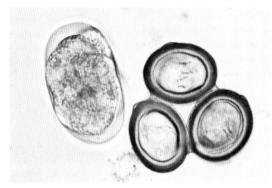

Fig. 34.7 Characteristic ova of the taeniid tapeworms are slightly oval. The dissimilar ovum is that of *Ancylostoma caninum*, the hookworm. (From Hendrix CM, Robinson E: *Diagnostic parasitology for veterinary technicians*, ed 4, St Louis, 2006, Mosby.)

proglottids have a single lateral pore located along the midpoint of either of their long edges (as opposed to the double-pore tapeworm). Dogs become infected by ingesting the cysticercus-infected intermediate host (Fig. 34.6). The intermediate hosts for *Taenia pisiformis* are rabbits and hares. *Taenia hydatigena* and *Taenia ovis* involve ruminant intermediate hosts.

As with *D. caninum*, if these fresh proglottids are teased or broken open, they may reveal thousands of hexacanth embryos. The proglottids of *Taenia* species also dry out in the external environment and resemble uncooked grains of rice. If reconstituted with water, they too usually assume their former single-pore appearance. If gravid proglottids of *Taenia* species are recovered from a dog's or cat's feces, the proglottid should be torn open or macerated in a drop of saline solution on a glass slide to reveal the characteristic eggs under the compound microscope.

The eggs of taeniid tapeworms are slightly oval. They are 43 μm to 53 μm by 43 μm to 49 μm in diameter *(T. pisiformis)*, 36 μm to 39 μm by 31 μm to 35 μm in diameter *(T. hydatigena)*, and 19 μm to 31 μm by 24 μm to 26 μm *(T. ovis)*. Eggs of *Taenia* species contain a single oncosphere with three pairs of hooks. The oncosphere is the hexacanth embryo. Fig. 34.7 shows the unique features of this taeniid tapeworm. The eggs are also similar to those of *Echinococcus* and *Multiceps* species.

Taenia taeniaeformis or *Hydatigera taeniaeformis* is called the "feline tapeworm" or the "feline taeniid." This tapeworm is observed infrequently in cats that are allowed to roam and prey on small mammals (Fig. 34.8). The egg of this tapeworm is 31 μm to 36 μm in diameter, and it contains a single oncosphere with three pairs of hooks. The oncosphere is often called a hexacanth embryo. As with the eggs of the canine taeniids, the eggs are similar to those of *Echinococcus* species.

Multiceps Species

Multiceps multiceps and *Multiceps serialis* are also tapeworms of the small intestine of canids. The eggs of *M. multiceps* are 29 μm to 37 μm in diameter, whereas those of *M. serialis* are elliptic and measure 31 μm to 34 μm by 29 μm to 30 μm. Both contain a single oncosphere with three pairs of hooks. As with the eggs of the canine and feline taeniids, the eggs of *Multiceps* species are similar to those of *Echinococcus* species.

Echinococcus Species

Echinococcus granulosus and *Echinococcus multilocularis* are tapeworms that are associated with unilocular and multilocular hydatid disease. *E. granulosus* is the hydatid cyst tapeworm of dogs, whereas *E. multilocularis* is the hydatid cyst tapeworm of cats. These are important parasites because of their extreme zoonotic potential (Fig. 34.9). The egg of *E. granulosus* is ovoid and measures 32 μm to 36 μm by 25 μm to 30 μm. It contains a single oncosphere with three pairs of hooks. The egg of *E. multilocularis* is ovoid and measures 30 μm to 40 μm. It contains a single oncosphere with three pairs of hooks. These eggs are similar in appearance to those of *Taenia* and *Multiceps* species.

> **TECHNICIAN NOTE** The hydatid cysts produced by *Echinococcus* species can develop in a variety of organs in the human intermediate host.

The adult *Echinococcus* is a tiny tapeworm that is only 1.2 μm to 7.0 μm in length. The entire tapeworm has only three

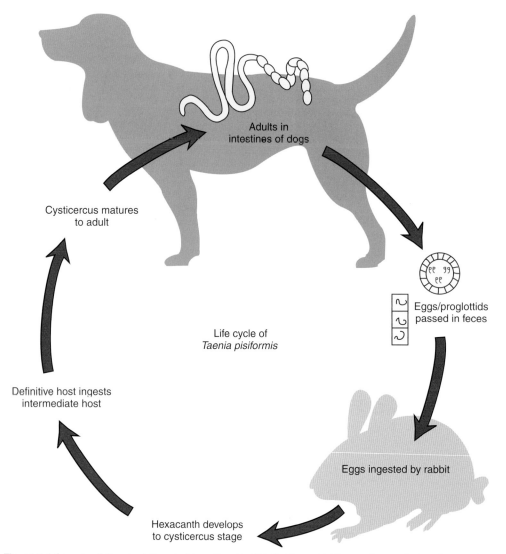

Life cycle of
Taenia pisiformis

Adults in
intestines of dogs

Eggs/proglottids
passed in feces

Eggs ingested by rabbit

Hexacanth develops
to cysticercus stage

Definitive host ingests
intermediate host

Cysticercus matures
to adult

Fig. 34.8 Life cycle of *Taenia pisiformis*. (From Hendrix CM, Robinson E: *Diagnostic parasitology for veterinary technicians*, ed 4, St Louis, 2012, Mosby.)

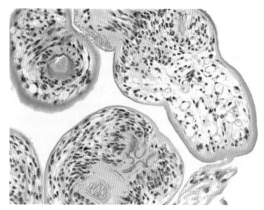

Fig. 34.9 Numerous *Echinococcus* protoscoleces in a hydatid cyst removed from human lung tissue (600×). (Photo from CDC website. In Sirois M: *Principles and practice of veterinary technology*, ed 3, St Louis, 2011, Mosby.)

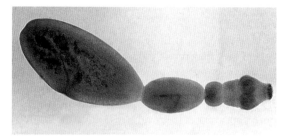

Fig. 34.10 The adult *Echinococcus* species is a tiny tapeworm that is only 1.2 mm to 7 mm in length. (From Hendrix CM, Robinson E: *Diagnostic parasitology for veterinary technicians*, ed 4, St Louis, 2012, Mosby.)

proglottids: one immature proglottid, one mature proglottid, and one gravid proglottid (Fig. 34.10). When passed, the tiny gravid proglottids are so small that they are often overlooked by the client, the veterinary technician, and the veterinarian. The definitive diagnosis of *Echinococcus* infection is best achieved by identifying adult tapeworms taken from the host's intestinal tract. In the rare instances in which *Echinococcus* infection is suspected, antemortem diagnosis is accomplished by purging the dog or cat with arecoline hydrobromide per os at 3.5 mg/kg and collecting the feces. This procedure is usually performed only when this infection is strongly suspected. Entire worms or their proglottids may be collected from the final clear mucus. Because of the severe zoonotic potential, all evacuated material should be handled with caution. Rubber gloves should be worn. After the feces have been examined, they should be incinerated.

Eucestodes of Ruminants and Horses

Equine Tapeworms

Anoplocephala perfoliata, Anoplocephala magna, and *Paranoplocephala mamillana* are the equine tapeworms. *A. perfoliata* is found in the small and large intestines and the cecum. *A. magna* is found in the small intestine and occasionally the stomach. *P. mamillana* is also found in the small intestine and occasionally in the stomach. The eggs of *A. perfoliata* have thick walls with one or more flattened sides, and they measure 65 μm to 80 μm in diameter. The eggs of *A. magna* are similar but slightly smaller, measuring 50 μm to 60 μm. The eggs of *P. mamillana* are oval and have thin walls that measure 37 μm to 51 μm. Eggs of all three species have a three-layer eggshell. The innermost lining is called the pyriform apparatus, which is pear-shaped. Eggs of all equine tapeworms can be recovered with standard fecal flotation. The prepatent period of all three species ranges from 28 to 42 days.

Ruminant Tapeworms

Moniezia species are tapeworms that are found in the small intestines of cattle, sheep, and goats. These tapeworms produce eggs with a characteristic cuboidal or pyramidal shape. When viewed with a compound microscope, these eggs appear square or triangular in silhouette. Two species are common: *Moniezia benedeni* in cattle and *Moniezia expansa* in cattle, sheep, and goats. The eggs of both species can be easily differentiated with standard fecal flotation procedures. Fig. 34.11 shows representative eggs of the *Moniezia* species. The eggs of *M. expansa* appear triangular and measure 56 μm to 67 μm in diameter.

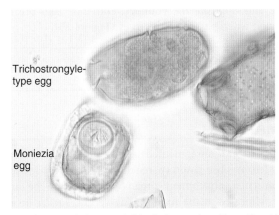

Trichostrongyle-type egg

Moniezia egg

Fig. 34.11 Characteristic ova of *Moniezia* species. (From Hendrix CM, Robinson E: *Diagnostic parasitology for veterinary technicians,* ed 3, St Louis, 2006, Mosby.)

The eggs of *M. benedeni* appear square, and they are approximately 75 μm in diameter. The prepatent period for these tapeworms is approximately 40 days.

Thysanosoma actinoides is the "fringed tapeworm" that is found in the bile ducts, pancreatic ducts, and small intestine of ruminants. Eggs of this tapeworm occur in packets of 6 to 12 eggs, with individual eggs measuring 19 μm by 27 μm.

Bladderworm of Ruminants

Cysticercus tenuicollis—the bladderworm (larval or metacestode stage) of *Taenia hydatigena*—may be found attached to the greater omentum within the abdominal cavity of many ruminants. These cysticerci are usually diagnosed during postmortem examination. *Cysticercus bovis*—the bladderworm (larval or metacestode stage) of *Taenia saginata,* which is the beef tapeworm of human beings—may be found within the musculature of the bovine intermediate host. These cysticerci are colloquially referred to as "beef measles," and they are usually diagnosed during postmortem meat inspection. Human beings become infected with the adult tapeworm by eating poorly cooked beef.

Bladderworm of Swine

Cysticercus cellulosae—the bladderworm (larval or metacestode stage) of *Taenia solium,* which is the pork tapeworm of human beings—may be found within the musculature of the porcine intermediate host. These cysticerci are colloquially referred to as "pork measles," and they are usually diagnosed during postmortem meat inspection. Human beings become infected with the adult tapeworm *T. solium* by eating poorly cooked pork containing cysticerci. Human beings may become infected with *C. cellulosae* in the muscles or within the nervous tissue (e.g., in the brain or the eye) by ingesting the eggs of *T. solium.*

Eucestodes of Small Mammals

Vampirolepis (also *Hymenolepis* or *Rodentolepis*) *nana* and *Hymenolepis diminuta* parasitize the small intestine of rodents and occasionally of dogs and humans. The parasite is unique in that it is able to complete its life cycle within a single individual. The eggs are found in the feces (Fig. 34.12), and the tailed larval cysticercoid develops in fleas, flour beetles, and other insects. Some of the eggs of *V. nana* may hatch within the intestine, and the hexacanth embryos burrow into the mucous membrane to form cysticercoids. These can later reenter the intestinal lumen to complete their development. The rest of the eggs pass out with the feces to await ingestion by flour beetles or fleas, in which the cysticercoids develop. *H. diminuta* infection requires the ingestion of an infected insect, so human infection with this tapeworm is unlikely.

> **TECHNICIAN NOTE** *Hymenolepis nana* is the only tapeworm that does not need an intermediate host to complete its life cycle.

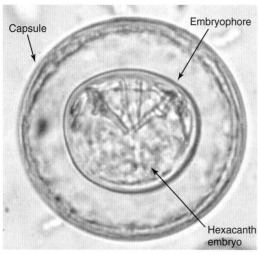

Fig. 34.12 Egg of *Hymenolepis diminuta* (Hymenolepididae), a common parasite of rodents. (From Bowman D: *Georgis' parasitology for veterinarians*, ed 9, St Louis, 2009, Saunders.)

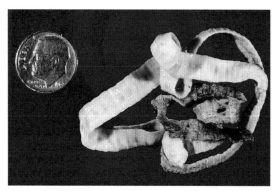

Fig. 34.13 Spent proglottids of *Spirometra mansonoides*, the "zipper tapeworm." (From Hendrix CM, Robinson E: *Diagnostic parasitology for veterinary technicians*, ed 3, St Louis, 2006, Mosby.)

PSEUDOTAPEWORMS

Zipper Tapeworms of Dogs and Cats

Spirometra species are often referred to as "zipper" tapeworms or sparganosis tapeworms (Fig. 34.13). These tapeworms are often found in the small intestines of both dogs and cats that live in Florida and along the Gulf Coast of North America. This tapeworm is unusual in that it produces an operculated egg. Each proglottid of *Spirometra* species has a central spiral uterus and an associated uterine pore through which eggs are released. These tapeworms characteristically release eggs until they exhaust their uterine contents. Gravid segments are usually not discharged into the pet's feces.

This tapeworm is unique because, although it is attached to the host's jejunum, the mature proglottids often separate along the longitudinal axis for a short distance. The tapeworm appears to "unzip," which is the origin of its common name, the "zipper tapeworm." Spent "zipped" and "unzipped" proglottids often appear in the feces of the pet.

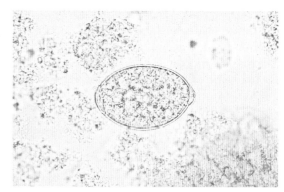

Fig. 34.14 Characteristic ovum of *Spirometra mansonoides*. (From Hendrix CM, Robinson E: *Diagnostic parasitology for veterinary technicians*, ed 3, St Louis, 2006, Mosby.)

The egg of *Spirometra* species resembles that of a fluke or digenetic trematode (Fig. 34.14). The egg has a distinct operculum at one end of the pole of the shell. The eggs are oval and yellowish-brown. They average 60 µm by 36 µm, they have an asymmetric appearance, and they are rather pointed at one end. When the eggs rupture, a distinct operculum is visible. The eggs are unembryonated when passed in the feces.

Broad Fish Tapeworms

Diphyllobothrium species are often referred to as "broad fish" tapeworms. This tapeworm may be 2 m to 12 m long; however, it probably does not grow as large as 12 m in dogs and cats. Each proglottid of this tapeworm has a central rosette-shaped uterus and an associated uterine pore through which eggs are released. These tapeworms continually release eggs until they exhaust their uterine contents. The terminal proglottids become senile rather than gravid, and they detach in chains rather than individually.

The eggs of the *Diphyllobothrium* species also resemble those of a fluke (digenetic trematode). The egg is oval, and it has a distinct operculum at one end of the shell. The eggs are light brown, and they average 67 µm to 71 µm by 40 µm to 51 µm. They tend to be rounded on one end. The operculum is present on the end opposite the rounded end. The eggs are unembryonated when passed in the feces (Fig. 34.15).

> **TECHNICIAN NOTE** Pseudotapeworms of veterinary importance include *Spirometra* and *Diphyllobothrium* species.

TREMATODES

Trematodes are unsegmented and leaflike. The organs are embedded in loose tissue (parenchyma), and they also possess two muscular attachment organs or suckers. The anterior sucker is located at the mouth. The ventral sucker or acetabulum is located on the ventral surface of the worm near the middle of the body or at the caudal end. There are three main groups of trematodes, but only the digenetic trematodes are parasites of domestic animals. Monogenetic trematodes are primarily external parasites of fish, amphibians, and reptiles.

Digenetic trematodes have an outer body wall or cuticle. They have a simple digestive tract that consists of a mouth, a pharynx, an esophagus, and an intestine that divides into two blind sacs (ceca). The main organs that are visible in

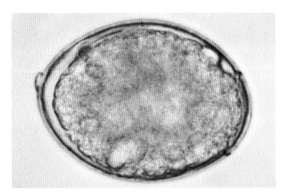

Fig. 34.15 The egg of *Diphyllobothrium* species resembles that of a fluke (digenetic trematode). (From Hendrix CM, Robinson E: *Diagnostic parasitology for veterinary technicians*, ed 4, St Louis, 2012, Mosby.)

trematodes are the reproductive organs. Most trematodes have both male and female reproductive organs in the same individual, but a few have separate sexes (e.g., *Schistosoma*). A nervous system and an excretory system are also present.

The life cycle of digenetic trematodes is complicated (Fig. 34.16). They pass through several different larval stages (miracidium, sporocyst, redia, cercaria, and metacercaria), and they typically require one or more intermediate hosts, one of which is nearly always a mollusk (e.g., snail, slug). Multiplication takes place in both the definitive (sexual) and intermediate (asexual) hosts. The eggs of digenetic trematodes are capped (operculated), and they contain a ciliated embryo called a miracidium. Through penetration or ingestion, the miracidium enters a suitable snail and develops through several stages that eventually give rise to a motile, tailed stage referred to as a cercaria. Cercariae are released from the snail and swim actively. Sometimes, depending on the species of fluke, the cercariae encyst on vegetation. This encysted stage, the metacercaria, is infective for the definitive host. In other species, the cercaria may penetrate the skin of the definitive host or encyst in another intermediate host. Table 34.2 summarizes the trematodes of veterinary importance.

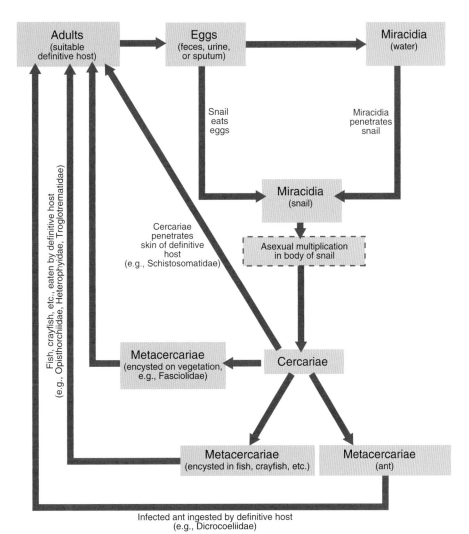

Fig. 34.16 Some life history variations of trematode parasites of domestic animals. (From Bowman D: *Georgis' parasitology for veterinarians*, ed 9, St Louis, 2009, Saunders.)

TABLE 34.2 Information About Some Trematodes of Veterinary Importance

Family	Genera and Species	Geographic Distribution	Hosts	Location in Host	Disease	Length of Adult	Length of Egg	Second Intermediate Host	Prepatent Period
Fasciolidae	Fasciola hepatica	Tropics and United States	Herbivorous mammals	Bile ducts	Hepatic fibrosis	3 cm	120 μm	Metacercariae on vegetation	60 days
	Fasciola gigantica	Africa	Humans	Bile ducts	Hepatic fibrosis	5 cm	120 μm	Metacercariae on vegetation	60 days
	Fasciolopsis buski	Asia	Pigs and humans	Intestine	Intestinal upset	8 cm	120 μm	Metacercariae on vegetation	90 days
	Fascioloides magna	United States and Europe	White-tailed deer	Liver (cysts)	Hepatitis, kills other cervids and small ruminants, nonpatent cysts in cattle	10 cm	120 μm	Metacercariae on vegetation	270 days
Paramphistomatidae	Paramphistomum and Cotylophoron	Worldwide	Ruminants	Rumen	Intestinal damage by immature flukes	10 mm	120 μm	Metacercariae on aquatic vegetation	80 days
Troglotrematidae	Nanophyetus salmincola	North Pacific Rim	Dogs and cats	Intestine	Transmits Neorickettsia helminthoeca	1 mm	80 μm	Fish	7 days
	Paragonimus kellicotti	Eastern United States	Minks, dogs, and cats	Lungs	Cysts in lungs	6 mm	90 μm	Crayfish	30 days
Heterophyidae	Cryptocotyle	United States, East Coast	Birds	Intestine	Enteritis	2 mm	30 μm	Fish	14 days
	Heterophyes	Middle East	Dogs and cats	Intestine	Enteritis	2 mm	30 μm	Fish	14 days
Opisthorchidae	Opisthorchis	Asia and Europe	Dogs and cats	Bile ducts	Very little	6 mm	30 μm	Fish	30 days
	Metorchis	United States	Foxes and pigs	Bile ducts	Very little	6 mm	30 μm	Fish	17 days
	Clonorchis	Asia	Dogs and cats	Bile ducts	Very little	6 mm	30 μm	Fish	60 days
Dicrocoelidae	Dicrocoelium dendriticum	New York, Quebec, British Columbia, Europe	Sheep, cattle, pigs, deer, and woodchucks	Bile ducts	Fibrosis with chronic disease	10 mm	40 μm	Ants	80 days
	Platynosomum fastosum	Caribbean and southern United States	Cats	Bile ducts and gall bladder	Hepatitis, fibrosis, vomiting, jaundice, and diarrhea	7 mm	45 μm	Lizards	30 days

Family	Species	Distribution	Definitive host	Location	Pathology	Size	Egg size	Intermediate/paratenic host	Prepatent period
Diplostomatidae	Alaria canis	Northern United States and Canada	Dogs and foxes	Intestine	Very little	4 mm	100 μm	Frogs (paratenic hosts)	35 days
	Alaria marcianae Fibricola texensis	Southern United States	Raccoons and opossums						
Schistosomatidae	Schistosoma mansoni	Worldwide	Humans	Mesenteric veins	Hepatic fibrosis	10–20 mm; sexes separate	55–145 μm; lateral spine	None; penetrate skin	60 days
	Schistosoma haematobium	Africa	Humans	Veins of urinary bladder	Erosion of bladder wall	10 mm; sexes separate	60 μm × 140 μm; terminal spine	None; penetrate skin	70–84 days
	Schistosoma japonicum	Asia	Humans, cats, and mammals	Mesenteric veins	Hepatic fibrosis	10 mm; sexes separate	58 μm × 85 μm; no spine	None; penetrate skin	35–42 days
	Schistosoma bovis	Africa	Cattle	Mesenteric veins	Hepatic fibrosis	10 mm; sexes separate	62 μm × 207 μm; terminal spine	None; penetrate skin	42 days
	Schistosoma margrebowiei	Africa	Horses and ruminants	Mesenteric veins	Hepatic fibrosis	10 mm; sexes separate	60 μm × 80 μm; no spine	None; penetrate skin	38 days
	Bivitellobilharzia loxodontae	Africa	Elephants	Mesenteric veins	Hepatic fibrosis	10 mm; sexes separate	71 μm × 87 μm; no spine	None; penetrate skin	Not known
	Heterobilharzia americana	United States	Raccoons, dogs, and opossums	Mesenteric veins	Hepatic fibrosis	10 mm; sexes separate	70 μm × 87 μm; no spine	None; penetrate skin	60 days
	Bird genera	Worldwide		Skin	Dermatitis in mammals	10 mm; sexes separate	Varied	None; penetrate skin	

Modified from Bowman D: *Georgis' parasitology for veterinarians*, ed 9, St Louis, 2009, Saunders.

Trematodes of Dogs and Cats

Lizard Poisoning Fluke of Cats

Platynosomum fastosum is the "lizard-poisoning fluke" of cats (Fig. 34.17). The adult flukes inhabit the liver, gallbladder, bile ducts, and, less commonly, the small intestine. The brownish operculated eggs are 34 μm to 50 μm by 20 μm to 35 μm.

Salmon Poisoning Fluke of Dogs

Nanophyetus salmincola is the "salmon-poisoning fluke" of dogs in the Pacific Northwest region of North America. The adult fluke inhabits the small intestine and serves as a vector for rickettsial agents, which produce "salmon poisoning" and "Elokomin fluke fever" in dogs. The eggs are unembryonated when laid and measure 52 μm to 82 μm by 32 μm to 56 μm (Fig. 34.18). They have an indistinct operculum and a small, blunt point at the end opposite the operculum.

Alaria of Dogs and Cats

Alaria species are intestinal flukes of dogs and cats, and they are found throughout the northern half of North America. Their ova are large, golden brown, and operculated (Fig. 34.19), and they measure 98 μm to 134 μm by 62 μm to 68 μm.

Canine Blood Fluke

Heterobilharzia americanum, the canine schistosome, is a blood fluke that parasitizes the mesenteric veins of the small and large intestines and portal veins of the dog. This fluke is enzootic in the Mississippi Delta and the coastal swampland of Louisiana. Although this fluke inhabits the vasculature, its presence is manifested by bloody diarrhea. Infected dogs also exhibit emaciation and anorexia. Diagnosis involves identification of the thin-shelled egg, which is approximately 80 μm by 50 μm and contains a miracidium. Fig. 34.20 shows the morphologic features of the egg of *H. americanum*. The prepatent period lasts for approximately 84 days.

Canine Lung Fluke

Paragonimus kellicotti is the "lung fluke" of dogs. Hermaphroditic adult flukes occur in cystic spaces within the lung parenchyma of both dogs and cats. These cystic spaces connect to the terminal bronchioles. The eggs are found in sputum or feces. The egg is yellowish-brown with an operculum, and it measures 75 μm to 118 μm by 42 μm to 67 μm (Fig. 34.21).

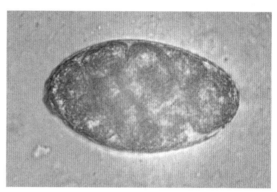

Fig. 34.18 Characteristic ovum of *Nanophyetus salmincola*. (From Hendrix CM, Robinson E: *Diagnostic parasitology for veterinary technicians*, ed 3, St Louis, 2006, Mosby.)

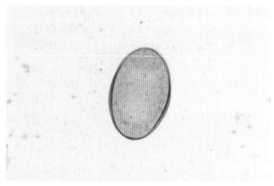

Fig. 34.19 Characteristic ovum of *Alaria* species, the intestinal flukes of dogs and cats. They are found throughout the northern half of North America. (From Hendrix CM, Robinson E: *Diagnostic parasitology for veterinary technicians*, ed 3, St Louis, 2006, Mosby.)

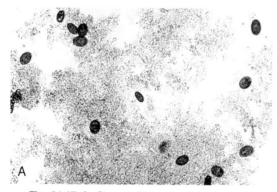 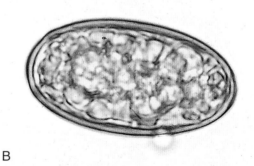

Fig. 34.17 A, Characteristic ova of *Platynosomum fastosum*, the "lizard-poisoning fluke" of cats. **B,** The brownish, operculated eggs are 34 μm to 50 μm by 20 μm to 35 μm. (From Hendrix CM, Robinson E: *Diagnostic parasitology for veterinary technicians*, ed 3, St Louis, 2006, Mosby.)

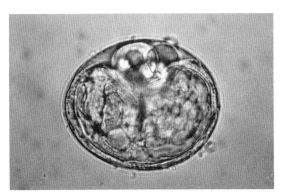

Fig. 34.20 Characteristic thin-shell ovum of *Heterobilharzia americanum.* These ova are approximately 80 µm by 50 µm, and they contain a miracidium. (From Hendrix CM, Robinson E: *Diagnostic parasitology for veterinary technicians*, ed 3, St Louis, 2006, Mosby.)

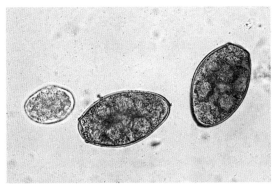

Fig. 34.21 The characteristic ovum of *Paragonimus kellicotti*, the lung fluke of dogs, which were recovered with standard fecal flotation. The eggs may be found in either sputum or feces, but they are often recovered with fecal flotation. There is also an *Ancylostoma caninum* egg on the left side of this image. (From Hendrix CM, Robinson E: *Diagnostic parasitology for veterinary technicians*, ed 3, St Louis, 2006, Mosby.)

Fluke eggs are usually recovered with fecal sedimentation techniques; however, the eggs of *P. kellicotti* may be recovered with standard fecal flotation solutions. The eggs of *P. kellicotti* may also be recovered in the sputum collected by tracheal washing. The adult flukes within the cystic spaces of the lung parenchyma can also be observed in thoracic radiographs. This fluke's prepatent period is 30 to 36 days long.

Trematodes of Ruminants
Liver Fluke

Fasciola hepatica is the "liver fluke" of cattle, sheep, and other ruminants. The hermaphroditic adult flukes are found in the bile ducts of the liver (Fig. 34.22). The eggs measure 140 µm by 100 µm, and they are yellowish-brown, oval, and operculated (Fig. 34.23). The prepatent period for *F. hepatica* is approximately 56 days long. *F. hepatica* has the greatest economic importance of all of the flukes that parasitize veterinary species. The life cycle of this species is quite complex (Fig. 34.24).

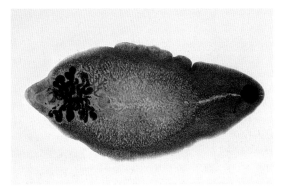

Fig. 34.22 Adult liver flukes *(Fasciola hepatica)* are broader in the anterior region, and they have a prominent anterior cone-shaped projection followed by prominent shoulders. (From Hendrix CM, Robinson E: *Diagnostic parasitology for veterinary technicians*, ed 4, St Louis, 2012, Mosby.)

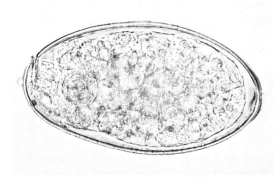

Fig. 34.23 Characteristic operculated ovum of *Fasciola hepatica*, the liver fluke of cattle, sheep, and other ruminants. (From Hendrix CM, Robinson E: *Diagnostic parasitology for veterinary technicians*, ed 3, St Louis, 2006, Mosby.)

Lancet Fluke

Dicrocoelium dendriticum is the "lancet fluke" of sheep, goats, and oxen. These tiny flukes reside within the fine branches of the bile ducts. The brown eggs have an indistinct operculum, and they measure 36 µm to 45 µm by 20 µm to 30 µm. Eggs of this and the aforementioned trematodes may be recovered from feces by fecal sedimentation or a commercially available fluke egg recovery test.

Rumen Flukes

"Rumen flukes" are composed of two genera: *Paramphistomum* and *Cotylophoron*. These adult flukes reside in the rumen and reticulum of cattle, sheep, goats, and many other ruminants. The eggs of *Paramphistomum* species measure 114 µm to 176 µm by 73 µm to 100 µm, whereas the eggs of *Cotylophoron* species measure 125 µm to 135 µm by 61 µm to 68 µm. The prepatent period of *Paramphistomum* species is 80 to 95 days.

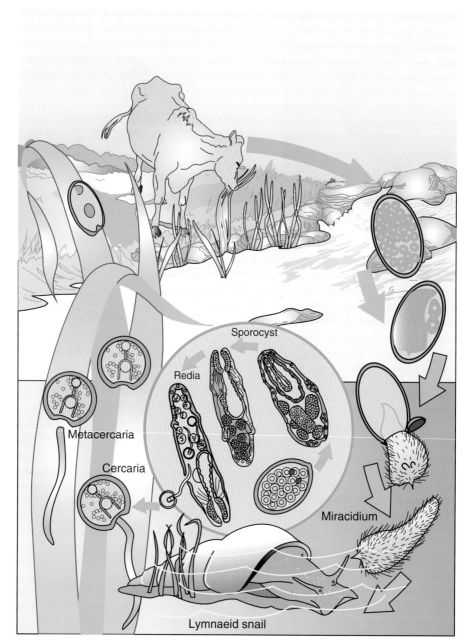

Fig. 34.24 Life history of *Fasciola hepatica*. The adult liver flukes produce fertile eggs that leave the host by way of the common bile duct and the intestinal tract. If these eggs are carried to water, a ciliated miracidium develops within them over a period of several weeks or months, depending on the temperature of the water. After hatching, the miracidia seek certain species of lymnaeid snails, in which they develop and multiply through one generation of sporocysts and two generations of rediae. The second generation of rediae produces free-swimming cercariae that leave the snail and encyst as metacercariae on various submerged objects, including aquatic vegetation. Ruminants and other animals become infected with *F. hepatica* when they ingest aquatic plants that have been contaminated with metacercariae. (From Bowman D: *Georgis' parasitology for veterinarians*, ed 9, St Louis, 2009, Saunders.)

Human Flukes

Schistosoma (Bilharzia) species are blood flukes of humans. Cercariae enter through the direct penetration of the skin. These flukes are similar to *Heterobilharzia americanum*, and they inhabit the blood vasculature of the mesenteric veins and the blood vasculature associated with major organs (i.e., the large and small intestines and the urinary bladder) of the abdominal cavities of humans.

ACANTHOCEPHALANS (THORNY-HEAD WORMS)

Acanthocephalans (thorny-head worms) are uncommon parasites with complicated life cycles. Like most nematodes, they have separate sexes. On the cranial end of these helminths is a spiny proboscis that is used to attach to the lining of the intestine wall. Thorny-head worms do not have a true gut; they absorb nutrients through their body wall. Acanthocephalans are usually recovered at necropsy (Fig. 34.25).

The most famous acanthocephalan is *Macracanthorhynchus hirudinaceus,* which is a parasite of pigs. This parasite has the dubious honor of possessing the longest scientific name among the parasites of domestic animals. *Oncicola canis* is an acanthocephalan that is found in the small intestine of dogs.

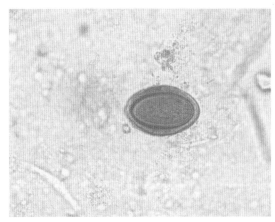

Fig. 34.25 Ova of an acanthocephalan recovered from a javelina.

■ KEY POINTS

- Phylum Platyhelminthes includes the flatworms that are commonly referred to as trematodes and cestodes.
- Members of the subclass Eucestoda are referred to as the true tapeworms.
- Members of the subclass Cotyloda are referred to as the pseudotapeworms.
- Tapeworms have an indirect life cycle that involves one or more intermediate hosts.
- A true tapeworm has two to four muscular suckers or acetabula that serve to attach the organism to the intestinal wall.
- The organs of attachment for pseudotapeworms are a pair of slitlike organs known as bothria, which are located on the lateral aspect of the scolex.
- *Dipylidium caninum* is the most common tapeworm found in the small intestines of dogs and cats.
- The intermediate host of *Dipylidium caninum* is the flea.
- Dogs and cats become infected with taeniid tapeworms by ingesting a cysticercus-infected intermediate host.
- *Echinococcus granulosus* and *Echinococcus multilocularis* are tapeworms that are associated with unilocular and multilocular hydatid cyst disease.
- *Anoplocephala perfoliata, Anoplocephala magna,* and *Paranoplocephala mamillana* are the equine tapeworms.
- Trematodes are flatworms with complex life cycles that include several different larval stages (i.e., miracidium, sporocyst, redia, cercaria, and metacercaria) and that typically require one or more intermediate hosts, one of which is nearly always a mollusk (e.g., snail, slug).
- Trematode parasites of dogs and cats include *Paragonimus kellicotti, Platynosomum fastosum, Nanophyetus salmincola, Alaria* species, and *Heterobilharzia americanum.*
- Trematodes of ruminants include *Fasciola hepatica, Dicrocoelium dendriticum, Paramphistomum,* and *Cotylophoron.*

35

Protozoa and Rickettsia

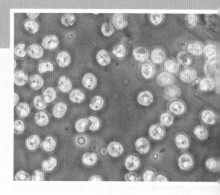

LEARNING OBJECTIVES

After studying this chapter, you will be able to:
- List the common protozoal parasites of veterinary importance and their definitive hosts.
- Describe the conditions under which protozoal parasites develop into cysts.
- Describe the life cycle of *Giardia*.
- Describe the general life cycle of sporozoans.
- Describe the life cycle of *Toxoplasma gondii* in feline and nonfeline hosts.
- List the common rickettsial parasites of veterinary importance.

KEY TERMS

Amastigote	Infectious enterohepatitis	Rickettsia
Bradyzoites	Merozoites	Tachyzoites
Cilia	Oocyst	Trophozoite
Coccidiosis	Promastigote	Trypomastigote
Flagella	Protozoa	Undulatory ridges
Hemoprotozoa	Pseudopodia	

There are about 65,000 known protozoans that can be found in a wide variety of habitats. Only a small percentage of protozoans are parasitic. Protozoa are single-celled organisms with one or more membrane-bound nuclei that contain DNA and specialized cytoplasmic organelles. Parasitic protozoa can be found in three primary phyla: (1) Sarcomastigophora, (2) Apicomplexa, and (3) Ciliophora. These protozoans can infect a variety of tissue sites within the definitive host. The most common sites for their detection are blood samples, in which they are called blood protozoa or hemoprotozoa, or fecal samples, in which they are called intestinal protozoa. Most hemoprotozoa seen in the United States are found in erythrocytes (red blood cells [RBCs]) within a stained blood smear. Ticks usually serve as intermediate hosts and transmit the RBCs that contain the hemoprotozoa from one animal to the next. The life cycles of protozoa can be simple or complex. Reproduction may be asexual (binary fission, schizogony, budding) or sexual (syngamy, conjugation). With certain groups of protozoa, reproductive stages are useful for identification. The trophozoite (also known as the vegetative form) is that stage of the protozoal life cycle that is capable of feeding, movement, and reproduction. Table 35.1 summarizes some common protozoal parasites of veterinary species.

TABLE 35.1 Select Protozoal Parasites of Veterinary Species

	Intermediate Hosts	Location in Final Host
Dogs		
Ciliates		
Balantidium coli		Cecum/colon
Sarcodines (Amoebas)		
Entamoeba histolytica		Large intestine
Flagellates		
Giardia species		Small intestine
Trypanosoma cruzi	Reduviid bugs	Peripheral blood
Leishmania species	Phlebotomine sand fly	Macrophages
Apicomplexans		
Babesia canis	Ticks	Erythrocytes
Cryptosporidium canis		Small intestine
Hepatozoon americanum	Ticks	Leukocytes
Hepatozoon canis	Ticks	Leukocytes
Cystoisospora canis (formerly *Isospora canis*)		Small intestine/cecum
Cystoisospora felis (formerly *Isospora felis*)		Small intestine/ileum
Cystoisospora ohioensis (formerly *Isospora ohioensis*)		Small intestine/cecum/colon
Cystoisospora rivolta (formerly *Isospora rivolta*)		Small intestine/cecum/colon
Cystoisospora burrowsi (formerly *Isospora burrowsi*)		Small intestine/cecum/colon
Sarcocystis species		Small intestine
Cats		
Flagellates		
Giardia species		Small intestine
Apicomplexans		
Cryptosporidium felis		Small intestine
Cytauxzoon felis	Ticks	Erythrocytes
Cystoisospora felis (formerly *Isospora felis*)		Small intestine/ileum
Cystoisospora rivolta (formerly *Isospora rivolta*)		Small intestine/cecum/colon
Sarcocystis species		Small intestine
Toxoplasma gondii		Intestinal mucosal cells
Horses		
Babesia caballi	Ticks	Erythrocytes
Babesia equi	Ticks	Erythrocytes
Eimeria leuckarti		Small intestine
Giardia equi		Small intestine
Sarcocystis neurona		Spinal cord, other central nervous system tissue
Ruminants		
Babesia bigemina	Ticks	Erythrocytes
Cryptosporidium species		Small intestine
Eimeria bovis		Small intestine
Tritrichomonas foetus		Reproductive system
Swine		
Eimeria species		Small intestine
Cryptosporidium species		Small intestine
Cystoisospora suis (formerly *Isospora suis*)		Small intestine

Continued

TABLE 35.1	**Select Protozoal Parasites of Veterinary Species—cont'd**	
	Intermediate Hosts	Location in Final Host
Rabbits		
Eimeria irresidua		Small intestine
Eimeria magna		Small intestine
Eimeria media		Small/large intestine
Eimeria perforans		Small intestine
Eimeria stiedai		Bile ducts

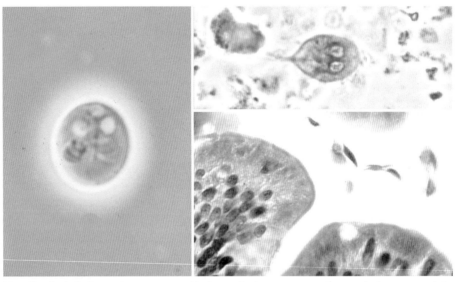

Fig. 35.1 *Giardia. Left,* A cyst that was passed in feces. A phase-contrast micrograph shows two of the four nuclei near the top of the image. *Top right, Giardia* trophozoite in a trichrome-stained fecal smear. *Bottom right,* Section through intestinal mucosa of an infected animal with detached trophozoites present within the lumen. (From Bowman D: *Georgis' parasitology for veterinarians,* ed 9, St Louis, 2009, Saunders.)

TECHNICIAN NOTE The term trophozoite refers to the motile, feeding stage of a protozoal parasite.

TECHNICIAN NOTE Protozoal parasites are usually transmitted to a new host during the cyst stage.

Organelles for locomotion consist of flagella (long, whiplike structures), cilia (short flagella, usually arranged in rows or tufts), pseudopodia (temporary extensions and retractions of the body wall), and undulatory ridges (small, snakelike waves that form in the cell membrane and move posteriorly). Locomotor organelles and modifications of them are frequently used to help identify the type of protozoa recovered from an animal. The trophozoite is often too fragile to survive transfer to a new host, and it is generally not infective. Transmission to a host often occurs when the protozoan is in the cyst stage. Most metabolic functions are suspended when the parasite is encysted. The cyst wall prevents desiccation. The cyst stage occurs under certain conditions that include the following:

- Lack of nutrients
- Low oxygen tension
- Lack of water
- Low pH
- Accumulation of waste
- Overcrowding

PHYLUM SARCOMASTIGOPHORA

The phylum Sarcomastigophora includes the amoebas and the flagellates. There are about 44,000 known species in this phylum, but only about 2300 are parasitic. The flagellates possess one or more flagella during their trophozoite life cycle stage. The trophozoite is the motile stage of the parasite. The amoebae move via pseudopods, and they have both a motile trophozoite form and a cyst stage. Genera of veterinary importance in this phylum include *Trypanosoma, Leishmania, Giardia, Trichomonas, Histomonas,* and *Entamoeba.*

Giardia

Giardia species are flagellated protozoans that are often recovered from the feces of dogs and cats with diarrhea, but they may also be recovered from animals with normal stools. This parasite occurs in two morphologic forms: (1) a motile feeding stage known as the trophozoite stage and (2) a resistant cyst stage (Fig. 35.1). Horses, cows, sheep, goats, and pigs are also susceptible to infection. The motile stage is pear-shaped and dorsoventrally flattened, and it contains four pairs of flagella. It measures 9 μm to 21 μm by 5 μm to 15 μm. Two nuclei and a prominent adhesive disk are present on the cranial portion of the cell, and they resemble a pair of eyes staring back at the observer.

The mature cysts are ovals that measure 8 μm to 10 μm by 7 μm to 10 μm. They have a refractile wall and four nuclei. Immature cysts, which represent recently encysted motile forms, contain only two nuclei. In dogs, diarrhea may begin as early as 5 days after exposure to Giardia, with cysts first appearing in the feces at 1 week. Fig. 35.2 summarizes the life cycle of Giardia.

> **TECHNICIAN NOTE** The trophozoites of *Giardia* species are typically seen in animals with diarrhea, whereas cysts are more commonly observed in formed stool.

Diagnosis is made with standard fecal flotation. Zinc sulfate (specific gravity, 1.18) is considered the best flotation medium for recovering cysts. Cysts are often distorted, with a semilunar appearance. The motile trophozoite occasionally may be found on a direct smear of fresh feces with isotonic saline. Lugol's iodine may be used to visualize the internal structures of cysts and trophozoites. Fecal immunodiagnostic tests are also commonly used.

Trypanosomes

Trypanosomes are a group of hemoprotozoans that are occasionally found in the southern United States. *Trypanosoma cruzi* is a parasite of humans and occasionally of dogs. Birds and cattle may also become infected. Rather than being found within RBCs, trypanosomes are extracellular and they "swim" within the blood. They are 3 to 10 times as long as an RBC is wide, and they are banana-shaped. They have a lateral undulating membrane and a thin, whiplike tail (flagellum) that is used for swimming (Fig. 35.3). The swimming stage is called a **trypomastigote**. The cyst stage, which is known as the **amastigote**, also exists, and it may be found within cardiac muscle and other tissues. These parasites are also transmitted by blood-feeding arthropods (reduviid bugs). Diagnosis of trypanosomes is by identification of the organism in blood, lymph node aspirate, or cerebrospinal fluid or sometimes by serologic tests.

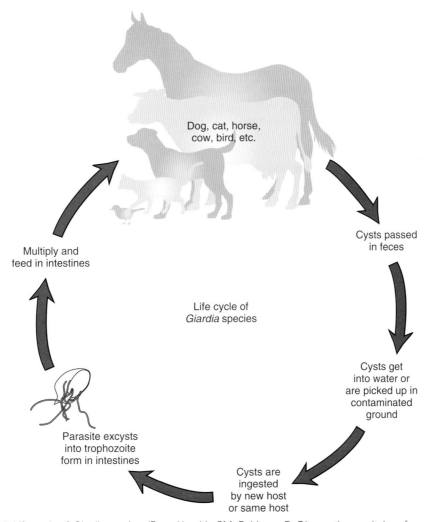

Dog, cat, horse, cow, bird, etc.

Cysts passed in feces

Life cycle of *Giardia* species

Multiply and feed in intestines

Cysts get into water or are picked up in contaminated ground

Parasite excysts into trophozoite form in intestines

Cysts are ingested by new host or same host

Fig. 35.2 Life cycle of *Giardia* species. (From Hendrix CM, Robinson E: *Diagnostic parasitology for veterinary technicians*, ed 4, St Louis, 2012, Mosby.)

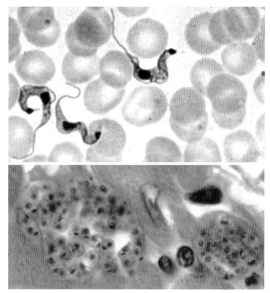

Fig. 35.3 *Trypanosoma cruzi.* The top image shows a trypomastigote in a Wright-stained buffy coat preparation from a naturally infected dog. The bottom image shows the amastigote stages in heart muscle. (Courtesy Dr. Steven S. Barr. In Bowman D: *Georgis' parasitology for veterinarians*, ed 9, St Louis, 2009, Saunders.)

Leishmania

Leishmania species are hemoprotozoans that can infect several mammal species, including dogs, cats, and humans. The parasite is transmitted by flies of the genus *Phlebotomus* and *Lutzomyia* (sand flies), but experimental infections have occurred with certain tick breeds. *Leishmania* species were long thought to be of concern only in pets that had traveled outside of North America. However, the parasites have been found in several U.S. states, most notably in Texas. Two forms of the disease leishmaniasis have been recognized. The mucocutaneous form, which is characterized by skin sores, is caused primarily by *Leishmania braziliensis.* The visceral form, which is primarily caused by *Leishmania donovani* and *Leishmania infantum* (also called *Leishmania chagasi*), affects several internal organs (e.g., spleen, liver, bone marrow).

The life cycle of these organisms is simple. The parasite is transmitted during its flagellated promastigote stage via a bite from its insect vector. The promastigotes are then phagocytized by the host's macrophages (Fig. 35.4). The promastigotes multiply by binary fission, develop into the amastigote stage, and are then released when the cell ruptures. The released amastigotes are then phagocytized by other macrophages. Large numbers of organisms can be present in a variety of tissues. The amastigotes are picked up by the sand fly when it takes a blood meal from the host. These then develop into promastigotes in the sand fly to complete the life cycle. Diagnosis generally requires fluorescent antibody testing or molecular diagnostics.

Trichomonads

Trichomonads are long, slender organisms with a single flagellum attached to the dorsal surface, thereby forming a sail-like structure that ripples as the organism glides through debris.

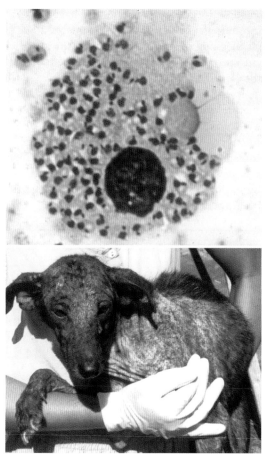

Fig. 35.4 *Leishmania infantum.* The top image shows a macrophage from the bone marrow of an infected dog that contains large numbers of amastigotes. The bottom image is of a dog from Brazil that is infected with *L. infantum (L. chagasi)* showing the typical cutaneous manifestation of a long-standing infection. (From Bowman D: *Georgis' parasitology for veterinarians*, ed 9, St Louis, 2009, Saunders.)

Tritrichomonas foetus is a parasite of the reproductive tract of cattle. The organism resides in the prepuce of bulls and the vagina, cervix, and uterus of cows. Infection manifests as infertility, spontaneous abortion, and pyometra. *T. foetus* is pear-shaped and approximately 10 µm to 25 µm long, and it has three anterior flagella. Diagnosis involves the demonstration of the motile trophozoite in the supernatant of centrifuged fluid from washings of the vagina or the prepuce.

Trichomonas gallinae is found in crop washes and crop swabs from pigeons, doves, and poultry. It is transmitted only by direct contact with an infected bird or with water that has been contaminated by an infected bird. *T. gallinae* causes necrotic ulcerations in the esophagus, crop, and proventriculus. Nonpathogenic species of trichomonads are also found in the cecum and colon of many domestic animals. Diagnosis involves the demonstration of the parasite in a direct saline smear of crop contents, and it is characterized by four anterior flagella. An air-dried smear can be stained with Wright's stain. The parasite assumes an oval shape, staining blue with a red axostyle.

Histomonas

Histomonas meleagridis infects turkeys, chickens, pheasants, and similar avian species. It is transmitted when the bird ingests the ova of the nematode transport host, *Heterakis gallinarum*. Earthworms serve as paratenic hosts for the nematode, and birds can also be infected with the protozoa when they ingest the nematode. The flagellated trophozoite is released from the nematode larvae in the cecal lumen. It then loses its flagella and enters the cecal epithelium and liver as an amoeboid form, where it reproduces and causes inflammation and tissue necrosis. In turkeys, the organism causes a fatal liver disease called infectious enterohepatitis, or "blackhead." Diagnosis requires histopathologic examination of the liver.

Entamoeba

Entamoeba histolytica is primarily a parasite of humans in tropical regions. Trophozoites and cysts of various amoeboid organisms are frequently demonstrated by fecal smears or standard fecal flotation tests of healthy cattle, sheep, goats, horses, and swine. These generally are of no clinical importance. *E. histolytica* may produce acute or chronic diarrhea in dogs. Other species of amoebas have been implicated in diseases of primates and tortoises.

PHYLUM APICOMPLEXA

Apicomplexans are the sporozoans. There are about 4600 species, and all are parasitic. Sporozoans are unique in that all of their life cycle stages are haploid except for the zygote. Fig. 35.5 contains a sample sporozoan life cycle. Sporozoal parasites are found within the host cells, and they commonly occur in the intestinal tract cells and blood cells. *Oocyst* is the name given to the cyst stage of this group of intestinal protozoa. The genera of greatest importance in veterinary species include the following intracellular parasites:

- *Cystoisospora (Isospora)*
- *Toxoplasma*
- *Cryptosporidium*
- *Cytauxzoon*

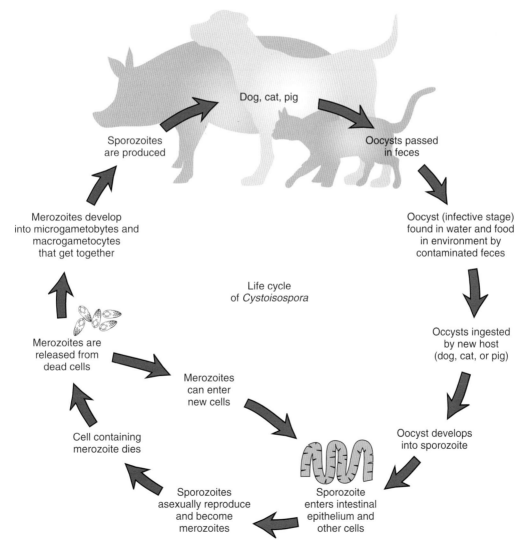

Fig. 35.5 Life cycle of *Cystoisospora* species. (From Hendrix CM, Robinson E: *Diagnostic parasitology for veterinary technicians*, ed 4, St Louis, 2012, Mosby.)

- *Sarcocystis*
- *Plasmodium*
- *Babesia*
- *Eimeria*

Cystoisospora

Cystoisospora species are protozoal parasites of the small intestine of both dogs and cats. They produce a clinical syndrome known as coccidiosis, which is one of the most commonly diagnosed protozoal diseases in puppies and kittens. Coccidiosis is rarely a problem in mature animals. The oocyst is the diagnostic stage that is observed in a fecal flotation of fresh feces. It is unsporulated in fresh feces, and it varies in size and shape among the common species (Fig. 35.6).

The canine coccidians and their oocyst measurements are as follows: *Cystoisospora canis,* 34 μm to 40 μm by 28 μm to 32 μm; *Cystoisospora ohioensis,* 20 μm to 27 μm by 15 μm to 24 μm; and *Cystoisospora wallacei,* 10 μm to 14 μm by 7.5 μm to 9.0 μm. The feline coccidians and their measurements are as follows: *Cystoisospora felis,* 38 μm to 51 μm by 27 μm to 29 μm and *Cystoisospora rivolta,* 21 μm to 28 μm by 18 μm to 23 μm. The prepatent period varies among species, but it is usually 7 to 14 days.

> **TECHNICIAN NOTE** Coccidians are among the most commonly diagnosed parasites in puppies and kittens.

Isospora suis is the coccidian that parasitizes the small intestine of swine, especially young piglets. Oocysts are usually found with fecal flotation of fresh feces. They are subspherical, they lack a micropyle, and they measure 18 μm to 21 μm. Postmortem diagnosis in piglets that exhibit clinical signs but that are not shedding oocysts can be achieved with histopathology using a direct smear of a jejunum that has been stained with Diff-Quik. Diagnosis is by observation of the banana-shaped merozoites. The prepatent period is 4 to 8 days long.

Toxoplasma

Toxoplasma gondii is another intestinal coccidian of cats. Its oocysts are usually diagnosed via standard fecal flotation.

Oocysts of *T. gondii* are unsporulated in fresh feces, and they measure 10 μm by 12 μm. Several immunodiagnostic tests that involve the use of whole blood or serum are available for the diagnosis of *T. gondii* infection. The prepatent period is highly variable. It ranges from 5 to 24 days, depending on the route of infection. The life cycle is complex and involves several different stages, including tachyzoites, bradyzoites, merozoites, microgametocytes, and macrogametocytes.

> **TECHNICIAN NOTE** Cats infected with *Toxoplasma gondii* generally only shed oocysts for less than 2 weeks of their entire lives.

Although cats are the definitive hosts of *T. gondii,* various life cycle stages of the parasite can infect other species, including humans (Fig. 35.7). Although this organism is usually not harmful to healthy humans, it can cause serious problems in the fetuses of pregnant women. Toxoplasmosis can be spread from cats to people by the ingestion of the infectious oocysts found in cat feces, but most humans contract the disease by eating undercooked meat. Pregnant women should avoid the cleaning of cat litter pans and wear gloves while gardening.

Cryptosporidium

Cryptosporidium is another coccidian parasite that parasitizes the small intestine of a wide variety of animals, including dogs, cats, and particularly young calves. The sporulated oocysts in the feces are oval to spherical and measure only 4 μm to 6 μm. Diagnosis is made by standard fecal flotation. The oocysts are extremely small and may be observed just under the coverslip, although they are not in the same plane of focus as other oocysts and parasite ova (Fig. 35.8). The examination of fresh fecal smears with special stains (i.e., modified acid-fast stains) is also helpful. Because people may become infected with *Cryptosporidium* species, feces that are suspected of harboring this protozoan should be handled with great care.

Sarcocystis

Sarcocystis is a coccidian parasite that is found in the small intestine. Several species infect dogs and cats. The identification of an individual species may be quite difficult. The oocysts of

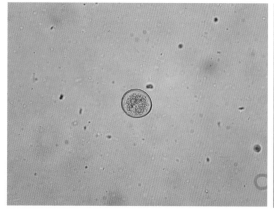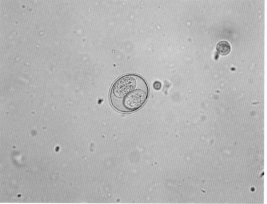

Fig. 35.6 *Cystoisospora felis* unsporulated oocyst *(left)* and sporulated oocyst *(right)*. (From Bowman D: *Georgis' parasitology for veterinarians,* ed 9, St Louis, 2009, Saunders.)

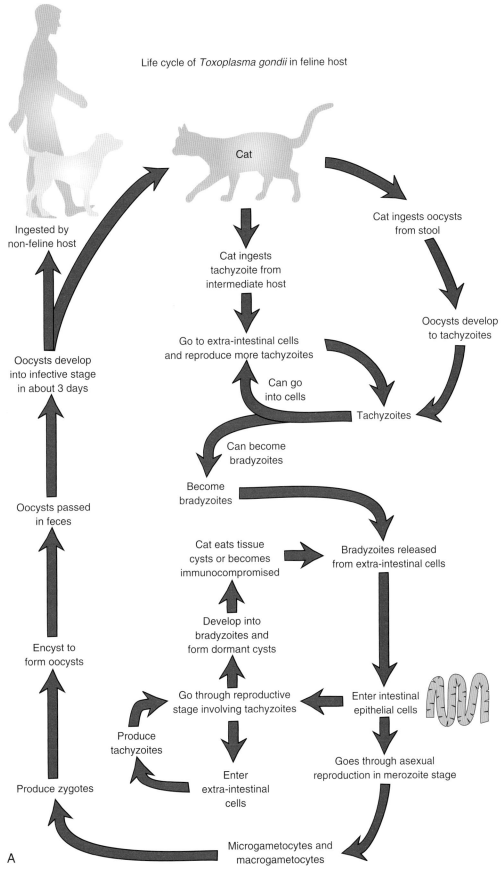

Fig. 35.7 A, Life cycle of *Toxoplasma gondii* for feline hosts. **B,** Life cycle of *Toxoplasma gondii* for nonfeline hosts. (From Hendrix CM, Robinson E: *Diagnostic parasitology for veterinary technicians*, ed 4, St Louis, 2012, Mosby.)

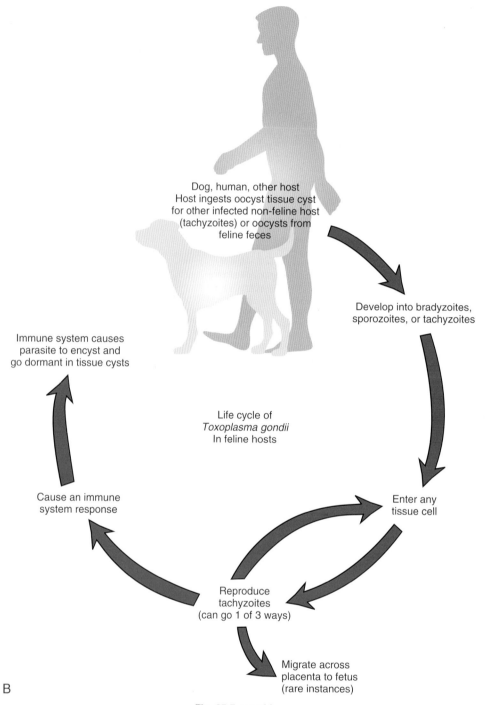

Dog, human, other host
Host ingests oocyst tissue cyst
for other infected non-feline host
(tachyzoites) or oocysts from
feline feces

Develop into bradyzoites,
sporozoites, or tachyzoites

Immune system causes
parasite to encyst and
go dormant in tissue cysts

Life cycle of
Toxoplasma gondii
In feline hosts

Enter any
tissue cell

Cause an immune
system response

Reproduce
tachyzoites
(can go 1 of 3 ways)

Migrate across
placenta to fetus
(rare instances)

B

Fig. 35.7, cont'd

Sarcocystis species are sporulated when they are passed in the feces. Each oocyst contains two sporocysts, each with four sporozoites. These individual oocysts measure 12 μm to 15 μm by 8 μm to 12 μm, and they may be recovered from a standard fecal flotation of fresh feces.

Babesia

Babesia canis is an intracellular parasite that is found within the erythrocytes of dogs, and it is also referred to as a piroplasm

because of its pear-shaped body (Fig. 35.9). Diagnosis involves the observation of the basophilic, pear-shaped trophozoites in RBCs on stained blood smears. *Babesia bigemina* is an intracellular parasite that is found within the RBCs of cattle. This parasite is a large piroplasm that is 4 μm to 5 μm long by approximately 2 μm wide. It is characteristically pear-shaped, and it occurs in pairs that form an acute angle within the erythrocyte. The intermediate host for this protozoan parasite is the tick *Boophilus annulatus*. *Babesia equi* and *Babesia caballi*

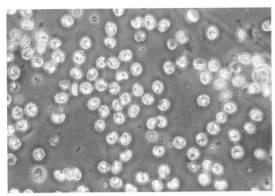

Fig. 35.8 Oocysts of *Cryptosporidium* species. (From Hendrix CM, Robinson E: *Diagnostic parasitology for veterinary technicians*, ed 3, St Louis, 2006, Mosby.)

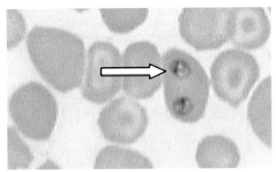

Fig. 35.9 Basophilic, pear-shaped trophozoites of *Babesia canis* within canine red blood cells on a stained blood smear. (From Hendrix CM, Robinson E: *Diagnostic parasitology for veterinary technicians,* ed 3, St Louis, 2006, Mosby.)

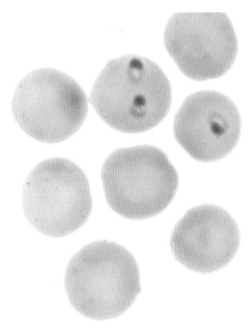

Fig. 35.10 Feline erythrocytes infected with the characteristic signet-ring-shaped *Cytauxzoon* piroplasms. (From Little S: *The cat*, Philadelphia, 2011, W. B. Saunders.)

are intracellular parasites that are found within the RBCs of horses. They are also referred to as the equine piroplasms. Diagnosis involves the observation of the basophilic, pear-shaped trophozoites in RBCs on stained blood smears. Trophozoites of *B. equi* may be round, amoeboid, or pyriform. Four organisms may be joined, which gives the effect of a Maltese cross. Individual organisms are 2 μm to 3 μm long. Trophozoites of *B. caballi* are pyriform, round, or oval and 2 μm to 4 μm long. They occur characteristically in pairs at acute angles to each other.

Cytauxzoon

Cytauxzoon felis is another intracellular parasite that has been sporadically reported in the RBCs of cats in various locales (e.g., Missouri, Arkansas, Georgia, Texas) throughout the United States. It is transmitted through the bite of *Dermacentor variabilis* and other tick species, including *Amblyomma americanum*. As the range of the tick vectors increases, the disease prevalence has expanded, and it has now been identified in the mid-Atlantic. The parasite infects wild and domestic felids. The vector ticks infect the host with the schizont form, which then enter macrophages. The schizonts undergo asexual reproduction within the macrophages, and the cells become large enough to occlude venous flow. The macrophages subsequently

rupture, releasing merozoites that infect erythrocytes. The erythrocyte form is called a piroplasm and has been described as being shaped like a "bejeweled ring" and which are referred to as the ring form in stained blood smears (Fig. 35.10). Piroplasms may also undergo asexual reproduction and lead to destruction of the erythrocyte, inducing anemia. Acute cytauxzoonosis occurs during the schizont phase and can lead to multiple-organ failure and death. Piroplasms may be seen during acute infection and in cats that survived the acute phase in the past. The piroplasm form occurs later in the course of disease. Fine-needle aspirates of the lymph nodes, liver, or spleen may demonstrate evidence of schizont-filled macrophages earlier in the course of the disease. Polymerase chain reaction (PCR) assays are available for confirmation of diagnosis.

> **TECHNICIAN NOTE** Infections with *Cytauxzoon felis* are usually fatal.

Hepatozoon

Hepatozoon canis and *Hepatozoon americanum* are intracellular, malaria-like parasites that affect dogs. The blood forms of the parasites (the gamonts) of these protozoan parasites are found in the leukocytes. Leukocytes that contain gamonts of *H. canis* are common in peripheral blood smears, whereas gamonts of *H. americanum* are rare. Schizonts are found in the endothelial cells of the spleen, the bone marrow, and the liver. The gamonts are surrounded by a delicate capsule, and they stain pale blue with a dark, reddish-purple nucleus. Numerous pink granules are found in the cytoplasm of the leukocyte. The "onion skin" tissue cysts of *H. americanum* are found in the skeletal muscle of dogs (Fig. 35.11). This is an unusual parasite in that the dog becomes infected after the ingestion of an infected tick, *Amblyomma americanum*. *H. canis* is well adapted to its canine host, and it varies from producing a subclinical to a mild disease. *H. americanum* produces a violent and frequently fatal course of disease; it is theorized to have crossed the species barrier from a wild animal host to the domestic dog.

Eimeria

Eimeria leuckarti is a coccidian that is found in the small intestine of the horse. This protozoan demonstrates unique large oocysts (80 μm to 87 μm by 55 μm to 60 μm) with thick walls, distinct micropyles, and a dark brown color. These oocysts can be recovered with fecal flotation, and they are the largest coccidian oocysts. They are frequently observed on histopathologic examination. The prepatent period ranges from 15 to 33 days.

Ruminants serve as host to many species of *Eimeria*. The identification of individual species of coccidia is often difficult because their oocysts are so similar in size and shape. The two

most common species of coccidia in cattle, *E. bovis* and *E. zuernii*, can be differentiated with standard fecal flotation. Oocysts of *E. bovis* are oval, they have a micropyle, and they measure 20 μm by 28 μm, whereas those of *E. zuernii* are spherical, they lack the micropyle, and they measure 15 μm to 22 μm by 13 μm to 18 μm. When oocysts are recovered with fecal flotation, the observation is usually noted as "coccidia." Several species of *Eimeria* are capable of infecting rabbits (Fig. 35.12), but one, *E. stiedai*, is of particular importance. Heavy infections can cause bile duct blockage and liver failure. Mortality is high among young rabbits.

> **TECHNICIAN NOTE** Heavy infections with *Eimeria stiedai* are often fatal, especially among young rabbits.

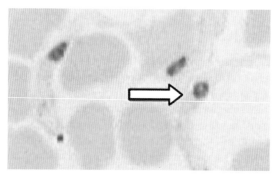

Fig. 35.11 The "onion skin" tissue cysts of *Hepatozoon americanum* are found in the skeletal muscle of dogs. (From Hendrix CM, Robinson E: *Diagnostic parasitology for veterinary technicians*, ed 3, St Louis, 2006, Mosby.)

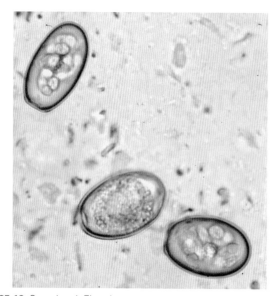

Fig. 35.12 Sporulated *Eimeria magna* oocysts from the feces of a domestic rabbit. (From Bowman D: *Georgis' parasitology for veterinarians*, ed 9, St Louis, 2009, Saunders.)

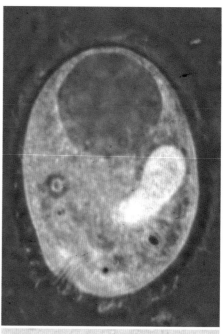

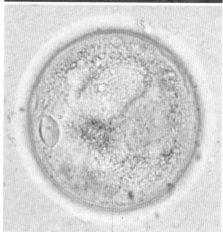

Fig. 35.13 *Balantidium coli. Top,* Trophozoite (electronic flash photograph) of motile ciliate. *Bottom,* Cyst. Trophozoites abound in the large intestine of normal swine, and cysts are passed in their feces. (From Bowman D: *Georgis' parasitology for veterinarians*, ed 9, St Louis, 2009, Saunders.)

Plasmodium

Various species of *Plasmodium* can cause malaria in mammals, birds, and reptiles. The organism is transmitted by mosquitoes, and it develops into merozoites within hepatocytes. The hepatocytes rupture, and the released merozoites then invade erythrocytes and reticulocytes. The diagnosis of infections with *Plasmodium* species can be accomplished by demonstrating the organisms on a blood smear or by organ impression smears and the histopathologic examination of the liver and the spleen. Molecular diagnostic tests are also available. *Leucocytozoon* and *Haemoproteus* are similar parasites that affect the blood cells of birds.

PHYLUM CILIOPHORA

There are about 7200 species in the phylum Ciliophora, of which about 2200 are parasitic. Only one genus, *Balantidium*, is of veterinary significance.

Balantidium coli is the ciliated protozoan that is found in the large intestine of swine. Although it is commonly observed during the microscopic examination of fresh diarrheic feces, it is generally considered nonpathogenic. Two morphologic stages may be found in feces: the cyst stage and the motile trophozoite stage (Fig. 35.13). Both stages may vary in size. This is a large protozoan parasite. The trophozoites may be 150 µm by 120 µm, with a sausage- to kidney-shaped macronucleus. The organism is covered with numerous rows of cilia, and it moves about the microscopic field with lively motility. The cyst is spherical to ovoid and 40 µm to 60 µm in diameter, with a slight greenish-yellow color. Both of these stages may be easily recognized by microscopic examination of the intestinal contents or of fresh diarrheic feces.

RICKETTSIAL PARASITES

The rickettsia are a group of obligate intracellular gram-negative bacteria. The major taxonomic families are the Rickettsiaceae (Table 35.2), which include the genera *Rickettsia*, *Orientia*, and *Coxiella*, and the Anaplasmataceae (Table 35.3), which include the genera *Anaplasma* (Fig. 35.14), *Ehrlichia* (Fig. 35.15), *Wolbachia*, and *Neorickettsia*. The organisms are transmitted via arthropod and helminth vectors.

TABLE 35.2 Pathogenic Rickettsiaceae That Affect Animals

Agent	Disease	Incidental Hosts	Reservoir Hosts	Vectors	Geographic Distribution
Rickettsia rickettsii	Rocky Mountain spotted fever	Humans, dogs	Rodents	*Dermacentor* spp. ticks, *Amblyomma cajennense*, *Rhipicephalus sanguineus*	Western Hemisphere
Rickettsia felis	Cat flea typhus	Humans	Norway rat, domestic cats, opossum	*Ctenocephalides felis* (cat flea)	Western Hemisphere, Europe
Rickettsia conorii	Boutonneuse fever Mediterranean spotted fever Israeli spotted fever Astrakhan fever	Humans	Rodents, dogs	*Rhipicephalus* spp. ticks	Southern Europe, Africa, Asia
Rickettsia typhi	Murine typhus	Humans	Rats, opossums, cats	*Xenopsylla cheopis* (rat flea)	Worldwide
Rickettsia prowazekii	Epidemic typhus	Domestic animals	Flying squirrels, humans	Human body louse, flying squirrel louse, squirrel flea	Worldwide
Orientia tsutsugamushi	Scrub typhus	Humans, dogs	Birds, rats	Mites	Eastern Asia, Northern Australia, Western Pacific Islands
Piscirickettsia salmonis	Piscirickettsiosis	Salmonid fish	Unknown	Unknown	Chile, Norway, Ireland, Canada

From Songer JG, Post KW: *Veterinary microbiology: bacterial and fungal agents of animal disease*, St Louis, 2005, Saunders.

TABLE 35.3 Anaplasmataceae of Veterinary Importance

Organisms	Hosts	Diseases	Vector Reservoirs	Infected Cells	Geographic Distribution
Aegyptianella spp.	Birds, reptiles, amphibians	Anemia, sudden death	*Argus, Amblyomma, Ixodes* spp., unknown	RBCs	Africa, Asia, South America, Southern Europe, South Texas
Anaplasma (Ehrlichia) bovis	Cattle	Bovine ehrlichiosis	*Rhipicephalus appendiculatus, Amblyomma variegatum, A. cajennense, Hyalomma excavatum* Rabbits, ruminants?	Mononuclear leukocytes	Africa, Asia, South America
Anaplasma caudatum, centrale, marginale, ovis	Ruminants	Anaplasmosis	*Boophilus, Dermacentor, Ixodes, Rhipicephalus* spp. Ruminants, wild cervids	RBCs	Worldwide
Anaplasma phagocytophilum (Ehrlichia equi, HGE agent, *E. phagocytophila)*	Humans, horses, small ruminants	Human and equine granulocytic ehrlichiosis, tick-borne fever	*Ixodes* spp. Deer, sheep, white-footed mice	Granulocytes	Worldwide
Anaplasma (Ehrlichia) platys	Dogs	Infectious cyclic thrombocytopenia	*Rhipicephalus sanguineus?* Ruminant?	Platelets	United States, Southern Europe, Middle East, Venezuela, Taiwan
Ehrlichia canis	Canidae	Canine monocytic ehrlichiosis	*Rhipicephalus sanguineus, Amblyomma americanum?* Canids	Mononuclear leukocytes	Worldwide
Ehrlichia chaffeensis	Humans, dogs, deer	Human monocytic ehrlichiosis	*Amblyomma americanum, Dermacentor variabilis,* domestic dogs, white-tailed deer	Mononuclear leukocytes	United States
Ehrlichia ewingii	Dogs, humans	Canine granulocytic ehrlichiosis	*Amblyomma americanum* Canids	Granulocytes	United States
Ehrlichia muris	Mice	Not named	*Haemaphysalis flava* Not known	Mononuclear leukocytes	Not known
Ehrlichia (Cowdria) ruminantium	Ruminants	Heartwater	*Amblyomma* ticks Ruminants	Granulocytes, endothelium, macrophages	Sub-Saharan Africa, Caribbean
Neorickettsia helminthoeca	Canidae	Salmon poisoning disease	Ingestion of fluke-infested salmonid fish Fluke-infested fish	Mononuclear leukocytes	U.S. Pacific Northwest
Neorickettsia (Ehrlichia) risticii	Horses	Potomac horse fever, equine monocytic ehrlichiosis	Ingestion of fluke-infested insects Flukes	Mononuclear leukocytes, enterocytes	North and South America
Neorickettsia (Ehrlichia) sennetsu	Humans	Sennetsu fever	Ingestion of fluke-infested fish Fluke-infested fish	Mononuclear leukocytes	Japan, Southeast Asia

HGE, Human granulocytic ehrlichiosis; *RBCs,* red blood cells.
From Songer JG: *Veterinary microbiology: bacterial and fungal agents of animal disease,* St Louis, 2005, Saunders.

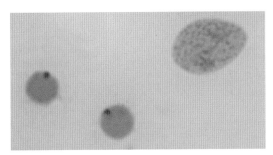

Fig. 35.14 Blood smear from cow with anaplasmosis showing two typically parasitized erythrocytes and an immature form. (Courtesy Raymond E. Reed. In Songer JG, Post KW: *Veterinary microbiology: bacterial and fungal agents of animal disease*, St Louis, 2005, Saunders.)

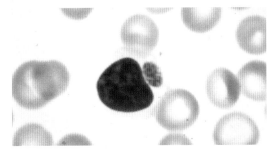

Fig. 35.15 *Ehrlichia canis*—infected lymphocyte. (Courtesy Raymond E. Reed. In Songer JG, Post KW: *Veterinary microbiology: bacterial and fungal agents of animal disease*, St Louis, 2005, Saunders.)

KEY POINTS

- Parasitic protozoa can be found in three primary phyla: (1) Sarcomastigophora, (2) Apicomplexa, and (3) Ciliophora.
- Protozoal parasites are usually transmitted to a new host during the cyst stage.
- *Giardia* species are common flagellates that can infect a variety of mammals, including humans.
- Trypanosomes and *Leishmania* species are zoonotic parasites that are primarily found in the southern United States.
- *Tritrichomonas foetus* is a parasite of the reproductive tract of cattle that can cause infertility, spontaneous abortion, and pyometra.
- Apicomplexans (sporozoans) are found within the host cells, and they commonly occur in intestinal tract cells and blood cells.
- Cats are the only definitive host for *Toxoplasma gondii*, but various life-cycle stages of the parasite can infect other species, including humans.
- *Cytauxzoon felis* is an intracellular parasite that is sporadically found in the RBCs of cats and is usually fatal.
- A variety of *Eimeria* species are capable of infecting ruminants and small mammals.
- Rickettsia are obligate intracellular parasites with two primary taxonomic families: Rickettsiaceae and Anaplasmataceae.

36

Arthropods

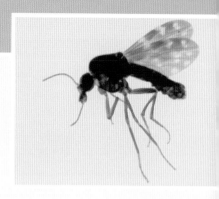

LEARNING OBJECTIVES

After studying this chapter, you will be able to:

- Describe the general characteristics of organisms in the phylum Arthropoda.
- Differentiate between insects and arachnids.
- Describe the general life cycle of the insects.
- Describe the general life cycle of the arachnids.
- Describe the general characteristics of fleas.
- List the species of fleas that are commonly encountered in veterinary species.
- Differentiate between Mallophaga and Anoplura species.
- Describe the life cycle of lice.
- List and describe the flies that may parasitize veterinary species.
- Describe the life cycle of ticks.
- Differentiate between hard ticks and soft ticks.
- List the commonly encountered species of ticks that parasitize veterinary species.
- Describe the general characteristic of sarcoptiform mites.
- Discuss the general life cycle of sarcoptiform mites.
- List the commonly encountered species of mites that parasitize veterinary species.

OUTLINE

KEY TERMS

Acariasis

Arachnids

Ectoparasite

Flea-bite dermatitis

Hirudiniasis

Hypostome

Instar

Mange

Myiasis

Nits

Nymphs

Pediculosis

Periodic parasite

Pupa

Tick paralysis

Warbles

Organisms in the phylum Arthropoda are characterized by the presence of jointed legs. They have a chitinous exoskeleton that is composed of segments. In the more advanced groups, some segments have fused together to form body parts, such as a head, thorax, and abdomen. Arthropods have a true body cavity (coelom), a circulatory system, a digestive system, a respiratory system, an excretory system, a nervous system, and a reproductive system. The sexes are separate, and reproduction is by means of eggs. Only certain groups of arthropods are parasitic. Members of other groups may act as intermediate hosts for the previously discussed endoparasites. When a parasite resides on the surface of its host, it is called an ectoparasite. Most ectoparasites are either insects (e.g., fleas, lice, flies) or arachnids (e.g., ticks, mites). A few larval nematodes are also ectoparasites. Leeches (bloodsucking annelids) are also considered to be ectoparasites. Infestation by leeches is referred to as hirudiniasis.

The following general characteristics differentiate the two major classes of arthropods of veterinary importance:

- Insects have three pairs of legs, three distinct body regions (head, thorax, and abdomen), and a single pair of antennae.

- Arachnids (adults) have four pairs of legs, a body divided into two regions (cephalothorax and abdomen), and no antennae.

Pentastomids (tongue worms) are another group of parasitic arthropods that is rarely encountered in the respiratory passages of vertebrates. These organisms resemble worms rather than arthropods during the adult stage. Adults have two pairs of curved, retractile hooklets near the mouth. Immature stages are mitelike, with two or three pairs of legs.

> **TECHNICIAN NOTE** The mouthparts of insects have adaptations for chewing/biting, sponging, or piercing/sucking.

The mouthparts of insects vary in structure, depending on feeding habits, with adaptations for chewing/biting, sponging (lapping up), or piercing/sucking. The thorax may have one or two pairs of functional wings in addition to the three pairs of jointed legs. The sexes are separate, and reproduction results in the production of eggs or larvae. Development often involves three or more larval stages called instars, which are followed by the formation of a pupa and a change in form or transformation (complete metamorphosis) to the adult stage. In other insects, development occurs from the egg through several immature stages (nymphs), which resemble the adult in form but are smaller (incomplete metamorphosis). Fleas and flies demonstrate complete metamorphosis, and lice demonstrate incomplete metamorphosis. Insects may produce harm to their definitive host as adults, larvae, or both.

The arachnids include ticks, mites, spiders, and scorpions. Ticks and mites are the more important groups of arachnids in veterinary medicine, although some spiders and scorpions can harm domestic animals by way of toxic venoms. Arachnids are generally small and may even be microscopic. Their mouthparts are borne on a structure called the basis capituli, and they consist of a pair of mobile digits adapted for cutting (chelicerae) and a pair of sensory structures (palps). The hypostome is a structure with recurved teeth that maintains attachment to the host and that bears a groove to permit the flow of arthropod saliva and host blood or lymph. The life cycle stages consist of egg, larva, nymph, and adult. There can be more than one nymphal instar. Nymphs resemble the adult in form, but they are smaller. There is usually only one larval stage, which differs from the nymphs and adults in size and has only three pairs of legs.

> **TECHNICIAN NOTE** Several serious diseases such as tularemia can be spread by arthropods.

ORDER: SIPHONAPTERA (FLEAS)

Fleas are blood-sucking parasites of dogs, cats, rodents, birds, and people. They are vectors of several diseases, such as bubonic plague and tularemia. More than 2000 species of fleas have been identified throughout the world. Adult fleas are always parasitic, feeding on both mammals and birds. Dogs and

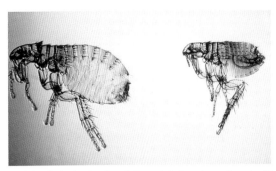

Fig. 36.1 Morphologic details of the adult female and male *Ctenocephalides felis*, the cat flea. (From Hendrix CM, Robinson E: *Diagnostic parasitology for veterinary technicians*, ed 4, St Louis, 2012, Mosby.)

cats are host to comparatively few species of fleas. Cat and dog fleas—*Ctenocephalides felis* and *Ctenocephalides canis*, respectively—can act as intermediate hosts for the common tapeworm, *Dipylidium caninum*. Heavy infestations with fleas, especially in young animals, produce anemia. Flea saliva is antigenic and irritating, and it causes intense pruritus (itching) and hypersensitivity. This condition is known as flea-bite dermatitis or miliary dermatitis.

Fleas are laterally compressed, wingless insects with legs that are adapted for jumping (Fig. 36.1). Adult fleas have piercing/sucking (siphonlike) mouthparts that are used to suck the blood of their hosts. They move rapidly on the host and from host to host. Flea infestations are encountered most frequently on dogs and cats. They can be detected around the base of the tail, on the ventral abdomen, and under the chin.

Fleas demonstrate complete metamorphosis (Fig. 36.2). Eggs deposited on the host fall off and develop into larvae in the environment. The larvae can occasionally be found in the host animal's bedding, on furniture, or in cracks and crevices of the host animal's environment. The larvae are maggotlike, with a head capsule and bristles (Fig. 36.3). Flea larvae feed on organic debris, including the excrement of adult fleas. Flea droppings are reddish-brown, comma-shaped casts of dehydrated blood (Fig. 36.4). Flea droppings in the animal's hair coat indicate flea infestation.

> **TECHNICIAN NOTE** If water is slowly dropped onto flea droppings on a gauze sponge, the droppings will reconstitute to blood.

The specific identification of fleas requires the expertise of an entomologist. Other fleas of veterinary importance are *Pulex irritans*, *Xenopsylla cheopis*, and *Echidnophaga gallinacea*. Fleas have preferred hosts, but they attack any source of blood if the preferred host is not available. Adult fleas can also survive for extended periods off of the host, and they can heavily infest premises.

Echidnophaga gallinacea is also known as the "stick-tight flea" of poultry. A common flea of chickens and guinea fowl, it also feeds on dogs and cats. This flea has unique feeding habits. The female flea inserts its mouthparts into the skin of the host and remains attached at that site. These specimens resemble attached ticks; however, they are fleas.

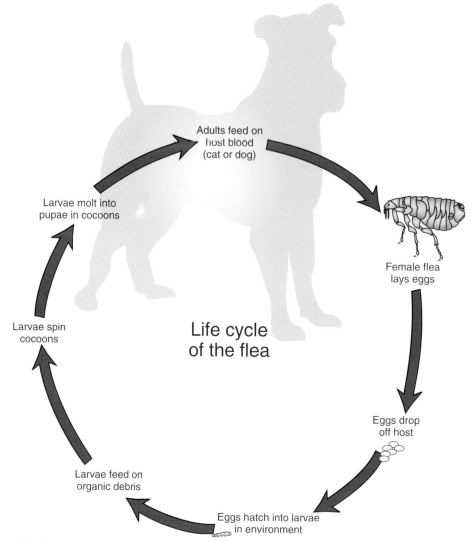

Life cycle
of the flea

Adults feed on
host blood
(cat or dog)

Larvae molt into
pupae in cocoons

Female flea
lays eggs

Larvae spin
cocoons

Eggs drop
off host

Larvae feed on
organic debris

Eggs hatch into larvae
in environment

Fig. 36.2 Life cycle of the flea. (From Hendrix CM, Robinson E: *Diagnostic parasitology for veterinary technicians*, ed 4, St Louis, 2012, Mosby.)

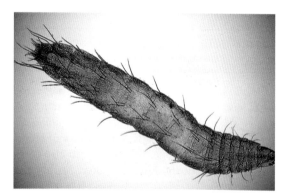

Fig. 36.3 Larva of *Ctenocephalides felis*, the cat flea. Flea larvae resemble tiny fly maggots; they are 2 mm to 5 mm long, white (after feeding, they become brown), and sparsely covered with hairs. (From Hendrix CM, Robinson E: *Diagnostic parasitology for veterinary technicians*, ed 4, St Louis, 2012, Mosby.)

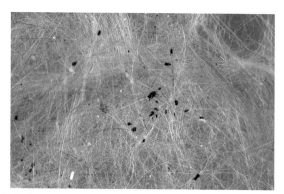

Fig. 36.4 Flea dirt (flea feces or flea frass) of *Ctenocephalides felis*, the cat flea. Flea dirt can be used to diagnose current or recent infestations by fleas. (From Hendrix CM, Robinson E: *Diagnostic parasitology for veterinary technicians*, ed 4, St Louis, 2012, Mosby.)

Fleas are not commonly found on horses or ruminants. In barns where feral cats abound and where excessive bedding is used, fleas have been found on calves in large numbers and can produce significant anemia. *Pulex irritans,* the human flea, has been recovered from dogs and cats, especially in the southeastern United States.

ORDERS: MALLOPHAGA AND ANOPLURA (LICE)

Lice are dorsoventrally flattened, wingless insects with clawed appendages for clasping to the host animal's hairs. They have three body divisions: the head, with its mouthparts and antennae; the thorax, with its three pairs of legs and its lack of wings; and the abdomen, which is the portion that bears the reproductive organs. Lice are separated into two orders on the basis of whether their mouthparts are modified for biting/chewing (Mallophaga) or sucking (Anoplura). Sucking lice feed on blood and move slowly on the host. They are larger than the chewing lice, and they are red to gray; their color usually depends on the amount of blood ingested from the host. They have a long, narrow head. Biting lice feed on epithelial debris and can move rapidly over the host. They have a broad, rounded head (wider than the widest portion of the thorax), they are smaller than the sucking lice, and they are generally yellow in color. Lice are host-specific, they remain in close association with the host, and they have preferred locations on the host (Table 36.1). Lice glue their eggs or nits (Fig. 36.5) to the hairs or feathers of the host. The nits are tiny: they are approximately 0.5 mm to 1.0 mm in length, oval, and white. Nits hatch approximately 5 to 14 days after being laid by the adult female louse. The nymphal stage is similar in appearance to the adult. However, it is smaller and lacks functioning reproductive organs and genital openings. The three nymphal stages are each progressively larger than their predecessors. The nymphal stage lasts from 2 to 3 weeks.

> **TECHNICIAN NOTE** Anoplurans are larger than Mallophagans and have narrow heads.

The adult stage is similar in appearance to the nymphal stage, but it is larger. It has functional reproductive organs. Male and female lice copulate, the female lays eggs and cements them to a hair or feather, and the life cycle begins again. It takes 3 to 4 weeks to complete the cycle. Nymphal and adult stages live no more than 7 days if they are removed from the host. Eggs hatch within 2 to 3 weeks during warm weather, but they seldom hatch off of the host. Transmission is usually by direct contact, but it can occur via equipment contaminated with eggs, nymphs, or adults.

Louse infestations (pediculosis) tend to be more severe in young, old, or poorly nourished animals, especially in overcrowded conditions and during the colder months. Sucking lice produce anemia, whereas biting lice are irritating and disturbing to the animal. Common biting lice of domestic animals

TABLE 36.1	**Lice Found on Domestic Animals and Humans**	
Host	**Anoplura**	**Mallophaga**
Dog	*Linognathus setosus*	*Trichodectes anis, Heterodoxus spiniger*
Cat	None	*Felicola subrostratus*
Cow	*Haematopinus eurysternus, Haematopinus quadripertusus, Haematopinus tuberculatus, Linognathus vituli, Solenopotes capillatus*	*Damalinia bovis*
Horse	*Haematopinus asini*	*Damalinia equi*
Pig	*Haematopinus suis*	None
Sheep	*Linognathus ovillus, Linognathus pedalis, Linognathus africanus*	*Damalinia ovis*
Goat	*Linognathus africanus, Linognathus stenopsis*	*Damalinia caprae, Damalinia crassipes, Damalinia limbata*
Rat	*Polyplax spinulosa*	None
Mouse	*Polyplax serrata*	None
Guinea pig	None	*Gliricola porcelli, Gyropus ovalis, Trimenopon hispidum*
Human	*Pediculus humanus capitis, Pediculus humanus, Pthirus pubis*	None

From Bowman D: *Georgis' parasitology for veterinarians,* ed 9, St Louis, 2009, Saunders.

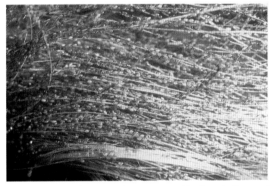

Fig. 36.5 Thousands of nits can be cemented by female lice to the hair coat of a domesticated animal. This calf's tail contains thousands of nits. (From Hendrix CM, Robinson E: *Diagnostic parasitology for veterinary technicians,* ed 4, St Louis, 2012, Mosby.)

include *Trichodectes canis* (dog) (Fig. 36.6), *Damalinia equi* (horse), *Damalinia bovis* (cow), *Damalinia ovis* (sheep), *Damalinia caprae* (goat), and *Felicola subrostratus* (cat). Common sucking lice of domestic animals include *Linognathus setosus* (dog) (Fig. 36.7), *Haematopinus asini* (horse), *Haematopinus vituli, Haematopinus eurysternus, Solenopotes capillatus, Haematopinus quadripertusus* (cow), *Linognathus ovillus, Linognathus pedalis* (sheep), and *Haematopinus suis* (pig).

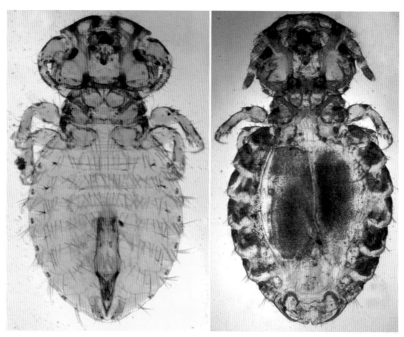

Fig. 36.6 *Trichodectes canis* (Mallophaga: Ischnocera) of the dog. The male is on the left, and the female is on the right. (From Bowman D: *Georgis' parasitology for veterinarians*, ed 9, St Louis, 2009, Saunders.)

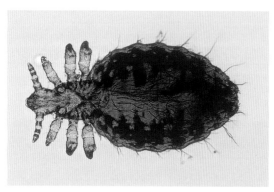

Fig. 36.7 Sucking louse *Linognathus setosus* of dogs. (From Hendrix CM, Robinson E: *Diagnostic parasitology for veterinary technicians*, ed 4, St Louis, 2012, Mosby.)

> **TECHNICIAN NOTE** Infestation with lice is referred to as pediculosis.

Diagnosis involves the careful examination of the hair coat or feathers of infested animals, which easily reveals lice and their accompanying nits. Hair clippings also serve as a good source for lice. The infestation of animals with thick hair coats may be easily overlooked. A handheld magnifying lens or a binocular headband magnifier may help with the observation of adult and nymphal lice crawling through or clinging to hair or feathers or tiny nits cemented to individual hairs. Any lice or nits observed may be collected with thumb forceps and placed in a drop of mineral oil on a glass microscope slide. The identification of lice beyond their order is difficult and not usually necessary.

ORDER: DIPTERA (FLIES)

Diptera are a large, complex order of insects. As adults, most members have one pair of wings, which is the origin of the ordinal name: *di-*, meaning "two," and *-ptera*, meaning "wing." Its members vary with regard to size, food source preference, and developmental stage that parasitizes an animal or produces lesions. Flies are a diverse group of insects that undergo complete metamorphosis. The wings may be scaled or membranous, and the insects possess a pair of balancing structures called halters. The mouthparts may be adapted for sponging or for piercing/sucking. Flies produce harm by inflicting painful bites, sucking blood, producing hypersensitive reactions, depositing eggs in sores, migrating during the larval stages through tissues of the host and escaping through holes in the skin (warbles), causing annoyance, and acting as vectors and intermediate hosts to other pathogenic agents. Adult Dipterans that make frequent visits to the vertebrate host to intermittently feed on blood are referred to as periodic parasites. When Dipteran larvae develop in the tissues or organs of vertebrate hosts, they produce a condition known as myiasis. As periodic parasites, blood-feeding Dipterans may be classified with regard to which sex feeds on vertebrate blood as well as food preference. In certain Dipteran groups only the females feed on vertebrate blood; these female flies require vertebrate blood for laying their eggs. In the second group of blood-feeding Dipterans, both male and female flies require a vertebrate blood meal.

> **TECHNICIAN NOTE** Flies produce harm by inflicting painful bites, sucking blood, producing hypersensitive reactions, depositing eggs in sores, larval migration through tissues of the host, and acting as vectors and intermediate hosts to other pathogenic agents.

Blackflies and Midges

Biting midges ("no-see-ums") are small *Culicoides* species flies, and they are 1 mm to 3 mm in length (Fig. 36.8). The females are bloodsuckers that inflict a painful bite. Some species cause allergic dermatitis, whereas others transmit helminths, protozoa, and viruses. Horses often become allergic to the bites of *Culicoides* gnats, and they will scratch and rub bitten areas, thereby causing alopecia, excoriations, and thickening of the skin. This condition has several names, including "Queensland itch," "sweat itch," "sweet itch," and "summer dermatitis" (the latter name because it is often seen during the warmer months of the year). These flies also serve as the intermediate host for *Onchocerca cervicalis*, a nematode with microfilariae that are found in the skin of horses. These flies also transmit the bluetongue virus of sheep.

Members of the genus *Simulium* (blackflies, buffalo gnats) are small flies that range from 1 mm to 6 mm in length and have a characteristic humped back. They have broad, unspotted wings with prominent veins along the cranial margins of the wings. These tiny flies have serrated, scissor-like mouthparts that inflict painful bites. They produce similar harm as no-see-ums, and, in great numbers, they can exsanguinate a host.

Because the females lay their eggs in well-aerated water, these flies are often found in the vicinity of swiftly flowing streams. They are swift fliers, and they move in great swarms, inflicting painful bites and sucking the host's blood. These flies may keep cattle from grazing or cause them to stampede. An animal's ears, neck, head, and abdomen are favorite feeding sites. These flies also feed on poultry, and they can serve as intermediate hosts for the protozoan parasite *Leukocytozoon*.

Sandflies and Muscid Flies

Sandflies (*Phlebotomus* and *Lutzomyia* species) are mothlike flies that are known primarily for their role in the transmission of leishmaniasis and viral diseases. The females suck blood.

Muscid flies include the housefly, the face fly, the horn fly, and the stable fly. The housefly and face fly do not suck blood, but they are annoyances, because they are attracted to excrement and secretions.

> **TECHNICIAN NOTE** Face flies spread the bacteria that causes pinkeye in cattle.

Both act as intermediate hosts for spirurid parasites (*Habronema* spp., *Thelazia* spp.) and they can mechanically transmit bacteria. The horn fly (*Haematobia irritans*) and the stable fly inflict painful bites and suck blood. Horn flies spend most of their lives on the host (cattle). The stable fly stays on the host for short periods, during which it obtains the blood meals. This is an outdoor fly; however, during the late fall and during rainy weather, it may enter barns.

> **TECHNICIAN NOTE** The intermediate host for *S. stilesi* is the female horn fly, *Haematobia irritans*.

The stable fly can spread bacterial and viral diseases to cattle and horses, and it is an intermediate host for the stomach worm of horses (*Habronema*). The stable fly, *Stomoxys calcitrans*, is often called the "biting housefly." It is approximately the size of *Musca domestica*, which is the common housefly. Rather than possessing sponging mouthparts, the stable fly has a bayonet-like proboscis that protrudes forward from the head (Fig. 36.9). The fly usually lands on the host with its head pointed upward. It is a sedentary fly in that it does not move on the host. The fly inflicts painful bites that puncture the skin and bleed freely. When large numbers of stable flies attack dairy

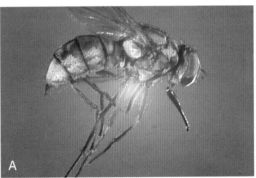
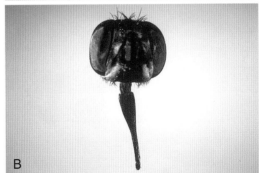

Fig. 36.9 A, Side of the stable fly. **B,** Head of the stable fly. *Stomoxys calcitrans*, the stable fly or biting housefly, is approximately the same size as the housefly, *Musca domestica*.

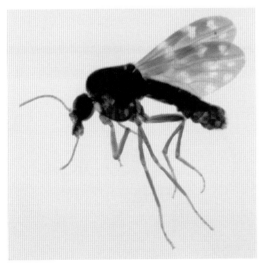

Fig. 36.8 *Culicoides* (Nematocera: Heleidae), a "no-see-um." (From Bowman D: *Georgis' parasitology for veterinarians*, ed 9, St Louis, 2009, Saunders.)

cattle, milk production can fall. Beef cattle may refuse to graze in the daytime when they are attacked by large numbers of flies; as a result, these cattle do not gain the usual amount of weight. These flies are found worldwide. In the United States, they are found in the central and southeastern states, where cattle are raised. Both male and female flies are avid blood feeders, feeding on any domestic animal. They usually attack the legs and ventral abdomen, and they may also bite the ears. These flies may feed on the tips of the ears of dogs with pointed ears, especially German Shepherds. The ears of dogs that have been bitten often demonstrate a loss of hair and the presence of dried, crusty blood on the ear tips.

Deer Flies and Horseflies

Chrysops species (deer flies) and *Tabanus* species (horseflies) are large, measuring up to 3.5 cm long. These are heavy-bodied, robust Dipterans with powerful wings and large eyes. Horseflies and deer flies are the largest flies in the Diptera group, in which only the females feed on vertebrate blood. Fig. 36.10 shows *Tabanus* species, the largest blood-feeding Dipterans. Horse flies are larger than deer flies. Deer flies have a dark band that passes from the cranial to the caudal margin of the wings.

Adult flies lay eggs in the vicinity of open water. Larval stages of these flies are found in aquatic to semi-aquatic environments, often buried deep in mud at the bottom of lakes and ponds. Adults are seen in the summer, and they are fond of sunlight. Female flies feed in the vicinity of open water and have reciprocating, scissorlike mouthparts. They use these sharp, bladelike mouthparts to lacerate tissues and lap up the oozing vertebrate blood. These flies feed primarily on large animals, such as cattle and horses. Preferred feeding sites include the underside of the abdomen around the navel, the legs, or the neck and withers. These flies generally feed a number of times at multiple feeding sites before they stop feeding. When disturbed by the animal's swatting tail or by the panniculus reflex (i.e., skin twitching), the flies leave the host, but the blood continues to ooze from the open wound. These fly bites are painful, and affected cattle and horses become restless. Because they often feed on multiple hosts, these flies may act as mechanical transmitters of anthrax, anaplasmosis, and the virus of equine infectious anemia. They are serious pests of livestock, they can transmit filarial nematodes, and they act as mechanical vectors of bacterial, viral, and rickettsial disease agents.

Sheep Keds

Hippoboscids or sheep keds (*Melophagus ovinus*) are dorso-ventrally flattened, wingless flies that resemble ticks. They suck blood, and they spend their entire lives on the host (sheep). They cause pruritus and damage the wool. Keds are hairy, leathery, and 4 mm to 7 mm in length. The head is short and broad, the thorax is brown, and the abdomen is broad and grayish brown. The legs are strong and armed with stout claws (Fig. 36.11). Some say that keds have a "louselike" appearance, but they are not related to lice.

Flies That Produce Myiasis

Blowflies, flesh flies, and screwworm flies are larger flies with bright coloration. The adults do not suck blood, but they deposit their eggs in decaying organic matter, septic wounds, or living flesh. The larvae of *Callitroga hominivorax* and *Wohlfahrtia opaca* are the only primary invaders of living tissue in North America. Other members are attracted to septic wounds and are known as secondary invaders. Botflies (Fig. 36.12) (*Gasterophilus* spp., *Hypoderma* spp., *Cuterebra* spp., *Oestrus ovis*) are beelike flies, the adults of which do not feed. The adult flies glue their eggs to the hairs of the host or deposit them at the entrance of animal burrows. The larvae hatch and penetrate the skin of the host. Some migrate extensively through the host's body, and others develop locally. The larval stage (bot) is present in the nasal passages of sheep (*Oestrus*), in the stomach of the horse (*Gasterophilus*), and in the dorsal subcutis of the cow (*Hypoderma*).

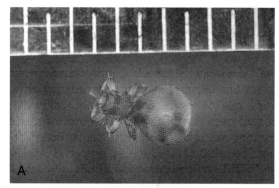
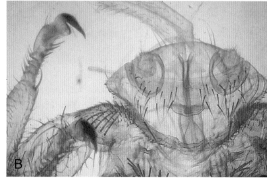

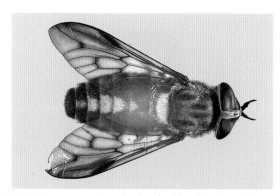

Fig. 36.10 *Tabanus* species, the largest blood-feeding Dipteran. This tabanid is approximately 2.5 cm in length.

Fig. 36.11 A, Body of the sheep ked. **B,** Head of the sheep ked. *Melophagus ovinus,* the sheep ked.

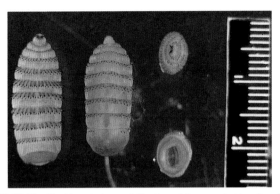

Fig. 36.12 The final larval stage of *Gasterophilus* species is often found within the feces of an equine host. Note the presence of anterior hooks, with larva attached to the gastric mucosa. (From Hendrix CM, Robinson E: *Diagnostic parasitology for veterinary technicians*, ed 4, St Louis, 2012, Mosby.)

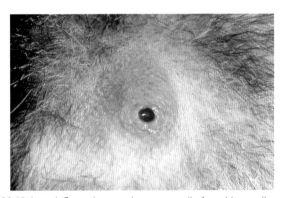

Fig. 36.13 Larval *Cuterebra* species are usually found in swollen, cyst-like, subcutaneous sites, with a fistula (pore or hole) that communicates with the outside environment. The larva breathes through the pore. (From Hendrix CM, Robinson E: *Diagnostic parasitology for veterinary technicians*, ed 4, St Louis, 2012, Mosby.)

Cuterebra are parasites of rabbits and rodents, but they may also infest cats, dogs, and humans. They produce large pockets in the subcutaneous tissues of the host as well as air holes in the skin and are known as warbles (Fig. 36.13).

Anopheles, Aedes, and *Culex* Species (Mosquitoes)

Although they are tiny, fragile Dipterans, mosquitoes are some of the most voracious blood feeders on domestic animals and human beings (Fig. 36.14). The females suck blood, and they are also notable for their role in the transmission of numerous protozoal, viral, and nematode diseases to both animals and people. Mosquitoes can plague livestock, and, in swarms, they have been known to keep cattle from grazing in certain areas or to cause them to stampede. The feeding of large numbers of swarming mosquitoes may cause significant anemia in domestic animals. Large numbers of mosquitoes may be produced from eggs that were laid in relatively small bodies of water. Mosquitoes spread malaria (*Plasmodium* species), yellow fever, and elephantiasis among people and serve as the intermediate host for the heartworm, *Dirofilaria immitis*.

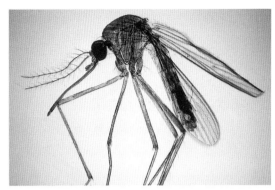

Fig. 36.14 Female *Culex* species. This is one genus from among several pathogenic genera of mosquitoes. (From Hendrix CM, Robinson E: *Diagnostic parasitology for veterinary technicians*, ed 4, St Louis, 2012, Mosby.)

CLASS: ACARINA (MITES AND TICKS)

Ticks

Infestation by mites or ticks is referred to as acariasis. Ticks are blood-sucking arachnids. They are dorsoventrally flattened in the unengorged state. The tick's head, which is known as the capitulum, serves as an organ of cutting and attachment. It is made of a penetrating, anchor-like sucking organ called the hypostome and four accessory appendages (two cutting chelicerae and two pedipalps) that act as sensors and supports when the tick fastens to the host's body. The mouthparts may be concealed under the tick's body, or they may extend from the cranial border. Most ticks are inornate; that is, they are reddish or mahogany, without markings. Some species are ornate and have distinctive white patterns on the dark scutum background. Adult ticks have eight legs, with claws on the ends of the legs. They may attach to and feed on one to three different hosts during a life cycle and are therefore referred to as one-host, two-host, or three-host ticks (Fig. 36.15).

There are two types of ticks: hard ticks (Ixodidae) and soft ticks (Argasidae). Hard ticks are important vectors of protozoal, bacterial, viral, and rickettsial diseases. The saliva of female ticks of some species is toxic, and it produces flaccid, ascending paralysis in animals and people (tick paralysis). Tick species that are commonly associated with tick paralysis are *Dermacentor andersoni* (the Rocky Mountain spotted fever tick), *Dermacentor occidentalis* (the Pacific Coast tick), *Ixodes holocyclus* (the Australian paralysis tick), and *Dermacentor variabilis* (the wood tick).

The adults, larvae, and nymphs attach to the host and feed on blood. Eggs are deposited in the environment. Hard ticks are dorsoventrally flattened, with well-defined lateral margins in the unengorged state. They have a hard, chitinous covering *(scutum)* on the dorsal surface of the body. Hard ticks may have grooves, margins, and notches (festoons) that are useful for identification purposes. Important hard ticks in North America include *Rhipicephalus sanguineus* (Fig. 36.16), *Dermacentor variabilis* (Fig. 36.17), *Dermacentor andersoni, Dermacentor occidentalis, Dermacentor albipictus, Ixodes scapularis, Ixodes*

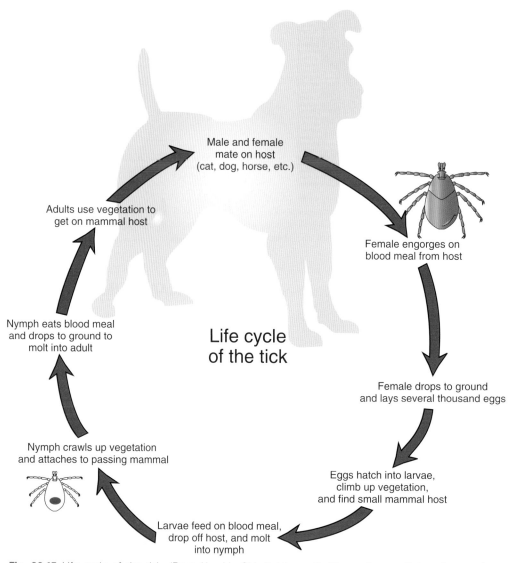

Fig. 36.15 Life cycle of the tick. (From Hendrix CM, Robinson E: *Diagnostic parasitology for veterinary technicians*, ed 4, St Louis, 2012, Mosby.)

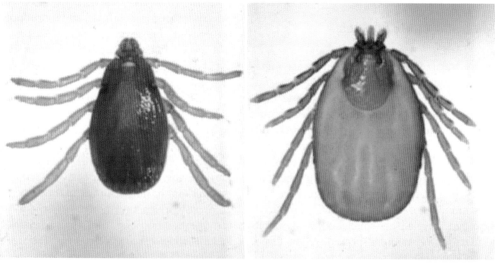

Fig. 36.16 *Rhipicephalus sanguineus* male *(left)* and female *(right)*. (From Bowman D: *Georgis' parasitology for veterinarians*, ed 9, St Louis, 2009, Saunders.)

cookei, Ixodes pacificus, Amblyomma americanum (Fig. 36.18), Amblyomma maculatum, Haemaphysalis leporispalustris, and Rhipicephalus annulatus. Rhipicephalus sanguineus is unusual in that it can become established in indoor dwellings and kennels.

> **TECHNICIAN NOTE** There are two families of ticks: hard ticks (Ixodidae) and soft ticks (Argasidae).

Soft ticks lack a scutum, and their mouthparts are not visible from the dorsal surface. The lateral edges of the body are rounded. The females feed often, and their eggs are laid off of the host. Soft ticks are more resistant to desiccation than hard ticks, and they can live for several years in arid conditions. There are three genera of veterinary importance: *Argas* species, *Otobius megnini*, and *Ornithodoros* species.

Argas species are ectoparasites of birds. The larvae, nymphs, and adults live in cracks and crevices of poultry houses and feed at night about once a month. They cause restlessness, loss of productivity, and severe anemia. They also serve as a vector for bacterial and rickettsial diseases of birds. *O. megnini*, the spinose ear tick, occurs on housed stock, dogs, and even people. Only the larval and two of the nymphal stages are parasitic (Fig. 36.19). They live in the external ear canal and suck blood, thereby causing inflammation and the production of a waxy exudate. *Ornithodoros* species live in sandy soils, in primitive

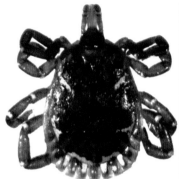

Fig. 36.17 Engorged, adult female *Dermacentor variabilis*. Unfed adults are approximately 6 mm long; engorged adult females are about 12 mm long and bluish gray in color. (From Hendrix CM, Robinson E: *Diagnostic parasitology for veterinary technicians*, ed 4, St Louis, 2012, Mosby.)

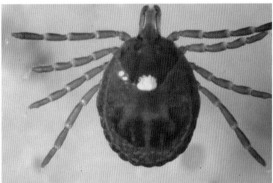

Fig. 36.18 *Amblyomma americanum*. The male *(left)* has an ornamented scutum with festoons. The scutum of the female *(right)* bears a single, large, light-colored dot, hence the name *lone-star tick*. (From Bowman D: *Georgis' parasitology for veterinarians*, ed 9, St Louis, 2009, Saunders.)

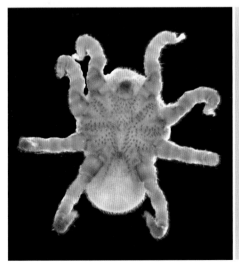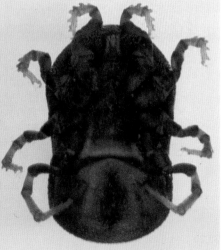

Fig. 36.19 *Otobius megnini*. *Left,* First nymph. *Right,* Second nymph. (From Bowman D: *Georgis' parasitology for veterinarians*, ed 9, St Louis, 2009, Saunders.)

housing, or in shady areas around trees. This genus is probably more important to people and rodents than to domestic animals, but *Ornithodoros coriaceus* is known to transmit the agent of foothill abortion in California. There are several diseases that can be transmitted by ticks, some of which include:

- Lyme disease
- Anaplasmosis
- Babesiosis
- Ehrlichiosis
- Borrelia
- Rocky Mountain spotted fever (RMSF)
- Tularemia
- Tick paralysis
- Tick-borne relapsing fever
- Bartonellosis
- Hepatozoonosis

Mites

Mites are arachnids that occur as parasitic and free-living forms, some of which act as intermediate hosts for cestodes. Most parasitic mites are obligate parasites, which spend their entire life cycle on the host and produce the dermatologic condition referred to as mange. A few species found on birds and rodents live off of the host and visit the host only to obtain a blood meal (e.g., *Dermanyssus gallinae*, *Ornithonyssus bacoti*). Most mite infestations are transmitted through direct contact with an infested animal. Burrowing mite infestations are diagnosed with deep skin scrapings at the periphery of lesions.

The first group of parasitic mites can be classified together as sarcoptiform mites. Sarcoptiform mites have several common key characteristics or features. These mites may produce severe dermatologic problems in a variety of domestic animals. The dermatitis produced by these mites is usually accompanied by a severe pruritus. Sarcoptiform mites are barely visible to the naked eye, and they are approximately the size of a grain of salt. Their bodies are round to oval. Sarcoptiform mites have legs with pedicels or stalks at the tip. The pedicels may be long or short. If the pedicel is long, it may be straight (unjointed) or jointed. At the tip of each pedicel may be a tiny sucker. The description of the pedicel (e.g., long or short, jointed or unjointed) may be used to identify these sarcoptiform mites. Another group of mites that is parasitic only as larvae is the trombiculid mites or "chiggers."

Sarcoptiform mites are divided into two basic families: Sarcoptidae, which burrow or tunnel within the epidermis, and Psoroptidae, which reside on the surface of the skin or within the external ear canal. The burrowing mites (Sarcoptidae) include the following: *Sarcoptes scabiei* (Fig. 36.20), *Notoedres cati* (Fig. 36.21), and *Knemidokoptes* species. These mites tunnel into the superficial layers of the epidermis and feed on tissue fluids. Infestations begin as localized areas of inflammation and hair loss, but they spread rapidly to become generalized. Over a 10- to 15-day period, the female deposits 40 to 50 eggs within the tunnel. After egg deposition, the female dies. Larvae emerge from the eggs within 3 to 10 days, and they exit the tunnel to wander on the skin surface. These larvae molt to the nymphal stage within minute pockets of the epidermis. Nymphs become sexually active adults within 12 to 17 days, and the life cycle begins again.

Sarcoptic mange caused by *S. scabiei* can affect most animal species, including people, but it is most commonly seen on dogs and pigs. It is characterized by a loss of hair and intense

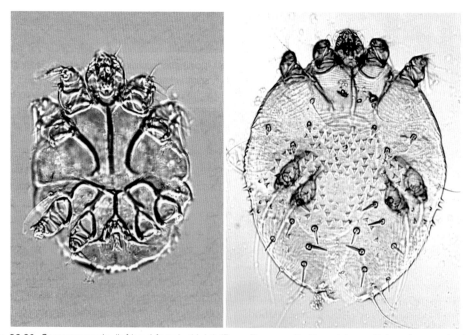

Fig. 36.20 *Sarcoptes* male *(left)* and female *(right)*. (From Bowman D: *Georgis' parasitology for veterinarians,* ed 9, St Louis, 2009, Saunders.)

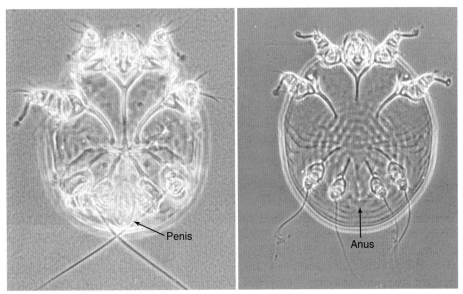

Fig. 36.21 *Notoedres* male *(left)* and female *(right)*. (From Bowman D: *Georgis' parasitology for veterinarians,* ed 9, St Louis, 2009, Saunders.)

pruritus. Each animal species has its own variety of *S. scabiei*, and cross-transmission does not occur. However, temporary infestation may take place without colonization of the skin. Notodectic mange (caused by *Notoedres*) is more restricted with regard to host range, and it occurs in cats and occasionally rabbits. Knemidokoptic mange (caused by *Knemidokoptes*) affects birds. This mite tunnels in the superficial layers of the epidermis of the pads and shanks of the feet. In severe cases, the beak and cere also may be affected. The mite characteristically produces a yellow to gray-white mass that resembles a honeycomb. This condition may be disfiguring. The parasites pierce the skin that underlies the scales, thereby causing an inflammation with exudate that hardens on the surface and that displaces the scales superficially. This process causes the thickened, scaly nature of the skin.

Demodex species are also burrowing mites that live in the hair follicles and sebaceous glands of the skin. They are considered part of the normal skin fauna of most mammals. Demodectic mange is most common among dogs, and it can be localized or generalized. *Demodex gatoi* is pruritic and contagious. It is the only Demodex spp that has these properties. Immunodeficiency—both genetic and induced by the mites—is necessary for an infestation to become clinically apparent. The disease is characterized by loss of hair, thickening of the skin, and pustule formation. Pruritus is not a manifestation of this type of mange. Deep skin scrapings are used to recover the cigar-shaped mites for diagnosis (Fig. 36.22).

> **TECHNICIAN NOTE** Immunodeficiency of the host is necessary for infestation with *Demodex* species to be clinically apparent.

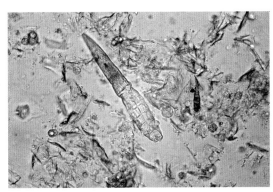

Fig. 36.22 Adult *Demodex canis*. *Demodex* mites resemble eight-legged alligators; they are elongated, with very short, stubby legs. The adult and nymphal stages have eight legs, whereas the larvae have six legs. (From Hendrix CM, Robinson E: *Diagnostic parasitology for veterinary technicians,* ed 4, St Louis, 2012, Mosby.)

Nonburrowing mites (Psoroptidae) include *Psoroptes*, *Chorioptes*, and *Otodectes*. These mites live on the surface of the skin and feed on keratinized scales, hair, and tissue fluids. *Psoroptes* species (Fig. 36.23), *Chorioptes* species, *Otodectes cynotis*, *Psorergates ovis*, and *Cheyletiella* species are examples of nonburrowing mites. Psoroptic mange is important in sheep. The mites are active in the superficial keratinized layer of the skin, but they also pierce the skin with their mouthparts. Vesicles develop, with crusting and intense pruritus. Chorioptic mange is less severe and tends to remain localized. *Chorioptes bovis* is the more important species, and it is a common parasite of cattle.

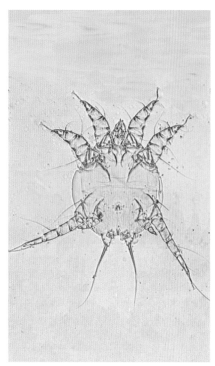

Fig. 36.23 An adult male *Psoroptes*. This species is commonly recovered from infested rabbit ears. (From Bowman D: *Georgis' parasitology for veterinarians*, ed 9, St Louis, 2009, Saunders.)

Cheyletiella and *Otodectes* species are parasites of dogs and cats. Members of the genus *Cheyletiella* produce a mild condition referred to as "walking dandruff." *Otodectes cynotis* (Fig. 36.24) live in the external ear canal of dogs and cats. A brownish, waxy exudate accumulates, with crust formation, ulceration, and secondary bacterial infections. Infested animals scratch frequently at the ears and shake their heads. Head shaking can result in the rupture of blood vessels and hematomas of the pinna. The mites can be found in the waxy exudate and crust within the ear canal.

PENTASTOMIDS (TONGUE WORMS)

Pentastomids (tongue worms) resemble helminths, but they are actually related to the arthropods. *Linguatula serrata* is the "canine pentastome" or the "canine tongue worm." Pentastomes are usually parasites of snakes and reptiles, but this tongue worm parasitizes the nasal and respiratory passages of dogs. It resembles a helminth, but it is classified as a type of

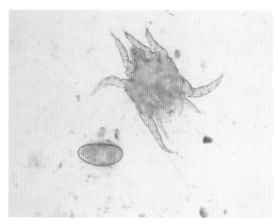

Fig. 36.24 Adult and ova of the ear mite, *Otodectes cynotis.*

arthropod, because it has a mitelike larval stage. The pentastome eggs measure 70 μm by 90 μm. On the inside of the egg, the mitelike larval stage with its jointed claws is often visible.

PHYLUM: ANNELIDA (SEGMENTED WORMS)

Hirudo Medicinalis (Medicinal Leech)

Leeches are annelids; they are not considered true helminths, but they are often described as parasitic worms. As ectoparasites of human beings, domestic animals, and wild animals, leeches are members of the phylum Annelida and the class Hirudinea. Leeches may have a pathologic or beneficial role in veterinary medicine.

The term *hirudiniasis* is derived from the classic Linnaean nomenclature, and it is defined as the invasion of the nose, mouth, pharynx, or larynx by leeches or the attachment of leeches to the skin. Leeches are voracious blood feeders; depending on the number that attach to the host, the host may become anemic and die from blood loss. Leeches have recently gained favor as postsurgical tools in reconstructive and microvascular surgery. *Hirudo medicinalis*, the medicinal leech, has been used in reconstructive and microvascular surgery in human beings; such use in veterinary medicine is forthcoming.

Leeches are segmented worms with slender, leaf-shaped bodies that are devoid of bristles. A typical leech has two suckers: a large and adhesive caudal sucker and a smaller cranial one that surrounds the mouth. Most leeches are found in fresh water, and a few are found in salt water; some are terrestrial varieties.

▌ KEY POINTS

- Ectoparasites of domestic animals include insects (e.g., fleas, lice, biting flies) and arachnids (e.g., mites, ticks).
- Immature or larval stages of nematodes and some adult stages of nematodes may parasitize an animal's skin or subcutaneous tissues.
- Insects that parasitize domestic animals are primarily members of the orders Hemiptera (true bugs), Mallophaga

(chewing lice), Anoplura (sucking lice), Diptera (two-winged flies), and Siphonaptera (fleas).
- Insects have three pairs of legs, three distinct body regions (head, thorax, and abdomen), and a single pair of antennae. Arachnids (adults) have four pairs of legs, a body that is divided into two regions (cephalothorax and abdomen), and no antennae.

- The life-cycle stages of ticks and mites consist of egg, larva, nymph, and adult. There can be more than one nymphal instar.
- Infestation by chewing or sucking lice is referred to as pediculosis.
- Infestation by larval dipterans is referred to as myiasis.
- Infestation by fleas is referred to as siphonapterosis.
- Infestation by mites or ticks is referred to as acariasis.
- *Ctenocephalides felis and Ctenocephalides* canis are the cat and dog fleas.
- Heavy infestations with fleas, especially in young animals, produce anemia.
- Flea saliva is antigenic and irritating. It causes intense pruritus (itching) and hypersensitivity, which is known as flea-bite dermatitis or miliary dermatitis.
- Lice are separated into two orders on the basis of whether their mouthparts are modified for biting/chewing (Mallophaga) or sucking (Anoplura).
- Flies produce harm by inflicting painful bites, sucking blood, producing hypersensitive reactions, depositing eggs in sores, larval migration through tissues of the host, and acting as vectors and intermediate hosts to other pathogenic agents.
- Adult ticks have eight legs, with claws on the ends of the legs, and they feed on one to three different hosts during a life cycle.
- Hard ticks (Ixodidae) are important vectors of protozoal, bacterial, viral, and rickettsial diseases.
- The saliva of female ticks of some species is toxic and produces flaccid, ascending paralysis in both animals and people (i.e., tick paralysis).
- Most parasitic mites are obligate parasites that spend their entire life cycles on the host and produce the dermatologic condition referred to as mange.
- Sarcoptiform mites are divided into two basic families: Sarcoptidae, which burrow or tunnel within the epidermis, and Psoroptidae, which reside on the surface of the skin or within the external ear canal.
- *Demodex* species are also burrowing mites that live in the hair follicles and sebaceous glands of the skin.
- Nonburrowing mites (Psoroptidae) include *Psoroptes, Chorioptes,* and *Otodectes.*

Cytology

Unit Outline

Unit Objectives

Describe the collection and handling of cytology samples.
Describe the preparation techniques that are used with cytology samples.
Discuss the general procedure for the evaluation of cytology samples.
Describe the general characteristics of samples taken from inflammatory lesions.
Describe the general characteristics of samples taken from neoplastic lesions.
Discuss the microscopic appearance of cells in cytology samples taken from a variety of sites.

Exfoliative cytology is the study of cells that have been shed from body surfaces. It refers to the examination of cells that are present in body fluids (e.g., cerebrospinal, peritoneal, pleural, and synovial fluids), on mucosal surfaces (e.g., in the trachea or vagina), or in secretions (e.g., semen, prostatic fluid, milk). The primary purpose of the cytology evaluation is to differentiate inflammation from neoplasia. The types and numbers of cells that are present in a properly collected and prepared cytology specimen can provide rapid diagnostic information to the clinician. Samples for cytology evaluation can be collected quickly and do not generally require specialized materials or equipment for proper evaluation. With careful attention to quality control—including the use of appropriate collection, preparation, and staining techniques—a high-quality cytology sample can be obtained. Such samples yield valuable results for the clinician and often preclude the need for more invasive procedures to determine a patient's diagnosis, treatment, and prognosis.

Cytology provides somewhat different information than a histopathologic evaluation. Histopathology observes cells in relation to their neighboring cells. The histopathologist evaluates the cellular architecture. The preparation of a sample for histopathology involves several complex steps and some specialized equipment. To prepare a sample for histopathology, the tissue is first immersed in fixative. Several steps are involved in dehydrating the tissue before it is imbedded in paraffin. The paraffin block is then sliced, and the slice is mounted on a glass slide before it is stained. Cytologic evaluations observe the cells individually or in small groups. The cells in a cytologic preparation are randomly distributed, with no evidence of their in vitro relationship to each other.

37

Sample Collection and Handling for Cytology

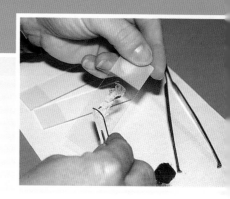

LEARNING OBJECTIVES

After studying this chapter, you will be able to:

- List techniques that can be used for the collection of cytology samples.
- Describe the procedure for collecting samples by swabbing.
- Describe the procedure for collecting samples by imprinting.
- Describe the techniques for fine-needle biopsy sample collection.
- Describe the techniques for transtracheal wash sample collection.
- Describe the general procedure for collecting samples by centesis.
- List the methods that can be used to concentrate cytology samples.

OUTLINE

KEY TERMS

Abdominocentesis
Arthrocentesis
Centesis
Fine-needle biopsy

Paracentesis
Punch biopsy
Thoracocentesis
Transtracheal wash

Tzanck preparation
Wedge biopsy

Cytology samples from solid masses on an animal's body or that are obtained from a surgical procedure can be collected by the swab, scrape, or imprint technique. Fine-needle biopsy can also be used for some solid samples as well as fluid samples. Centesis refers to fluid samples that are collected from body cavities.

SWABS

Swabs are generally collected only when imprints, scrapings, and aspirates cannot be made, such as with fistulous tracts and vaginal collections. The area is swabbed with a moist, sterile cotton or rayon swab (Fig. 37.1). Sterile isotonic fluid (e.g., 0.9% saline) should be used to moisten the swab. Moistening the swab helps to minimize cell damage during sample collection and smear preparation. For the collection of vaginal swabs, restrain the animal in a standing position with the tail elevated. Clean and rinse the vulva, and then insert a lubricated speculum or smooth plastic tube to a point just cranial to the urethral orifice in the vagina. The cells collected are those that have exfoliated, or shed, from the vaginal wall (epithelial cells and neutrophils) and those passing through the vagina from the uterus, especially erythrocytes during proestrus and estrus in the bitch. If collecting a sample from a moist

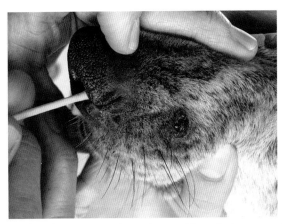

Fig. 37.1 A moist cotton swab can be used to collect some cytology samples.

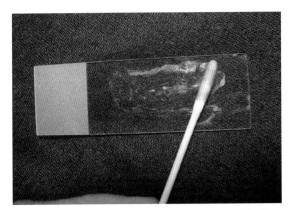

Fig. 37.2 The swab is rolled on a clean glass slide to make the smear.

lesion, the swab need not be moistened. After sample collection, the swab is gently rolled along the flat surface of a clean glass microscope slide (Fig. 37.2). The swab should not be rubbed across the slide surface, because this causes excessive cell damage.

> **TECHNICIAN NOTE** Swabs must be moistened with sterile saline before the collection of samples.

Ear swabs samples may contain excess amounts of wax. This may interfere with the evaluation of the sample. To minimize this effect, gentle heating of the slide may be necessary. Passing the slide briefly through a flame or gentle heat from a warm hair dryer may be used to dissolve the wax. Excess heat must be avoided, because it will destroy the cellular components of the sample. Aside from the Gram staining procedure, this is the only circumstance under which cytology samples may require heat application.

SCRAPINGS

Smears of scrapings may be prepared from tissues that are collected during necropsy or surgery or from external lesions

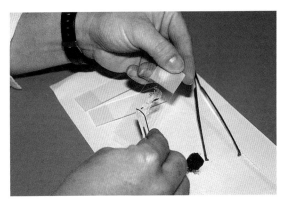

Fig. 37.3 A scalpel blade can be used to collect cells from solid masses.

on the living animal. Scraping has the advantage of collecting many cells from the tissue, so it is therefore advantageous when the lesion is firm and yields few cells. The major disadvantages of scrapings are that they are more difficult to collect and that they collect only superficial samples. As a result, scrapings from superficial lesions often reflect only a secondary bacterial infection or inflammation-induced tissue dysplasia, which markedly hinders their use for the diagnosis of neoplasia.

To obtain a scraping, localize the lesion and hold the scalpel blade perpendicular to the lesion's cleaned and blotted surface. Pull the blade across the lesion several times. The material collected on the blade is transferred to the middle of a glass microscope slide (Fig. 37.3) and spread by one or more of the techniques described later in this chapter for the preparation of smears from aspirates of solid masses.

IMPRINTS

Imprints, which are also referred to as impression smears, may be prepared from external lesions on the living animal or from tissues removed during surgery or necropsy. These are easy to collect and require minimal restraint, but they collect fewer cells than scrapings and usually contain a greater amount of contamination (bacterial and cellular) as compared with fine-needle biopsies. As a result, imprints from superficial lesions often reflect only a local secondary bacterial infection or inflammation-induced tissue dysplasia. In many instances, the bacteria and tissue dysplasia markedly hinder the making of an accurate diagnosis of neoplasia.

The Tzanck preparation is a type of imprint collection that can be used on external lesions. To perform this procedure, prepare at least six clean glass slides. The lesion is imprinted before it is cleaned, and that first slide designated as Number 1. The lesion should then be cleaned with a saline-moistened surgical sponge and reimprinted with the slide marked as imprint Number 2. The lesion is then debrided and reimprinted with the slide, which is marked as imprint Number 3. If a scab is present, the underside of the scab should be imprinted and the slide marked as imprint Number 4 (Fig. 37.4). Imprints from the tissue exposed by removal of the

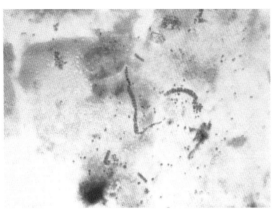

Fig. 37.4 This sample was prepared with an imprint of the underside of a scab. Squamous epithelial cells and chains of coccoid organisms *(Dermatophilus congolensis)* are present.

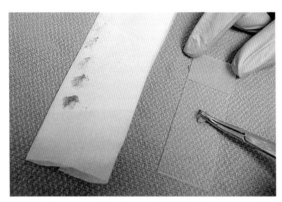

Fig. 37.5 The tissue must be thoroughly blotted to remove blood and tissue fluid before the imprint slide is prepared.

scab and scrapings or swabs from that exposed tissue can both be collected.

> **TECHNICIAN NOTE** Multiple small imprints should be made on a clean glass microscope slide.

To collect imprints from tissues collected during surgery or necropsy, blood and tissue fluid first should be removed from the surface of the lesion being imprinted by blotting with a clean, absorbent material (Fig. 37.5). Excessive blood and tissue fluids inhibit tissue cells from adhering to the glass slide, thereby producing a poor cellular preparation. In addition, excessive fluid inhibits cells from spreading and assuming the size and shape that they usually have on air-dried smears. If a delay occurs from the time of sample collection until the imprint is taken, a scalpel blade should be used to expose a fresh surface before blotting and sampling the surface. The middle of a clean glass microscope slide is then touched against the blotted surface of the tissue to be imprinted. Multiple imprints are generally made on each slide (Fig. 37.6). Several slides may be imprinted so that slides are available for special stains, if necessary.

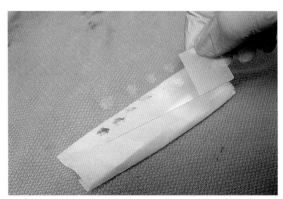

Fig. 37.6 Multiple imprints should be made for each tissue. Blot the sample again if tissue fluid and blood begin to reappear on the imprint slide.

FINE-NEEDLE BIOPSY

Fine-needle biopsies (FNBs) may be collected from masses, including lymph nodes, nodular lesions, and internal organs. For cutaneous lesions, they provide an advantage over other methods by avoiding superficial contamination (i.e., bacterial and cellular). However, fewer cells are usually collected than with other methods, such as scrapings. Fine-needle biopsy can be performed by either an aspiration or nonaspiration method.

Preparation of the Site for Fine-Needle Biopsy

If microbiologic tests are to be performed on a portion of the sample collected or if a body cavity is to be penetrated (e.g., the peritoneal and thoracic cavities and joints), then the area of aspiration is surgically prepared. Otherwise, the preparation is essentially that required for a vaccination or venipuncture. An alcohol swab may be used to clean the area.

Selection of Syringe and Needle

For the aspiration method of fine-needle biopsy, use a 21- to 25-gauge needle and a 3- to 20-mL syringe. The softer the aspirated tissue is, the smaller the needle and syringe to be used. The use of a needle larger than 21-gauge for aspiration is seldom advantageous, even for firm tissues such as fibromas. When larger needles are used, tissue cores tend to be aspirated, thereby resulting in a poor yield of free cells that are suitable for cytologic preparation. In addition, larger needles tend to cause greater blood contamination.

The size of syringe used is influenced by the consistency of the tissue being aspirated. Softer tissues, such as lymph nodes, often may be aspirated successfully with a 3-mL syringe. Firm tissues, such as fibromas and squamous cell carcinomas, require a larger syringe to maintain adequate suction for the sufficient collection of cells. Because the ideal size of the syringe is not known for many masses before aspiration, a 12-mL syringe is a useful size.

> **TECHNICIAN NOTE** Fine-needle biopsy can be performed with an aspiration or nonaspiration technique.

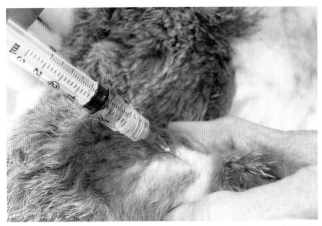

Fig. **37.7** Collection of a nonsterile sample by the fine-needle biopsy aspiration technique.

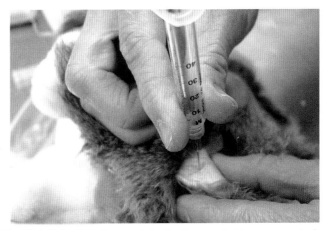

Fig. **37.8** Collection of a sample by the fine-needle biopsy nonaspiration technique.

Aspiration Procedure

The mass to be aspirated is held firmly to help with penetration of the skin and mass and to control the direction of the needle. The needle, with the syringe attached, is introduced into the center of the mass, and strong negative pressure is applied by withdrawing the plunger to approximately three fourths of the volume of the syringe (Fig. 37.7). Several areas of the mass should be sampled, but aspiration of the sample into the barrel of the syringe and contamination of the sample by aspiration of the tissue that surrounds the mass must be avoided. To accomplish this, when the mass is large enough to allow the needle to be redirected and moved to several areas in the mass without danger of the needle's leaving the mass, negative pressure is maintained during the redirection and movement of the needle. However, when the mass is not large enough for the needle to be redirected and moved without danger of the needle leaving the mass, negative pressure is relieved during the redirection and movement of the needle. In this situation, negative pressure is applied only when the needle is static. High-quality collections often do not have aspirate material visible in the syringe and sometimes not even in the hub of the needle.

When material is observed in the hub of the needle or after several areas are sampled, the negative pressure is relieved from the syringe, and the needle is withdrawn from the mass and the skin. Next, the needle is removed from the syringe, and air is drawn into the syringe. The needle is then replaced onto the syringe, and some of the tissue in the barrel and hub of the needle is expelled onto the middle of a glass microscope slide by rapidly depressing the plunger. When possible, several preparations should be made, as described in the following sections of this chapter.

Nonaspirate Procedure (Capillary Technique, Stab Technique)

This technique is easier to perform than aspiration, because it does not involve directing the syringe and needle and pulling the plunger with the same hand. The mass to be sampled is held firmly to help with the penetration of the skin and mass and to help direct the needle. A 22-gauge needle is introduced into the mass. A syringe with the plunger removed may be left attached to the needle to facilitate handling (Fig. 37.8). The needle is moved rapidly back and forth through the mass five to six times along the same tract. The cells are collected by shearing and capillary action. The needle is removed from the mass and attached to a 10-mL syringe that has been prefilled with air. The material is expelled onto a clean glass microscope slide by rapidly depressing the plunger (Fig. 37.9). The expelled material should be smeared using one of the techniques described for the preparation of smears.

Generally, enough material is collected to make only one smear. Therefore, the procedure should be repeated two or three times in different sites of the mass to ensure adequate slide numbers and areas of the mass to evaluate.

TISSUE BIOPSY

Tissue biopsy is the sampling of a piece of tissue for cytologic or histopathologic examination or both. Many organs and tissues—including kidney, liver, lung, lymph node, prostate, skin, spleen, and thyroid—and masses (tumors) may be biopsied. Biopsies can often be classified as excisional vs incisional. When the entire tumor is removed, the procedure is called an excisional biopsy. If only a portion of the tumor is removed, the procedure is referred to as an incisional biopsy. Biopsy techniques include gentle abrasion with a blade, needle aspiration, and excision, including punch biopsy and endoscope-guided biopsy. The technique used varies with the tissue to be biopsied. Considerations include the location, accessibility, and nature of the tissue. Prospective skin biopsy sites are clipped of hair, with care taken to avoid skin irritation and the inducement of an inflammatory artifact. Cleansing of the site is neither recommended nor necessary. The lesion must not be scrubbed, and any scales, crusts, or surface debris should not be disturbed, because they may offer valuable diagnostic clues.

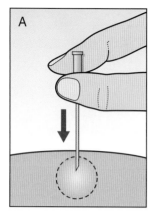
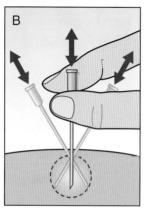
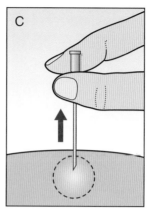
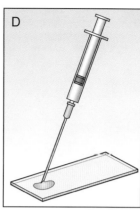

Fig. 37.9 Fine-needle biopsy nonaspiration technique; diagrammatic stepwise illustration of a biopsy procedure. **A,** The needle is inserted into the target tissue. **B,** The needle is moved back and forth inside the target to vary the angle. **C,** The needle is withdrawn. **D,** The needle is attached to the syringe, and the sample is blown onto the microscope slide. (From Raskin R, Meyer D: *Canine and feline cytology*, ed 2, St Louis, 2010, Saunders.)

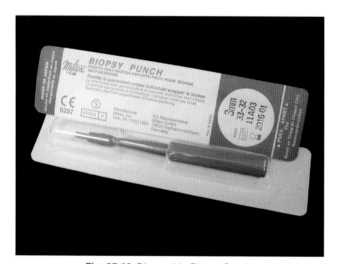
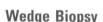

Fig. 37.10 Disposable Biopsy Punch.

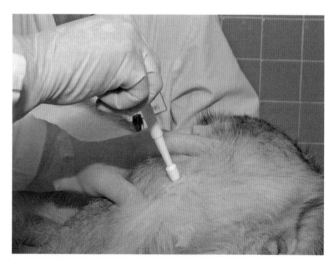

Fig. 37.11 The biopsy punch is pressed into the skin while rotational motion is applied in one direction. (From Taylor SM: *Small animal clinical techniques*, St Louis, 2010, Saunders.)

Wedge Biopsy

Elliptic wedge biopsy specimens are commonly obtained with a scalpel. The wedge biopsy offers the advantages of a large, variably sized specimen that is easily oriented by the pathology technician. Solitary lesions are often best removed with this technique. When a wedge biopsy specimen is taken, a sharp scalpel blade is used to excise the entire lesion, or the wedge is taken from an area of the lesion, through a transition zone, to normal tissue. The pathology technician can then trim the specimen on its long axis to provide the pathologist with a slide that shows abnormal tissue, a transition zone, and normal tissue.

Punch Biopsy

The punch biopsy technique has a number of advantages over wedge biopsy, particularly the ease and speed of the procedure. Keyes cutaneous biopsy punches (3-, 4-, 6-, and 8-mm disposable skin biopsy punches) are most commonly used (Fig. 37.10).

With the biopsy punch, 4-mm specimens require no sutures, and 6- or 8-mm biopsy specimens require only one or two sutures. Ideally, two or three punch biopsy specimens of various lesions should be collected. A local anesthetic should be infiltrated around the site. The punch is gently rotated in one direction until the punch blade has sectioned the tissue (Fig. 37.11). The punch is rotated in only one direction, because back-and-forth rotation increases the likelihood of specimen damage as a result of shearing forces.

Tissue samples for histopathologic examination often are fixed in 10% neutral phosphate-buffered formalin. To ensure adequate fixation, slabs of tissue no more than 1 cm wide should be placed in fluid-tight jars that contain formalin at approximately 10 times the specimen's volume. With large tissues, the sample can be removed to a smaller jar with less formalin content after it has been fixed for 24 hours.

TECHNICIAN NOTE Punch biopsy specimens are collected by gently pressing the biopsy punch into the skin while applying rotational motion in one direction.

After the specimen has been collected by either the wedge or punch method, the specimen should be gently removed by grasping the margin of the tissue with a pair of fine forceps. Fresh, unfixed tissue is extremely fragile. Specimens collected by endoscopy can be gently flushed from the tip of the endoscope with sterile saline (Fig. 37.12). The specimen is then blotted gently on a paper towel to remove excess blood and placed on a small piece of wooden tongue depressor or cardboard (Fig. 37.13). Skin specimens should be placed with the subcutaneous side down. Gently pressing the biopsy specimen flat facilitates adherence and allows for the proper anatomic orientation of the specimen in the laboratory. Allow the tissue to dry onto the "splint."

Specimens with the attached "splint" are then immersed or floated specimen side down in the fixative. The timely placement of the specimen in the fixative is critical, because artifactual changes may begin to occur within 1 minute after the biopsy specimen is obtained. Adequate specimen fixation requires at least 24 hours before processing. Formalin freezes at −11° F (−24° C), and this freezing may cause substantial artifactual damage in unfixed specimens. Therefore, to ensure proper fixation without freezing artifact, specimens should remain at room temperature for at least 6 hours before exposure to possible extreme cold.

CENTESIS

Centesis refers to the introduction of a needle into any body cavity or organ for the purpose of removing fluid. The collection of fluid from the peritoneal cavity (abdominocentesis or paracentesis) and the thoracic cavity (thoracocentesis) are commonly performed in small animal practice. Cystocentesis (the percutaneous aspiration of urine from the urinary bladder) is discussed in Unit 5. Fluid samples for cytologic evaluation may also be collected from around the spinal column, from within joints (arthrocentesis), and from the eye. General anesthesia is required for the collection of cerebrospinal fluid, synovial fluid, and aqueous and vitreous humor.

Before the collection of peritoneal or pleural fluid, the site should be aseptically prepared and all equipment and supplies should be gathered. Preparing several smears from the fluid as soon as it is collected is helpful, so a plentiful supply of glass slides should be ready. A portion of the fluid should be collected in an ethylenediaminetetraacetic acid (EDTA) tube. A 21-gauge needle is most commonly used and should be attached to a 60-mL syringe. For small animal patients, thoracocentesis is usually performed with the animal in a standing position and the needle inserted in the seventh or eighth intercostal space along the cranial aspect of the rib. Abdominocentesis may be performed in a standing animal or with the patient in lateral recumbency (Fig. 37.14). The needle is introduced into the ventral abdomen to the right of the midline approximately 1- to 2-cm caudal to the umbilicus. The procedure is slightly different for exotic and farm animals.

Ease of collection may reflect the volume of fluid present or the pressure within that body cavity. It also is influenced by the technical proficiency of the operator and, in the case of conscious animals, the cooperation of the animal. The total volume collected must be recorded at the time of collection. Certain gross characteristics of body fluids should be recorded at collection, including sample color and turbidity. Subsequently, total nucleated cell counts, cell types, and morphologic features are determined.

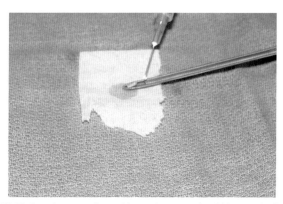

Fig. 37.12 Specimens collected by endoscopy should be gently flushed from the tip of the endoscope.

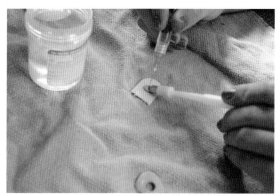

Fig. 37.13 A sterile needle can be used to remove a punch biopsy specimen onto a splint.

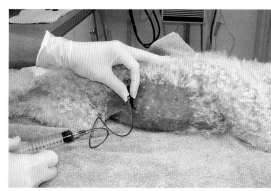

Fig. 37.14 Collection of peritoneal fluid by abdominocentesis.

Color and Turbidity

Color and turbidity are influenced by protein concentration and cell numbers. Gross discoloration with increased turbidity may be caused by iatrogenic contamination with peripheral blood, recent or old hemorrhage, inflammation, or a combination of these conditions.

The perforation of superficial vessels during collection may result in contamination with peripheral blood. Such admixture of blood with the sample may be obvious as a streak of blood in otherwise clear fluid at some stage during collection. Blood-tinged fluid may also be the result of recent or old hemorrhage into the body cavity being sampled. Both peripheral blood contamination and recent hemorrhage result in a clear supernatant and red (erythrocyte-rich) sediment after centrifugation. Recent hemolysis imparts a reddish discoloration to the supernatant. Hemorrhage that occurred at least 2 days previously generally causes a yellowish supernatant (as a result of hemoglobin breakdown products), usually with little erythrocytic sediment (Fig. 37.15).

Cytologic examination of the fluid also may assist with determining the time of hemorrhage. Clumps of platelets may be observed in recent and often iatrogenic (operator-induced) hemorrhage. These clumps are not obvious after approximately 1 hour. Blood must be present in the cavity for several hours before macrophage ingestion of erythrocytes becomes evident. If the hemorrhage occurred a day or so before collection, hemoglobin breakdown products such as hemosiderin may be seen in the macrophages. Inflammation may also discolor body fluids, with the degree of turbidity reflecting leukocyte numbers. Color may vary from an off-white or cream to a red-cream or dirty brown, depending on the number of erythrocytes involved and the integrity of the cells present.

Consistent terminology must be used when describing cell types. Specific details of the morphologic features of each cell type also assist the clinician in making the diagnosis. Neutrophils and macrophages should be evaluated for the presence of vacuoles or phagocytized material. Neoplastic cells should be evaluated for malignant changes, such as mitotic figures and basophilic cytoplasm.

TRANSTRACHEAL/BRONCHIAL WASH

The cytologic evaluation of samples obtained from the trachea, bronchi, or bronchioles may assist with the diagnosis of

pulmonary disease in animals. Transtracheal washes may be performed by passage of a catheter through an endotracheal tube in an anesthetized animal (orotracheal approach), through the nasal passages (nasotracheal approach), or through the skin and trachea (percutaneous approach) in a conscious sedated animal. The transtracheal route minimizes pharyngeal contamination of the specimen, but it is an invasive procedure and consequently requires aseptic technique. These procedures are commonly used in both small and large animals.

> **TECHNICIAN NOTE** Transtracheal wash can be performed with an endotracheal or percutaneous technique.

Percutaneous Technique

The percutaneous method requires the use of an 18- to 20-gauge through-the-needle (jugular) catheter. The laryngeal area is clipped of hair and aseptically prepared. A small amount (usually 0.5 to 1.0 mL) of 2% lidocaine is injected into the cricothyroid membrane and the surrounding skin. The needle is inserted into the trachea through the cricothyroid membrane, and the catheter is advanced into the lumen of the trachea (Fig. 37.16). Sterile physiologic saline solution is infused through the catheter at a rate of 0.5 mL to 1.0 mL per kilogram of body weight. When the animal coughs, the syringe plunger should be retracted several times and the fluid collected should be placed into a plain sterile tube. Samples should be processed immediately.

Orotracheal Technique

This technique may be preferred in very small or fractious animals. The patient must be lightly anesthetized, and an appropriately sized endotracheal tube should be placed. A polypropylene urinary or jugular catheter is then placed through the endotracheal tube, and saline is infused as described for the percutaneous method. A red rubber catheter may be used, but care must be taken to ensure that the catheter does not collapse during aspiration, which may occur with highly viscous samples (Fig. 37.17). Depending on the level of anesthesia, the animal will often not cough, so the saline should

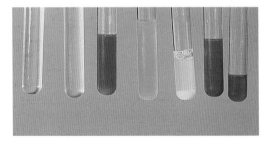

Fig. 37.15 Gross appearance of various effusions *(left to right):* clear and colorless, yellow and slightly turbid, hemolyzed and slightly turbid, orange and turbid, sedimented fluid, bloody and turbid, and brown and slightly turbid.

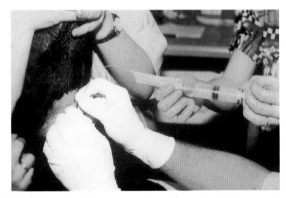

Fig. 37.16 Collection of transtracheal wash sample by the percutaneous method.

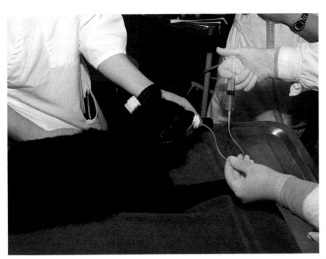

Fig. 37.17 Collection of transtracheal wash sample by the orotracheal method. (From Taylor SM: *Small animal clinical techniques*, St Louis, 2010, Saunders.)

be withdrawn within a few seconds and evaluated. Bronchoalveolar lavage (BAL) is an orotracheal technique that is used to collect samples specifically from the lower respiratory tract. Bronchoscopy is the preferred method for performing a BAL, but specialized equipment (e.g., a bronchoscope) is required.

With either method, only a small amount of the saline that is infused will be harvested with the initial collection. Subsequent coughing of the animal may also contain cells of interest, so all fluid released during coughing subsequent to the initial collection should be collected after the animal has been returned to its cage. This fluid should be placed in a sterile tube, with a notation made of the site of collection. Such fluids are often contaminated, but they can sometimes be used for evaluation when the initial collection yields insufficient information.

Samples with little mucus (that generally correspond to small numbers of cells) should be centrifuged at low speed, and smears should be prepared from the sediment. Samples that contain much mucus (and usually numerous cells) may not need to be centrifuge concentrated before a smear is made. Total nucleated cell counts are usually not performed on tracheal wash fluids. Cell numbers are subjectively recorded from the evaluation of the smear. A tracheal wash smear from a normal animal contains few cells, usually with a small amount of mucus. The mucus often appears microscopically as eosinophilic to purple strands that may enmesh the cells. Epithelial cells are the principal cell type present.

The cytologic evaluation of samples obtained from the nasal cavity may be useful during the investigation of diseases that affect the upper airway. Fluid (normal saline) may be infused into the nasal cavity through the nose with a syringe and tubing and then aspirated. This procedure is referred to as a nasal flush. Such specimens are processed as are those for a tracheal wash. Various abnormalities may be demonstrated with this

procedure, such as inflammation secondary to sepsis, fungi and yeasts, and neoplasia. These should not be confused with glove powder, which may be present in some specimens.

CONCENTRATION TECHNIQUES

When a cytologic smear is to be made of fluid with a cell count of less than 500/μL, the concentration of cells is mandatory. (Such concentration may be helpful even at higher cell counts.) Four methods are described.

Low-Speed Centrifugation

To concentrate fluids by centrifugation, the fluid is centrifuged for 5 minutes at 165 g to 360 g with a centrifuge with a radial arm length of 14.6 cm (this is the arm length of most urine centrifuges) at 1000 rpm to 1500 rpm. After centrifugation, the supernatant is separated from the sediment and analyzed for total protein concentration. The sediment is resuspended in a few drops of supernatant by gently thumping the side of the tube. A drop of the resuspended sediment is placed on a slide, and a smear is made by the blood smear or compression preparation technique. When possible, several smears should be made using each technique. The addition of plasma may help cells to adhere to the microscope slide. After air drying, the slide may be stained with a Romanowsky stain.

Gravitational Sedimentation

Gravitational sedimentation is another method that is used to concentrate cells. It is most commonly used for cerebrospinal fluid (CSF) evaluations. One method uses a glass cylinder (which can be made by cutting the end off of a test tube) attached to a microscope slide with paraffin wax. (The smooth tube end is dipped in melted wax and placed on a warm slide.) The cells in approximately 1 mL of CSF are allowed about 30 minutes to settle. The supernatant is then carefully removed with a pipette, and the tube is detached. (Excess CSF may be gently removed with absorbent paper.) The slide is air dried, and residual paraffin is carefully scraped off. The slide may be stained with a Romanowsky stain.

Membrane Filtration

The membrane filtration of alcohol-diluted CSF may also be used to concentrate cells. A membrane pore size of 5 is usually satisfactory. Filter holders that attach to a syringe are available. The CSF is permitted to gravity feed from the syringe barrel, or it is gently injected through the filter at no more than 1 drop/sec. The filter paper must be kept horizontal to distribute the cells evenly. Increased resistance to filtration suggests that the pores are becoming obstructed by cells or protein, and no more CSF should be forced through the filter. The filtration of another, smaller volume of CSF through fresh filter paper results in a less-crowded preparation.

After removal from the syringe holder, the filter is fixed in 95% ethanol for at least 30 minutes. Holders are available for easy handling of the filter paper during fixation and staining. A trichrome-type stain must be used. Romanowsky stains are unsuitable because they stain the filter paper too intensely. A satisfactory staining procedure can be performed by immersing the filter paper for 2 minutes in each specific substance in the following order: 80%, 70%, 50%, and 30% ethanol and then distilled water. This is followed by 4 minutes in hematoxylin, 5 minutes in running tap water, 4 minutes in Pollak's stain, 1 minute in 0.3% acetic acid, 1 minute in 95% ethanol, 2 minutes in N-propyl alcohol (propanol), and 2 minutes in a 1:1 mixture of propanol and xylene. The sample finally undergoes three rinses of 2 minutes each in xylene. At all stages, the filter must be treated gently to avoid dislodging cells. Depending on the size of the filter, it may need to be cut to a suitable size before placement on a microscope slide (cell side up). The filter is then flooded with a mounting medium with a refractive index similar to that of filter paper (approximately 1.5), and a coverslip is applied.

Cytologically, the cells trapped by the membrane filter are rounder than those seen after sedimentation (and therefore may be harder to distinguish), and they are in slightly different planes of focus. Furthermore, the filter produces a patterned background that may be distracting. This distraction is minimized by ensuring that the sample is not overstained and by using the appropriate mounting medium. The pore size that is generally used is far too large to trap free bacteria. Quantitatively, more cells are collected by filtration than by the two sedimentation methods.

Cytocentrifugation

As with any fluid of low cellularity, a cytocentrifuge can be used for the preparation of CSF cytologic smears. Such equipment is generally too expensive for a veterinary practice to justify purchasing. However, it often is used in a referral laboratory. This technique allows cells to be concentrated within a small circular area on the slide.

▌ KEY POINTS

- Cytology samples from solid masses on an animal's body or that are obtained from a surgical procedure can be collected by the swab, scrape, or imprint technique.
- Fine-needle biopsy can also be used for some solid samples as well as fluid samples.
- Fine-needle biopsy can be performed by either an aspiration or nonaspiration method.
- Centesis refers to the collection of fluids from body cavities.

- The collection of samples for evaluation of the trachea, bronchi, and bronchioles can be performed with the transtracheal wash technique.
- Transtracheal wash can be performed with either a percutaneous or endotracheal technique.
- Concentration techniques may be needed for samples with low cellularity.

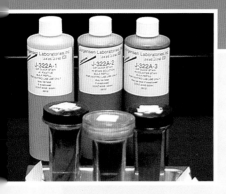

38

Preparation of Cytology Smears

LEARNING OBJECTIVES

After studying this chapter, you will be able to:
- List the methods that can be used to prepare cytology samples for evaluation.
- Describe the technique for performing the compression smear.
- Describe the technique for performing the line smear.
- Describe the technique for performing the starfish smear.

- Describe the technique for performing the modified compression smear.
- Describe the procedure for fixing and staining cytology samples.
- List potential problems with staining that may be encountered, and describe possible solutions.

OUTLINE

KEY TERMS

Compression smears
Fixative
Impression smears

Line smears
Modified compression preparations
New methylene blue (NMB)

Romanowsky stains
Starfish smears

Cytology samples may be processed by a variety of techniques, including impression smears, compression smears, modified compression preparations, line smears, starfish smears, or wedge smears. The exact type of preparation depends on the characteristics of the sample. Some samples may also require concentration by centrifugation. Fluid samples may require anticoagulants or preservatives. Several different preparations are usually made from each sample. This allows for additional diagnostic testing without additional collection. A variety of staining techniques are also available for cytology specimens. Some samples require processing with more than one staining procedure.

SMEAR PREPARATION

Preparation of Smears From Solid Masses

Several methods may be used to prepare smears for the cytologic evaluation of solid masses, including lymph nodes and internal organs. The experience of the person preparing the smears and the characteristics of the sample influence the choice of smear preparation technique. A combination of slide preparation techniques is therefore suggested. Some cytologic preparation techniques are described in the following sections.

Compression Preparation

The compression technique, which is sometimes referred to as the "squash prep," can yield excellent cytologic smears. However, in less experienced hands, it often yields unreadable cytologic smears, because too many cells are ruptured or the sample is not sufficiently spread. A compression preparation is made by expelling the aspirate onto the middle of one slide and then gently placing a second slide (the spreader slide) over the aspirate horizontal with and at a right angle to the first slide (the prep slide) (Figs. 38.1 and 38.2). The spreader slide is then quickly and smoothly slid across the prep slide. Downward pressure should not be placed on the spreader slide, because

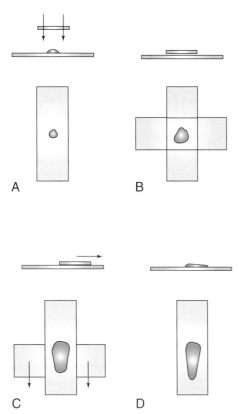

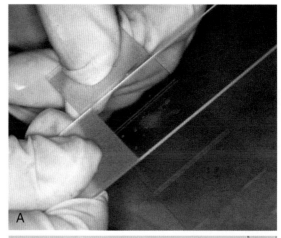

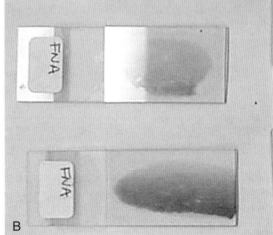

Fig. 38.1 Compression Preparation. **A,** A portion of the aspirate is expelled onto a glass microscope slide. **B,** Another slide is placed over the sample, thereby spreading the sample. If the sample does not spread well, gentle digital pressure can be applied to the top slide. Care must be taken not to place excessive pressure on the slide, which could cause the cells to rupture. **C,** The slides are smoothly slid apart, which usually produces well-spread smears **(D),** but this may also result in excessive cell rupture.

Fig. 38.2 **A,** Preparation of a compression smear. **B,** Completed compression smear.

this may cause excessive cell rupturing, making the sample unable to be interpreted.

> **TECHNICIAN NOTE** Compression smears are useful for a wide variety of cytology samples.

A modification of the compression preparation that has less tendency to rupture cells is to lay the second slide over the aspirate, rotate the second slide 45 degrees, and then lift it upward (Fig. 38.3).

Combination Technique

One combination procedure involves spraying the aspirate onto the middle of a clean glass microscope slide or prep slide. Place the prep slide on a flat, solid, horizontal surface, and pull the spreader slide backward at a 45-degree angle to the first slide until it makes contact with approximately one third of the aspirate. The spreader slide should be slid smoothly and rapidly forward, as if making a blood smear. Next, the spreader slide is placed horizontally over the back third of the aspirate at a right

angle to the prep slide. The weight of the spreader slide is usually sufficient to spread the material. Avoid the temptation to compress the slides manually. Keep the spreader slide flat and horizontal, and use a quick, smooth motion to slide the spreader slide across the prep slide (Fig. 38.4).

This procedure makes a compression preparation of the back third of the aspirate. The middle third of the aspirate is left untouched. This procedure leaves the front third of the aspirate gently spread. If the aspirate is of fragile tissue, this area should contain sufficient intact cells for evaluation. The back third of the aspirate has been spread with the shear forces of a compression preparation. If the aspirate contains clumps of cells that are difficult to spread, some clumps should be sufficiently spread in the back third of the preparation. If the aspirate is of low cellularity, the middle third remains more concentrated and is the most efficient area to study.

Starfish Smear

Another technique for spreading aspirates is to drag the aspirate peripherally in several directions with the point of a syringe needle, producing a starfish shape (Fig. 38.5). This technique

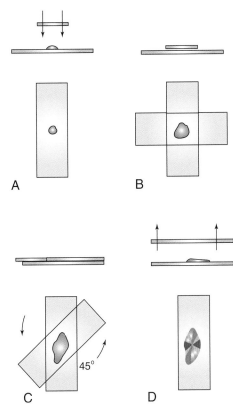

Fig. 38.3 Modification of the compression preparation. **A,** A portion of the aspirate is expelled onto a glass microscope slide. **B,** Another slide is placed over the sample, causing the sample to spread. If necessary, gentle digital pressure can be applied to the top slide to spread the sample more. Care must be taken not to place excessive pressure on the slide, which could cause the cells to rupture. **C,** The top slide is rotated approximately 45 degrees and lifted directly upward to produce a squash preparation with subtle ridges and valleys of cells **(D).**

tends to not damage fragile cells, but it does allow a thick layer of tissue fluid to remain around the cells. Sometimes the thick layer of fluid prevents the cells from spreading well and interferes with the evaluation of cell detail. Usually, however, some acceptable areas are present.

> **TECHNICIAN NOTE** The starfish smear, which is also called the needle-spread technique, is ideal for the preparation of viscous samples.

Preparation of Smears From Fluid Samples

Cytologic smears should be prepared immediately after fluid collection. When possible, fluid samples for cytologic examination should be collected in ethylenediaminetetraacetic acid (EDTA) tubes. Smears may be prepared directly from fresh, well-mixed fluid or from the sediment of a centrifuged sample by wedge (blood) smear, line smear, or compression preparation techniques. The cellularity, viscosity, and homogeneity of the fluid influence the selection of the smear technique.

Line Smear

When the fluid cannot be concentrated by centrifugation or the centrifuged sample is of low cellularity, the line smear technique may be used to concentrate cells in the smear (Fig. 38.6). A drop of fluid is placed on a clean glass slide, and the blood smear technique is used, except the spreading slide is raised directly upward approximately three fourths of the way through the smear, yielding a line that contains a much higher concentration of cells than the rest of the slide. Unfortunately, an excessive amount of fluid may also remain in that line and prevent the cells from spreading well.

The compression preparation technique often spreads viscous samples and samples with flecks of particulate material better than the blood smear and line smear techniques. The blood smear technique usually produces well-spread smears of sufficient cellularity from homogeneous fluids that contain at least 5000 cells/μL, but it often produces smears of insufficient cellularity from fluids containing less than 5000 cells/μL. The line smear technique may be used to concentrate fluids of low cellularity, but often it does not sufficiently spread cells from highly cellular fluids. In general, translucent fluids are of low to moderate cellularity, whereas opaque fluids usually have high cellularity. Therefore, translucent fluids often require concentration, either by centrifugation or by the line smear technique. When possible, concentration by centrifugation is preferred.

> **TECHNICIAN NOTE** Samples with low cellularity and small volume should be prepared with the line smear technique.

To prepare a smear by the wedge (blood smear) technique, a small drop of the fluid is placed on a glass slide approximately 1.0 to 1.5 cm from the end. Another slide is pulled backward at a 30- to 40-degree angle until it makes contact with the drop. When the fluid flows sideways along the juncture between the slides, the second slide is quickly and smoothly pushed forward until the fluid has all drained away from the second slide. This procedure makes a smear with a feathered edge.

FIXING AND STAINING THE CYTOLOGY SAMPLE

Although many stains incorporate a cellular fixative, accomplishing this as a separate step in the procedure is advantageous to ensure the highest-quality preparation. The preferred fixative for cytology specimens is 95% methanol. The methanol must be fresh and not contaminated with stain or cellular debris. Methanol containers must be protected from evaporation and dilution that results from environmental humidity, which will introduce humidity artifacts onto the slide. The prepared cytology slides should remain in the fixative for 2 to 5 minutes. Longer fixative times will improve the quality of the staining procedure and not harm the samples.

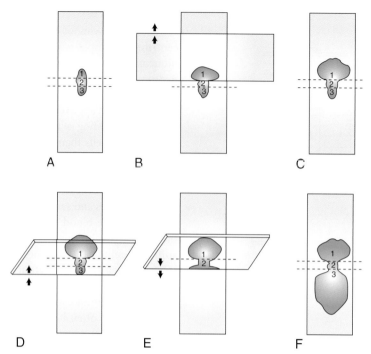

Fig. 38.4 Combination cytologic preparation. **A,** A portion of the aspirate is expelled onto a glass microscope slide (the prep slide). **B,** Another glass microscope slide (the spreader slide) is placed over approximately one third of the preparation. If additional spreading of the aspirate is needed, gentle digital pressure can be used. Excessive pressure should be avoided. **C,** The spreader slide is slid smoothly forward. This procedure makes a compression preparation of approximately one third of the aspirate *(1)*. The spreader slide also contains a squash preparation (not depicted). Next, the edge of a tilted glass microscope slide (a second spreader slide) is slid backward from the end opposite the compression preparation until it makes contact with approximately one third of the expelled aspirate **(D and E)**. **F,** The second spreader slide is then slid rapidly and smoothly forward. These steps produce an area *(3)* that is spread with mechanical forces like those of a blood smear preparation. The middle area *(2)* is left untouched, and it contains a high concentration of cells.

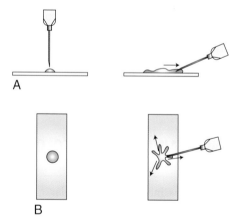

Fig. 38.5 Needle spread or "starfish" preparation. **A,** A portion of the aspirate is expelled onto a glass microscope slide. **B,** The tip of a needle is placed in the aspirate and moved peripherally to pull a tail of the sample with it. This procedure is repeated in several directions, which results in a preparation with multiple projections.

TECHNICIAN NOTE Prepared cytology slides should remain in fixative for a minimum of 2 to 5 minutes before staining.

Several types of stains have been used for cytologic preparations. The two general types that are most commonly used are the Romanowsky-type stains (e.g., Wright's, Giemsa, Diff-Quik, DipStat) and Papanicolaou stain and its derivatives (e.g., Sano's trichrome). The advantages and disadvantages of both types of stains are discussed. However, because the Romanowsky-type stains are more rewarding, practical, and readily available in practice situations, the remainder of this discussion deals predominantly with Romanowsky-stained preparations.

Romanowsky Stains

Romanowsky stains are inexpensive, readily available, and easy to prepare, maintain, and use. They stain organisms and the cytoplasm of cells excellently. Although nuclear and nucleolar detail cannot be perceived as well with Romanowsky stains as with Papanicolaou stains, nuclear and nucleolar detail is usually sufficient for differentiating neoplasia from inflammation and for evaluating neoplastic cells for cytologic evidence of malignant potential (criteria of malignancy).

Smears to be stained with Romanowsky stains are first air dried. Air drying partially preserves (fixes) the cells and causes

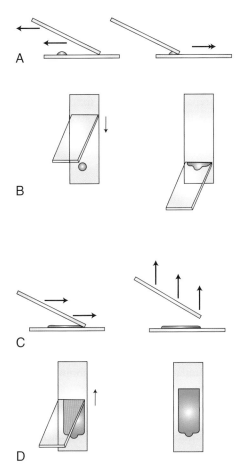

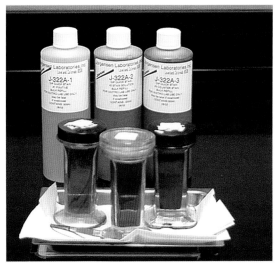

Fig. 38.7 A three-step Romanowsky stain suitable for cytology samples.

Fig. 38.6 Line smear concentration technique. **A,** A drop of fluid sample is placed on a glass microscope slide close to one end. **B,** Another slide is slid backward to make contact with the front of the drop. When the drop is contacted, it rapidly spreads along the juncture between the two slides. **C,** The spreader slide is then smoothly and rapidly slid forward. **D,** After the spreader slide has been advanced approximately two thirds to three fourths of the distance required to make a smear with a feathered edge, the spreader slide is raised directly upward. This procedure produces a smear with a line of concentrated cells at its end rather than a feathered edge.

cause a problem after evaluators become familiar with the stains that they routinely use.

Each stain usually has a unique recommended staining procedure. These procedures should be followed in general, but they should be adapted to the type and thickness of the smear being stained and to the evaluator's preference. The thinner the smear and the lower the total protein concentration of the fluid, the less time needed in the stain. The thicker the smear and the greater the total protein concentration of the fluid, the more time needed in the stain. As a result, fluid smears with low protein and low cellularity (e.g., abdominal fluid) may stain better in half or less of the recommended time. Thick smears (e.g., those of neoplastic lymph nodes) may need to be stained for twice the recommended time or longer. Each technician tends to have a different preferred staining technique. By trying variations in the recommended time intervals for stains, the evaluator can establish which times produce the preferred staining characteristics.

them to adhere to the slide so that they do not fall off during the staining procedure.

Many Romanowsky stains are commercially available, including Diff-Quik (Dade Behring, Deerfield, IL), DipStat (Medichem, Inc., Santa Monica, CA), and other quick Wright's stains (Fig. 38.7). Most—if not all—Romanowsky stains are acceptable for the staining of cytologic preparations. Diff-Quik stain does not undergo the metachromatic reaction. As a result, granules of some mast cells do not stain. When mast cell granules do not stain, the mast cells may be misclassified as macrophages, which may lead to confusion during the examination of some mast cell tumors. Increasing the fixative time to approximately 15 minutes may alleviate this problem. In addition, during the evaluation of blood smears or bone marrow aspirates, Diff-Quik does not stain polychromatophilic red blood cells well and occasionally does not stain basophils. The variations among different Romanowsky stains should not

New Methylene Blue Stain

New methylene blue (NMB) stain is a useful adjunct to Romanowsky stains (Fig. 38.8). It stains cytoplasm weakly, if at all, but it provides excellent nuclear and nucleolar detail. Because NMB stains cytoplasm weakly, the nuclear detail of cells in cell clumps may be better visualized. Generally, red blood cells do not stain with NMB, but they may develop a pale blue tint. As a result, marked red blood cell contamination of smears does not obscure nucleated cells.

> **TECHNICIAN NOTE** New methylene blue stain provides excellent nuclear detail, but it stains cytoplasm weakly.

Papanicolaou Stains

The delicate Papanicolaou stains give excellent nuclear detail and delicate cytoplasmic detail. They allow the viewer to see through

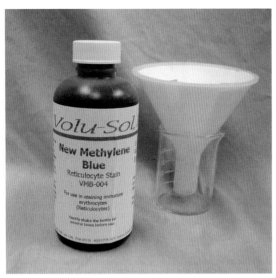

Fig. 38.8 New methylene blue stain is used when critical nuclear detail must be visualized.

layers of cells in cell clumps and to evaluate nuclear and nucleolar changes well. They do not stain cytoplasm as strongly as Romanowsky stains and therefore do not demonstrate cytoplasmic changes as well. They also do not demonstrate bacteria and other organisms as well as Romanowsky stains do.

Papanicolaou staining requires multiple steps and considerable time. In addition, the necessary reagents are often difficult to locate, prepare, and maintain in practice. Papanicolaou stains and their derivatives require the specimen to be wet fixed (i.e., the smear must be fixed before the cells have dried). Wet fixing requires spraying the smear with a cytologic fixative or placing it in ethanol immediately after preparation. When the smear is to be placed in ethanol, it should be made on a protein-coated slide, which prevents the cells from falling off the slide when the slide is immersed.

Staining Problems

Poor stain quality often perplexes both novice and experienced cytologists. Most staining problems can be avoided if the following precautions are taken:

- Always use new, clean slides. Even "precleaned" slides should be wiped with alcohol before use to remove residue.
- Fresh, well-filtered (if periodic filtration is required) stains and fresh buffer solution (if a buffer is required) should be used.
- Cytologic preparations should be fixed immediately after air drying unless they are being sent to an outside laboratory. The outside laboratory should be consulted before the slides are fixed.
- The surface of the slide or smear should not be touched at any time by human hands.

Occasionally a sample may be contaminated with a foreign substance (e.g., lubrication jelly) that alters the specimen's staining. Table 38.1 shows some of the problems that can occur with Romanowsky stains and some proposed solutions to these problems.

SUBMISSION OF CYTOLOGIC PREPARATIONS AND SAMPLES FOR INTERPRETATION

When the in-house evaluation of a cytologic preparation does not furnish sufficient reliable information for the management of a case, the preparation may be submitted to a veterinary clinical pathologist or cytologist for interpretation, or an alternative procedure (e.g., biopsy and histopathologic evaluation) may be performed. If possible, the person to whom the cytologic preparation is sent should be contacted, and specifics concerning sample handling should be discussed (e.g., the number of smears to send, whether to fix or stain the smears before mailing).

When possible, two or three air-dried unstained smears and two or three air-dried Romanowsky-stained smears should be submitted. Pathologists may stain the air-dried unstained smears with the Romanowsky or NMB stains of their choice. The Romanowsky-stained smears are a safety factor. Some tissues stain poorly when they are air dried but not stained for several days. In addition, slides occasionally are shattered during transport and cannot be stained on receipt. Sometimes the microscopic examination of shards from the broken prestained smears allows for diagnosis. If only a few smears can be prepared from the sample, one should be submitted air dried and

TABLE 38.1	Problems That Can Occur With Romanowsky Stains and Proposed Solutions
Problem	Solution
Excessive Blue Staining (RBCs May Be Blue-Green)	
Prolonged stain contact	Decrease staining time
Inadequate wash	Wash longer
Specimen too thick	Make thinner smears, if possible
Stain, diluent, buffer, or wash water too alkaline	Check with pH paper and correct pH
Exposure to formalin vapor	Store and ship cytologic preparations separate from formalin containers
Wet fixation in ethanol	Air dry smears before fixation
Delayed fixation	Fix smears sooner, if possible
Surface of the slide was alkaline	Use new slides

TABLE 38.1 Problems That Can Occur With Romanowsky Stains and Proposed Solutions—cont'd

Problem	Solution
Excessive Pink Staining	
Insufficient staining time	Increase staining time
Prolonged washing	Decrease duration of wash
Stain or diluent too acidic	Check with pH paper and correct pH; fresh methanol may be needed
Excessive time in red stain solution	Decrease time in red stain solution
Inadequate time in blue stain solution	Increase time in blue stain solution
Mounting coverslip before preparation is dry	Allow preparation to dry completely before mounting coverslip
Weak Staining	
Insufficient contact with one or more of the stain solutions	Increase staining time
Fatigued (old) stains	Change stains
Another slide covered specimen during staining	Keep slides separate
Uneven Staining	
Variation of pH in different areas of slide surface (may be caused by slide surface being touched or slide being poorly cleaned)	Use new slides and avoid touching their surfaces before and after preparation
Water allowed to stand on some areas of the slide after staining and washing	Tilt slides close to vertical to drain water from the surface or dry with a fan
Inadequate mixing of stain and buffer	Mix stain and buffer thoroughly
Precipitate on Preparation	
Inadequate stain filtration	Filter or change the stains
Inadequate washing of slide after staining	Rinse slide well after staining
Dirty slides used	Use new, clean slides
Stain solution dries during staining	Use sufficient stain and do not leave it on slide too long
Miscellaneous	
Overstained preparations	Destain with 95% methanol and restain; Diff-Quik—stained smears may have to be destained in the red Diff-Quik stain solution to remove the blue color; however, this damages the red stain solution
Refractile artifact on RBC with Diff-Quik stain (usually a result of moisture in the fixative)	Change the fixative

RBC, Red blood cell.

unstained and the other submitted air dried, fixed, and stained. Smears should be well labeled with alcohol-resistant ink or another permanent labeling method. If a Papanicolaou stain is to be used, several wet-fixed smears should be submitted. When biopsies or aspirates are not obtainable or warranted, swabs are useful for sample collection, especially swabs of mucosal surfaces and those from deep within soft-tissue lesions.

Fluid samples should have smears prepared from them immediately. Direct smears and concentrated smears should be submitted. In addition, an EDTA tube (lavender top) and a sterile serum tube (red top) fluid sample should be submitted. A total nucleated cell count and total protein concentration can be performed on the EDTA tube sample, and, if necessary, chemical analyses can be performed on the serum tube sample.

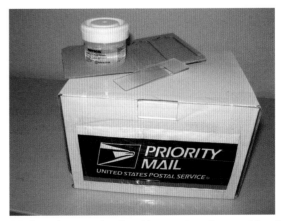

Fig. 38.9 Preparing samples for shipment to reference laboratories. Unfixed slides must not be in proximity to formalin containers.

Slides must be protected when they are mailed. Simple cardboard mailers do not provide sufficient protection to prevent slide breakage if they are mailed in unpadded envelopes. Marking the envelope with phrases such as "Fragile," "Glass," "Breakable," and "Please hand cancel" has little effect. Placing a pad of bubble wrap or polystyrene on each side of the slide holder usually prevents slide breakage. Slides may also be mailed in plastic slide holders or innovative holders, such as small pill bottles.

Unfixed slides should not be mailed with samples that contain formalin, and they should be protected against moisture. Formalin fumes alter the staining characteristics of smears, and water causes cell lysis (Fig. 38.9).

KEY POINTS

- Commonly performed methods for the preparation of solid samples for cytologic evaluation include the compression smear, the starfish smear, and combination methods.
- Fluid samples can be prepared with the compression smear or the line smear.
- Preparation methods are based on the characteristics of the sample and the volume of sample obtained.
- A variety of preparation methods may be needed, and multiple preps are usually made.

- The compression preparation is the most commonly used method.
- Line smears are preferred when sample volume is small and cellularity is low.
- Cytology slides are fixed with methanol before they are stained.
- Most cytology samples can be stained with Romanowsky stain.

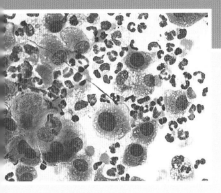

39

Microscopic Evaluation of Cytology

LEARNING OBJECTIVES

After studying this chapter, you will be able to:

- Describe the general procedure for the evaluation of cytology samples.
- Describe the general appearance of samples from inflammatory lesions.
- Describe the general appearance of samples from neoplastic lesions.

- State the nuclear criteria of malignancy.
- Differentiate between suppurative, granulomatous, pyogranulomatous, and eosinophilic inflammation.
- Describe the general tumor types.
- State the characteristics of samples from each of the general categories of tumors.

OUTLINE

Inflammation, 305

Neoplasia, 308

KEY TERMS

Anisokaryosis
Anisonucleoliosis
Benign
Carcinoma
Discrete round cell tumors
Eosinophilic
Epithelial cell tumors
Granulomatous
Histiocytoma

Karyolysis
Karyorrhexis
Lymphoma
Malignant
Mast cell tumors
Melanoma
Mesenchymal cell tumors
Neoplasia
Nuclear molding

Plasma cell tumors
Pleomorphism
Pyknosis
Pyogranulomatous
Sarcoma
Suppurative
Transmissible venereal tumors

The primary purpose of the cytology evaluation is to differentiate inflammation from neoplasia. The evaluation should proceed in a systematic manner and is focused initially on determining the predominant cell types present. Any morphologic abnormalities present are also noted and quantified. The presence of any infectious agents is also noted. Fig. 39.1 summarizes the steps in the evaluation of cytology specimens. The initial evaluation of the cytology preparation should be performed with low magnification (100×) to determine whether all areas are adequately stained and to detect any localized areas of increased cellularity. To improve resolution by decreasing light refraction, a drop of oil can be placed on the smear and a coverslip added. A consistent approach to examination helps to ensure high-quality results. Large objects such as cell clusters, parasites, crystals, and fungal hyphae are normally evident during the low-power examination. This initial evaluation should be used to characterize the cellularity and composition of the sample by recording the types of cells present and the relative

numbers of each type. A high-power examination (400× to 450×) should then be performed to evaluate and compare individual cells and to further characterize the types of cells present. Oil immersion must be used to identify specific nuclear criteria of malignancy and cytoplasmic abnormalities that are indicative of malignancy and various inflammatory reactions. The cytology report should indicate the cell types present, their appearance, and their relative proportions.

> **TECHNICIAN NOTE** Always examine the entire slide under low magnification to determine if it is adequately stained and to detect any localized areas of increased cellularity.

INFLAMMATION

Inflammation is a normal physiologic response to tissue damage or invasion by microorganisms. This damage releases

305

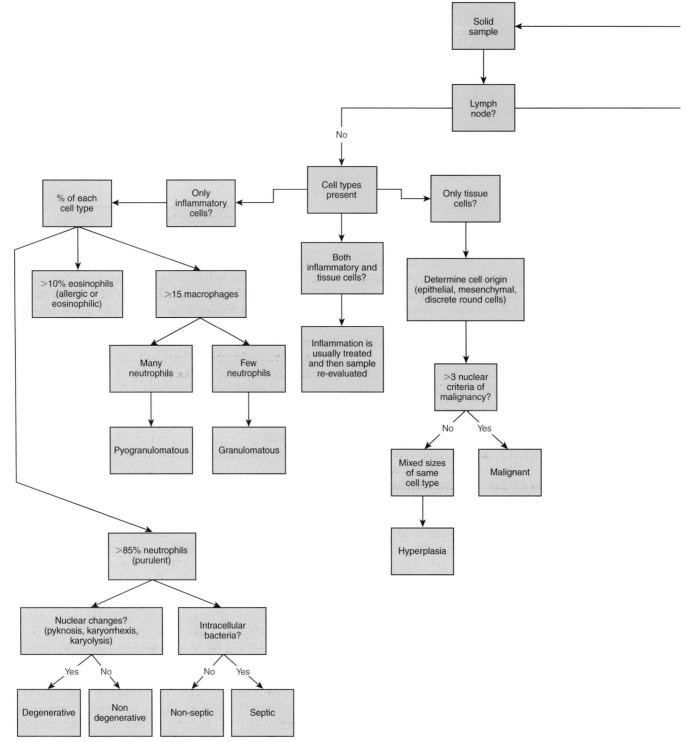

Fig. 39.1 Flow chart for the examination of cytology specimens.

substances that have a chemotactic effect on certain white blood cells. These chemotactic factors are therefore involved in attracting white blood cells to the site of inflammation. The first white blood cells to arrive are the neutrophils. Neutrophils phagocytize dead tissue and microorganisms. The process of phagocytosis creates pH changes both within the neutrophils and in the site. As the pH changes, neutrophils become unable

to phagocytize any further, and the cells quickly die. At this point, macrophages move in to the site and pick up the phagocytic activity. Cytology samples from inflammatory sites are therefore characterized by the presence of white blood cells, particularly neutrophils and macrophages. Occasionally eosinophils or lymphocytes may also be present. In fluid samples, total nucleated cell counts of more than 5000/µL are common

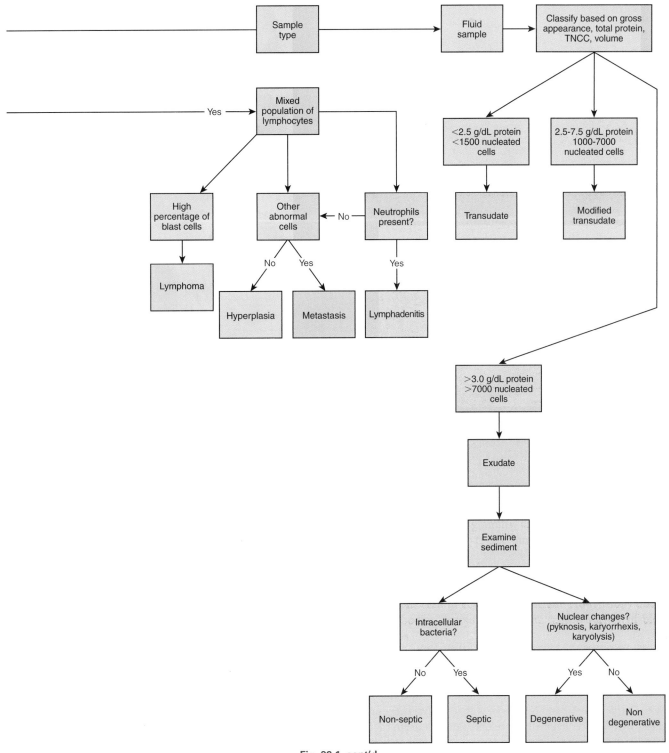

Fig. 39.1, cont'd

findings with inflammation. The fluid is often turbid, and it may be white or pale yellow. The total protein count is often more than 3 g/dL.

Inflammation can be categorized as suppurative (purulent), granulomatous, pyogranulomatous, or eosinophilic on the basis of the relative numbers of the various cell types present.

> **TECHNICIAN NOTE** Samples from inflammatory lesions are characterized by a predominance of leukocytes.

Suppurative (purulent) inflammation (Fig. 39.2) is characterized by the presence of large numbers of neutrophils that

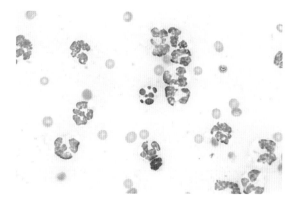

Fig. 39.2 Suppurative inflammation as evidenced by a large number of neutrophils. Note the presence of karyorrhexis in the center cell.

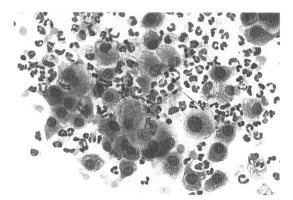

Fig. 39.3 Pyogranulomatous inflammation. Macrophages represent more than 15% of the cells present.

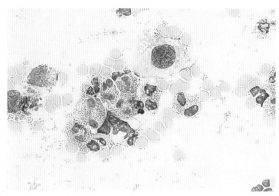

Fig. 39.4 Eosinophilic inflammation. Note the single macrophage and the numerous free eosinophilic granules.

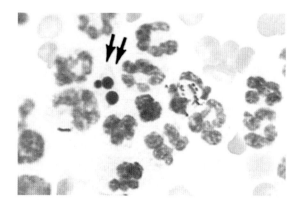

Fig. 39.5 Septic inflammation. Note the degenerated neutrophils with phagocytized bacterial rods. A pyknotic cell *(double arrow)* is also present.

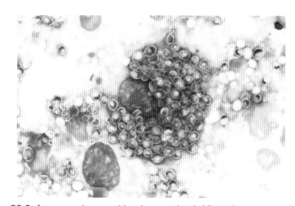

Fig. 39.6 A macrophage with phagocytized *Histoplasma capsulatum* organisms. Numerous organisms are also free in this sample.

> **TECHNICIAN NOTE** Karyolysis, karyorrhexis, and pyknosis are common nuclear changes that may be seen in inflammatory cells.

NEOPLASIA

Unlike inflammation, neoplastic specimens normally contain rather homogeneous populations of a single cell type.

usually make up more than 85% of the total nucleated cell count. When significant numbers of macrophages are present (i.e., more than 15% of the total count), the sample is classified as granulomatous or pyogranulomatous (Fig. 39.3). Fungal and parasitic infections often manifest with this presentation. The presence of more than 10% of eosinophils in addition to increased numbers of neutrophils indicates an eosinophilic inflammation (Fig. 39.4). This is usually found with parasitic infections, but it may also be present with some neoplastic disorders.

After they have been designated as inflammatory, the cells must also be evaluated for evidence of degeneration and for the presence of microorganisms. Nuclear changes that may be found in inflammatory cells (e.g., neutrophils) include karyolysis, karyorrhexis, and pyknosis, with karyolysis having the greatest significance. Pyknosis represents slow cell death (aging) and refers to a small, condensed, dark nucleus that may fragment (karyorrhexis). Karyolysis represents rapid cell death, as occurs with some septic (bacterial) inflammatory reactions. It appears as a swollen, ragged nucleus without an intact nuclear membrane and with reduced staining intensity. Cells should also be evaluated for the presence of bacteria. Inflammatory cells that contain phagocytized microorganisms are referred to as septic (Fig. 39.5). Additional phagocytized material may include erythrocytes, parasites, and fungal organisms (Fig. 39.6).

Although mixed cell populations are sometimes seen, these usually involve a neoplastic area with a concurrent inflammation. Neoplasia is indicated when the cells that are present are of the same tissue origin. After cells have been identified as neoplastic, the technician should identify the tissue origin and evaluate the cells for the presence of malignant characteristics (Table 39.1).

> **TECHNICIAN NOTE** Samples from neoplastic lesions are characterized by a homogenous population of cells of the same tissue origin.

Neoplasia must first be differentiated as either benign or malignant. Benign neoplasia is represented by hyperplasia with no criteria of malignancy present in the nucleus of the cells. The cells are of the same type, and they are relatively uniform in appearance. Cells that display at least three abnormal nuclear configurations are identified as malignant. The nuclear criteria of malignancy can include any of the following:

- Anisokaryosis: Any unusual variation in the overall size of the cell nucleus
- Pleomorphism: Variability in the size and shape of the same cell type
- High or variable nucleus-to-cytoplasm ratio
- Increased mitotic activity: Mitosis is rare in normal tissue, and cells usually divide evenly in two. Any increase in the presence of mitotic figures or cells that are not dividing equally is considered a malignancy criterion.
- Coarse chromatin pattern: The chromatin pattern is coarser than normal and may appear ropy or cordlike.
- Nuclear molding: A deformation of nuclei by other nuclei within the same cell or adjacent cells
- Multinucleation: Multiple nuclei within a cell
- Nucleoli that vary in size (anisonucleoliosis), shape (angular nucleoli), and number (multiple nucleoli)

In general, if three or more nuclear criteria of malignancy are present, the specimen is identified as malignant. Exceptions to this general rule are indicated if inflammation is also present or if only a few cells display malignant characteristics. The histopathologic verification of cytologic findings is important for most tumors, whether they are cytologically benign or malignant. In addition, cytologically benign cells may be obtained from malignant tumors. Histopathologic examination offers the advantage of enabling the assessment of factors, such as local tissue infiltration and vessel or lymphatic invasion by tumor cells. These characteristics of malignant tumors are not evident cytologically.

> **TECHNICIAN NOTE** Cells that display at least three abnormal nuclear configurations are identified as malignant.

TABLE 39.1   Nuclear Criteria of Malignancy

Criteria	Description	Schematic Representation
Macrokaryosis	Increased nuclear size. Cells with nuclei >10 μ in diameter suggest malignancy.	
Increased nucleus-to-cytoplasm (N:C) ratio	Normal nonlymphoid cells usually have an N:C of 1:3 to 1:8, depending on the tissue. Ratios ≥1:2 suggest malignancy.	See *Macrokaryosis*
Anisokaryosis	Variation in nuclear size. This is especially important if the nuclei of multinucleated cells vary in size.	
Multinucleation	Multiple nucleation in a cell. This is especially important if the nuclei vary in size.	
Increased mitotic figures	Mitosis is rare in normal tissue.	
Abnormal mitosis	Chromosomes are improperly aligned.	See *Increased mitotic figures*
Coarse chromatin pattern	The chromatin pattern is coarser than normal. It may appear ropy or cordlike.	
Nuclear molding	Nuclei are deformed by other nuclei within the same cell or adjacent cells.	
Macronucleoli	Nucleoli are increased in size. Nucleoli ≥5 μ strongly suggest malignancy. For reference, RBCs are 5 to 6 μ in cats and 7 to 8 μ in dogs.	
Angular nucleoli	Nucleoli are fusiform or have other angular shapes instead of their normal round to slightly oval shape.	
Anisonucleoliosis	Nucleolar shape or size varies. This is especially important if the variation is within the same nucleus.	See *Angular nucleoli*

RBC, Red blood cell.

TABLE 39.2   General Appearance of the Three Basic Tumor Categories

Tumor Type	General Cell Size	General Cell Shape	Schematic Representation	Cellularity of Aspirates	Clumps or Clusters Common
Epithelial	Large	Round to caudate		Usually high	Yes
Mesenchymal (spindle cell)	Small to medium	Spindle to stellate	Mast cell Lymphosarcoma	Usually low	No
Discrete round cell	Small to medium	Round	Transmissible veneral tumor Histocytoma	Usually high	No

From Sirois M: *Principles and practice of veterinary technology,* ed 3, St Louis, 2011, Mosby.

Specimens that have been classified as malignant should be further evaluated to determine the cell type involved. The primary types of tumors that are encountered in veterinary medicine are categorized as epithelial cell tumors, mesenchymal cell tumors, and discrete round cell tumors. The overall characteristics of samples from each of these cell types are summarized in Table 39.2.

Epithelial cell tumors are also referred to as carcinoma or adenocarcinoma. The samples tend to be highly cellular, and they often exfoliate in clumps or sheets (Fig. 39.7). Mesenchymal cell tumors are also referred to as sarcoma, and they are usually less cellular. The cells tend to exfoliate singly or in wispy spindles (Fig. 39.8). Discrete round cell tumors exfoliate very well, but are usually not in clumps or clusters. Round cell tumors include histiocytoma, lymphoma, mast cell tumors, plasma cell tumors, transmissible venereal tumors, and melanoma. Histiocytoma and transmissible venereal tumors appear somewhat similar except that histiocytoma is not usually highly cellular (Fig. 39.9). Plasma cell tumors can be recognized by the presence of large numbers of cells with an eccentrically located nucleus and a prominent perinuclear clear zone (Fig. 39.10). Mast cells can be recognized by their prominent purple/black granules (Fig. 39.11). Melanoma is characterized by cells with prominent dark black granules (Fig. 39.12). Occasionally, cells from poorly differentiated tumors may contain few or no granules (amelanotic melanoma). A variety of terminology is used to describe these various tumor types, and some references may differ with regard to their classification of specific types of tumors.

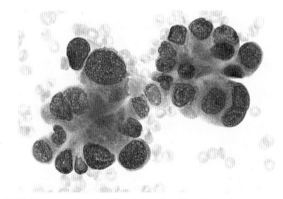

Fig. 39.7 Lung carcinoma. Clusters of cells with anisokaryosis, binucleation, and high and variable nucleus-to-cytoplasm ratios are present.

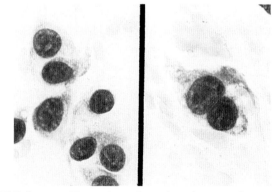

Fig. 39.8 Sarcoma. The aspirate shown here from a malignant spindle cell tumor includes cells that demonstrate anisokaryosis; anisonucleoliosis; and large, prominent, and occasionally angular nucleoli.

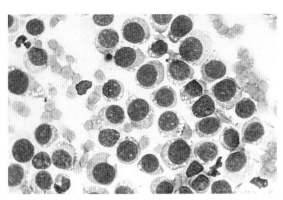

Fig. 39.9 Large numbers of round cells from an imprint of a transmissible venereal tumor.

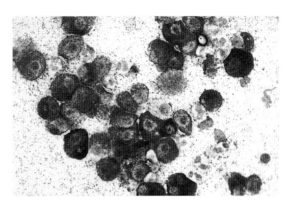

Fig. 39.11 Aspirate from a highly granular mast cell tumor. Several eosinophils are also present.

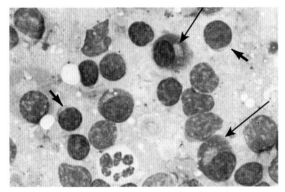

Fig. 39.10 Several plasma cells are evident in this sample taken from a hyperplastic lymph node. Small lymphocytes are also present *(arrows)*.

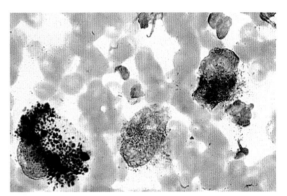

Fig. 39.12 A melanophage *(uppermost cell)* and two melanocytes.

KEY POINTS

- Samples that appear inflammatory can be categorized as suppurative (purulent), granulomatous, pyogranulomatous, or eosinophilic on the basis of the relative numbers of the various cell types present.
- Neoplastic specimens normally contain homogeneous populations of a single cell type.
- Benign neoplasia is described as hyperplasia with no criteria of malignancy present in the nucleus of the cells.
- Nuclear criteria of malignancy can include anisokaryosis; pleomorphism; a high or variable nucleus-to-cytoplasm ratio; increased mitotic figures; a coarse chromatin pattern;
- nuclear molding; multinucleation; and nucleoli that vary with regard to size, shape, and number.
- Samples from epithelial cell tumors tend to be highly cellular, and they often exfoliate in clumps or sheets.
- Samples from mesenchymal cell tumors tend to have low cellularity, and they exfoliate singly or in wispy spindles.
- Samples from discrete round cell tumors tend to exfoliate very well, but they are usually not in clumps or clusters.
- Plasma cell tumors can be recognized by the presence of large numbers of cells with an eccentrically located nucleus and a prominent perinuclear clear zone.

40

Cytology of Specific Sites

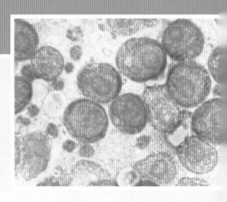

LEARNING OBJECTIVES

After studying this chapter, you will be able to:

- Describe the characteristics of samples of normal peritoneal and pleural fluid.
- State the criteria that are used to classify a sample as an exudate, a transudate, or a modified transudate.
- List and describe the cell types that are seen in normal lymph nodes.
- Describe the appearance of a sample from a reactive lymph node.
- Describe the characteristics of samples of normal synovial fluid.
- Describe the appearance of samples collected via tracheal wash.
- Describe the appearance of vaginal cytology samples from a normal female.
- Describe the evaluations that are performed on semen samples.

OUTLINE

KEY TERMS

Cornified	Modified transudate	Reactive lymph node
Curschmann's spirals	Parabasal	Synovial fluid
Exudate	Peritoneal fluid	Transudate
Lymphoma	Pleural fluid	Wave motion

EAR SWABS

Evaluation of samples from the ear canal aids in the diagnosis of otitis externa. Samples are collected prior to initiation of treatment using cotton swabs, with a separate swab used for each ear. The swab is introduced into the ear either directly or through an otoscope (Fig. 40.1). The secretions collected are

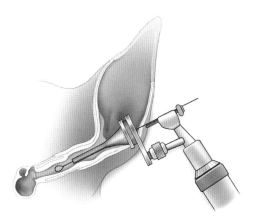

Fig. 40.1 Smears of horizontal ear canal secretions may be collected by passing a cotton-tipped swab through the cone of an otoscope after otoscopic examination. (From Valenciano A, Cowell R: *Cowell and Tyler's diagnostic cytology and hematology of the dog and cat*, ed 4, St Louis, 2014, Mosby.)

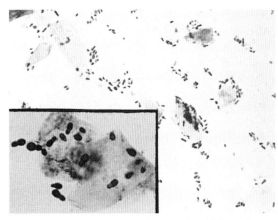

Fig. 40.2 Sample from an ear swab that contains *Malassezia* organisms.

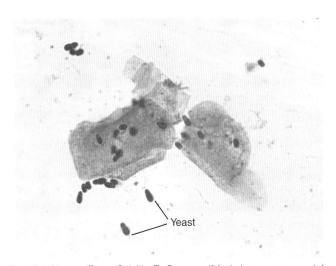

Fig 40.3 Yeast. (From Colville T, Bassert JM: *Laboratory manual for clinical anatomy and physiology for veterinary technicians*, ed 4, 2024, Elsevier Inc.)

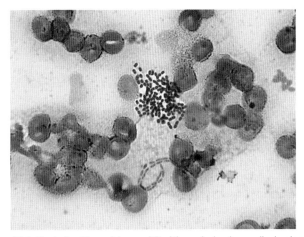

Fig. 40.4 Bacteria. (From Murray PR: *Murray's basic medical microbiology: Foundations and clinical cases*, ed 2, 2024, Elsevier Inc.)

then rolled onto a clean glass slide. Ideally, two slides should be prepared from each swab. The first one is left unstained and a small amount of mineral oil added to the sample. A coverslip is added and the slide evaluated under low power and low light to identify any parasites present. The second slide is air-dried and stained with any routine hematology stain or with Gram stain. If excessive cerumen is present, the slide can be gently heat fixed to partially remove the cerumen, although this is not a requirement. The stained slide is best used for identification of bacteria and yeasts. Separate stain jars should be maintained for ear cytology so that any bacteria or yeasts from samples don't contaminate the stain jars used for hematology.

Samples from normal patients contain cornified squamous epithelial cells, with negligible evidence of inflammation and few microorganisms. Common abnormal findings are bacteria and yeasts, with or without inflammatory cells. Infections involving cocci primarily involve *Staphylococcus* spp. while infections with bacterial rods usually involve *Pseudomonas*. Common parasites that may be found include *Otodectes cynotis* and *Otobius megnini*.

The organism *Malassezia*, which is a potential cause of chronic skin lesions and ear infections, will stain with Gram stain, Diff-Quik, or even new methylene blue for a quick "wet prep." Look for the characteristic peanut-shaped organisms (Fig. 40.2). Some controversy exists among specialists regarding whether the presence of *Malassezia* in small numbers is significant. Some believe that any organisms found are grounds for treatment, whereas others claim that low numbers may be found in normal ears. When bacteria, yeasts, or mites are identified, the veterinary technician should report results as an average number seen per high power field (Figs. 40.3 and 40.4).

> **TECHNICIAN NOTE** Yeasts, squamous epithelial cells, and *Malassezia* organisms are commonly isolated from ear swabs.

PERITONEAL AND PLEURAL FLUID

Under normal circumstances, the peritoneal and thoracic cavities contain only enough fluid to adequately lubricate the surfaces of the organs and the cavity walls. Fluid is collected in ethylenediaminetetraacetic acid (EDTA) tubes for total nucleated cell counts (TNCCs), cytologic examination, and refractometric protein measurements and in plain tubes for the determination of the total protein concentration. Other clinical chemistry determinations are performed infrequently on the peritoneal and pleural fluids.

Color, Turbidity, and Odor

Normal peritoneal and pleural fluids are colorless to straw yellow and transparent to slightly turbid. Both fluids should be odorless. Gross discoloration and increased turbidity may be the result of increased cell numbers or protein concentrations. The collection of malodorous peritoneal fluid from an abdominocentesis may indicate a necrotic segment of bowel within the peritoneal cavity, a ruptured segment of bowel with free gut contents in the cavity, or accidental enterocentesis. These conditions may be distinguishable cytologically and by reference to other clinical findings. Although not commonly seen, chylothorax may be evident as a "milky" fluid, especially if the animal has recently eaten, because of the chylous effusion's high fat content and large number of mature lymphocytes. In fasted animals, the fluid may be tan. Unlike fluids with high leukocyte counts (which also may have a whitish color), chylous fluid does not have a clear supernatant after centrifugation. The fat in chylous fluid is present as small droplets (chylomicrons), which can be stained with Sudan III or IV. The fat in chylous fluid may be dissolved with ether after the fluid has been alkalinized with sodium hydroxide or sodium bicarbonate. If significant numbers of erythrocytes are present, the fluid may have a reddish color.

Total Nucleated Cell Count

A TNCC is performed using the same methods that are used for a complete blood count (see Unit 2). As a cross-species generalization, normal peritoneal and pleural fluids have less than 10,000 nucleated cells/µL (usually 2000/µL to 6000/µL). Mononuclear cells may be visible as clusters of cells, which can make counting individual cells difficult.

A differential count of at least 100 nucleated cells should be performed, with cell types and morphologic characteristics noted. Nucleated cells are categorized as neutrophils, large mononuclear cells (a collective grouping of mesothelial cells and macrophages), lymphocytes, eosinophils, and any other nucleated cells. Notes on cell morphologic characteristics should include comments about the nuclear and cytoplasmic appearance. If bacteria are present, their morphologic features (i.e., bacilli, coccobacilli, or cocci) and location (i.e., free or phagocytized) must be recorded. In such cases, another smear can be stained with Gram stain and the fluid cultured.

> **TECHNICIAN NOTE** Peritoneal and pleural fluids are evaluated for color, transparency, odor, and TNCC.

Cellular Elements

Normal peritoneal and pleural fluids contain few erythrocytes. The number present on a smear should be estimated. Suitable categories include rare, few, many, and large numbers. The number present varies with the method of sample preparation. Iatrogenic contamination and acute and chronic hemorrhage are distinguished grossly, as previously outlined. If erythrocytes have been present in the fluid for several hours, they may be phagocytized by macrophages (erythrophagocytosis) (Fig. 40.5).

Peritoneal and pleural fluid samples should also be evaluated for cellularity. The TNCC and total protein values for the sample allow it to be classified as transudate, modified transudate, or exudate (Table 40.1). Published normal values for the peritoneal and pleural fluid cytology of dogs and cats are scarce. Normal horses generally have an average of approximately 55% to 60% neutrophils, 25% to 30% large mononuclear cells, 10% to 20% lymphocytes, and an occasional eosinophil (less than 1%). Values for cattle are somewhat similar, but normal animals often have comparable numbers of neutrophils and lymphocytes.

Exudates are fluids with increased cellularity and protein concentration as a result of inflammation. The following cross-species generalization can be made. Suppurative inflammatory reactions increase the total cell count, the percentage, and the absolute numbers of neutrophils to more than 85% of the nucleated cells. Suppurative inflammatory reactions usually cause high-normal to elevated TNCCs, with elevated neutrophil percentages and numerous mesothelial cells, macrophages, or both. Mesothelial cells line the body cavities. In the presence of increased fluid within the cavities, these cells may become reactive (i.e., multinucleate, with anisocytosis and anisokaryosis, prominent nucleoli, and basophilic cytoplasm) (Fig. 40.6). Reactive mesothelial cells may be difficult to distinguish from some neoplastic cells. Some mesothelial cells may be present as clusters or rafts of cells. These clusters result from the proliferation and exfoliation of cells from the peritoneal lining, or the mesothelium, in response to a decrease in contact inhibition between cells on opposing surfaces of the peritoneum as a result of the effusion. Macrophages may

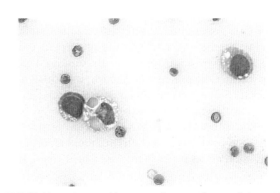

Fig. 40.5 Fluid aspirate with macrophages. One cell is exhibiting erythrophagia.

TABLE 40.1	Characteristics of Fluid Samples			
	Transudate	**Exudate**	**Normal**	**Modified Transudate**
Origin	Noninflammatory hypoalbuminemia Vascular stasis Neoplasia	Inflammatory Infection Necrosis		Feline infectious peritonitis Chylous effusion Lymphatic fluid
Amount of fluid	Large	Variable	Small	Variable
Color	Clear, colorless, or red-tinged	Turbid, white, or slightly yellow	Clear, colorless	Variable; usually clear
Protein	<3.0 g/dL	>3.0 g/dL	<2.5 g/dL	2.5–7.5 g/dL
Total nucleated cell count	<1500/μL	>5000/μL	<3000/μL	1000-7000/μL
Cell types	Mixture of monocytes, macrophages, lymphocytes, and mesothelial cells*	Inflammatory: neutrophils, macrophages, lymphocytes[†], and eosinophils[†]	Same as transudate	Lymphocytes, nondegenerate neutrophils, mesothelial cells, macrophages, and neoplastic cells

*Normal, reactive.
[†]Variable numbers.

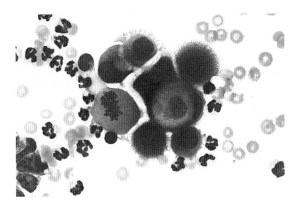

Fig. 40.6 A cluster of reactive mesothelial cells. Note the mitotic figure.

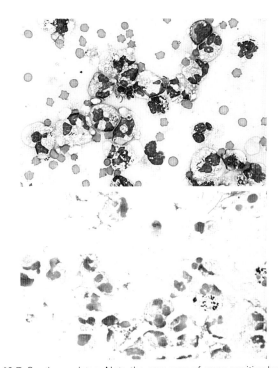

Fig. 40.7 Septic exudates. Note the presence of gram-positive bacterial rods.

phagocytize degenerate cells or cellular debris. Migrating parasite larvae can cause increased neutrophil and eosinophil percentages, with or without an elevated TNCC.

Cellular morphologic features depend on the microorganisms present. They may vary from cytoplasmic vacuolation with few nuclear changes evident to marked cytoplasmic vacuolation, marked nuclear swelling and disruption (karyolysis), and general cellular degeneration or fragmentation. Bacteria may be evident within the cytoplasm of neutrophils and macrophages (Fig. 40.7). Cases of simple peritonitis may have a single type of bacterium evident, or the bacterial population may be mixed as a result of devitalization or rupture of the bowel. Accidental penetration of the bowel during abdominocentesis may also result in a mixed population of bacteria in the smear. However, in the latter case, leukocyte numbers and morphologic characteristics are usually normal, and the bacteria are frequently not phagocytized. Large ciliated organisms may also be noted in large-bowel enterocentesis in horses.

Transudates (ascitic effusions) typically have low protein concentrations and low TNCCs (less than 500/μL), with fairly normal differential counts or possibly an increase in the percentage of large mononuclear cells (Fig. 40.8). The mononuclear cells are principally mesothelial cells, which may be in clusters or rafts and may be quite reactive in appearance. Transudates are frequently secondary to congestive heart failure, or they may occur in animals with low blood albumin concentrations.

Modified transudates are characterized by relatively low to moderate TNCCs, predominantly as a result of the leakage of lymphatics. This leakage is responsible for the high total protein concentration of modified transudates. Cells that are present include low numbers of inflammatory cells

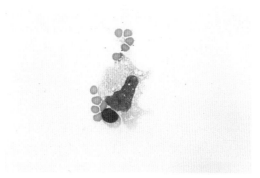

Fig. 40.8 Macrophage, small lymphocyte, and several red blood cells. This sample is characteristic of normal fluid and transudates.

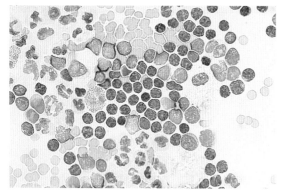

Fig. 40.9 Smear from a chylous effusion. A mixture of mature lymphocytes, neutrophils, and an eosinophil are present. This is characteristic of a modified transudate.

TABLE 40.2 Cell Types Found in Lymph Node Aspirates	
Cell Type	**Characteristics**
Lymphocytes, small	Similar in appearance to the small lymphocyte seen on a peripheral blood film; slightly larger than an RBC; scanty cytoplasm; dense nucleus
Lymphocytes, intermediate	Nucleus approximately twice as large as an RBC; abundant cytoplasm
Lymphoblasts	Two to four times as large as an RBC; usually contain a nucleolus; diffuse nuclear chromatin
Plasma cells	Eccentrically located nucleus, trailing basophilic cytoplasm, and perinuclear clear zone; vacuoles and/or Russell bodies may be present
Plasmablasts	Similar to lymphoblasts with more abundant basophilic cytoplasm; may contain vacuoles
Neutrophils	May appear similar to neutrophil in peripheral blood or show degenerative changes
Macrophages	Large phagocytic cells; may contain phagocytized debris, microorganisms, and so on; abundant cytoplasm
Mast cells	Round cells that are usually slightly larger than lymphoblasts; distinctive purple-staining granules may not stain adequately with Diff-Quik
Carcinoma cells	Epithelial tissue origin; usually found in clusters; pleomorphic
Sarcoma cells	Connective tissue origin; usually occur singly with spindle-shaped cytoplasm
Histiocytes	Large, pleomorphic, and single or multinuclear; nuclei are round to oval

RBC, Red blood cell.

(nondegenerate), mostly small mature lymphocytes, few macrophages, and some mesothelial cells (Fig. 40.9).

Intra-abdominal tumors may exfoliate cells into the peritoneal fluid. The cytologic diagnosis of such neoplasia may be difficult, and it is often a task for a specialist cytologist. However, the technician should be able to recognize abnormal lymphocytes by using the criteria of malignancy previously outlined and should be suspicious of clusters of pleomorphic, secretory-type cells. The presence of unexpected cells (e.g., mast cells) must also be noted.

> **TECHNICIAN NOTE** The evaluation of the cellular elements of fluid samples allows the samples to be classified as exudates, transudates, or modified transudates.

LYMPH NODES

The cytologic evaluation of lymph node tissue is performed to diagnose causes of lymph node enlargement and to differentiate among hyperplasia, inflammation, primary neoplasia (lymphoma), and metastatic neoplasia. Lymph nodes may show evidence of inflammation (lymphadenitis), hyperplasia (benign neoplasia), mixed (both inflammatory and neoplastic cells present), neoplasia (lymph node cells with abnormal nuclear features), and metastasis (neoplastic cells from other body tissues that spread to lymph nodes). Each of these has specific cell types that are associated with the abnormality.

Lymph node tissue is normally collected from the periphery of an enlarged lymph node by fine-needle biopsy. In patients with generalized lymphadenopathy, samples should be obtained from two lymph nodes. Because lymph nodes that drain the oral cavity and the gastrointestinal tract are antigenically stimulated under normal conditions, these should be avoided. Samples are then prepared by the compression technique and stained with standard Romanowsky-type stains.

A variety of cell types may be found in lymph node aspirates. These include lymphocytes, plasma cells, white blood cells, and neoplastic cells. Microorganisms, lymphoglandular bodies, and bacteria may also be present. Lymphoglandular bodies are small cytoplasmic fragments that may be seen between cells and that are not a pathologic feature. Table 40.2 contains a summary of the cell types that may be found in lymph node aspirates.

In a normal lymph node, the predominant cell type is the small, mature lymphocyte. These tend to comprise more than three fourths of the total cells present. Smaller numbers of intermediate lymphocytes and lymphoblasts as well as macrophages are also present. Plasma cells may occasionally be seen (Fig. 40.10). Mast cells are usually rare in cytologic preparations

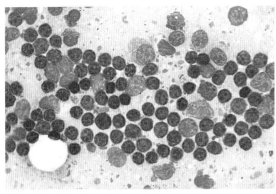

Fig. 40.10 Aspirate from a normal lymph node. Small, mature lymphocytes predominate.

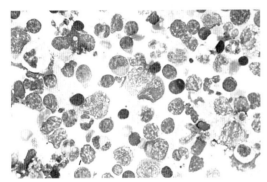

Fig. 40.11 Pyogranulomatous lymphadenitis. Numerous macrophages and neutrophils are evident, along with a mixture of lymphocyte types.

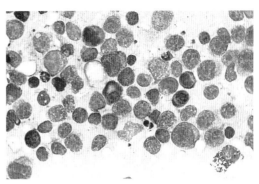

Fig. 40.12 An imprint of a reactive lymph node. Note the mixed population of small, medium, and large lymphocytes, plasma cells, and a mast cell *(lower right)*.

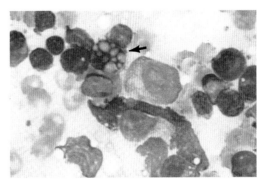

Fig. 40.13 The plasma cell that appears vacuolated *(arrow)* is a Mott cell that contains Russell bodies. Small lymphocytes and lymphoblasts are also present.

of lymph node tissue. Lymph nodes with evidence of inflammation (lymphadenitis) will have a predominance of phagocytic leukocytes (Fig. 40.11).

> **TECHNICIAN NOTE** Normal lymph nodes are characterized by a predominance of small, mature lymphocytes.

Reactive Lymph Nodes

Lymph nodes that are responding to antigenic stimulation also contain predominantly small, mature lymphocytes and are referred to as reactive lymph nodes. However, plasma cells, lymphoblasts, and intermediate lymphocytes are more abundant than they are in a normal lymph node (Fig. 40.12). Occasional Mott cells (plasma cells that contain secretory vesicles of immunoglobulin) may also be seen (Fig. 40.13). Antigenic stimulation can also cause an inflammatory response and would be characterized by the presence of neutrophils, macrophages, or both.

> **TECHNICIAN NOTE** Reactive lymph nodes contain predominantly small, mature lymphocytes as well as plasma cells, lymphoblasts, and intermediate lymphocytes.

Malignant Neoplasia

Primary lymphoid neoplasia, or lymphoma, is characterized by a predominance of lymphoblasts, and mitotic figures are common. Macrophages are also present, and plasma cells are scarce. Other neoplastic cells that may be present in lymph node aspirates include mast cells, carcinoma cells, sarcoma cells, and histiocytes. Cells that display at least three abnormal nuclear configurations are usually identified as malignant (Fig. 40.14). Lymph node samples may also contain metastatic cells from other body parts (Fig. 40.15).

CEREBROSPINAL FLUID

As a cross-species generalization, normal cerebrospinal fluid (CSF) contains no erythrocytes and less than 25 nucleated cells per microliter (usually 0 to 10 per µL). Pleocytosis is an elevated CSF nucleated cell count. Normal CSF contains 95% to 100% mononuclear cells, almost all of which are lymphocytes. Bacterial infections that involve CSF generally cause marked pleocytosis, mostly as a result of neutrophils. Inflammation associated with viruses, fungi, neoplasia, or degenerative conditions generally causes less dramatic pleocytosis, with a significant proportion of mononuclear cells (often lymphocytes). Eosinophils are sometimes seen, especially with parasitic

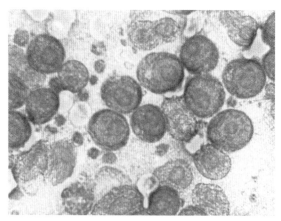

Fig. 40.14 Immature, neoplastic lymphocytes are present in this sample from a dog with malignant lymphoma.

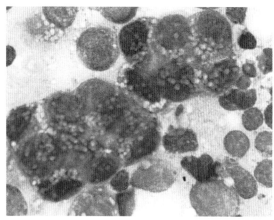

Fig. 40.15 An epithelial cell cluster from a transitional cell carcinoma that metastasized to a local lymph node.

inflammatory responses. In general, the causative agent often is not cytologically apparent. Neoplastic cells are seldom observed in CSF.

Normal CSF contains virtually no erythrocytes. Erythrocytes may be counted by charging a hemocytometer with a well-mixed sample of undiluted and unstained CSF. All cells in the entire boxed area of one side are counted. With this method, both erythrocytes and nucleated cells are observed. Distinguishing between these two groups of cells is usually possible, but not to subcategorize the nucleated cells. Cell counts for undiluted CSF are multiplied by 1.1 to give the total number of cells per microliter. (If ethanol-diluted CSF is used, the cell counts are multiplied by 2.2.) If distinguishing erythrocytes from nucleated cells in unstained CSF is difficult, the total number of cells counted by the latter method can be subtracted from the number of nucleated cells counted to calculate the erythrocyte count.

The use of various correction factors has been advocated to adjust CSF nucleated cell counts for any peripheral blood leukocytic contamination. Because normal CSF contains no erythrocytes, the observed nucleated cell count may be corrected if the number of erythrocytes per microliter of CSF is known. The simplest approach is to consider that each 500 to 1000 erythrocytes would be accompanied by a single leukocyte.

In addition to the cytology evaluation, a variety of chemical and immunologic tests are performed on CSF samples.

AQUEOUS AND VITREOUS HUMOR

Fluid from the eye is similar to CSF in that it has low cellularity. It is composed mostly of small mononuclear cells and essentially no erythrocytes, and it has a low protein concentration. The interpretation of changes in aqueous humor is similar to that of CSF.

SYNOVIAL FLUID ANALYSIS

If only one or two drops can be obtained, as in some normal joints of cats and dogs, the gross assessment of fluid color and turbidity as well as the cytologic examination of a direct smear (possibly with concurrent subjective assessment of viscosity) may be all that is practical. If 0.5 mL to 1 mL is collected, a TNCC and a refractometric protein measurement (on EDTA-preserved fluid) may be added to the list of tests. The collection of larger volumes allows for the performance of additional tests, such as the mucin clot test (see Chapter 24).

> **TECHNICIAN NOTE** Minimal evaluation of synovial fluid involves the assessment of color, turbidity, and examination of a direct smear.

Color and Turbidity

Normal synovial fluid is clear to straw yellow and nonturbid. Yellow synovial fluid is common in large animals, especially horses. Turbidity, when present, is caused by cells, protein (or fibrin), or cartilage.

Normal synovial fluid contains few erythrocytes. Iatrogenic contamination during arthrocentesis is common. The differentiation between contamination and recent or old hemorrhage is performed as previously described.

Viscosity

Viscosity reflects the quality and concentration of hyaluronic acid, which is part of the synovial fluid–mucin complex. The function of mucin is joint lubrication. Viscosity may be quantitated with a viscometer; however, subjective assessment is most often used.

Normal synovial fluid is sticky. If a drop is placed between the thumb and the forefinger, as the digits are separated, it forms a 1- to 2-inch strand before breaking. Similarly, when gently expressed through a needle on a horizontally held syringe, it hangs in a 1- to 2-inch strand before it separates from the needle tip.

In general, viscosity is not decreased in normal joints and in samples from patients with degenerative problems. It frequently is decreased in joints with bacterial inflammation as a result of mucin degradation by bacterial hyaluronidase and in joints with significant effusion (including hydrarthrosis) as a result of the dilution of mucin and hyaluronic acid.

Because EDTA may degrade hyaluronic acid, both viscosity and mucin clot formation usually are assessed on fluid to which no anticoagulant has been added. If anticoagulation is necessary as a result of a high fluid fibrinogen concentration, heparin is the preferred anticoagulant.

Slides for cell counts may be prepared on EDTA-preserved fluid or fluid without anticoagulant (the latter especially if only a few drops are obtained and the smear is made immediately). Thin smears are made by slowly advancing the spreader slide. Because of the high viscosity of normal synovial fluid, cells usually do not accumulate at the feathered edge of the smear. The margination of cells increases as the viscosity of the fluid decreases. At low cell counts (i.e., less than 500/µL), concentration of cells by centrifugal sedimentation and the subsequent resuspension of cells in a small volume of supernatant fluid produces a more cellular smear. Slides are usually stained with a Romanowsky stain. Table 40.3 summarizes the classification of synovial fluid.

Normal synovial fluid generally contains at least 90% mononuclear cells and less than 10% neutrophils (Fig. 40.16). Eosinophils are rarely observed. Mononuclear cells comprise about equal numbers of lymphocytes and monocytic/macrophage-type cells, which are nonvacuolated and nonphagocytic. Large vacuolated or phagocytic mononuclear cells comprise less than 10% of the differential count of normal synovial fluid. Macrophages become vacuolated in normal synovial fluid that is not processed soon after collection; therefore, the prompt preparation of smears is important to prevent this artificial finding.

Cells in synovial fluid with good viscosity tend to align in a linear fashion in the direction of the smear, giving a "windrow" appearance (Fig. 40.17). Mucin precipitation produces an eosinophilic granular background in Romanowsky-stained smears, the density of which reflects smear thickness. Cells in

smears from viscous fluid may not spread out well on the slide, which can make their identification difficult. Such fluid may be diluted 1:1 with saline-reconstituted hyaluronidase (150 U/mL).

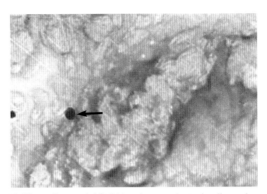

Fig. 40.16 Normal synovial fluid has low nucleated cell numbers with a thick, granular to ropy background material separating the cells. The low cellularity generally means that fewer than one to two small to medium-sized mononuclear cells are seen on high-power examination *(arrow)*. (From Raskin R, Meyer D: *Canine and feline cytology*, ed 2, St Louis, 2010, Saunders.)

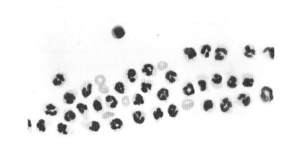

Fig. 40.17 Synovial fluid from a patient with inflammatory joint disease. These neutrophils are in the typical "windrow" arrangement that is commonly seen in synovial fluid. (From Raskin R, Meyer D: *Canine and feline cytology*, ed 2, St Louis, 2010, Saunders.)

TABLE 40.3 Classification of Synovial Fluid

	Normal	Hemarthrosis	Degenerative Arthropathy	Inflammatory Arthropathy
Appearance	Clear to straw-colored	Red, cloudy, or xanthochromic	Clear	Cloudy
Protein	<2.5 g/dL	Increased	Normal to decreased	Normal to increased
Viscosity	High	Decreased	Normal to decreased	Normal to decreased
Mucin clot	Good	Normal to poor	Normal to poor	Fair to poor
Cell count (/µL)	<3000 (dogs) <1000 (cats)	Increased red blood cells	1000 to 10,000	5000 to >100,000
Neutrophils	<5%	Relative to blood	<10%	>10% to 100%
Mononuclear cells	>95%	Relative to blood	>90%	10% to <90%
Comments	Only a small amount should be present (<0.5 mL in most joints).	Erythrophagia helps to confirm previous hemorrhage.	Synoviocytes are typically macrophages or synovial lining cells that are found in thick sheets.	Septic and nonseptic etiologies; bacteria are rarely observed in infected joints.

From Raskin R, Meyer D: *Canine and feline cytology*, ed 2, St Louis, 2001, Saunders.

This decreases sample viscosity after a few minutes, allowing for more accurate cell morphology when smeared.

As a generalization, mononuclear cells predominate in samples from patients with traumatic and degenerative arthropathies, usually with increased numbers of large vacuolated or phagocytic cells. Occasionally, when joint erosion has progressed through to subchondral bone, osteoclasts may be observed. By contrast, neutrophils predominate in samples from patients with infectious arthropathies (e.g., as a result of bacteria, viruses, and mycoplasmas) and many noninfectious conditions (e.g., rheumatoid arthritis, systemic lupus erythematosus). When cells are clumped together in a smear, new methylene blue stain may demonstrate interlocking fibrin strands. Rarely the causative organism in septic joint fluid may be observed cytologically, especially when phagocytized. Culture is recommended when an infectious process is suspected. A chronic–active type of arthropathy is suggested when neutrophils and vacuolated/phagocytic macrophages are both increased in number. Lupus erythematosus cells, which are neutrophils that contain phagocytized nuclear chromatin, are seen occasionally in the synovial fluid of animals with systemic lupus erythematosus.

TRACHEAL WASH

TNCCs are usually not performed on tracheal wash fluids. Cell numbers are subjectively recorded from the evaluation of the smear. A tracheal wash smear from a normal animal contains few cells, usually with a small amount of mucus. The mucus often appears microscopically as eosinophilic to purple strands that may enmesh the cells. Epithelial cells are the principal cell type. If the sample is collected from the level of the trachea, ciliated epithelial cells predominate. These cells are columnar to cuboidal, with a polar nucleus on the border opposite the cilia (Fig. 40.18). If the specimen is collected from the bronchi, bronchoalveolar epithelial cells are also fairly common. They are round, nonciliated cells with basophilic cytoplasm, and they may occur in clumps. A few goblet cells (secretory epithelial cells) may also be observed.

If the sample is a bronchoalveolar wash, alveolar macrophages may predominate. These are large individual cells with a large round to oval nucleus and a moderate amount of basophilic cytoplasm. If they become reactive or activated, the cytoplasm increases in volume and becomes more granular and vacuolated. Neutrophils, lymphocytes, eosinophils, plasma cells, mast cells, and erythrocytes are rarely seen in specimens from normal animals.

Abnormal tracheal washes are generally exudates. These samples contain numerous mucus strands, and they are cellular. Eosinophilic spiral casts from small bronchioles (Curschmann's spirals) suggest a chronic bronchiolar problem (Fig. 40.19). Cell morphology is highly variable both among and within samples. Many cells may be unidentifiable. Neutrophils and macrophages are numerous. With acute inflammation, neutrophils are the predominant cell type, and they may represent more than 95% of nucleated cells (Fig. 40.20). As the process becomes more chronic, mononuclear macrophages increase in number. The causative agent, which is possibly bacterial or fungal, may be noted—whether free, phagocytized, or both—in the smear. Tracheal wash samples can be cultured using routine microbiologic procedures.

> **TECHNICIAN NOTE** Abnormal tracheal washes are generally exudates.

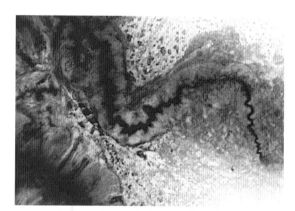

Fig. 40.19 Tracheal wash sample from a dog with chronic bronchial disease. A large Curschmann's spiral and several macrophages are present. The eosinophilic background represents mucus.

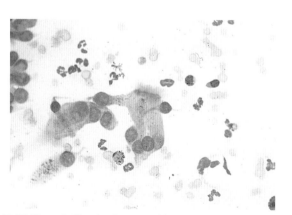

Fig. 40.18 Normal ciliated columnar epithelial cells in a normal tracheal wash sample.

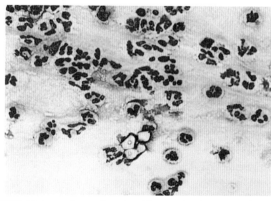

Fig. 40.20 High numbers of neutrophils, an alveolar macrophage, and a cluster of four granules of cornstarch from glove powder in a tracheal wash sample.

The presence of bacteria or fungi in a tracheal wash does not necessarily mean that the organism is pathogenic. Plant or fungal spores sometimes contaminate tracheal washes from herbivores (i.e., inhaled from feed), and they may be phagocytized by macrophages. Oral or pharyngeal contamination of the collection apparatus or increased inspiratory effort with contamination of the upper tracheal mucosa by pharyngeal microflora may cause inclusion of bacteria in a tracheal wash specimen. Such bacteria are frequently associated with or adherent to squamous epithelial cells of the pharyngeal mucosa.

Eosinophils are prominent (i.e., possibly more than 10% of nucleated cells) in inflammatory reactions with an allergic or parasitic component. Because cell preservation is often only fair, free eosinophil granules rather than intact eosinophils may be noted. Rarely, parasite eggs or larvae may be noted in the smear.

Erythrocytes are rarely seen in normal tracheal wash specimens. Recent hemorrhage may be evidenced by numerous intact erythrocytes in the smear. By contrast, with old hemorrhage, few erythrocytes may be noted and many of the macrophages may contain hemosiderin granules (i.e., dark blue or red cytoplasmic granules).

Neoplastic cells may be detected in tracheal wash specimens. Criteria for malignancy are as previously described. Neoplastic cells are frequently found in clusters. They are generally epithelial in origin, and they are frequently secretory in appearance (i.e., their cytoplasm is basophilic and vacuolated).

NASAL FLUSH

A nasal flush from a normal animal contains cornified and noncornified squamous epithelial cells, often with adherent bacteria and negligible evidence of hemorrhage or inflammation. Various abnormalities may be demonstrated with this procedure, such as inflammation secondary to sepsis, fungi and yeasts, and neoplasia (Fig. 40.21). These should not be confused with glove powder, which may be present in some specimens (see Fig. 40.20).

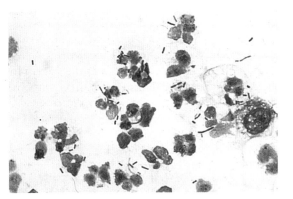

Fig. 40.21 Nasal wash from a patient with bacterial rhinitis. Note the large numbers of degenerate neutrophils and bacteria that are present both intracellularly and extracellularly.

VAGINAL CYTOLOGY

Exfoliative vaginal cytology is a useful adjunct to the history and clinical examination for determining the stage of the estrous cycle in bitches and queens. It assists with the optimal timing of mating or artificial insemination in small animals, but it is not of practical value for these purposes in mares, cows, does, ewes, or sows. Cytologic findings must be interpreted in conjunction with the history and clinical signs. The findings at each stage of the canine estrous cycle are detailed in the following sections. These stages are convenient divisions of a continuum of change, and they are brought about by variations in blood estrogen and progesterone concentrations. Because the determination of the stage of the estrous cycle may be difficult on the basis of a single examination, repeat examinations every few days may be necessary. Unlike the bitch, the queen ovulates after coital stimulation. Cytologic findings at different stages of the estrous cycle are similar to those of the bitch for epithelial cells and neutrophils; however, erythrocytes are not present at any stage.

Cell Types Seen on Vaginal Cytology Sample Preparations

Some variation exists in the terminology used to describe the cell types that are commonly seen in vaginal cytology preparations. In addition to neutrophils and erythrocytes, a variety of squamous epithelial cells are also seen in vaginal cytology preparations (Fig. 40.22). These cells are further categorized on the basis of their size and degree of cornification. The epithelial cells present may include the small basal cells, the slightly larger parabasal epithelial cells (Fig. 40.23), and the largest-sized noncornified squamous epithelial cells, which are sometimes referred to as intermediate (Fig. 40.24). At some stages of the estrous cycle, these intermediate cells may contain pyknotic nuclei (Fig. 40.25). Cornified epithelial cells are angular in appearance. They usually have no nuclei (Fig. 40.26), or they may contain a pyknotic nuclei. Bacteria may be present in vaginal smears at any stage of the estrous cycle (especially during estrus), but they usually have no pathologic significance (i.e., they are part of the normal vaginal microflora).

> **TECHNICIAN NOTE** Vaginal swabs may contain a variety of epithelial cells in addition to neutrophils and erythrocytes.

Anestrus

The anestrual bitch has no vulvar swelling and does not attract male dogs. A vaginal smear reveals predominantly noncornified squamous epithelial cells (i.e., large cells with a rounded border, abundant basophilic cytoplasm, and a large round nucleus). On the basis of size, these cells may be categorized as intermediate, parabasal, or basal epithelial cells. The smear may also contain some neutrophils but no erythrocytes. Anestrus is variable in length, but it generally lasts less than 4.5 months. Some reference materials refer to this stage as diestrus.

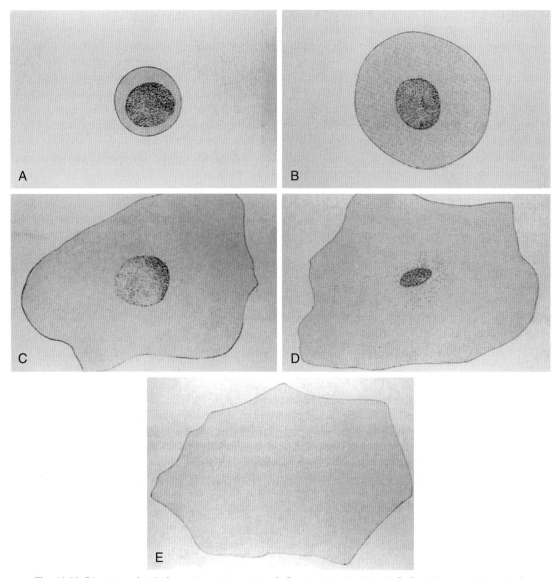

Fig. 40.22 Diagrams of cells from the canine vagina. **A,** Parabasal epithelial cell. **B,** Small intermediate cell. **C,** Large intermediate cell. **D,** Superficial cell with pyknotic nucleus. **E,** Anuclear superficial cell.

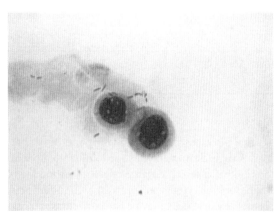

Fig. 40.23 Parabasal vaginal epithelial cells from a dog.

Proestrus

A bitch in proestrus has a swollen vulva, with a reddish vulvar discharge. The bitch attracts but does not accept male dogs that are attempting to breed. Proestrus may last 4 to 13 days, with an average of 9 days. Proestrus is often further subdivided into early proestrus and late proestrus. Gradual changes in physiology and cellular morphology are seen as the stages progress. During early proestrus, high numbers of erythrocytes are present along with basal and parabasal epithelial cells (Fig. 40.27). As proestrus continues, the numbers of erythrocytes gradually decrease, and the epithelial cells begin to show signs of cornification (e.g., pyknotic nuclei). During late proestrus, nearly all epithelial cells present are intermediate cells with pyknotic nuclei. Small numbers of neutrophils are

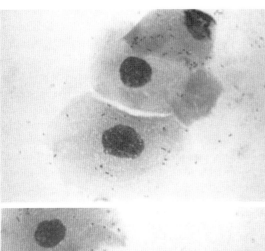

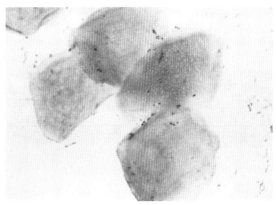

Fig. 40.26 Anuclear superficial (cornified) vaginal epithelial cells from a dog.

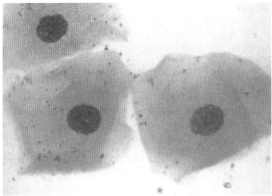

Fig. 40.24 Small and large intermediate vaginal epithelial cells from a dog.

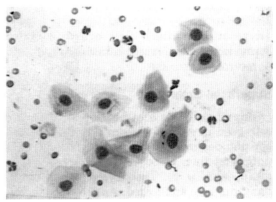

Fig. 40.27 Vaginal smear from a dog in proestrus. Intermediate epithelial cells predominate. Red blood cells and a few neutrophils are also present.

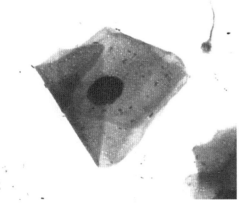

Fig. 40.25 Superficial epithelial cell with a slightly pyknotic nucleus and folded angular cytoplasm.

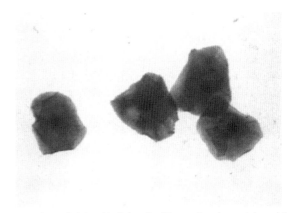

Fig. 40.28 Superficial epithelial cell with a pyknotic nuclei and folded angular cytoplasm from a dog in estrus.

sometimes seen in proestrus samples, especially during the earlier stage.

Estrus

The estrual bitch has a history of recent proestrus and a swollen vulva, with possibly a pinkish to straw-colored discharge that becomes whiter as metestrus approaches. Bitches in estrus accept male dogs that are attempting to mate. A vaginal smear reveals that all squamous epithelial cells are cornified and usually anuclear (Fig. 40.28), that neutrophils are absent, and that small numbers of erythrocytes may be present. At the end of estrus, erythrocyte numbers decrease further, and neutrophil numbers increase rapidly. Estrus generally lasts 4 to 13 days, with an average of 9 days (Fig. 40.29).

Metestrus

A bitch in metestrus has a history of recent estrus. The vulvar swelling and discharge have decreased, and she no longer attracts or is receptive to male dogs. Cornified squamous epithelial cells are replaced by noncornified squamous epithelial cells and abundant cytologic debris. By approximately the 10th day after estrus, all epithelial cells are noncornified. Neutrophils increase in number until approximately the third day of metestrus and then decrease to a few by about the 10th day. Erythrocytes are generally absent throughout metestrus. Metestrus may last for 2 to 3 months. Cytologically, metestrus and anestrus are often difficult to differentiate. Pregnancy is not cytologically distinguishable from metestrus or anestrus. Figs. 40.30 and 40.31 summarize the purpose of vaginal cytology in practice.

> **TECHNICIAN NOTE** The evaluation of the relative numbers of each cell type on the vaginal swab smear helps with determining the stage of estrous when used in combination with the animal's behavioral history and clinical presentation.

Vaginitis and Metritis

Inflammation of the vagina or uterus results in a pinkish-white vulvar discharge, usually without vulvar swelling or clinical signs of proestrus or estrus. A vaginal swab reveals noncornified squamous epithelial cells and massive numbers of neutrophils, possibly with free or phagocytized bacteria (Fig. 40.32).

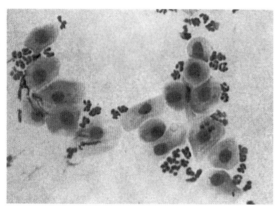

Fig. 40.29 Numerous neutrophils and intermediate cells from the vaginal smear of a dog in metestrus.

FECAL CYTOLOGY

Dry-mount fecal cytology is sometimes used in conjunction with fecal flotation and other diagnostic tests for evaluation of patients with signs of gastrointestinal disease. Samples must be evaluated within 5 minutes after collection. The type of sample collected may vary but can include swabs of voided feces, rectal saline lavage, and rectal scraping. A fecal loop can also be used to collect samples. Voided samples are least desirable because they tend to only provide a sample that represents the intestinal lumen rather than the mucosal surface. Slight dilution of the feces may be needed and can be accomplished by placing a drop of sterile saline on a clean glass microscope slide and mixing a small amount of fecal material into the saline using a sterile wooden applicator. Rectal scraping can be performed with a sterile swab or a blunt spatula.

Dry-mount fecal cytology samples are prepared as thin films. They must be thoroughly air dried before staining. Any standard Romanowsky stain can be used.

The slide is examined under the oil immersion objective. Fecal cytology slides from normal samples generally contain a variety of bacilli and rare cocci. Yeast may be present in normal samples as well. The smear is examined for pathogens such as *Cryptosporidium, Giardia, Entamoeba, Campylobacter, Trichomonas,* and *Balantidium. Clostridium perfringens* or *Clostridium difficile* may be present in low numbers in fecal cytology samples from normal animals. Increased numbers of these or other bacterial organisms would require additional diagnostic testing.

Campylobacter are gram-negative, small, slender, spiral to curved rods that may form chains. Their presence is considered abnormal. The presence of leukocytes in the fecal sample is an abnormal finding that requires further diagnostic testing. Epithelial cells are present when samples are collected traumatically. When samples are collected atraumatically, the presence of large numbers or sheets of epithelial cells may indicate mucosal pathology.

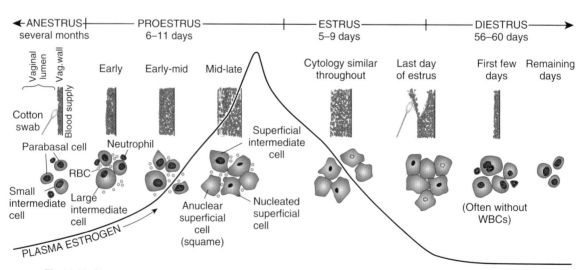

Fig 40.30 Changes in vaginal wall thickness, cell cytology, and estrous cycle relative to blood estrogen levels in dogs. RBC, Red blood cell; WBC, white blood cell. (Modified from Feldman EC, Nelson RW: Ovarian cycle and vaginal cytology. In Feldman EC, Nelson RW, editors: Canine and feline endocrinology and reproduction, ed 3, Philadelphia, 2004, Elsevier, p 755.)

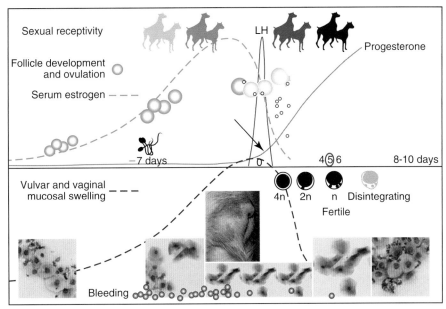

Fig 40.31 Breeding management (canine) diagram outlines the hormonal, behavioral, and cytologic changes occurring during estrus. Sexual receptivity, vaginal cytology, and hemorrhagic discharge are not accurate indicators of the optimal time to breed. However, vaginal cytology should be monitored initially. As soon as there is a significant cornification (50% superficial cells), serum progesterone testing should begin. Samples are collected on Mondays, Wednesdays, and Fridays to monitor for the initial rise in serum progesterone (twice baseline in the range of 1.5–3 ng/mL) because this event is temporally associated with the luteinizing hormone (LH) surge. (Courtesy Dr. Rob Lofstedt.)

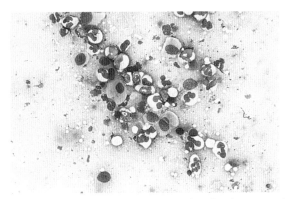

Fig. 40.32 Degenerate neutrophils in an imprint of a tissue scraping of vaginal papules. A few parabasal and intermediate epithelial cells are also present.

URINE CYTOLOGY

Urine cytology can be both a complementary component of urinalysis and a standalone diagnostic tool for characterization of a number of urinary tract and systemic diseases. It can be a minimally invasive and cost-effective procedure, providing a rapid and accurate diagnosis. Urine cytology improves identification and correct characterization of a number of infectious agents and may allow for differentiation of benign versus neoplastic processes. To perform a urine cytology add a drop of urine sediment to a slide, spread the drop of urine on slide, let it air dry, and, finally, stain with Diff-Quick or Gram stain.

SEMEN EVALUATION

The evaluation of semen is an important part of the assessment of male animals for breeding soundness. Avoid exposing semen samples to marked changes in temperature (especially cold), water, disinfectants, or variations in pH. All laboratory equipment used for semen collection and examination should be clean and dry and warmed to approximately 37° C (98.6° F). This equipment includes microscope slides, coverslips, and pipettes. Stains and diluents should also be warmed to approximately 37° C. Samples should be processed in a warm room as soon as possible after collection.

The following characteristics are readily determined in the laboratory: volume of ejaculate, gross appearance, wave motion, microscopic motility, spermatozoal concentration, ratio of live-to-dead spermatozoa, assessment of morphologic features, and presence of foreign cells or material. It is important to record the animal's species, breed, age, brief history with salient clinical findings, and suspected abnormalities as well as the method of semen collection (e.g., artificial vagina, electroejaculation, massage).

Volume of Ejaculate

The volume of ejaculate is measured with a volumetric flask, which may be incorporated into the collection receptacle. Marked species variations occur, and the method of collection greatly influences the volume obtained, its gross appearance, and the spermatozoal concentration. As a generalization, ejaculate volume is larger but spermatozoal concentration lower (and the specimen apparently more dilute) when collected by electroejaculation than when collected with an artificial vagina. In addition, repeated ejaculation—whether it is associated with semen collection or sexual activity—decreases the volume and concentration of semen obtained at subsequent collections. Semen volume tends to be greater if collection is preceded by a period of sexual arousal (i.e., "teasing").

The ejaculate is composed of three portions: a sperm-free watery secretion, a sperm-rich fraction, and a sperm-poor fraction. The first and third fractions are derived from accessory sex glands. In bucks, bulls, rams, and toms, all three fractions are collected together. However, with boars, dogs, and stallions, the third fraction conveniently may be collected separately, which is advisable, because the third fraction is voluminous in these three animals and is therefore an unnecessary encumbrance during the subsequent evaluation of the semen sample. In these three species, the first two fractions (collected together) are used in the other procedures that follow.

The approximate average total ejaculate volumes (all three fractions) are as follows: boar, 250 mL; buck and ram, 1 mL; bull, 5 mL; dog, 10 mL; stallion, 65 mL; and tom, 0.04 mL. Ejaculate volume does not necessarily correlate with fertility. In general, spermatozoal number, motility, and morphologic characteristics are better guides to fertility. However, small ejaculates may be of concern in species that should have voluminous ejaculates. Knowledge of the ejaculate volume is necessary to determine total spermatozoal numbers if the sample is to be divided (and possibly diluted) for artificial insemination procedures.

Gross Appearance of Ejaculate

The opacity and color of the sample should be recorded. Opacity subjectively reflects the concentration of spermatozoa. Categories used include thick, creamy, opaque; milky opaque; opalescent milky; and watery white. This generalization works best for semen from bucks, bulls, and rams, which normally have opaque, creamy-white semen because of a high spermatozoal concentration. As the density of spermatozoa decreases, the specimen becomes more translucent and milkier in appearance. Semen from boars, dogs, and stallions is normally fairly translucent and white to gray. Contaminants, especially intact or degenerate erythrocytes, cause the discoloration of semen.

Sperm Motility

Sperm motility (movement) is subjectively assessed and depends on the careful handling of the sample for meaningful results. Variations in temperature and exposure to nonisotonic fluids or destructive chemicals (including detergents) must be avoided. Motility is correlated with fertility; however, improper specimen handling adversely affects its assessment. If other tests (especially sperm morphology) suggest that the semen is normal but the sperm motility is poor, another sample should be examined to ensure that technical errors were not responsible for the poor motility. Motility may be conveniently assessed in two ways.

Wave Motion

Wave motion is a subjective assessment of the gross motility of sperm. Four general classifications are used—very good, good, fair, and poor—on the basis of the amount of swirling activity observed in a drop of semen on a microscope slide at low power (40×) magnification. These categories respectively correspond to distinct vigorous swirling, moderate slow swirling, barely discernible swirling, and a lack of actual swirling but with motile sperm present, which may cause the sample to have an irregular oscillating appearance. Wave motion depends on high sperm density and is therefore best in samples from bucks, bulls, and rams, which normally have high sperm concentrations. Wave motion decreases as sperm concentration decreases. Consequently, normal boars, dogs, stallions, and toms may have fair or poor wave motion. As a guide, if wave motion is very good or good, the sample should be diluted for evaluation of the percentage of motile sperm and their rate of motility.

Motility

The progressive motility of individual spermatozoa is determined on a relatively dilute drop of semen under a coverslip that is examined at 100× magnification. Because the motility of individual spermatozoa is difficult to appreciate in dense samples, such concentrated samples should be diluted before examination. Warm physiologic saline or fresh buffered 2.9% sodium citrate solutions are suitable diluents.

A drop of semen is placed on a slide and diluted until a satisfactory concentration of spermatozoa is observed. A coverslip is placed on top to produce a monolayer of cells. Excessive dilution of the sample makes the evaluation of motility difficult. The rate of motility is generally subjectively classified as very good, good, fair, or poor, which corresponds to rapid linear activity, moderate linear activity, slow linear or erratic activity, and very slow erratic activity, respectively. The percentage of motile spermatozoa is broadly categorized as very good, good, fair, or poor, which corresponds to approximately 80% to 100%, 60% to 80%, 40% to 60%, and 20% to 40% motile cells, respectively. Satisfactory samples should have at least 60% moderately active spermatozoa.

Sperm Concentration

Several solutions are satisfactory for semen dilution before sperm numbers are counted, including 5 g of sodium bicarbonate or 9 g of sodium chloride with 1 mL of formalin in 1 L of distilled water; 3% chlorazene; or 12.5 g of sodium sulfate with 33.3 mL of glacial acetic acid in 200 mL of distilled water (Gower's solution). A 1 : 200 dilution is made, and the sample is counted using a hemocytometer. The number of spermatozoa in the central grid area of one side of the chamber is counted at 400× magnification. The number of spermatozoa per milliliter of semen is calculated by multiplying the number observed by 2 million. If the spermatozoal concentration is high (e.g., in bucks, bulls, and toms), fewer squares may be counted and the multiplication factor adjusted accordingly. Spermatozoal concentration may also be determined by colorimetric and electronic particle counter techniques.

Depending on the collection method, average sperm concentrations (in millions per milliliter) are approximately 150 for boars and stallions, 3000 for bucks and rams, 1200 for bulls, 300 for dogs, and 1700 for toms.

Live-to-Dead Sperm Ratio

Staining with a vital dye allows for discrimination between live and dead spermatozoa. An eosin/nigrosin mixture is popular for this purpose, and it also permits the examination of sperm morphologic features. The stain is prepared by adding 1 g of eosin B and 5 g of nigrosin to a 3% solution of sodium citrate dihydrate. This solution is stable for at least 1 year.

A small drop of warm stain is gently mixed with a small drop of semen on a warm microscope slide. After several seconds of contact between the specimen and the dye, the mixture is smeared (as when making a blood smear) and then rapidly dried. After the smear is dried, microscopic examination may be delayed. Live sperm resist staining and appear white (clear) against the blue-black nigrosin background. By contrast, dead sperm passively take up the eosin and are stained a pinkish red. The ratio of live-to-dead sperm, which is expressed as a percentage, is determined by examination at 400× or 1000× magnification and preferably after the observation of 200 cells.

Unfortunately, this procedure is susceptible to technical problems. Conditions that kill sperm, especially temperature changes, produce misleading results. Findings should always be interpreted with regard to other results, such as sperm concentration, motility, and morphology.

Sperm Morphology

Sperm morphology is readily assessed on a smear stained with Wright's or Romanowsky stain. Species differences exist regarding the fine points of sperm morphology, but all sperm have the same basic structure (Fig. 40.33). The percentage of abnormal spermatozoa and their types are recorded after observing 100 to 500 cells. Counting the lower number of cells (i.e., 100) is usually adequate after the technician has become proficient. Abnormalities are conveniently divided into head, midpiece, and tail problems. Abnormalities are often categorized as primary or secondary.

Primary defects occur during spermatozoal production and include heads that are double, too large, too small, or oddly shaped (e.g., pyriform, round, twisted, knobby) (Fig. 40.34); midpieces that are swollen, kinked, twisted, double, or eccentrically attached to the head (abaxial); and tails that are coiled (Fig. 40.35). Primary abnormalities are generally considered more serious than secondary ones. Their percentage is fairly consistent if another semen sample is collected within several days. Slightly abaxial midpiece attachment in boars is probably not as significant as it is in other species, because it may be found in numerous spermatozoa of apparently normal boars.

Secondary defects may occur at any time from storage in the epididymis until the smear is made. Therefore, because secondary abnormalities may be artifactual, careful specimen handling is mandatory. The minimization of technique-induced secondary abnormalities allows for easier sample interpretation. Secondary defects include tailless heads, protoplasmic droplets on the midpiece, and bent or broken tails (Fig. 40.36). For every tailless head, there is a headless tail, so the latter need not be counted. Protoplasmic droplets are distinct from swollen midpieces. Protoplasmic droplets are normally present while spermatozoa are in the epididymis. The droplets migrate caudally along the midpiece while the sperm

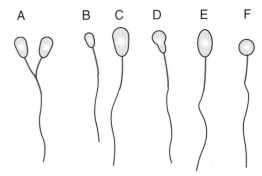

Fig. 40.34 Diagrammatic representation of primary spermatozoal abnormalities involving the head. **A,** Double head (bicephaly). **B,** Small head (microcephaly). **C,** Large head (macrocephaly). **D,** Pear-shaped head (pyriform). **E,** Elongated head. **F,** Round head.

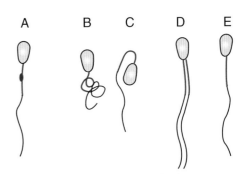

Fig. 40.35 Diagrammatic representation of primary spermatozoal abnormalities involving the midpiece and tail. **A,** Swollen midpiece. **B,** Coiled midpiece and coiled tail. **C,** Bent midpiece. **D,** Double midpiece. **E,** Abaxial midpiece.

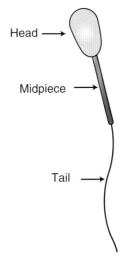

Fig. 40.33 Diagram of a normal spermatozoa.

Head →

Midpiece →

Tail →

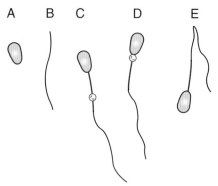

Fig. 40.36 Diagrammatic representation of secondary spermatozoal abnormalities involving the midpiece and tail. **A,** Tailless head. **B,** Headless tail. **C,** Distal protoplasmic droplets. **D,** Proximal protoplasmic droplets. **E,** Bent tail.

cells mature in the epididymis. The droplets are usually shed before the spermatozoa leave the epididymis.

As a broad generalization, less than 20%—and usually less than 10%—of spermatozoa are abnormal in a normal animal. Higher percentages of abnormal spermatozoa may compromise fertility. However, the total number of normal spermatozoa is important rather than just the percentage of abnormal sperm.

Other Cells in Semen

Normal semen contains few (if any) leukocytes, erythrocytes, or epithelial cells and no bacteria or fungi. If present, their approximate quantity should be noted. If bacteria or fungi are observed without an inflammatory response, sample contamination by the normal preputial microflora should be suspected. Attention to preputial sanitation before sample collection should remedy the problem. If indicated, a semen sample may be submitted for microbiologic examination.

Cells from the germinal layers of the testis are an unusual finding in semen and represent severe testicular damage. Such cells include spermatids, spermatocytes, and large ciliated cells (often called medusa heads). Precise categorization is unimportant as long as these cells are classified as immature sperm cells.

EVALUATION OF PROSTATIC SECRETIONS

Disorders of the prostate are not uncommon in dogs, but they are rare in other domestic animals. Cells of prostatic origin may be collected by urethral catheterization in combination with prostatic massage (or penile massage) performed per rectum to stimulate prostatic secretion. Prostatic tissue may be aspirated by transcutaneous needle biopsy.

An enlarged prostate may be the result of prostatic hypertrophy, hyperplasia, metaplasia, neoplasia, or inflammation. Prostatic cells may occur singly or in clusters. Spermatozoa may be present in some fluid samples, especially those that are collected by penile massage.

Normal prostatic cells have a uniform size and shape, with a fairly high nucleus-to-cytoplasm ratio, transparent to gray cytoplasm, homogeneous nuclear chromatin, and no obvious nucleoli. Normal prostatic fluid or tissue contains few leukocytes. Prostatic hypertrophy is gland enlargement that results from the increased size of individual cells without increased cell numbers. A hypertrophic prostate is not cytologically distinguishable from a normal prostate. The distinction is made on the basis of gland size at palpation or radiography. Prostatic hyperplasia is gland enlargement that results from increased numbers of cells. The cells are uniform in size and appearance and have a high nucleus-to-cytoplasm ratio; basophilic cytoplasm that is often vacuolated; and a nucleus with a "roughened" chromatin pattern and a uniform, small, single nucleolus. Few leukocytes are present. Metaplasia is a change (from normal) in the population of prostatic cells. Exfoliated or biopsied cells have the appearance of noncornified squamous epithelial cells. Consequently, they have a low nucleus-to-cytoplasm ratio and a somewhat pyknotic nucleus. Prostatic neoplasia is characterized by a pleomorphic population of cells with a high nucleus-to-cytoplasm ratio and very basophilic cytoplasm. Nuclear size varies among cells, and nuclei contain variable numbers of large, irregular (angular), and pleomorphic nucleoli. A cytologic diagnosis of prostatic abscessation is based on finding large numbers of neutrophils in fluid or tissue samples. Macrophages and lymphocytes may also be present in variable numbers.

EXAMINATION OF MILK

Subclinical and clinical bovine mastitis (mammary gland infection) is an important economic concern for dairy farmers. Mastitis may be detected by several laboratory procedures. Those most frequently used indirectly or directly reflect milk somatic cell counts or bacterial counts. Tests are performed on milk samples from individual quarters, on milk samples from all four quarters pooled together, or on bulk milk (from several cows together, usually the whole herd).

When individual animals are being screened, foremilk (i.e., the sample obtained before milking begins) is generally used. It has more cells than a sample obtained in the middle of milking but fewer cells than one collected at the end of milking. Cell counts also vary with the stage of lactation. Milk samples from normal cows within the first week and at the end of lactation have higher cell counts than those obtained in the interim.

Somatic cell counts of normal milk are generally less than 300,000 cells/mL to 500,000 cells/mL. Counts of more than 500,000 cells/mL indicate mastitis. Information on the California Mastitis Test is located in Chapter 47.

Differential cell counts are sometimes performed. Nucleated cells are categorized as neutrophils or mononuclear cells. Normal milk obtained during mid-lactation generally has less than 10% neutrophils, whereas, with severe acute mastitis, the milk may have up to 95% neutrophils.

KEY POINTS

- Peritoneal and pleural fluids are evaluated for color, transparency, odor, and TNCC.
- Cells are counted and classified from samples of peritoneal and pleural fluids.
- The evaluation of cellular elements in fluid samples allows the samples to be classified as exudates, transudates, or modified transudates.
- In a normal lymph node, the predominant cell type is the small, mature lymphocyte.
- Reactive lymph nodes contain predominantly small, mature lymphocytes as well as plasma cells, lymphoblasts, and intermediate lymphocytes.
- Evaluations performed on synovial fluids include the assessment of fluid color and turbidity; the cytologic examination of a direct smear; the subjective assessment of viscosity; and a TNCC, mucin test, and refractometric protein measurement.
- Abnormal tracheal washes are generally exudates.
- Yeasts, squamous epithelial cells, and *Malassezia* organisms are commonly isolated from ear swabs and may not indicate pathology.
- Vaginal swabs may contain a variety of epithelial cells in addition to neutrophils and erythrocytes.
- Epithelial cells that are present in vaginal cytology samples may include small basal cells, slightly larger parabasal epithelial cells, noncornified squamous epithelial cells (intermediate cells), and cornified epithelial cells.

UNIT 8

Microbiology

Unit Outline

Unit Objectives

List and describe the supplies and equipment needed for microbiology testing.
Describe the general characteristics of bacteria and fungi.
Discuss sample collection procedures for bacterial and fungal samples.
Describe commonly used staining procedures for bacterial and fungal samples.
Describe proper techniques for culturing bacterial and fungal samples.
Describe the proper procedure for antimicrobial sensitivity testing.
Describe the procedure for performing the California Mastitis Test.
List and describe common biochemical tests performed on bacterial samples.

Microbiology refers to the study of microbes. Microbes are organisms that are too small to be seen with the unaided eye. Bacteria, fungi, and viruses are all microbes. Some parasites are also considered microbes. The fields of study of bacteria, fungi, and viruses are referred to as bacteriology, mycology, and virology, respectively. Virology evaluations in the veterinary clinical laboratory are usually performed with immunologic methods. Bacteria and fungi can be evaluated with a number of routine microbiology procedures. Although some practices send all microbiology work to a reference laboratory, most practices do some testing in-house. Bacterial and fungal samples can be collected quickly, easily, and inexpensively, and tests do not require much in the way of specialized equipment. Careful attention to quality control is vital to ensure the diagnostic value of results.

Most microbes found on and in the body are nonpathogenic (i.e., they are normal flora). The intestinal and respiratory tracts, the skin, and parts of the urinary and reproductive tracts all have known normal flora. Samples collected from some locations, such as the spinal column, the blood, and the urinary bladder, should be free of normal flora. Microbes that are considered normal flora and nonpathogenic when found in one location can produce significant disease if they are found in a site where they should not reside.

41

Introduction to Microbiology

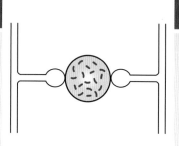

LEARNING OBJECTIVES

After studying this chapter, you will be able to:

- Describe the general characteristics of bacteria, fungi, and viruses.
- Discuss bacteria growth characteristics and requirements for growth.
- Describe the characteristic shapes and arrangements of bacteria.
- Discuss the significance of spore formation in bacteria and fungi.

- Describe the reproduction of fungal organisms.
- Differentiate among the four groups of pathogenic fungi.
- Discuss general methods for viral specimen collection and handling.
- List the methods for the evaluation of samples with suspected viral pathogens.

OUTLINE

KEY TERMS

Ascospores
Bacilli
Basidiospores
Capnophilic
Cocci
Conidia
Endospores
Facultative anaerobes

Fastidious microbes
Flagella
Hyphae
Mesophiles
Microaerophilic
Mycelium
Obligate aerobes
Obligate anaerobes

Prokaryotic
Psychrophiles
Spirochetes
Sporangiospores
Thermophiles
Yeast
Zygospores

A basic understanding of the characteristics of bacteria, fungi, and viruses will help the veterinary technician with the collection, preparation, and evaluation of samples for analysis. The identification of bacterial pathogens is the primary purpose of microbiology examinations. Fungal organisms are also encountered with relative frequency in veterinary practice. Viral pathogens are numerous, but techniques for the evaluation of samples for viral pathogens are generally performed in specialty reference laboratories and government-sponsored testing locations.

CLASSIFICATION AND NOMENCLATURE OF BACTERIA

The living world is divided into five main kingdoms:

- Plantae—Plants
- Animalia—Animals
- Monera—Procaryotae
  - These are procaryotic cells in which the nuclei are not membrane bound.
  - All bacteria are included in this kingdom.

- Protista
  - These are eucaryotic, unicellular microorganisms with membrane-bound nuclei.
  - This includes the protozoa and algae.
- Fungi
  - These are eucaryotic, multicellular, multinucleated microorganisms.

There are several differences between eucaryotes and procaryotes that are outlined in Table 41.1.

The classification of bacteria can be performed as follows:
- Part
  - This is a grouping of bacteria based on certain basic characteristics, such as shape, Gram reaction, and oxygen requirement.
- Order
  - This is a grouping related to families. They have an ending: "ales."
- Family
  - These are closely related genera.
- Genus
  - These are closely related species.
- Species
  - These are organisms that share a set of biologic characteristics and will also react the same way to biochemical tests.
- Subspecies
  - These are strains within a species. They are bacteria subdivided on the basis of small but consist differences within a species.

When we name bacteria we refer to this as nomenclature. The nomenclature gives the bacteria the names we use to refer to the bacteria when working in the field of science. When naming bacteria we use a binomial system of nomenclature. Each bacterial species name is given two words, Latin or Greek. The name need not be descriptive. The first word begins with a capital letter and describes the genus name. The second word begins with a small letter and describes the species. Both words are always italicized or underlined, for example, *Staphylococcus intermedius*.

BACTERIAL CELL MORPHOLOGY

Bacteria are small prokaryotic cells that range in size from 0.2 to 2.0 μm. The bacteria that are most frequently studied in the laboratory range from 0.5 to 1 μm in width and from 2 to 5 μm

TABLE 41.1 Differences in Eucaryotic and Procaryotic cells

	Eucaryotic	Procaryotic
Nuclear membrane	Contains	Doesn't have
Nucleus	Contains	Doesn't have
Mitochondria	Contains	Doesn't have
Chloroplast	Contains	Doesn't have
Golgi apparatus	Contains	Doesn't have

in length. Most cellular organelles are absent except cell walls, plasma membranes, and ribosomes. Microbial structures that may or may not be present include:
- Capsules
  - These are the outermost coverings of many bacteria. A capsule consists of a slimy or jelly-like material. It functions to protect bacteria against phagocytosis and promotes bacterial attachment. It promotes pathogenicity, or the ability to produce disease. Some bacteria are pathogenic if they can form a capsule; others are not. The capsule also helps prevent nutrient loss and dehydration. It can also be useful in serological identification of bacteria.
- Cell Walls
  - A cell wall is composed of a base layer and an outside layer. Both layers are present in gram-negative and gram-positive bacteria. It is the difference in these layers that allows us to differentiate gram-negative from gram-positive bacteria. The cell wall gives rigidity to the cell and helps maintain the cell shape and size. Medications like penicillin interfere with the cell wall synthesis to kill the bacteria. Penicillins are not effective against mycoplasma bacteria because they lack cell walls.

> **TECHNICIAN NOTE** All bacteria except mycoplasmas and spirals have cell walls.

- Cell Membranes or Cytoplasmic Membranes
  - This is the innermost layer separating the cytoplasm from the cell wall. It selectively controls the passage of materials in and out of the cell. It functions similar to a mitochondria. It has no function in the shape of the bacteria.
- Cytoplasm
  - Cytoplasm is a complex fluid mass that contains two sections. The cytoplasmic area contains ribosomes, which are RNA protein particles that synthesize particles. It also contains granular inclusions, which are the primary storage granules. The nuclear area of the cytoplasm is rich in DNA. The nuclei of bacteria are not surrounded by nuclear membranes and lack discrete chromosomes, mitotic apparatus, and nucleoli. It has general control of cell functions and is responsible for cellular reproduction.
- Mesosomes
  - These are the cytoplasmic membrane invaginations. They increase the cell surface area for the purposes of secretion and cell division.
- Flagella
  - These are long whiplike appendages that protrude through the cell wall from a basal body beneath the cell membrane. Not all bacteria have flagella. These organs allow for movement.
- Pili (Fimbriae)
  - These are long whiplike hollow tubes that protrude through the cell wall from the basal body. They are mainly present in gram-negative bacteria. They have no

function in motility. Their purpose is for the attachment of viruses and mammalian cells. They allow bacteria to stick to one another and to other organisms as well as inanimate objects. They contribute to the adhesiveness of the bacteria, which contributes to their pathogenicity.
- Plasmid
  - This is a small piece of self-replicating DNA that contains a limited number of genes. It controls conjugation and is called F factor. Many gram-negative bacteria contain F factor, which enables them to form pairs and mate by conjugation. It also contains genes for transferable drug resistance known as R factor.
- Endospores
  - These are intracellular refractile bodies. They are commonly called spores. Organisms in the genera *Bacillus and Clostridium* are spore forming. They have a low rate of metabolism and can survive for decades. Spores vary in size, shape, and location. They are highly refractile, resistant to staining and chemicals, and heat resistant.

Bacteria have specific requirements for temperature, pH, oxygen tension, and nutrition. These requirements must be considered when collecting and preparing microbiology samples. In addition, the identification of some bacteria can be aided by using these characteristics. The majority of clinically significant bacterial species require a pH in the range of 6.5 to 7.5.

Oxygen requirements for bacteria can vary and bacteria can be classified by those differences. The following are common classifications of bacteria based on oxygen requirements.
- Obligate aerobes
  - Bacteria that require oxygen to survive
- Obligate anaerobes
  - Bacteria that are killed in the presence of oxygen or those with growth that is inhibited in the presence of oxygen
- Facultative anaerobes
  - Organisms that can survive in the absence of oxygen, but their growth is limited
- Microaerophilic
  - Bacteria that prefer reduced oxygen tension
- Capnophilic
  - Bacteria that require high levels of carbon dioxide

TECHNICIAN NOTE Bacteria can be described on the basis of their requirements for oxygen as obligate aerobes, obligate anaerobes, facultative anaerobes, microaerophilic organisms, or capnophilic organisms.

Nutritional requirements vary among bacteria, and culture media types are chosen on the basis of these requirements. Some bacteria have strict requirements and are referred to as fastidious microbes.

Temperature requirements also vary among different bacteria. However, nearly all bacteria that are pathogenic to animals grow best at 20° C to 40° C. Bacteria classified by temperature can be broken into the following categories.

- Mesophiles
  - Bacteria that grow best between 20° C to 40° C
- Psychrophiles
  - Bacteria with lower temperature requirements to as −20° C (−4° F) to 20° C (68° F)
- Thermophiles
  - Bacteria with higher temperature requirements

TECHNICIAN NOTE Most pathogenic bacteria thrive at temperatures of 20° C to 40° C.

Methods of identification are directed toward characterizing bacteria on the basis of a variety of criteria. These criteria include size, shape, arrangement, and chemical reactivity. These characteristics are often used for the differentiation of specific bacterial pathogens.

Bacteria may be organized into the following groups according to their shape (Fig. 41.1):
- Coccus (pl., cocci):
  - Spherical cells, such as *Staphylococcus aureus,* which is the causative agent of mastitis in animals
- Bacillus (pl., bacilli):
  - Shaped like rods or cylinders, such as *Bacillus anthracis,* which is the causative agent of anthrax in animals and human beings
- Spiral (spirochetes):
  - Usually occur singly and can be subdivided into loose spirals, such as *Borrelia anserina,* which causes avian borreliosis; tight spirals, such as *Leptospira pomona,* which causes red water disease in cattle; and comma-shaped spirals, such as *Campylobacter fetus,* which causes abortion in cattle
- Coccobacillus (pl. coccobacilli):
  - Some small rod-shaped bacteria, such as some strains of *Escherichia coli,* may stain in a polar fashion so that they take on the appearance of two cocci in a pair.
- Pleomorphic:
  - Shapes that range from cocci to rods

TECHNICIAN NOTE Bacteria are classified according to their shape and arrangement.

Bacteria are found in a variety of arrangements. Some grow as single cells while others remain attached after dividing and form chains or clusters. Many exhibit patterns of arrangement,

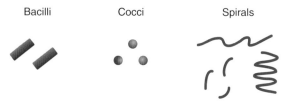

Bacilli   Cocci   Spirals

Fig. 41.1 Bacterial cell shapes.

such as the following, that are important for their identification (Fig. 41.2):
- Single:
  - Some bacteria occur singly, such as spirilla (sing., spirillum) and most bacilli (sing., bacillus).
- Pairs:
  - Some bacteria occur in pairs, such as *Streptococcus pneumoniae* (diplococcus).
- Clusters or bunches:
  - Some bacteria occur in clusters, bunches, or groups. For example, *Staphylococcus aureus* forms grapelike clusters.
- Chains:
  - Some organisms grow in short or long chains, such as the *Streptococcus* species.
- Palisades:
  - Some organisms can be arranged in a palisade or "Chinese letter" pattern, such as *Corynebacterium* species.

With a pleomorphic organism (e.g., a member of the *Corynebacterium* species), judging whether the organism is a coccus or a bacillus may be difficult. If the Gram-stained smear was made from a pure culture and if any of the cells present are definitely rod shaped, then the organism must be regarded as a bacillus for purposes of identification.

Spores

When cultured, a few genera of bacteria form intracellular refractile bodies called endospores or, more commonly, spores. Organisms of the genera *Bacillus* and *Clostridium* are spore formers. Bacterial spores are resistant to heat, desiccation, chemicals, and radiation.

Spores vary in the size, shape, and location within the cell. They may be classified as follows (Fig. 41.3):
- Central:
  - Present in the center of the cell, such as *Bacillus anthracis*
- Subterminal:
  - Present near the end of the cell, such as *Clostridium chauvoei*
- Terminal:
  - Present at the end or pole of the cell, such as *Clostridium tetani*

Performing a special spore stain may not be necessary, because the endospores can usually be visualized as nonstaining bodies in Gram-stained samples.

> **TECHNICIAN NOTE** The presence and location of spores can help with the identification of bacterial species.

BACTERIAL GROWTH

Bacterial cells contain a single DNA strand and reproduce primarily by binary fission. When bacteria colonize any media, such as living tissue or a culture plate in a laboratory, bacteria growth proceeds through four distinct phases (Fig. 41.4).

Lag Phase

The initial phase, which is referred to as the lag phase, represents the time during which the bacteria are adapting their metabolism to use the resources found on their new media, assuming that the media contains the appropriate growth factors and conditions for the particular bacterial species.

Exponential Growth Phase

The lag phase is followed by the exponential growth phase. The rate of growth during this phase is often referred to as the doubling time or generation time. The generation time is variable with different species and under different environmental conditions. The exponential growth phase continues until essential nutrients are depleted, toxic waste products accumulate, or space becomes limiting.

Stationary Phase

The colony then enters the stationary phase, which is the time during which the total numbers of cells show no net increase or decrease. The length of this phase is also variable for different bacterial species.

Death or Decline Phase

The final phase is the logarithmic decline phase, or the death phase. The rate of death is not necessarily the same as the rate

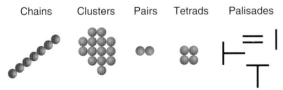
Fig. 41.2 Bacterial cell arrangements.

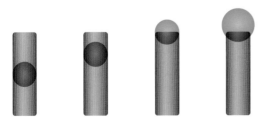
Fig. 41.3 Bacterial endospores.

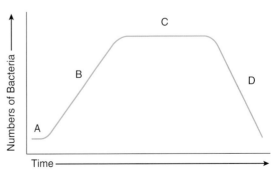
A – Lag phase
B – Exponential growth phase
C – Stationary phase
D – Log decline phase

Fig. 41.4 Generalized bacterial growth curve.

of initial growth. Spore formation usually occurs during this phase.

FACTORS THAT INFLUENCE INFECTION

Infection develops when microorganisms enter the body, multiply, and produce a reaction to disrupt normal body function. There are numerous factors that affect whether an infection will actually occur when an animal is exposed to bacteria in the environment. The factors that influence infection include:

- Infective dose
  - This is the number of organisms required to cause a disease. It varies with the virulence of the organism involved and the resistance of the host.
- Tissue affinity
  - Depending on which tissues the bacteria comes in contact with, certain bacteria infect and destroy certain types of tissues; for example, rabies affects nervous tissue.
- Portal of entry
  - Some types of bacteria must enter via a certain route to become infective; for example, *Clostridium tetani* must enter through a puncture wound to cause tetanus.
- Toxic factors
  - Some bacteria produce toxins to cause disease. There are two kinds:
    - Exotoxins
      - They are excreted from the bacteria into its environment, and their potency can vary greatly.
    - Endotoxins
      - Produced within the cell and are released when the cell dies. They are produced by gram-negative bacteria and are a toxic component of the cell wall.
- Enzymatic factors
  - Enzymes that can be produced by some bacteria can affect they types of diseases they produce; for example, coagulase, which causes coagulation of fibrinogen in serum, causing fibrin formation protecting the bacteria from phagocytosis.

Other factors that influence whether an infection will occur when exposed to a bacteria include the host's defense mechanisms that a bacteria must overcome to become infective and include:

- Physical barriers
- Chemical barriers
- Biological barriers

FUNGAL CHARACTERISTICS

Fungi are heterotrophs, and they may be parasitic or saprophytic. Most are multicellular, except yeasts. They contain eukaryotic cells with cell walls composed of chitin. Fungal organisms consist largely of webs of slender tubes called hyphae, which grow toward food sources. Fungi digest their food externally, through the release of digestive enzymes, and then

bring the resulting small molecules into the hyphae. Hyphae make up a branching web called a mycelium. Hyphae can be described as septate or nonseptate. Septate hyphae have cross-walls within the hyphae. The presence or absence of those cross-walls can aid in the identification of the organism. Fungal organisms may also have a reproductive structure called a fruiting body that produces and releases reproductive cells called spores. Different groups of fungi produce different types of spores. Yeasts reproduce by budding rather than spore formation.

Most fungi rely on both sexual and asexual reproductive systems. Asexual spores produced by some fungi are either sporangiospores or conidia (Fig. 41.5). Sexual spores include ascospores, basidiospores, and zygospores (Fig. 41.6). Fungi can be differentiated on the basis of the structure of the hyphae and the presence of spores.

Pathogenic fungal organisms can be categorized into one of the following four groups on the basis of the type of reproductive structures present:

- Basidiomycetes: mushrooms or club fungi
- Ascomycetes: cup fungi
- Zygomycetes: molds
- Deuteromycetes: also known as *Fungi imperfecti*, because no known sexual stage occurs

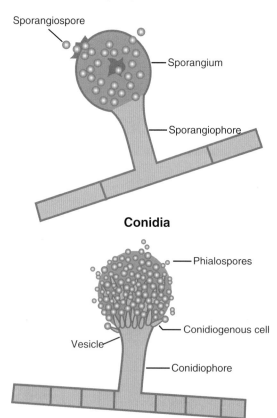

Fig. 41.5 Sporangiospores and conidia, which are the two main types of asexual spores. (Courtesy Ashley E. Harmon. From Songer JG, Post KW: *Veterinary microbiology: bacterial and fungal agents of animal disease*, St Louis, 2005, Saunders.)

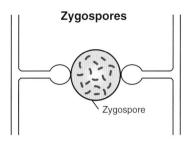

Zygospores

Zygospore

Basidiospores

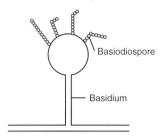

Basiodiospore

Basidium

Ascospores

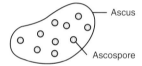

Ascus

Ascospore

Fig. 41.6 Sexual spores (zygospores, basidiospores, and ascospores) are produced through the fusion of the protoplasm and nuclei of two cells by meiosis.

TECHNICIAN NOTE The structure of the hyphae and the presence of spores can aid in the identification of fungal species.

VIROLOGY

Most virologic techniques are performed in specialized laboratories. They include histopathologic and serologic examination, electron microscopy, and the attempted isolation and identification of the virus. The veterinary technician should contact the diagnostic laboratory to check which facilities are available, which samples are preferred, and whether a transport medium is necessary. If an exotic reportable disease is suspected, the proper authorities should be notified, and no clinical material should be removed from the facility.

Many of the viral diseases encountered may be diagnosed on clinical and pathologic grounds. Serologic tests are available for most viral diseases. Some may require paired serum samples that are collected 2 to 3 weeks apart, starting during the early stages of the disease. A rising antibody titer indicates recent infection by the virus.

Virus isolation is expensive and time-consuming, and it may provide only a diagnosis after the animals have recovered or died. However, in some instances, the isolation and identification of a virus should be attempted, such as to establish the identity of a viral disease not previously seen in a practice, to discover the exact agent when serologic and other tests have given equivocal results, to find the immunologic type of a virus in an epizootic, and to verify the etiologic agent if a public health problem is involved.

The isolation of a virus from a diseased animal does not necessarily mean that the virus caused the disease, because many viruses can persist in animals without clinical signs of illness. Some other pathogen or condition could have been responsible for the disease. Virus isolation is most successful when specimens are collected early during the active infectious phase of the disease.

Viruses vary greatly with regard to their ability to remain viable in tissues and exudates. Contamination with bacteria greatly decreases the success of attempted virus isolation. Specimens are selected on the basis of their likelihood to contain large numbers of virus particles. Samples for virology testing must be collected aseptically, kept at 4° C, and taken to a laboratory in the shortest time possible.

Cell Culture

To demonstrate the presence of a virus in a specimen, the virus is grown (isolated) in the laboratory, or the virus antigens or antibodies are assayed. Unlike bacteria, which can be grown on nutrient agar, viruses need living cells in which to grow and replicate. The tissue cells are placed into a suitable glass bottle or chamber containing a medium that is rich in nutrients. The cells settle and begin to grow in a confluent monolayer across the surface of the container. Various types of cells have been used for the tissue culture of viruses. Most animal cells can be grown in vitro for some generations, but some cells divide indefinitely and are used for virus isolation. These cells are called continuous cell lines, and they are of a single type of cell. Continuous cell lines, such as those from fetal kidney, embryonic trachea, skin, and other cells, are derived from monkeys, dogs, cattle, pigs, cats, mice, hamsters, rabbits, and other animals. The virus specimen is commonly inoculated into a primary culture of cells derived from the same species of animal from which the specimen was taken.

After the cell culture has been inoculated with the virus specimen and incubated, it is examined. If the virus is present, cell damage may be visible as the virus particles invade the tissue cells. This damage is referred to as a cytopathic effect. Different types of cytopathic effects are used to identify viruses. Some viruses cause cell lysis, and others cause the cells to fuse and form syncytiae (sheets) and giant cells. An inclusion body is another type of cytopathic effect that may be seen.

Immunologic and Molecular Diagnostics Examination

Clinical signs and cell culture examination may identify the virus to a family level and perhaps to the genus and species level, but definitive identification requires serologic procedures that are based on immunologic principles. Sometimes these serologic procedures may be used on the specimens directly, which saves the time and expense of cell culture. In-house diagnostic tests are available to detect the presence of some common viral pathogens. Unit 4 contains more details about the immunologic tests used for the detection of viral antigens and antibodies.

Molecular diagnostic tests (e.g., polymerase chain reactions) are also routinely used for the identification of pathogens. These are discussed in Unit 4.

KEY POINTS

- Bacterial morphologic characteristics are described on the basis of the shape and arrangement of the cells.
- Bacteria vary with regard to their requirements for oxygen, temperature, and nutrients.
- Some bacteria contain specialized structures (e.g., capsules, spores) that can aid in their identification.

- Different groups of fungi produce different types of spores.
- Yeasts reproduce by budding rather than spore formation.
- Fungi are classified into different groups on the basis of the type of reproductive structures that are present.
- Viral culture is performed in specialized reference laboratories.

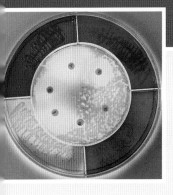

42

Equipment and Supplies for Microbiology

LEARNING OBJECTIVES

After studying this chapter, you will be able to:

- List the supplies needed for collecting and evaluating bacterial and fungal samples.
- Discuss the safety concerns related to the microbiology laboratory.
- Describe the types of media available for culturing bacteria.

- List the commonly used culture media, and state the characteristics of the media.
- Describe commonly available modular test media.
- Describe the culture media used for the evaluation of fungal samples.

OUTLINE

KEY TERMS

Agar
Alpha-hemolysis
Beta-hemolysis
Blood agar
Culture medium
Culturette

Differential media
Enriched media
Enterotubes
Fastidious
Gamma-hemolysis
Inoculating loops

MacConkey agar
Mueller-Hinton agar
Sabouraud dextrose agar
Selective media
Thioglycollate

THE IN-HOUSE MICROBIOLOGY LABORATORY

Ideally, the practice facility should have a separate room away from the main traffic areas of the clinic for microbiologic procedures. The room must have adequate lighting and ventilation; a washable floor and limited traffic; at least two work areas (one for processing the samples and one for culture work) with smooth surfaces that are easily disinfected; electrical outlets; ample storage space; and easy access to an incubator and a refrigerator.

LABORATORY SAFETY

Most of the microorganisms encountered in the microbiology laboratory are potentially pathogenic, and many are zoonotic. All specimens should be treated as potentially zoonotic. The safety of every person working in the laboratory depends on the strict observance of rules. Aseptic technique is always observed when transferring or working with infectious agents or specimens.

Veterinary technicians must wear personal protective equipment when handling patient specimens, including a clean, long-sleeved, knee-length, white laboratory coat or clean, long-sleeved surgical scrubs to prevent the contamination of street clothes and the dissemination of pathogens to the general public. Disposable gloves are always worn in the microbiology laboratory, and face masks may be needed if the production of aerosol particles is likely. Laboratory coats should be washed at least weekly in hot water and strong bleach. If the coat becomes soiled during daily diagnostic procedures, it is removed immediately and placed in a receptacle designated for dirty linens. All laboratory coats should be washed together. At no time should laboratory coats be mixed with other laundry from the veterinary clinic or with laundry from outside of the laboratory.

> **TECHNICIAN NOTE** All specimens should be treated as potentially zoonotic.

All personal protective equipment should be removed before leaving the laboratory. The veterinary technician must wash his or her hands thoroughly before leaving the laboratory.

Materials that have been contaminated with potentially infectious agents must be decontaminated before disposal. Scissors, forceps, and scalpel blade holders can be sterilized in an autoclave. Potentially hazardous materials (i.e., plates, test tubes, slides, pipettes, and broken glass) are placed in appropriate containers for disposal. If these materials must be discarded in the trash receptacles, they must first be autoclaved to eliminate any infectious agents. Bench tops are cleaned with disinfectant (70% ethanol or dilute bleach solution) at the beginning and end of the work period. Spilled cultures are treated with disinfectant and allowed contact for 20 minutes before they are cleaned up. The surfaces of all other equipment, such as incubators and refrigerators, should be wiped down with disinfectant on a daily basis. Nondisposable wire loops that have been contaminated with microbes must be flamed immediately after use.

Eating, drinking, smoking, handling contact lenses, and applying cosmetics are not permitted in the laboratory. Appropriate signage should state this rule. Personnel who wear contact lenses in the laboratory should also wear goggles or a face shield. Long hair must be tied back or tucked inside the laboratory coat. Labels should be moistened with water rather than with the technician's tongue. No food is stored in the laboratory; instead, it is stored outside of the laboratory in designated cabinets or refrigerators. All accidents must be reported promptly to the laboratory supervisor or to the veterinarian.

EQUIPMENT AND SUPPLIES NEEDED FOR THE MICROBIOLOGY LABORATORY

A good-quality incubator that is capable of maintaining constant temperature and humidity is the primary piece of equipment needed in the microbiology laboratory. More information about incubators is available in Unit 1. The supplies that are needed for collecting and preparing bacterial and fungal samples include the following:

- Sterile cotton-tipped swabs
- Dull scalpel blades
- 3- to 20-mL syringes and 21- to 25-gauge needles
- Sterile endotracheal tube or jugular or urinary catheter
- Collection tubes and preservatives
- Rayon swab in transport media, such as Culturette (BD, Franklin Lakes, NJ) (Fig. 42.1)
- High-quality glass slides and coverslips
- Inoculating loops or wires; reusable metal or single-use disposable plastic loops (Fig. 42.2) and 10-mL calibrated loops
- Bunsen burner (natural gas or propane gas) or alcohol lamp (Fig. 42.3)

- Candle jar or anaerobe jar
- A variety of culture media, including plates and broth
- Antibiotic disks and dispensers (Fig. 42.4)
- Gram stain and other stains as needed
- Scissors, forceps, and scalpel with blades (stored in 70% alcohol and flamed to sterilize)
- "Discard jar" containing disinfectant for contaminated instruments
- Wooden tongue depressors for handling fecal specimens
- Racks to hold tubes and bottles
- Refrigerator "cold packs" and polystyrene shipping containers for samples that must be sent to reference laboratories

CULTURE MEDIA

A culture medium (pl., media) is any material—solid or liquid—that can support the growth of microorganisms. For bacteriology, culture media may be purchased as dehydrated powder or as prepared agar plates or ready-to-use liquid media for biochemical tests. All of the commonly used media may be obtained already prepared from supply houses. Large reference and research laboratories may prepare and sterilize their own media from dehydrated powder. Solidifying agents used in the

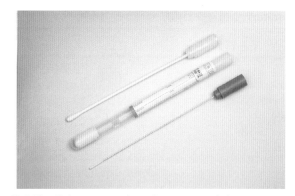

Fig. 42.1 The Culturette consists of a rayon swab in transport media. (Courtesy B. Mitzner, DVM.)

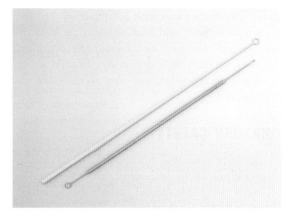

Fig. 42.2 Disposable plastic inoculating loops. (Courtesy B. Mitzner, DVM.)

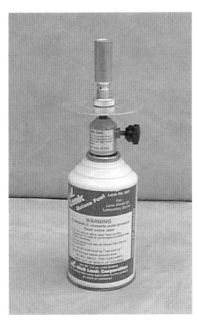

Fig. 42.3 Propane burner for sterilizing metal inoculating loops. (Courtesy B. Mitzner, DVM.)

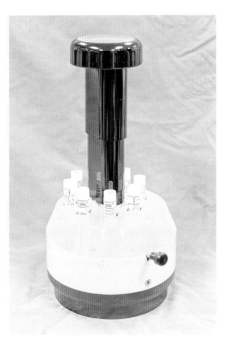

Fig. 42.4 Antibiotic disks with dispenser.

preparation of solid media include agar and gelatin. Agar is a dried extract of sea algae known as agarophytes. Gelatin is a protein that is obtained from animal tissues.

For maximum life, agar plates should be kept refrigerated at 5° C to 10° C. Plates must be kept away from the internal walls of the refrigerator, because contact with the jacket can freeze and ruin the media.

Types of Media

Six general types of culture media are available: transport media, general purpose media, enriched media, selective media, differential media, and enrichment media. Some culture media contain characteristics of more than one type. There are hundreds of different types of culture media available, but the average veterinary practice needs just a few (Fig. 42.5). In many veterinary practices, modular media that contain multiple types of media in a single culture plate are common. General purpose media, which are sometimes referred to as nutrient media, are not commonly used in veterinary practice. Enriched media are formulated to meet the requirements of the most fastidious pathogens. They are basic nutrient media with extra nutrients added, such as blood, serum, or egg. Examples include blood agar and chocolate agar. Selective media contain antibacterial substances, such as bile salts or antimicrobials, that inhibit or kill all but a few types of bacteria. They facilitate the isolation of a particular genus from a mixed inoculum. MacConkey agar is a type of selective media. Differential media allow bacteria to be differentiated into groups based on their biochemical reactions on the medium. Simmons citrate is a differential medium. Enrichment media are liquid media that favor the growth of a particular group of organisms. They contain nutrients that encourage the growth of the desired organisms or that contain inhibitory substances that suppress competitors. Examples include tetrathionate broth and selenite broth. Transport media are designed to keep microbes alive while not encouraging growth and reproduction. The Culturette used for specimen collection contains prepared transport media. More specific details about some of the commonly used culture media are presented in the next sections of this chapter. What is presented is not meant to be an all-inclusive list; dozens of additional types of media are available. However, many of those not listed here are found only in large reference or research laboratories.

> **TECHNICIAN NOTE** Types of culture media include transport media, general purpose media, enriched media, selective media, differential media, and enrichment media.

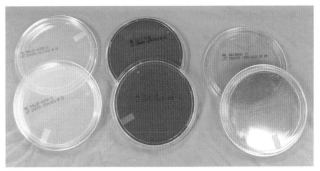

Fig. 42.5 Commonly used culture media. From left to right, Mueller-Hinton agar, blood agar, and MacConkey agar.

Blood Agar

This enriched medium supports the growth of most bacterial pathogens. Although several types of blood agar are available, trypticase soy agar with sheep blood is the most commonly used type. Blood agar acts as an enrichment medium and a differential medium, because four distinct types of hemolysis can be detected on blood agar:

1. Alpha-hemolysis: partial hemolysis that creates a narrow band of greenish or slimy discoloration around the bacterial colony (Fig. 42.6)
2. Beta-hemolysis: complete hemolysis that creates a clear zone around the bacterial colony
3. Gamma-hemolysis: hemolysis that produces no change in the appearance of the medium and no hemolysis around colonies
4. Delta-hemolysis: a zone of hemolysis surrounded by a narrow zone of hemolysis around a bacterial colony; also called double-zone hemolysis

---

TECHNICIAN NOTE Bacteria can be classified on the basis of their patterns of hemolysis in blood agar.

MacConkey Agar and Eosin-Methylene Blue Agar

MacConkey and eosin-methylene blue (EMB) agars are selective and differential media. MacConkey agar contains crystal violet (which suppresses the growth of gram-positive bacteria), bile salts that are selective for lactose-fermenting *Enterobacteriaceae*, and a few other bile-salt—tolerant gram-negative bacteria. Growth or no growth on MacConkey agar may be used as a test for the primary identification of gram-negative genera. EMB media performs the same function and may also be used to identify lactose-fermenting organisms.

The indicators in MacConkey agar are lactose and neutral red. Lactose-fermenting organisms such as *Escherichia coli* and *Enterobacter* and *Klebsiella* species produce acid from lactose and grow as pinkish-red colonies on this medium. Bacteria that cannot ferment lactose attack the peptone in MacConkey agar, producing an alkaline reaction and colorless colonies.

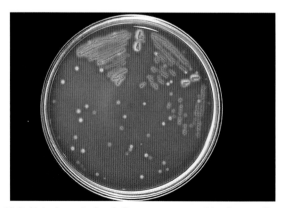

Fig. 42.6 Alpha-hemolysis of *Streptococcus* on blood agar. (Courtesy Public Health Image Library, PHIL#8170, Richard R. Facklam, Atlanta, 1977, Centers for Disease Control and Prevention.)

Clinical specimens for routine isolation are usually cultured separately on both blood and MacConkey agars. The examination of both blood and MacConkey agar cultures that have been inoculated with the same clinical specimen can yield considerable information. For example, no growth on the MacConkey agar plate but good growth on the blood agar plate suggests that the isolated pathogen is probably a gram-positive organism.

Chromogenic Agar

A wide variety of chromogenic agars are available that are both selective and differential media. These are designed to provide sufficient information to definitively identify some bacterial species. In most cases, the use of chromogenic agar allows for more rapid identification of bacteria and thus saves time and costs because additional biochemical tests may not be needed. Some chromogenic agars are divided into sections, whereas others are single plates. Examples of chromogenic agar include several types designed to identify certain resistant bacteria based on their color and colony appearance on the specific chromogenic agar (Fig. 42.7). Another type is used to identify and differentiate *Escherichia coli* from other enteric bacteria. For example, on an *E. coli* chromogenic agar, if colonies of *E. coli* are present, they will appear dark blue-green whereas other enteric bacteria will be magenta. Nonenteric bacteria are inhibited on the media, but if they do grow, the colonies will be colorless.

Thioglycollate Broth

Thioglycollate is a liquid medium that is used to culture anaerobic bacteria to determine the oxygen tolerance of microbes. The medium contains a stable oxygen gradient, with high concentrations of oxygen near the surface of the agar and anaerobic conditions near the bottom.

Obligate aerobes will grow only in the oxygen-rich top layer, whereas obligate anaerobes will grow only in the lower part of the tube. Facultative anaerobes can grow throughout the medium, but they will primarily grow in the middle of the tube, between the oxygen-rich and oxygen-free zones. The primary use of thioglycollate broth in veterinary practice is as an enrichment media and for blood cultures.

Urea Tubes

Urea slants are streaked with inoculum and incubated overnight at 37° C. Urea medium is a peach color. If the bacteria hydrolyze the urea in the medium, ammonia production turns the medium to a pink color. A negative result produces no color change (Fig. 42.8).

Sulfide-Indole Motility Tubes

The tube of sulfide-indole motility (SIM) medium is inoculated with a straight stab to a depth of approximately 1 inch. Care is

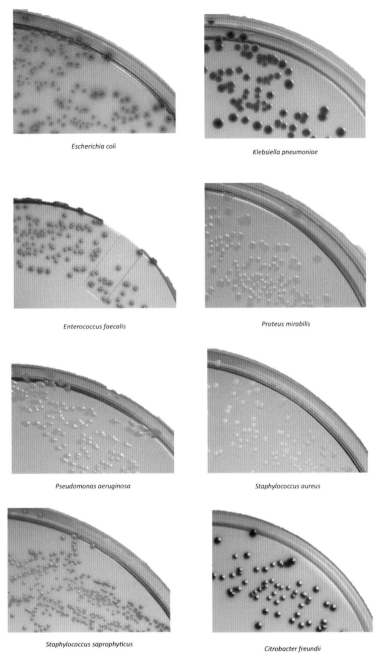

Fig. 42.7 Chromogenic agar. (Courtesy Microvet Diagnostics.)

taken to withdraw the wire out along the same line as was used for entry. Hydrogen sulfide production is indicated by the blackening of the medium. Indole production requires the addition of 5 drops of Kovac's reagent to the top of the medium. If tryptophan has been broken down to indole by the bacteria in the tube, a red ring immediately forms on top of the medium.

Simmons Citrate Tubes

Simmons citrate medium differentiates bacteria according to their use of citrate. Only the slant surface is inoculated. If bacteria use the citrate in the medium, a deep blue color develops. The unchanged medium is green.

Triple Sugar Iron Agar

Triple sugar iron agar medium is used for the presumptive identification of salmonellae and the initial differentiation of enteric bacteria. The medium contains an indicator system for hydrogen sulfide production as well as a pH indicator, phenol red, that colors the uninoculated medium red. All *Enterobacteriaceae* ferment glucose, and the small amount that is present (0.1%) is attacked preferentially and rapidly. At an early stage of

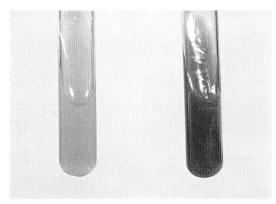

Fig. 42.8 Urea tubes. The pink coloration indicates a positive reaction (urea hydrolysis). The yellow color indicates a negative reaction. (Courtesy Public Health Image Library, PHIL#6711, Atlanta, 1976, Centers for Disease Control and Prevention.)

incubation, both the slant and the butt turn yellow as a result of acid production. However, after the glucose is metabolized under aerobic conditions and if the organism cannot ferment lactose or sucrose, the slope reverts to the red (alkaline) condition. The butt, under anaerobic conditions, remains yellow (acidic) (Fig. 42.9). To allow this reaction, the triple sugar iron agar always must be used in tubes with loose caps or plugged with sterile cotton.

If the organism can ferment lactose, sucrose, or both in addition to the glucose, the lactose and sucrose are then attacked with resulting acid production, and the medium turns yellow (acidic) throughout. Lactose and sucrose are present in 1% quantities to maintain acidic conditions in the slant, which remains yellow. With organisms that produce hydrogen sulfide, blackening of the medium is partly superimposed on the other reactions. The triple sugar iron slants should be read after about 16 hours of incubation at 37° C. After longer incubation, the blackening tends to reach the bottom of the tube and obscures the yellow butt.

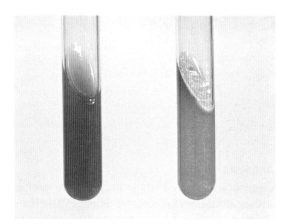

Fig. 42.9 Triple sugar iron agar is used to classify bacteria according to their ability to ferment glucose, lactose, or sucrose as well as to produce hydrogen sulfide. A yellow result indicates fermentation; the reddish result indicates no fermentation. (Courtesy Public Health Image Library, PHIL#6710, Atlanta, 1976, Centers for Disease Control and Prevention.)

The following summarizes the reactions of *Salmonella* species in triple sugar iron agar:

- Alkaline (red) slant and alkaline (red) butt: none of the sugars attacked
- Alkaline (red) slant and acidic (yellow) butt: glucose fermentation only
- Acidic (yellow) slant and acidic (yellow) butt: glucose attacked in addition to lactose, sucrose, or both
- Blackening along the stab line and through the medium: hydrogen sulfide production

The triple sugar iron slant is stab inoculated with a single colony from the selective medium with a straight inoculating wire. The wire is pushed down to the bottom of the agar, and when withdrawing the wire, the agar slant is streaked. The inoculating wire still contains enough bacteria to inoculate a tube of lysine decarboxylase broth. During the search for salmonellae, at least two suspicious colonies should be individually tested in triple sugar iron agar per brilliant green plate. The triple sugar iron tubes should be incubated, with loose caps, at 37° C for 16 to 24 hours.

Brain–Heart Infusion Broth

Brain–heart infusion broth is a useful general-purpose broth that is used to increase the number of organisms (preenrichment) before they are plated on solid medium. The broth is inoculated with the patient sample, and subcultures are taken as needed for additional testing.

For culture of blood samples, approximately 1 mL of the patient's blood sample is added to nutrient broth or to a special blood culture medium that can be obtained commercially. Because a patient's blood contains many substances that are inhibitory to bacteria, adding the blood sample directly to broth dilutes the effect of these natural inhibitors.

Mannitol Salt Agar

Mannitol salt agar is not routinely used, but it is a highly selective medium for staphylococci, and it could be used to isolate *Staphylococcus aureus* from contaminated specimens. The medium has a high salt content (7.5%), and it contains mannitol and the pH indicator phenol red. Staphylococci are salt tolerant. *S. aureus* (but usually not *Staphylococcus epidermidis*) ferments mannitol. The resulting acid turns *S. aureus* colonies and the surrounding medium yellow.

Bismuth Sulfite Agar

In this selective medium, freshly precipitated bismuth sulfite acts with brilliant green to suppress the growth of coliforms while permitting the growth of salmonellae. Sulfur compounds provide a substrate for hydrogen sulfide production. The metallic salts in the medium stain the colony and the surrounding medium black or brown in the presence of hydrogen sulfide.

Atypical colonies may appear if the medium is heavily inoculated with organic matter. This situation may be prevented by suspension of the sample in sterile saline and the use of the supernatant for inoculation.

The freshly prepared medium has a strong inhibitory action, and it is suitable for heavily contaminated samples. Storing the poured plates at 4° C for 3 days causes the medium to change color to green, thereby making it less selective, with small numbers of salmonellae being recovered.

The following summarizes the typical appearance of the more important bacterial organisms on bismuth sulfite agar and the appearance of their colonies:

- *Salmonella typhi:* black "rabbit eye" colonies, with a surrounding black zone and metallic sheen after 18 hours; uniformly black after 48 hours of incubation
- Other *Salmonella* species: variable colony appearance after 18 hours (black, green, or clear and mucoid); uniformly black colonies seen after 48 hours, often with widespread staining of the medium and a pronounced metallic sheen
- Other organisms (coliforms, *Serratia* and *Proteus* species): usually inhibited but occasionally dull green or brown colonies with no metallic sheen or staining of the surrounding medium

Mueller-Hinton Agar

Mueller-Hinton agar is a general-purpose medium that is primarily used for the performance of the agar diffusion antimicrobial sensitivity test. The chemical composition of the media does not interfere with the diffusion of the antimicrobials through the agar.

Sabouraud Dextrose and Bismuth—Glucose—Glycine—Yeast Media

Both of these media are used specifically for the culture of fungi and yeasts. Bismuth—glucose—glycine—yeast agar is commonly referred to as "biggy." Dermatophyte test media found in most veterinary clinics is composed of Sabouraud dextrose agar.

Combination and Modular Culture Media

Several modular culture systems are available for use in the veterinary practice laboratory. Spectrum CS (Vetlab Supply, Palmetto Bay, FL) (Fig. 42.10) systems are multi-chambered agar plates that contain both selective and nonselective media. The Bullseye plate also contains a central area with Mueller-Hinton agar for sensitivity testing. "Dipslides" or "paddle" media such as Uricult (Orion Diagnostics) (Fig. 42.11) are useful tools for urinary tract infection (UTI) screening. They consist of a two-sided agar paddle that is attached to the cap of a screw-top plastic tube. They are made with a variety of media combinations, although the most

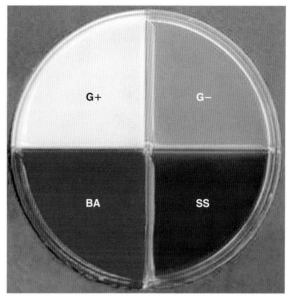

Fig. 42.10 Spectrum CS plate showing gram-positive, gram-negative, *Staphylococcus* select, and blood agar areas. (Courtesy Vetlab Supply.)

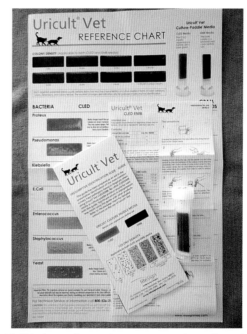

Fig. 42.11 Uricult media used to screen patients for urinary tract infections.

common ones have either MacConkey or EMB and cystine lactose electrolyte—deficient (CLED) agar. After incubation, a colony count is performed, and the color of the CLED agar is compared with a chart for presumptive identification. Positive cultures that meet quantitation criteria for UTI should be sent to an outside laboratory for confirmation and susceptibility testing.

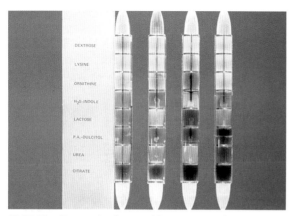

Fig. 42.12 The Enterotube is a multitest system that contains eight different agar preparations. (Courtesy Public Health Image Library, PHIL#5421, Theo Hawkins, Atlanta, 1977, Centers for Disease Control and Prevention.)

TECHNICIAN NOTE Commonly used modular media include the Bullseye system, Uricult, and Spectrum plates.

Enterotubes (BD, Franklin Lakes, NJ) (Fig. 42.12) are one type of commercially available microbiology test kit that incorporates multiple types of media. The kit is designed to provide for the differentiation of enteric bacteria on the basis of their biochemical reactions on the media. It tends to be relatively expensive, and it may not be financially justified unless large numbers of microbiology tests are performed on a variety of species.

Dermatophyte Test Media

Several products are available for the culturing of dermatophytes. The most common is standard dermatophyte test medium (DTM), which contains an indicator that turns red in the presence of most dermatophytes as well as antimicrobial agents to inhibit bacterial growth (Fig. 42.13). Rapid sporulation medium (RSM) or enhanced sporulation media (ESM) with color indicators can be used in conjunction with standard DTM to accelerate the formation of macroconidia used for identification and confirmation. DTM formulations are available in plate and tube formats. Standard Sabouraud dextrose agar will also promote the earlier formation of macroconidia, but it contains no color indicator.

TECHNICIAN NOTE Dermatophyte test media contains Sabouraud dextrose agar as well as antimicrobials and color indicators.

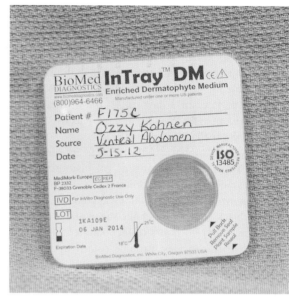

Fig. 42.13 InTray DM Enriched Dermatophyte Medium. This is a commonly used dermatophyte test medium.

Quality Control Cultures

Some cultures are required in a laboratory for quality control purposes. Various procedures and supplies must be monitored for quality and accuracy, including antibacterial susceptibility tests, media, biochemical tests, and certain tests for identification, such as the zone of beta-hemolysis around *S. aureus* for the cyclic adenosine monophosphate test. A selection of control organisms can be obtained on disks. Media that do not contain fermentable sugars, such as trypticase soy agar, are suitable for maintaining fewer fastidious organisms, such as *S. aureus* and *Enterobacteriaceae*. The bacteria can be stab inoculated into a tube of medium and subcultured approximately every 2 months.

Streptococcus, Pasteurella, and *Actinobacillus* species die quickly on culture plates. Streptococci may be kept in a tube of cooked meat broth and subcultured approximately every 4 weeks. *Pasteurella* and *Actinobacillus* species remain viable if mixed with approximately 0.5 mL of sterile whole blood in a small tube and stored in a deep freeze at −10° C or lower. Otherwise, these two genera should be subcultured on blood agar approximately every 3 days. Control cultures may be kept at room temperature in screw-capped tubes but preferably in a refrigerator at 4° C, which reduces the metabolic rate of the organisms.

KEY POINTS

- Equipment and supplies that are needed to perform microbiology testing in the practice laboratory include an incubator, sample collection materials, culture media, and staining supplies.
- Culture media can be obtained in tubes or plates. Tube media can be solid or liquid.
- A variety of culture media are available, but most veterinary practice laboratories require only a few types.

- Commonly used culture media includes blood agar, MacConkey agar, Mueller-Hinton agar, and dermatophyte test media.
- A variety of modular systems are available that contain more than one type of culture media to help with the identification of organisms.

43

Sample Collection and Handling for Microbiology

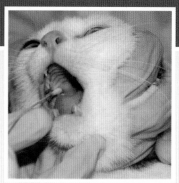

Photo from August JR: *Consultations in feline internal medicine*, vol 6, St Louis, 2010, Saunders.

LEARNING OBJECTIVES

After studying this chapter, you will be able to:

- Discuss the general guidelines for the collection of bacterial samples.
- List the methods that can be used to collect samples for microbiology testing.
- Describe the methods of collecting samples for fungal evaluations.
- List and describe aspects of sample collection for specific samples in a variety of sites.

OUTLINE

KEY TERMS

Aspiration
Culturette

Imprint
Swabbing

Transport media

Samples for microbiologic evaluation can be collected quickly, and most do not require specialized materials or equipment for proper evaluation. Microbiological examination can provide valuable diagnostic information if the process is begun with proper collection of specimens. Improper collection of specimens affects the results of microbiologic examination and may render culture and identification worthless. Specimens are commonly collected by various methods, including aspiration and swabbing. Imprints of tissues or external lesions can also provide suitable samples. Aspiration is generally used to collect samples from hollow organs (e.g., the bladder) and external lesions (e.g., pustules). The specific techniques used depend on the type of lesion and its location on the animal's body. Careful attention to aseptic technique is critical to the achievement of diagnostic-quality results. More information about aspiration, swabbing, and imprints is located in Unit 7.

> **TECHNICIAN NOTE** Samples for microbiology testing can be collected with a variety of techniques, including swabbing, aspiration, and imprints.

Samples that are to be immediately processed can usually be collected using sterile cotton swabs. However, this is the least suitable method of collection, because contamination risk is high, and cotton can inhibit microbial growth. Oxygen can also be trapped in the fibers, making the recovery of anaerobic bacteria less likely. Rayon or Dacron swabs are preferred. If delays in processing the sample are expected, a rayon swab in transport media (e.g., Culturette) must be used to preserve the quality of the sample.

The specimen selected must contain the organism that is causing the problem. Normal flora and contaminants may complicate sample collection and the subsequent interpretation of results. Better results will be obtained if specimens are collected from sites that would normally be sterile, because infections are likely to be caused by a single predominant organism. Good examples are urine (collected by cystocentesis) or intact skin pustules. Ears and fecal samples do not lend themselves well to in-house microbiology testing because of the number of commensal and secondary organisms that typically populate such exposed areas.

> **TECHNICIAN NOTE** Aseptic technique must be used when collecting samples for microbiology testing.

GENERAL GUIDELINES

The following general guidelines apply to proper specimen collection:

1. A complete history and sufficient clinical data must be obtained to help select the procedures that are most appropriate to isolate any organisms that may be present. Required data include the owner's name and the clinic's name, address, and phone number. Species, name, age, sex, the number of animals affected or dead, the duration of the problem, and the major signs observed should also be included. The tentative diagnosis, the organism suspected, any treatment given, and the type of laboratory investigation required should be included in the record.
2. It is best practice to collect specimens in early acute stages of viral disease and also later in the convalescent stages of disease. Ideally, specimens should be collected before the animal is treated or after it has been off medication for an appropriate time. If the animal has died, take samples as soon as possible after death to avoid postmortem contamination by bacteria that invade tissues.
3. The specimen must be collected aseptically. Specimen contamination is the most common cause of diagnostic failure. The importance of aseptic collection of microbiologic specimens cannot be overemphasized. Samples should be collected as soon as possible after the onset of clinical signs.
4. Ensure you are using the appropriate transfer medium to keep the organism alive until it is inoculated onto culture medium. Special transport medium should be used if anaerobic organisms are suspected. Fluid specimens can be submitted in the syringe if the needle cover is replaced.
5. Multiple specimens must be kept separate to avoid cross-contamination. This practice is essential for intestinal specimens because of the flora normally present there.
6. Keep specimens cool until they are in the laboratory ready for culture.
7. The specimen container is labeled, especially if a zoonotic condition is suspected, such as anthrax, rabies, leptospirosis, brucellosis, or equine encephalitis. Tissues from suspected zoonoses should be submitted in a sealed, leak-proof, unbreakable container.
8. Adequate time should be taken. Obtaining results quickly at the expense of accuracy is counterproductive.

Table 43.1 summarizes sample collection guidelines for microbiology specimens.

When collecting specimens for dermatophyte culture, clean the skin lesion to remove some of the surface contamination and collect specimens from the lesion periphery. Broken hair shafts and dry scale are most likely to contain viable organisms. Hairs and skin scales can be plucked from the area, or a toothbrush can be used to obtain hair and skin samples. To collect samples with a toothbrush, obtain a new human toothbrush and brush the suspected lesion for 1 to 2 minutes. Hairs should be visible in the bristles after brushing.

Table 43.2 summarizes sample collection guidelines for fungal testing.

TABLE 43.1 Sample Collection Guidelines for Microbiology Specimens

Site	Acceptable Specimen	Transport Device	Comments
Central nervous system	Spinal fluid	Blood culture medium	Hold, ship at RT
Blood	Whole, unclotted blood Minimum of 3 mL	Blood culture medium	Hold, ship at RT Submit ≤3 samples per 24 hr, collected during febrile spike
Eye	Conjunctival swab Corneal scrapings Ocular fluid	Amies or semisolid reducing medium Syringe	Hold, ship at RT Inoculate plated media directly with corneal scrapings if fungal keratitis suspected
Bone and joints	Joint aspirate Bone marrow aspirate, bone	Blood culture medium Sterile tube	Hold, ship at RT
Urinary tract	Urine by cystocentesis Catheterized urine	Sterile tube	Hold, ship under refrigeration
Upper respiratory tract	Nasopharyngeal swab Sinus washings Biopsy specimen	Semisolid reducing medium Sterile tube	Ship refrigerated except washings, biopsies (RT)
Lower respiratory tract	Transtracheal wash Lung aspirate or biopsy	Sterile tube Semisolid reducing medium	Hold, ship at RT
Gastrointestinal tract	Feces Rectal swab	Sterile cup or bag Cary-Blair or semisolid reducing medium	Feces: hold, ship at RT; refrigerate *Campylobacter, Brachyspira* suspects
Skin	Aspirate or swab, if superficial Deep swab of draining tract Tissue biopsy Scabs, hairs, scrapings	Sterile syringe Semisolid reducing medium Sterile tube with saline Paper envelope	Anaerobe suspects not refrigerated

Continued

TABLE 43.1 **Sample Collection Guidelines for Microbiology Specimens—cont'd**

Site	Acceptable Specimen	Transport Device	Comments
Milk	Remove milk from teat cistern; collect 5 to 10 mL aseptically	Sterile tube	Freeze
Necropsy tissue	Lesions, including adjacent normal tissue Minimum of 1 cm^3 to maximum of 35 cm^3 Include one serosal or capsular surface intact	Whirl-Pak bags Screw-capped jars	Individual containers to prevent cross-contamination; ship refrigerated
Reproductive tract	Prostatic fluid Raw semen Uterus Vagina Abortion	Sterile tube Biopsy Swab Fetal lung, liver, kidney, stomach contents, placenta in separate Whirl-Pak bags or screw-capped containers	Guarded swabbing for uterine cultures; hold, ship at RT Ship refrigerated

RT, Room temperature.
From Songer JG, Post KW: *Veterinary microbiology: bacterial and fungal agents of animal disease,* St Louis, 2005, Saunders.

TABLE 43.2 **Sample Collection for Fungal Testing**

Specimen	Container	Comments
Hair	Paper envelope (dry conditions inhibit overgrowth of bacterial or saprophytic fungal contaminants)	Wash and dry the affected area with soap and water. With forceps, epilate hairs from the periphery of an active lesion. Pull hairs in the direction of growth to include the root. Look for broken, stubby hairs, which are often infected. Useful for the diagnosis of dermatophytosis.
Skin	Paper envelope	Clean skin with an alcohol gauze sponge (cotton leaves behind too many fibers). Scrape the periphery of an active lesion with a sterile scalpel blade, and obtain crusts and scabs. Useful for the diagnosis of dermatophytosis.
Nails	Paper envelope	Proven nail infections in animals are rare. Cleanse the affected nail with alcohol gauze. Scrape the area with a scalpel blade so that fine pieces are collected, and collect debris from under the nail. Useful for the diagnosis of onychomycosis.
Biopsy	Sterile tube in sterile saline or water	Normal and affected tissue should be included. It is important to prevent specimen desiccation.
Urine	Sterile tube	Centrifuge and use sediment for direct examination and culture. Useful for the diagnosis of histoplasmosis.
Cerebrospinal fluid	Sterile tube	Useful for the diagnosis of cryptococcosis. Make an India ink preparation to observe encapsulated yeasts.
Pleural/abdominal fluid	Sterile tube	If fluid contains flakes or granules, they should be included, because these are actual colonies or organisms.
Transtracheal/bronchial washings	Sterile tube	Centrifuge and use sediment for direct examination and culture. Useful for the diagnosis of systemic mycoses.
Nasal flush	Sterile tube	Centrifuge and use sediment for direct examination and culture. Useful for the diagnosis of nasal aspergillosis and guttural pouch mycosis.
Ocular fluid	Sterile tube or syringe	Examine directly. Inoculate onto plated fungal media immediately after collection. Useful for the diagnosis of ocular blastomycosis.

From Songer JG, Post KW: *Veterinary microbiology: bacterial and fungal agents of animal disease,* St Louis, 2005, Saunders.

> **TECHNICIAN NOTE** Samples for dermatophyte testing are usually obtained by plucking hair and skin scales from the suspected lesion.

COLLECTION OF VIRAL SPECIMENS

Viruses are often present in the nasal or pharyngeal secretions early in the acute stage of respiratory diseases. Mucosal scrapings rather than swabs of the secretions should be taken. Sterile wooden tongue depressors are useful for mucosal scrapings. Attempted isolation from blood samples may be considered for generalized catarrhal diseases, which tend to have a viremic stage. Poxviruses are often demonstrated by electron microscopy in fluid from early vesicular lesions and sometimes in scabs from early lesions.

Specimens should also be selected for indirect studies, such as serologic, hematologic, histologic, and bacteriologic examinations. Viral diseases are often complicated by pathogenic bacteria that act as secondary invaders, which can turn a mild viral infection into a serious disease. Specimens for histopathologic examination should consist of thin sections of tissue placed immediately in 10% formalin. Sections for histologic examination must never be frozen, because this causes tissue artifacts that may be difficult to differentiate from a pathologic process.

Tissue samples for attempted virus isolation should be 2-inch cubes that contain both diseased and normal tissue, if possible. Mucosal scrapings should be obtained instead of swabs. Sterile screw-capped containers should be used for collection, with a separate container used for each sample. Veterinary technicians must use strict aseptic technique and label the containers carefully.

Submission of Samples

Specimens should be refrigerated (4° C) when possible, because virus titers decrease as temperature increases. If the specimens are to be delivered to the virology laboratory within 24 hours, they may be stored at 4° C and packed with coolant packs or ice in a polystyrene-insulated carton for shipment. If the time delay will be more than 24 hours, snap freezing at −70° C and shipping on dry ice is desirable, except for specimens of suspected parainfluenza and influenza virus, in which case the integrity of these viruses is best preserved at −20° C. Specimens must be shipped in airtight containers to prevent the entry of carbon dioxide into the container. Carbon dioxide gas from the dry ice can lower the pH of fluid and kill any pH-labile viruses.

Small pieces of tissue, fecal material, or mucus can be preserved in vials filled with 50% glycol and stored at 4° C. A virus transport medium is available commercially (NCS Diagnostics, Mississauga, ON, Canada). Because viruses vary in their longevity, a reference laboratory should be contacted for recommendations regarding appropriate transport medium and sampling procedure.

Fecal materials and fluids are often submitted for electron microscopic examination. A fixative (e.g., 10% buffered neutral formalin) should be added to the sample at a maximum fixative-to-sample ratio of 1 : 1 to prevent the overdilution of virus particles.

For urine samples, approximately 5 mL of urine is sent in a sterile container. Virus transport medium should not be used. The specimen must be kept chilled if it is to arrive at the laboratory within 24 hours of collection; otherwise, it should be shipped frozen.

If blood samples have been collected for serologic examination, they should be collected and processed as described in Unit 4.

■ KEY POINTS

- Samples for microbiologic evaluation can be collected quickly, and most do not require specialized materials or equipment.
- Careful attention to aseptic technique is crucial to the production of diagnostic-quality results.
- Microbiology samples can be collected by swabbing, aspiration, imprint, biopsy, and a variety of other techniques.
- Samples for dermatophyte testing are usually collected by plucking hairs and skin from the suspected lesion.
- Normal flora and contaminants may complicate sample collection and the subsequent interpretation of results.

44

Staining Specimens in Microbiology

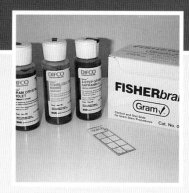

LEARNING OBJECTIVES

After studying this chapter, you will be able to:

- List the stains that are commonly used for microbiology specimens.
- Describe the components used in the Gram staining procedure.
- Describe the procedure for performing Gram staining.
- Describe the use of potassium hydroxide when evaluating bacterial and fungal samples.
- List and describe the staining procedures used for specific samples.

OUTLINE

KEY TERMS

Acid-fast stain
Capsule stain
Endospore stain
Flagella stain

Giemsa stain
Gram stain
Lactophenol cotton blue
Potassium hydroxide

Simple stain
Ziehl-Neelsen stain

A variety of stains are available for the preparation of bacterial and fungal samples. The two most commonly used stains are Gram stain and Ziehl-Neelsen (acid-fast) stain. Samples taken directly from patients are often Gram stained before the sample is cultured. Information obtained from a direct smear may help to determine the suitability of the specimen for identification, the predominant organism in a mixed specimen, the appropriate medium for culture, and the appropriate antibacterials for sensitivity testing. Staining kits for Gram (Fig. 44.1) and Ziehl-Neelsen (acid-fast) stains are available commercially. Commercially prepared staining solutions may require filtering if a precipitate forms. Simple stains, such as crystal violet or methylene blue, are typically used for yeasts. Lactophenol cotton blue stain is used to confirm the identity of fungal organisms. Many other types of stains are available for microbiology, but most are performed only in large reference or research laboratories. Standard hematology stains should not be used for evaluation of bacteria. Hematology stains will impart a purple color to all bacteria and other formed elements that may appear to be bacteria, and this can lead to misclassification of the organisms.

GRAM STAIN

Gram staining is used to categorize bacteria as gram positive or gram negative on the basis of cell wall structure. The Gram stain procedure requires a primary stain, a mordant, a decolorizer, and a counterstain. A mordant is a substance that fixes a dye to a structure. In this case, it fixes the primary stain to the bacterial cell wall. Depending on the manufacturer, the primary stain is usually a solution of crystal violet, the mordant is Gram's iodine solution, the decolorizer is either 95% ethanol or acetone, and the counterstain is either basic fuchsin or safranin.

> **TECHNICIAN NOTE** The components of the Gram stain are the primary stain, the mordant, the decolorizer, and the counterstain.

Procedure

The sample should be applied thinly on the slide. Swab specimens may be rolled lightly onto the slide. Touching the sterile wire to one colony on the plate is usually sufficient to obtain enough bacteria for application to the slide. The colonies

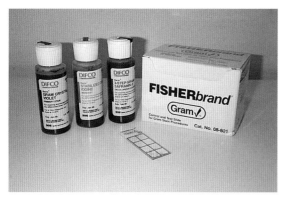

Fig. 44.1 Gram staining kit. (Courtesy B. Mitzner, DVM.)

PROCEDURE 44.1 Gram Staining Procedure

1. Draw a circle with a wax pencil in the center of a clean glass slide.
2. Place a drop of saline in the circle on the slide, and transfer a small amount of the specimen, as appropriate (e.g., inoculating loop, swab, wire).
3. Allow the slide to air dry.
4. Heat fix the slide by passing it through a flame two or three times, with the specimen side up.
5. Place the slide over a staining rack.
6. Pour crystal violet over the sample area, and allow it to sit for 30 seconds.
7. Rinse the slide with water.
8. Pour the iodine solution onto the area, and allow it to sit for 30 seconds.
9. Rinse the slide with water.
10. Flood the slide with decolorizer until no more purple color washes off (generally about 10 seconds).
11. Rinse the slide with water.
12. Add the basic fuchsin or safranin stain to the sample area, and allow it to sit for 30 seconds.
13. Rinse the slide with water.
14. Air dry the slide or blot it dry between paper towel sheets.

---

should be young (i.e., 24-hour culture), because older colonies may not yield proper results, and the stained bacteria often become excessively decolorized.

Bacterial samples from plates are gently mixed in a drop of water or saline on the slide. If the sample is obtained from inoculated broth, two to three loopfuls are spread onto the slide. A sample may also be smeared directly onto a slide, such as from a tissue or an abscess. Regardless of how the specimen is transferred onto the slide (e.g., swab, pipette, wire), care must be taken not to destroy the organisms.

The sample droplet on the slide may be encircled by using a wax pencil to help find the area after staining. After the material has dried on the slide, it is heat fixed by passing the slide through a flame two or three times, with the specimen side up. The technician should be careful to not overheat the slide. The temperature may be tested on the back of the hand, and the slide should feel warm but not hot. Heat fixing prevents the sample from washing off. It helps to preserve cell morphology, and it kills the bacteria and renders them permeable to stain. Procedure 44.1 contains the step-by-step Gram staining procedure. The decolorizer step is a critical step in the process. It is possible to over-decolorize or under-decolorize, yielding ambiguous or erroneous results. Note that slight variations may exist with different test kits. Always consult the materials provided by the kit manufacturer.

> **TECHNICIAN NOTE** Heat fixing before Gram staining prevents the sample from washing off, helps to preserve cell morphology, kills the bacteria, and renders them permeable to stain.

Interpretation

Bacteria that retain the crystal violet—iodine complex and stain purple are called gram-positive organisms (Fig. 44.2). Those that lose the crystal violet or purple color and stain red with safranin or basic fuchsin are classified as gram-negative organisms (Fig. 44.3). The morphology of the bacteria on the smear is also important to note.

Determining the Gram stain reaction is an important step in the identification process. Performing the procedure properly and interpreting the results correctly require practice. To ensure

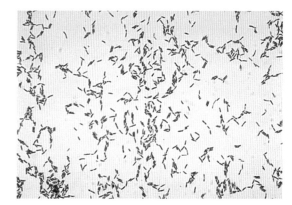

Fig. 44.2 Typical staining pattern of gram-positive *Actinomyces* bacteria. (Courtesy Public Health Image Library, PHIL#6711, William A. Clark, Atlanta, 1977, Centers for Disease Control and Prevention.)

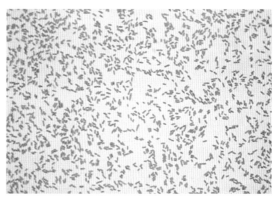

Fig. 44.3 Typical staining pattern of gram-negative *Yersinia* bacteria. (Courtesy Public Health Image Library, PHIL#6711, Atlanta, 1980, Centers for Disease Control and Prevention.)

proper staining quality, known (control) gram-positive and gram-negative organisms should be stained at least once a week and with each new batch of stain. These control organisms may be kept growing in the laboratory.

> **TECHNICIAN NOTE** Gram-positive bacteria appear purple when they are viewed microscopically, while gram-negative bacteria appear red.

POTASSIUM HYDROXIDE TEST

Sometimes an organism may stain both gram positive and negative, which is called a gram-variable reaction. This may occur as a result of excessive decolorization, an overly thick smear, excessive heat fixation, old cultures, or a poor-quality stain.

If a gram-variable reaction occurs, a quick way to check the reaction is with the potassium hydroxide (KOH) test. The procedure for this is as follows:

1. A loopful (or two, if necessary) of 3% KOH solution is placed on a slide.
2. A generous quantity of surface growth is removed from the culture and transferred to the drop of KOH.
3. The specimen is stirred into the KOH drop with a loop; the loop is then lifted slowly and gently. After a maximum of 2 minutes of stirring (usually 30 seconds), gram-negative organisms develop a mucoid appearance and produce a sticky strand when the drop is lifted with the loop. If the organisms are gram positive, the mixture stays homogeneous and does not form a strand when lifted.
4. The reaction is recorded as gram negative (i.e., a sticky strand and a mucoid mass formed) or gram positive (i.e., no sticky strand or mucoid mass formed).

> **TECHNICIAN NOTE** The KOH test is used to help with bacterial classification when gram-variable results are obtained.

A 10% to 20% KOH solution is used for the evaluation of fungal samples. Several versions of the procedure are performed. Some add dimethyl sulfoxide (DMSO) to the KOH to speed up the activity of the KOH, whereas others involve heating the slide. Additional components may involve counterstaining with India ink or Romanowsky stain.

ZIEHL-NEELSEN STAIN

This stain is primarily used to detect the acid-fast organisms of *Mycobacterium* and *Nocardia* species. Numerous types of acid-fast stains are available, and some are not configured for easy use in the veterinary practice laboratory. Acid-fast stains contain several solutions, including a primary stain, typically DMSO and carbol fuchsin; an acid-alcohol decolorizer; and a counterstain such as methylene blue. The slide is air dried and heat fixed by passing the slide, specimen side up, through a

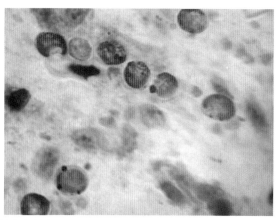

Fig. 44.4 Acid-fast stain of *Mycobacterium*. (Courtesy Marc Kramer, DVM, Avian and Exotic Animal Medical Center, Miami, FL.)

flame. The primary stain is used to flood the slide. The slide is then heated over the flame until the stain steams. The slide is cooled for 5 minutes and then rinsed with tap water. Acid alcohol is used to decolorize the slide for 1 to 2 minutes until the red color is gone, and the slide is rinsed again. The counterstain is added, and then the slide is rinsed with water and dried. Agents such as DMSO that are included in the initial staining procedure allow the stain to penetrate stain-resistant cells such as *Mycobacterium*. The subsequent addition of acid alcohol removes the stain. If the stain is not removed, the organism is "acid fast" and appears red, whereas non–acid-fast microorganisms stain blue (Fig. 44.4).

GIEMSA STAIN

Giemsa stain is used to detect spirochetes and rickettsiae as well as to demonstrate the capsule of *Bacillus anthracis* and the morphology of *Dermatophilus congolensis*. The smear is fixed in absolute methanol for 3 to 5 minutes and air dried. It is then dipped in diluted stain for 20 to 30 minutes. The staining time may be extended as indicated by the results. For *Borrelia anserina*, the smear is gently heated while it is covered with Giemsa stain and stained for 4 to 5 minutes. The smear is then rinsed, air dried, and examined for the purplish-blue–stained bacteria.

SPECIALIZED STAINS

Flagella stains, capsule stains, endospore stains, and fluorescent stains are also available, but they have limited application in the average veterinary practice laboratory. Fluorescent stains tend to be quite expensive, and they are used primarily for the identification of *Legionella* and *Pseudomonas*. Flagella stains usually contain crystal violet, and they are used to detect and characterize bacterial motility. These tend to be somewhat expensive for the small veterinary practice laboratory. Other methods that can be used to test motility include the hanging drop preparation and the use of motility test media. Capsule stains are used for the detection of pathogenic bacteria. All

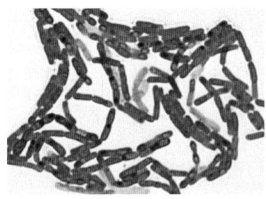

Fig. 44.5 Malachite green endospore stain of *Bacillus anthracis*. (From Songer JG, Post KW: *Veterinary microbiology: bacterial and fungal agents of animal disease*, St Louis, 2005, Saunders.)

bacteria that contain capsules are pathogenic. However, not all pathogenic bacteria contain capsules. Capsule stains often require the use of bright-field phase contrast microscopy.

Bacterial spores contain protein coats of keratin that are resistant to most normal staining procedures. Endospore stains detect the presence, location, and shape of spores, and they can aid in the differentiation of bacteria. Endospore staining is done on an older culture (i.e., more than 48 hours old), because spore formation occurs during the logarithmic decline phase. The procedure involves the addition of malachite green to the specimen on the slide and then heating the slide. The slide is washed and counterstained with safranin or basic fuchsin. Spores appear dark blue and green, with the remainder of the bacterial cell being pink or red (Fig. 44.5). Spores may also be found free from cells.

QUALITY CONTROL

Each time a clinical specimen is stained, a sample from a control culture should also be stained. This verifies the quality of the staining procedures and materials. Specialized Gram staining control slides are commercially available.

KEY POINTS

- The Gram stain is the most common staining procedure performed in the microbiology laboratory.
- Gram staining requires a primary stain, a mordant, a decolorizer, and a counterstain.
- Gram-positive organisms appear purple when viewed under the microscope, and gram-negative organisms are red.
- Samples with gram-variable reactions can be evaluated with the KOH test.
- Flagella stains, capsule stains, endospore stains, and fluorescent stains are primarily used in reference laboratories.
- The Ziehl-Neelsen stain is used to identify acid-fast organisms.

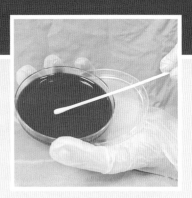

45

Culture Techniques in Microbiology

LEARNING OBJECTIVES

After studying this chapter, you will be able to:

- Describe the general sequence used when identifying bacteria.
- Describe the quadrant streak method of inoculation.
- Describe the procedure for the inoculation of slant tubes.
- Differentiate between presumptive identification and definitive identification.
- Discuss aspects of the incubation of culture plates.
- List colony characteristics that are evaluated on bacterial colonies.
- Describe methods for the culture of anaerobes.

OUTLINE

KEY TERMS

Candle jar
Filamentous
Incubation

Mucoid
Presumptive identification
Quadrant streak

Rhizoid
Slant tube
Undulate

A systematic approach is needed for the identification of pathogenic bacteria. Procedure 45.1 shows the typical sequences used to process microbiologic specimens. The practice laboratory should develop flow charts for use in the clinic that represent the bacteria seen most often as well as the tests used to differentiate those bacteria. There are often several options that can be used to determine the bacterial species. Fig. 45.1 is an example of a flow chart that can be used for the differentiation of microbes. Specimens are first streaked onto a primary medium, such as blood agar and MacConkey agar. The plates are incubated for 18 to 24 hours and then examined for growth. Suspected pathogens on the incubated plate should be further identified regarding their genus or species with the use of the flow chart. Determining the genus of a pathogenic organism is often possible by using just the staining and culture characteristics. This is referred to as a presumptive or tentative identification. Definitive identification usually requires additional biochemical testing. It is important to note that the veterinarian may make a decision regarding the initial treatment based on the presumptive identification, and additional testing may not affect therapeutic options. With comparatively few tests, an organism may be identified to the genus level with

a fair degree of certainty. Table 45.1 summarizes the identifying characteristics of common bacterial pathogens in veterinary species. Table 45.2 summarizes bacterial pathogens of veterinary importance, the species that are affected, the resultant diseases or lesions, and the specimens required for diagnosis. Appendix O, Bacterial Pathogens of Veterinary Importance, contains a summary of characteristics of and diseases produced by microbial pathogens seen in mammals and birds.

> **TECHNICIAN NOTE** Each practice laboratory should develop flow charts that represent the bacteria seen most often and the tests that will be used to differentiate those bacteria.

Most gram-positive and gram-negative organisms grow on blood agar. Gram-positive organisms usually do not grow on MacConkey agar, but this agar supports the growth of most gram-negative organisms. Selection of the colony from the routine blood agar plate is preferable to selecting it from MacConkey agar. The danger inherent in subculturing from a selective medium such as MacConkey agar is that inhibited organisms may be present as microcolonies on the plate. One of these could inadvertently be the colony of interest.

PROCEDURE 45.1   Typical Sequence of Testing of Microbiology Specimens

1. Collect specimen.
2. Direct Gram stain of specimen.
3. Inoculate culture media.
4. Incubate for 18 to 24 hours.
5. Check for growth.
   a. Negative (no growth)
      1. Reincubate.

    2. Recheck.
    3. If no growth, report as "no growth."
  b. Positive (colonies on media)
    1. Select representative colonies.
    2. Perform Gram staining.
    3. Continue with identification procedures (e.g., additional media, biochemical testing).

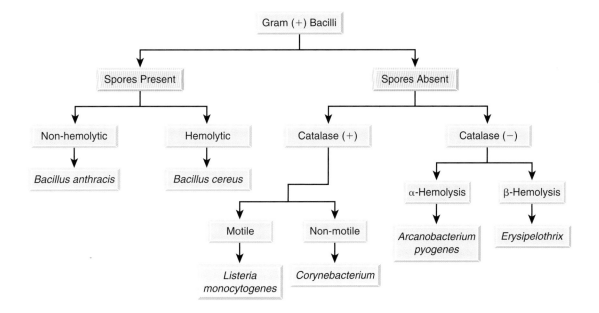

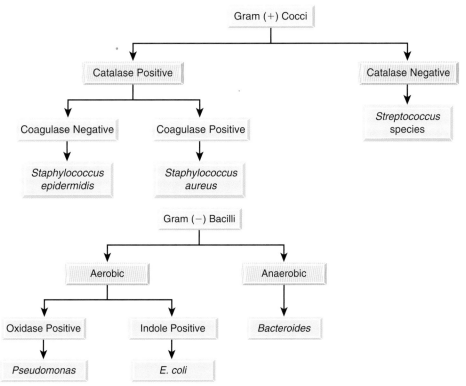

Fig. 45.1 Examples of flow charts that are used for the differentiation of bacteria.

TABLE 45.1   Common Bacterial Pathogens in Veterinary Specimens

	Blood Agar	MacConkey Agar	Other Characteristics
Gram Positive			
Staphylococcus	Smooth, glistening, white to yellow pigmented colonies	No growth	Catalase-positive glucose fermenter; double-zone hemolysis usually indicates coagulase positive; coagulase activity is a useful differential test
Streptococcus	Small, glistening colonies; hemolysis	No growth except some enterococci	Catalase negative; usually identified by type of hemolysis; beta-hemolytic strains more likely to be pathogens; others are often part of flora; Streptococcus agalactiae cAMP positive
Arcanobacterium pyogenes	Small, hemolytic, streplike colonies	No growth	Catalase negative; slow growth, often requiring 48 hr for distinct colonies; growth enhanced in candle jar
Corynebacterium pseudotuberculosis	Slow-growing, opaque, dry, crumbly colonies; usually hemolytic	No growth	Catalase positive; weak urease positive
Corynebacterium renale	Small, smooth, glistening colonies (24 hr); become opaque and dry later	No growth	Catalase positive; urease positive
Rhodococcus equi	Small, moist, white (24 hr); become large, pink colonies; no hemolysis	No growth	Catalase positive; delayed urease positive
Listeria monocytogenes	Small, hemolytic, glistening colonies	No growth	Catalase positive; motile at room temperature
Erysipelothrix rhusiopathiae	Small colonies after 48 hr; greenish (alpha) hemolysis	No growth	Catalase negative; hydrogen sulfide positive
Nocardia	Slow-growing, small, dry, granular, white to orange colonies	No growth	Partially acid fast; colonies tenaciously adhere to media
Actinomyces	Slow-growing, small, rough, nodular, white colonies	No growth	Require increased carbon dioxide or anaerobic incubation; not acid fast
Clostridium	Variable, round, ill-defined, irregular colonies; usually hemolytic	No growth	Obligate anaerobes
Bacillus	Variable, large, rough, dry, or mucoid colonies	No growth	Usually hemolytic; large rods with endospores
Gram Negative			
Escherichia coli	Large, gray, smooth, mucoid colonies; hemolysis variable	Hot pink to red colonies; red cloudiness in media	Hemolysis frequently associated with virulence
Klebsiella pneumoniae	Large, mucoid, sticky, whitish colonies; not hemolytic	Large, mucoid, pink colonies	Nonmotile; require biochemical tests to differentiate from Enterobacter
Proteus	Frequently swarming without distinct colonies	Colorless; limited swarming	Produces hydrogen sulfide in TSI
Other enterics	Gray to white, smooth, mucoid colonies	Colorless colonies	Biochemical tests for identification; serotyping indicated for Salmonella
Pseudomonas	Irregular, spreading, grayish colonies; variable hemolysis; may show a metallic sheen	Colorless, irregular colonies	Oxidase positive; fruity odor; may produce yellow to greenish soluble pigment in clear media
Bordetella bronchiseptica	Very small, circular, dew-drop colonies; variable hemolysis	Small, colorless colonies	May require 48 hr for distinct positive; rapid colonies; oxidase urease positive; citrate positive
Brucella canis	Very small, circular, pinpoint colonies after 48 to 72 hr; not hemolytic	No growth	Oxidase positive; catalase positive; urease positive
Moraxella	Round, translucent, grayish-white colonies; variable hemolysis	No growth	Oxidase and catalase positive; often nonreactive in routine biochemical tests; colonies may pit media
Actinobacillus	Round, translucent colonies; variable hemolysis	Variable growth; colorless colonies	Glucose fermenter; nonmotile; urease positive; sticky colonies
Mannheimia haemolytica	Round, gray, smooth colonies; hemolysis under the colony	Variable growth; colorless colonies	Glucose fermenter in TSI; weak oxidase positive
Pasteurella multocida	Gray, mucoid, round to coalescing colonies; no hemolysis	No growth	Glucose fermenter in TSI; weak oxidase and indole positive

cAMP, Cyclic adenosine monophosphate; TSI, triple sugar iron agar.

TABLE 45.2 **Bacterial Pathogens of Veterinary Importance**

Group	Genera	
Spirochetes	Leptospira	Borrelia
	Treponema	Brachyspira
Spiral and curved bacteria	Campylobacter	
	Helicobacter	
Gram-negative aerobic bacilli	Pseudomonas	Francisella
	Brucella	Neisseria
	Bordetella	
Gram-negative facultative bacilli	Escherichia	Proteus
	Shigella	Yersinia
	Salmonella	Citrobacter
	Klebsiella	Aeromonas
	Enterobacter	Actinobacillus
	Serratia	Haemophilus
		Pasteurella
Gram-negative anaerobic bacilli	Bacteroides	
	Fusobacterium	
Gram-positive bacilli	Bacillus	Listeria
	Clostridium	Erysipelothrix
	Lactobacillus	
Gram-negative pleomorphic	Rickettsia	Mycoplasma
	Ehrlichia	Eperythrozoon
	Anaplasma	Chlamydia
	Mycoplasma	
Gram-positive cocci	Staphylococcus	
	Streptococcus	
	Enterococcus	

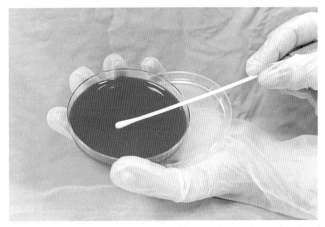

Fig. 45.2 Samples that are collected with a sterile swab can be directly inoculated.

PROCEDURE 45.2 **Quadrant Streak Method for Isolating Bacteria**

1. Use a sterile bacteriologic loop to remove a small amount of the bacterial colony from the culture plate or to take a loopful from a broth culture.
2. Optional: Divide a plate into four quadrants by marking the bottom of the Petri dish with a black marker.
3. Hold the loop horizontally against the surface of the agar to avoid digging into the agar when streaking the inoculum.
4. Lightly streak the inoculating loop over one quarter (Quadrant A) of the plate using a back-and-forth motion; keep each streak separate.
5. Pass the loop through a flame, and allow it to cool.
6. Place the inoculating loop on the edge of Quadrant A, and extend the streaks into Quadrant B using a back-and-forth motion.
7. Pass the loop through a flame, and allow it to cool.
8. Place the inoculating loop on the edge of Quadrant B, and extend the streaks into Quadrant C using a back-and-forth motion.
9. Pass the loop through a flame, and allow it to cool.
10. Place the inoculating loop on the edge of Quadrant C, and extend the streaks into Quadrant D using a back-and-forth motion.

INOCULATION OF CULTURE MEDIA

Care must be taken to prevent contamination when inoculating media and handling the specimen. Aseptic (sterile) technique must be used at all times. Before obtaining samples from a cadaver or an excised organ, sear the surface of the organ or tissue with a flamed spatula before it is cut open for sample collection. Culture plates are kept closed unless inoculating or removing colony specimens for testing. When transferring samples from or to a tube, pass the tube neck through a flame before and after the transfer of material and avoid putting down the cap. Instead, the cap should be held between the last two fingers. When flaming an inoculation loop or wire, place the near portion of the wire in the flame first, and then work toward the contaminated end. Placing the contaminated end into the flame first could result in the splattering of bacteria, resulting in aerosol contamination. When the specimen collected is a liquid, a small quantity of well-mixed samples is inoculated at the edge of the plate with a sterile swab or a bacteriologic loop. Some laboratories use presterilized glass rods for streaking samples, because Bunsen burners are not always available and glass rods can be autoclaved. Disposable inoculating loops and wires are also available. If the specimen has initially been collected on a sterile swab, this is streaked directly onto the plate (Fig. 45.2).

Streaking Culture Plates

The preferred method of streaking an agar plate is the quadrant streak method (Procedure 45.2 and Fig. 45.3). The goal when using this method is to obtain well defined and isolated bacterial colonies for further testing. Fig. 45.3, A, shows the primary streak or "well" of the plate. The bacteriologic loop may or may not be flamed and cooled before making streaks shown in parts B, C, and D of this figure. This depends on the estimated number of bacteria present in the specimen. The use of two loops—one of which is flamed and cooling while the other is being used—is a practical technique.

> **TECHNICIAN NOTE** The quadrant streak method is designed to help with the isolation of pure bacterial cultures.

Each streaked area is overlapped only once or twice to avoid depositing excessive numbers of bacteria in an area. Otherwise, the resultant colonies are not discrete and isolated. Isolated

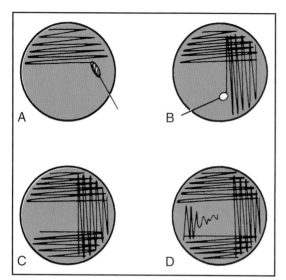

Fig. 45.3 The quadrant streak method for the isolation of bacteria. (From McCurnin DM, Bassert JM: *Clinical textbook for veterinary technicians,* ed 6, St Louis, 2006, Saunders.)

colonies typically grow in the area shown in Fig. 45.3, *D*. The use of the entire plate is important, and the streak lines should be kept close together to include as many streaks as possible, with care taken to not overlap the other streak lines. If several types of colonies grow on the plate, each colony is subcultured onto separate plates and the procedure repeated until a pure culture of discrete isolated colonies is obtained.

Inoculation of Slants

If agar slants are used, only the surface of the slant may be inoculated, or the butt and the surface may be inoculated. To inoculate only the surface of the slant, a straight flamed wire is used to obtain a colony of bacteria from the primary isolation plate. The surface of the slant tube is streaked in an S shape. To inoculate both the butt and slant, the butt of the slant is stabbed with the tip of the inoculating wire and then carefully withdrawn up the same insertion path. The surface of the slant is then streaked in an S shape (Procedure 45.3 and Fig. 45.4). Enough bacteria should be on the wire to inoculate the surface, even after the butt has been stabbed. The tube's cap should be replaced loosely.

TECHNICIAN NOTE The slanted surface of the slant tube is inoculated in an S shape.

INCUBATION OF CULTURES

For pathogens that can invade the internal organs of an animal, the optimal growth temperature is usually near 37° C. For some fish pathogens, skin pathogens (e.g., dermatophytes), and environmental organisms, the optimal growth temperature is

---

PROCEDURE 45.3   Inoculating Agar Slant and Butt

1. Use a sterile bacteriologic needle to remove a small amount of the bacterial colony from the culture plate or to take a loopful from a broth culture.
2. Stab the needle directly into the center of the agar, and push the needle all the way down to the bottom of the tube.
3. Withdraw the inoculating needle through the same path in the agar.
4. Streak the slant using a back-and-forth motion starting at the bottom of the slant.

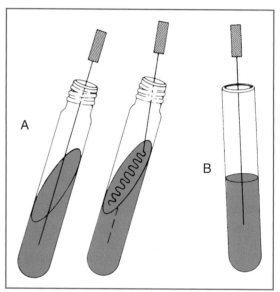

Fig. 45.4 Inoculation procedure for tube media. **A,** Inoculation of agar slant and butt, such as would be performed with triple sugar iron agar. **B,** Inoculation of motility test media. (From McCurnin DM, Bassert JM: *Clinical textbook for veterinary technicians,* ed 6, St Louis, 2006, Saunders.)

lower. Care should be taken to maintain the incubator temperature at 37° C, which is the optimal temperature, because bacterial growth for most pathogenic bacteria cannot occur above this temperature.

Incubation time depends on the generation time of individual bacterial species and the type of medium on which they are growing. For routine cultures, plates should be incubated for 48 hours, with plates examined after 18 to 24 hours of incubation. Organisms such as *Nocardia* species may take 72 hours of incubation before colonies are visible. The culture plates should be inverted during incubation so that moisture does not collect on the surface of the agar, which may cause the clumping of colonies.

TECHNICIAN NOTE Examine cultures 18 to 24 hours after the start of incubation.

Some pathogens require carbon dioxide for growth in the culture atmosphere. A candle jar may be used for this purpose. The plates are placed in a large jar, a lit candle is put on top of the plates, and the jar is sealed. The candle flame soon dies, leaving a decreased amount of oxygen and increased carbon dioxide in the jar's atmosphere. (This does not create an anaerobic condition.) The plates are incubated for 18 to 24 hours and then checked for growth. If no growth occurs, the plates are reincubated in the candle jar for another 18 to 24 hours and rechecked for growth. Larger laboratories may have incubators that automatically monitor temperature, carbon dioxide and oxygen levels, and humidity.

COLONY CHARACTERISTICS

An experienced technician can recognize several bacteria on the basis of gross observation of the colonies. Various colony characteristics, including the following, may help to identify the bacterium involved (Fig. 45.5):

- Size (in millimeters or described as pinpoint, medium, or large)
- Pigment
- Density (e.g., opaque, transparent)
- Elevation (e.g., raised, flat, convex, droplike)
- Form (e.g., circular, irregular, rhizoid, filamentous, undulate)
- Texture (e.g., glassy, smooth, mucoid, buttery, brittle, sticky)
- Odor (e.g., pungent, sweet)
- Any hemolysis (e.g., alpha, beta, gamma)

TECHNICIAN NOTE Colony morphology is assessed on pure cultures and may help with the presumptive identification of bacteria.

Many of the modular systems are provided with detailed color charts that can be used to identify the bacterial species based in part on their colony morphology (Fig. 45.6).

CULTURE OF ANAEROBES

Because most anaerobes survive exposure to air for less than 20 minutes, the collection of samples for anaerobic culture on swabs is not acceptable. Preferred anaerobic specimens include blocks of tissue (with a 2-inch-cube minimum) in a closed, sterile container as well as pus and exudate collected in a sterile syringe, with the air expelled and the needle plugged with a rubber stopper or bent backward on itself. Specialized anaerobic specimen collection systems are also available.

Specimens should be cultured as soon as possible after collection. The specimen is inoculated onto a blood agar plate and into thioglycollate broth. The blood agar plates are put into an anaerobe jar, which provides an anaerobic environment during incubation. A self-contained system, such as a Gas Pack (Oxoid, Columbia, MD), may also be used.

Conditions in which the isolation of anaerobes may be significant include soft-tissue abscesses, postoperative wounds, peritonitis, septicemia, endocarditis, endometritis, gangrene, pulmonary infection, and foot rot in cattle, sheep, and swine. The isolated anaerobe may be the sole etiologic agent, or it may be a partner in a synergistic relationship with another bacterium. For example, liver abscesses seen at slaughter in otherwise healthy feedlot cattle commonly yield the anaerobe *Fusobacterium necrophorum* and the aerobe *Actinomyces pyogenes*. For conditions that involve *Clostridium chauvoei*, *Clostridium septicum*, *Clostridium novyi*, and *Clostridium sordellii*, most laboratories use the fluorescent antibody technique for diagnosis. Specimens include affected muscle and a rib that contains bone marrow.

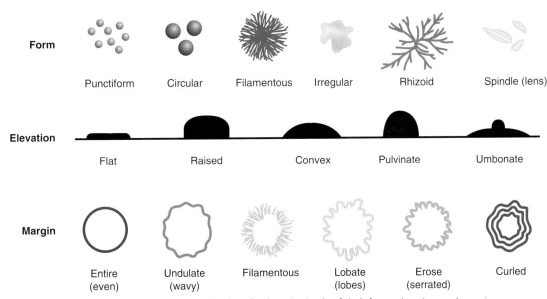

Fig. 45.5 Bacterial colonies may be described on the basis of their form, elevation, and margins.

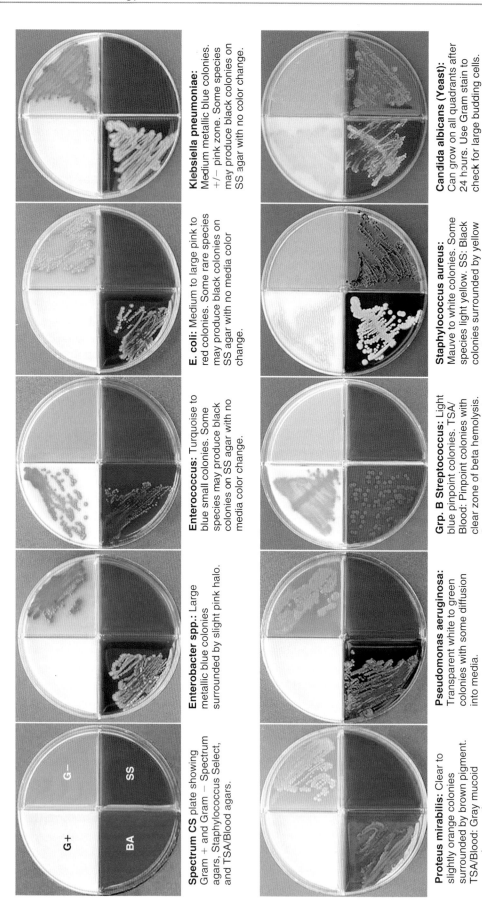

Spectrum CS plate showing Gram + and Gram − Spectrum agars, Staphylococcus Select, and TSA/Blood agars.

Proteus mirabilis: Clear to slightly orange colonies surrounded by brown pigment. TSA/Blood: Gray mucoid swarming growth.

Enterobacter spp.:: Large metallic blue colonies surrounded by slight pink halo.

Pseudomonas aeruginosa: Transparent white to green colonies with some diffusion into media.

Enterococcus: Turquoise to blue small colonies. Some species may produce black colonies on SS agar with no media color change.

Grp. B Streptococcus: Light blue pinpoint colonies. TSA/Blood: Pinpoint colonies with clear zone of beta hemolysis. Some species non-hemolytic.

E. coli: Medium to large pink to red colonies. Some rare species may produce black colonies on SS agar with no media color change.

Staphylococcus aureus: Mauve to white colonies. Some species light yellow. SS: Black colonies surrounded by yellow media.

Klebsiella pneumoniae: Medium metallic blue colonies. +/− pink zone. Some species may produce black colonies on SS agar with no color change.

Candida albicans (Yeast): Can grow on all quadrants after 24 hours. Use Gram stain to check for large budding cells.

Note: All organisms shown have been grown in pure culture. Mixed cultures should be interpreted with caution. The Spectrum CS Culture System and Spectrum-IV plate are for veterinary use only and is intended as an aid to the identification of certain common pathogens. Presumptive results should be verified using traditional culture methods.

* Also for use with Spectrum IV Quad plate

Fig. 45.6 Spectrum CS Interpretation Guide. Modular culture systems usually have interpretation guides that are based on colony morphology. (Courtesy Barry Mitzner, DVM.)

KEY POINTS

- A systematic approach is needed for the proper evaluation of cultures.
- The quadrant streak method is used to isolate a pure culture.
- Slant tubes can be inoculated on the slant surface, in the butt area, or in both areas.
- High-carbon-dioxide environments can be achieved with a candle jar.

- Cultures are incubated at 37° C and initially examined after 18 to 24 hours.
- Presumptive identification can often be achieved with the evaluation of colony morphology.
- The evaluation of colony morphology includes colony size, density, pigmentation, elevation, form, texture, and odor as well as determining the presence of any hemolysis.

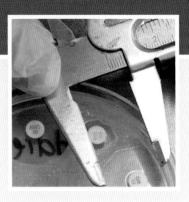

46

Antimicrobial Sensitivity Testing

LEARNING OBJECTIVES

After studying this chapter, you will be able to:

- Discuss the indications for performing antimicrobial sensitivity testing.
- Describe the procedure for performing an antimicrobial sensitivity test with the agar diffusion method.

- Describe the procedure for measuring the zone of inhibition and the significance of the measurement.
- Discuss the methods that are used to perform colony counts.

OUTLINE

KEY TERMS

Antimicrobial disks
Antimicrobial susceptibility test
Bauer-Kirby technique

Beta-lactamase
Direct sensitivity testing
Indirect sensitivity testing

McFarland suspension
Minimum inhibitory concentration
Zone of inhibition

ANTIBIOTIC RESISTANCE

Antibiotic resistance has been called one of the world's most pressing public and animal health problems. Antibiotic resistance occurs when a microbe changes or mutates in some way that reduces or eliminates the effectiveness of drugs, chemicals, or other agents designed to cure or prevent infections. Nearly every type of bacteria has become stronger and less responsive to antibiotic treatment when it is most needed. Antibiotics kill or inhibit the growth of susceptible bacteria. Sometimes one of the bacteria survives because it has the ability to neutralize or escape the effect of the antibiotic. That one bacterium can then multiply and replace all the bacteria that were killed off. Exposure to antibiotics therefore provides selective pressure, which makes the surviving bacteria more likely to be resistant. In addition, bacteria that were at one time susceptible to an antibiotic can acquire resistance through mutation of their genetic material or by acquiring pieces of DNA that code for the resistance properties from other bacteria. The DNA that codes for resistance can be grouped in a single easily transferable package. This means that bacteria can become resistant to

many antimicrobial agents because of the transfer of one piece of DNA. Some bacteria develop the ability to neutralize the antibiotic before it can do harm, others can rapidly pump the antibiotic out, and still others can change the antibiotic attack site so that it cannot affect the function of the bacteria.

These antibiotic-resistant bacteria can quickly spread to other animals and even family members and threaten the community with a new strain of infectious disease that is more difficult to cure and more expensive to treat. For this reason, antibiotic resistance is among the CDC's and USDA's top concerns. Antibiotic resistance can cause significant danger and suffering for those with common infections, once easily treatable with antibiotics. Microbes can develop resistance to specific medicines. A common misconception is that the animal becomes resistant to specific drugs. However, it is microbes, not animals, that become resistant to the drugs.

When an organism is resistant to many drugs, treating the infections it causes can become difficult or even impossible. An animal with an infection that is resistant to a certain medicine can pass that same resistant infection to another animal. In this way, a difficult-to-treat infection can be spread from one animal to another, and even to humans. In some cases, the infection can lead to serious disability or even death.

> **TECHNICIAN NOTE** Bacteria that produce β-lactamases are resistant to β-lactam antibiotics.

The most common mutation and form of antimicrobial resistance involves extended-spectrum beta (β)-lactamase (ESBL). β-Lactamases (also known as penicillinase) are enzymes produced by some bacteria that provide multiresistance to β-lactam antibiotics. These antibiotics are typically used to treat infections with a broad spectrum of gram-positive and gram-negative bacteria and include penicillins, cephalosporins, and cephamycins. β-Lactamase provides antibiotic resistance by breaking the antibiotics' structure. β-Lactam antibiotics all have a common element in their molecular structure: a four-atom ring known as a β-lactam. Through hydrolysis, the lactamase produced by the bacteria cleaves the β-lactam ring, deactivating the antibacterial properties of the medication. ESBLs are commonly found in *Escherichia coli*, *Klebsiella* spp., and *Proteus mirabilis* but can be found in other gram-negative rods. These organisms can cause serious infection and are a common source of nosocomial infection. They are also often resistant to other classes of antimicrobials (e.g., aminoglycosides, fluoroquinolones).

ANTIMICROBIAL SENSITIVITY TESTING

When bacteria are isolated from a patient, an antimicrobial sensitivity test may be performed to determine the bacterium's susceptibility or resistance to specific antimicrobial drugs.

The sensitivity test results allow the veterinarian to choose the most appropriate antimicrobial treatment for the patient. The specimen used for antimicrobial susceptibility testing must be obtained from the animal before treatment begins. The veterinarian may begin treatment before obtaining susceptibility results but then may change to a more appropriate drug when the results are available.

> **TECHNICIAN NOTE** Results of antimicrobial sensitivity testing allow for the selection of the most appropriate antimicrobial for the treatment of the patient.

AGAR DIFFUSION METHOD

The agar diffusion test is the most commonly performed method for antimicrobial susceptibility testing. It uses paper disks that have been impregnated with antimicrobials. This is a quantitative test that requires the measurement of inhibitory zone sizes to give an estimate of antimicrobial susceptibility. The concentration of drug in the disk is chosen to correlate with therapeutic levels of the drug in the treated animal. Diffusion methods that are in common use include the U.S. Food and Drug Administration (FDA) method; the standardized disk susceptibility method, which is a modified

Bauer-Kirby technique; and the International Collaborative Study standardized disk technique. The most commonly used method of antibiotic susceptibility testing is the Bauer-Kirby technique.

> **TECHNICIAN NOTE** The agar diffusion method is the most commonly performed type of sensitivity test.

Although cultures can be performed in the classic manner by using individual Mueller-Hinton agar plates, modular culture systems or specialized media are more commonly used in the veterinary practice. Some organisms, such as streptococci, do not grow sufficiently well on plain Mueller-Hinton agar for a test to be read. In these cases, Mueller-Hinton agar plus 5% blood must be used. However, having departed from the standardized method, the inhibitory zone sizes must be interpreted with caution. For example, the zone sizes for novobiocin are smaller if the medium contains blood. Most streptococci are still susceptible to penicillin.

A supply of antibiotic disks is needed that corresponds with the antibiotics that are commonly used in the clinic and the dosages that are most often needed. The antimicrobial content in a disk is indicated in Table 46.1. Only one disk that is representative of the tetracyclines and one that is representative of the sulfonamides are necessary because of the phenomenon of cross-resistance. For example, if the bacterial species is resistant to one of the tetracyclines, it is usually resistant to all members of the group.

Antimicrobial disks should always be kept in the refrigerator (4° C) when not being used and replaced as soon as possible after use. Outdated disks should never be used. The potency of the antimicrobial disks can be monitored with control organisms of known sensitivity patterns. A disk dispenser and a caliper or clear overlays for measuring inhibitory zones are also required. Disk dispensers should be obtained from the same manufacturer as the disks. Not all products are interchangeable. Inoculation of a thioglycollate or trypticase soy broth tube is recommended at the same time that plates are streaked. If the in-house culture results prove inconclusive, the broth culture can then be sent to an outside laboratory for confirmation.

Indirect sensitivity testing requires that colony samples be taken from the culture plate, subcultured in broth media, and incubated to achieve a turbidity that matches a standardized 0.5 McFarland suspension (Fig. 46.1). The broth suspension is then applied to Mueller-Hinton media with a swab or loop to cover the plate evenly. To obtain the broth solution, just the surfaces of three or four colonies should be touched with a sterile loop. The loop should be placed in saline or broth to make a suspension. If bacteria are taken from just the surface of the colony, there is less likelihood of picking up an unseen contaminant growing at the base of the colony. More than one colony of a bacterial species should always be taken, because a single colony may represent a variant that has a susceptibility pattern that is different from that of the parent strain. A correct density is an important aspect of getting

TABLE 46.1   Chart of Inhibitory Zones to Determine the Relative Resistance of the Bacterium to the Antibiotics Being Tested

Antimicrobial Agent	Disk Content	Susceptible (mm)	Intermediate (mm)	Resistant (mm)
Amikacin	30 µg	≥17	15—16	≤14
Amoxicillin/clavulanic acid (staphylococci)	20/10 µg	≥20		≤19
Amoxicillin/clavulanic acid (other organisms)	20/10 µg	≥18	14—17	≤13
Ampicillin* (gram-negative enteric organisms)	10 µg	≥17	14—16	≤13
Ampicillin* (staphylococci)	10 µg	≥29		≤28
Ampicillin* (enterococci)	10 µg	≥17		≤16
Ampicillin* (streptococci)	10 µg	≥26	19—25	≤18
Cefazolin	30 µg	≥18	15—17	≤14
Ceftiofur (respiratory pathogens only)	30 µg	≥21	18—20	≤7
Cephalothin†	30 µg	≥18	15—17	≤14
Chloramphenicol	30 µg	≥18	13—17	≤12
Clindamycin‡	≥2 µg	≥21	15—20	≤14
Enrofloxacin	5 µg	≥23	17—22	≤16
Erythromycin	15 µg	≥23	14—22	≤13
Florfenicol	30 µg	≥19	15—18	≤14
Gentamicin	10 µg	≥15	13—14	≤12
Kanamycin	30 µg	≥18	14—17	≤13
Oxacillin§ (staphylococci)	1 µg	≥13	11—12	≤10
Penicillin G (staphylococci)	10 U	≥29		≤28
Penicillin G (enterococci)	10 U	≥15		≤14
Penicillin G (streptococci)	10 U	≥28	20—27	≤19
Penicillin/novobiocin	10 U/30 µg	≥18	15—17	≤14
Pirlimycin‖	2 µg	≥13		≤12
Rifampin	5 µg	≥20	17—19	≤16
Sulfonamides	250 or 300 µg	≥17	13—16	≤12
Tetracycline¶	30 µg	≥19	15—18	≤14
Ticarcillin (*Pseudomonas aeruginosa*)	75 µg	≥15		≤14
Ticarcillin (gram-negative enteric organisms)	75 µg	≥20	15—19	≤14
Tilmicosin	15 µg	≥14	11—13	≤10
Trimethoprim/sulfamethoxazole**	1.25/23.75 µg	≥16	11—15	≤10

*Ampicillin is used to test for susceptibility to amoxicillin and hetacillin.
†Cephalothin is used to test all first-generation cephalosporins, such as cephapirin and cefadroxil. Cefazolin should be tested separately with the gram-negative enteric organisms.
‡Clindamycin is used to test for susceptibility to clindamycin and lincomycin.
§Oxacillin is used to test for susceptibility to methicillin, nafcillin, and cloxacillin.
‖Available as an infusion product for treatment of bovine mastitis during lactation.
¶Tetracycline is used to test for susceptibility to chlortetracycline, oxytetracycline, minocycline, and doxycycline.
**Trimethoprim/sulfamethoxazole is used to test for susceptibility to trimethoprim/sulfadiazine and ormetoprim/sulfadimethoxine.
From McCurnin DM, Bassert JM: *Clinical textbook for veterinary technicians*, ed 6, St Louis, 2006, Saunders.
Modified from National Committee for Clinical Laboratory Standards document M31-A2, Table 2, pp 55-59, 2002.

reproducible results. The "lawn" of cells that grows after inoculation should be evenly distributed. Extremes in concentration must be avoided.

> **TECHNICIAN NOTE** Indirect testing is more precise than direct testing, but results are not available as quickly.

The application of undiluted samples (e.g., urine) directly to the Mueller-Hinton plate is referred to as direct sensitivity testing. Although not as precise as indirect testing, reasonable results can be expected when only one organism is present. Antibiotic susceptibility should be interpreted with caution when the culture shows multiple organisms.

The antimicrobial disks are placed on the inoculated agar surface with a disk dispenser or sterile forceps that have been flamed and cooled between each use. The disks should be no closer than 10 mm to 15 mm to the edge of the plate and sufficiently separated from each other to avoid overlapping of any zone of inhibition. Unless the disks were placed with a self-tamping dispenser, use a second sterile swab to gently press the antibiotic disks into the agar. The plates are incubated aerobically at 37° C, and they should be placed in the incubator within 15 minutes after placing the disks on the inoculated agar. Inoculated plates should be inverted before they are placed in the incubator to avoid condensation collecting on the surface of the agar. The plates should be kept in stacks of four or fewer,

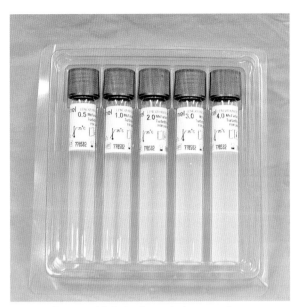

Fig. 46.1 McFarland standard suspensions.

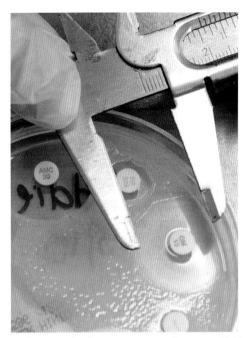

Fig. 46.2 The use of calipers to measure the zone of inhibition.

because plates in the center of a tall stack take longer to reach the incubation temperature.

> **TECHNICIAN NOTE** Measure the zone of inhibition and compare it against a standard chart to identify the susceptibility of the bacterium to the antibiotics being tested.

Whether testing is performed by the direct or indirect method, antibiotic susceptibility must be determined by the physical measurement of the inhibitory zones (Fig. 46.2). That measurement is then compared with a chart of inhibitory zones to determine the relative resistance of the bacterium to the antibiotics being tested (see Table 46.1).

Reading the Zones of Inhibition

The plates should be read after a constant period, most satisfactorily after overnight incubation (i.e., 18 to 24 hours). Prolonged incubation may alter the size of the zone of inhibition with antimicrobials that are not stable at 37° C or, at best, make the zones hard to read. If rapid results are imperative, the diameters of the zones of inhibition may be read after 6 to 8 hours of incubation. These results should be confirmed by reading them again after overnight incubation. The diameter of each inhibition zone (including the diameter of the disk) is measured from the underside of the plate using calipers, a transparent ruler, or a template. The zones are measured and recorded to the nearest millimeter. If Mueller-Hinton agar with blood has been used, the zone size must be read from the top surface, with the lid of the plate removed.

Interpretation of Zone Sizes

Table 46.1 lists some of the commonly used antimicrobials and gives the suggested interpretation of zone sizes with the FDA standardized disk method. The zone sizes are divided into two major categories: resistant or susceptible to the particular

antimicrobial agent. The latter category is subdivided into intermediate susceptibility and susceptible. For predictive purposes, a resistant organism is not likely to respond to therapy with the drug. A susceptible organism is susceptible to ordinary doses of the antimicrobial. Intermediate susceptibility implies that the organism is susceptible to ordinary doses when the drug is concentrated in the urine or tissues. The antimicrobial may be used for the treatment of systemic infections if a high dosage is safe.

The zone size alone is not indicative of the efficacy of an antimicrobial. Some drugs, such as vancomycin and colistin, do not readily diffuse through agar and give small inhibition zones, even when the test organism is fully susceptible. Therefore, direct comparisons with zone diameters produced by unrelated antimicrobials are misleading and should not be made.

Control Organisms

Susceptible reference organisms such as *Staphylococcus aureus*, American Type Culture Collection 25923, and *Escherichia coli*, American Type Culture Collection 25922, should be tested regularly, preferably in parallel with each batch of antimicrobial susceptibility tests. These control organisms are used to check such factors as the growth-supporting capability of the medium, the potency of the antimicrobial disks, and other variable conditions that can affect results.

Limitations of the Test

The FDA method is designed for rapidly growing bacteria. Caution is needed for tests of anaerobes or slow-growing organisms for which the criteria for the interpretation of zone diameters have not yet been established with certainty. In general, the zone diameters are somewhat larger for an equivalent minimal inhibitory concentration with slow-growing organisms as compared with rapid growers.

Some rare strains of staphylococci are resistant to methicillin and other penicillinase-stable penicillins. The routine test cannot be relied on to detect these strains, but they may be detected by incubation of an additional susceptibility test plate that contains a methicillin disk at 30° C. A reduced zone diameter or no zone surrounding the methicillin disk on the plate that has been incubated at 30° C is presumptive evidence of methicillin resistance.

MINIMUM INHIBITORY CONCENTRATION

A method similar to the agar diffusion method for sensitivity testing can be used to determine the minimum inhibitory concentration (MIC) of an antimicrobial. This is the lowest concentration of the specific antimicrobial that can inhibit the growth of a given bacteria. The choice of a specific concentration of antimicrobial is based on the MIC, the site of infection, and the breakpoint of the antimicrobial. Breakpoint refers to the dilution of the antimicrobial where the specific bacteria begins to show resistance. Other considerations for specific antimicrobials include patient characteristics, such as age, species, and overall health, as well as possible side effects, costs, ease of use, and frequency and route of administration.

To perform the test with the agar diffusion method, paper disks or strips with varying concentrations of the chosen antimicrobial are placed on a freshly inoculated culture plate and incubated. Measuring the zones of inhibition around each of these disks will help the veterinarian choose an appropriate concentration of medication to be given to the patient.

Alternately, the MIC can be determined using microwells with multiple known concentrations of the antimicrobial being tested (Fig. 46.3). A standard suspension of 10^5 CFU/mL of the bacteria is prepared from a pure colony, and the suspension is inoculated into the wells. The MIC number is the lowest concentration (in µg/mL) of an antibiotic that inhibits the growth of a given strain of bacteria. The breakpoint and range of dilutions differ by drug and bacterial species. Therefore, comparing MICs of different antibiotics is not based solely on the numerical value but on how far the MIC is from the breakpoint, the site of the infection, and other considerations.

For example, assume that a strain of *E. coli* has an MIC of 2 µg/mL for amoxicillin and an MIC of 8 µg/mL for cephalexin. For the dilutions for amoxicillin, at 2 µg/mL, this strain of *E. coli* is four dilutions away from the breakpoint. For cephalexin, the same strain of *E. coli* at an MIC of 8 µg/mL is two dilutions away from the breakpoint. So, based on the MIC number, this strain of *E. coli* is more susceptible to amoxicillin than cephalexin. The further away from the breakpoint that the organism will grow, the more effective the antibiotic will be.

Limitations of the Test

In order for an antimicrobial agent to cure an infection, the drug must be able to get to the site of the infection and attain a concentration at the infection site that is greater than the MIC of the infecting bacterium. Sometimes the concentration of bacteria at the infection site is greater than the amount used in routine testing. The MIC generally increases for an ESBL-producing isolate when challenged with greater than 10^5 CFU/mL. At the higher concentration of bacteria, the drug cannot overcome the increased concentration of ESBL that is present. Other factors may also contribute to clinical failures, such as the concentration of drug at the infection site compared with the MIC of the infecting bacteria and how long that concentration stays above the MIC. All organisms of the genus and species *E. coli*, *Klebsiella* spp., and *P. mirabilis* should be tested for ESBL. These are the most common organisms exhibiting ESBL production; however, other organisms have been found to produce ESBL. In monitoring clinical findings and evaluating the effectiveness of antimicrobial therapy, consideration should be given to the possibility that ESBL may negatively impact effective treatment.

COLONY COUNT

The presence of pathogenic bacteria does not necessarily indicate infection. For example, although normal urine is considered sterile, small numbers of organisms may occasionally be found, even after collection by cystocentesis. A colony count on cultured urine samples can help to support a diagnosis of urinary tract infection. Colony counts can be performed by streaking a blood agar or another nonselective agar plate with a calibrated loop that contains 10 µL of urine (Fig. 46.4). After incubation, all colonies are counted and

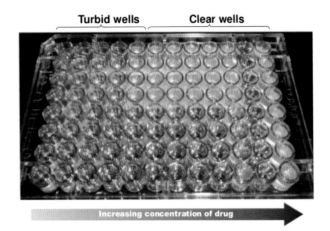

Fig. 46.3 Microwells with varying concentrations of antimicrobials used for determination of MIC.

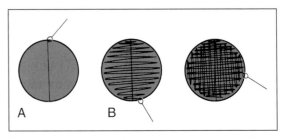

Fig. 46.4 The procedure for inoculating media for semiquantitative bacterial colony counts when culturing urine. **A,** Primary inoculation with a calibrated loop. **B,** A streak made at right angles to the previous streak. (From McCurnin DM, Bassert JM: *Clinical textbook for veterinary technicians,* ed 6, St Louis, 2006, Saunders.)

multiplied by 100 to determine the number of colony-forming units (CFUs) per milliliter of urine. Although they only serve as guidelines, significant numbers of CFUs are more than 1000 CFUs for samples collected by cystocentesis and more than 10,000 CFUs for those collected by catheter. Voided samples (although not recommended for culture) should have more than 100,000 CFUs in dogs and more than 10,000 CFUs in cats to be deemed significant.

KEY POINTS

- Antibiotic resistance occurs when a microbe changes or mutates in some way that reduces or eliminates the effectiveness of drugs, chemicals, or other agents designed to cure or prevent infections.
- Bacteria that produce β-lactamases are resistant to β-lactam antibiotics.
- Antibiotic sensitivity testing is performed to determine the resistance or susceptibility of bacteria to specific antimicrobials.
- The application of undiluted samples directly to the Mueller-Hinton plate is referred to as direct sensitivity testing.
- Indirect sensitivity testing requires that colony samples be taken from the culture plate, subcultured in broth media, and incubated to achieve a turbidity that matches a standardized 0.5 McFarland suspension.

- Antimicrobial disks are placed on the inoculated agar surface with a disk dispenser or a sterile forceps that has been flamed and cooled between each use.
- For the sensitivity test, the diameter of each inhibition zone (including the diameter of the disk) is measured from the underside of the plate with the use of calipers, a transparent ruler, or a template.
- The MIC should be determined to ensure that the most effective antimicrobial will be chosen and used at the appropriate dosage.
- The presence of pathogenic bacteria does not necessarily indicate infection.
- A colony count on cultured urine samples can help support a diagnosis of urinary tract infection.

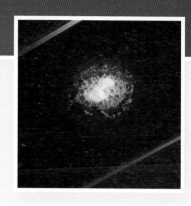

47

Additional Testing in Microbiology

LEARNING OBJECTIVES

After studying this chapter, you will be able to:
- List and describe methods for testing the motility of bacteria.
- List the commonly performed biochemical tests.
- Describe the commonly performed biochemical tests.
- Describe the procedure for performing the California Mastitis Test.

OUTLINE

KEY TERMS

California Mastitis Test
Catalase
Coagulase

Hanging drop
Indole
Kovac's reagent

Motility media
Oxidase

The presumptive identification of bacteria often gives the veterinarian enough information to develop a diagnostic and treatment plan. However, some organisms must be further differentiated to the species level and require additional testing for positive identification. A partial list of commonly performed tests follows.

MOTILITY

Several methods are commonly used to test motility: the hanging drop prep, the wet prep, and motility media. For a wet prep, a young broth culture is used. A moderately heavy suspension of the bacterial sample is made in a few milliliters of nutrient broth that are incubated for 2 to 3 hours at room temperature. A loopful of this culture is placed on a microscope slide under a coverslip and examined with the high dry objective lens. If the bacteria are obviously motile, with individual cells moving backward or forward among other cells, the answer has been obtained. Brownian movement should not be mistaken for true motility. Brownian movement is the shifting of cells or particles, with little movement relative to each other.

Wet preps tend to evaporate rapidly under the microscope, and some bacteria may not appear obviously motile unless provided with additional liquid. The hanging drop prep can

eliminate these problems. Special slides are available that contain concave depressions in the center. The slide should be cleaned with alcohol and wiped dry. A small ring of petroleum jelly is placed around the concave area of the slide just before use. To prepare the hanging drop prep, place a drop of bacterial suspension on a coverslip and invert the coverslip onto the concave area of the slide. Press the coverslip down slightly so that the petroleum jelly seals the concavity. The suspension will be left hanging upside down into the well of the concave slide. This preparation does not tend to dry out quickly, and it can be observed for a fairly long period.

If the organisms are nonmotile on microscopic examination, motility media should be used. Two tubes of a motility medium (e.g., sulfide indole motility [SIM] medium) are stab inoculated. One tube is incubated at 37° C and the other at room temperature for 24 to 48 hours. If growth is restricted to the stab inoculation line, the organism is nonmotile. Diffuse growth throughout the medium means that the bacterium is motile. To interpret the results, the tubes are held against a good light, and the inoculated tubes are compared with an uninoculated one. The SIM medium is unsuitable for the motility testing of organisms that produce hydrogen sulfide in this medium, because the blackening that results may make the motility test difficult to read. The SIM media is also capable of

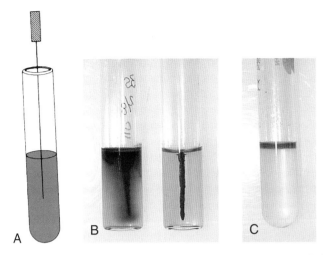

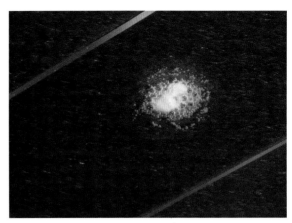

Fig. 47.2 A positive catalase test is indicated by the production of bubbles after hydrogen peroxide has been added to a sample on a slide. (From McCurnin D, Bassert J: *McCurnin's clinical textbook for veterinary technicians,* ed 7, St Louis, 2010, Saunders.)

Fig. 47.1 **A,** Inoculation of motility test media. The inoculation needle is stabbed into the medium and withdrawn along the same tract. **B,** Motile bacterial growth in the left tube and nonmotile growth in the right tube. **C,** Kovac's reagent added to detect the production of indole. (From McCurnin D, Bassert J: *McCurnin's clinical textbook for veterinary technicians,* ed 7, St Louis, 2010, Saunders.)

providing results for the indole test. The test evaluates the ability of the organism to produce indole. Kovac's reagent is added to the incubated tube. The reagent turns red if the bacteria produce indole (Fig. 47.1).

INDOLE TEST

Although the indole test can be performed using Kovac's reagent and an SIM tube as described earlier, it is more commonly performed as a spot test. There are several methods for performing the test. A small amount of a colony can be picked up from a pure culture with a cotton swab and a drop of Kovac's reagent added to it. A positive result is indicated by the development of a red to pink color on the swab. No color development indicates a negative test. Alternately, several drops of the indole reagent can be applied to a piece of filter paper, and a loop of the bacterial colony can be rubbed onto the reagent-saturated area. Kovac's reagent is not suitable for testing anaerobic bacteria. Other reagents can be used with the spot test on anaerobic and aerobic bacteria. The color change may differ depending on the specific reagent chosen. Development of a blue color indicates a positive test with the DMACA reagent.

CATALASE TEST

The catalase test is performed on gram-positive cocci and small gram-positive bacilli. It tests for the enzyme catalase, which acts on hydrogen peroxide to produce water and oxygen. A small amount of a colony from a blood agar plate is placed on a microscope slide, and a drop of catalase reagent (3% hydrogen peroxide) is added. If the colony is catalase positive, gas bubbles are produced (Fig. 47.2). No bubble production indicates a negative result.

No blood agar should be transferred with the colony, because blood agar can produce a slightly positive reaction. A positive reaction also may occur if a mixed colony is sampled (i.e., one with both catalase-positive and catalase-negative organisms growing together). The plate must be carefully streaked to obtain isolated colonies. Staphylococci can be used as catalase-positive controls, and streptococci can be used as catalase-negative controls.

COAGULASE TEST

The coagulase test is performed on catalase-positive, gram-positive cocci. *Staphylococcus aureus* produces coagulase, which is an enzyme that coagulates plasma. Two versions of the test are available: the slide coagulase test and the tube coagulase test. The coagulase test is used to differentiate among coagulase-positive *S. aureus*, *Staphylococcus intermedius*, and coagulase-negative *Staphylococcus* (e.g., *Staphylococcus epidermidis* or *Staphylococcus saprophyticus*).

The tube coagulase test uses lyophilized plasma (purchased from a medical supply house) that has been diluted according to the manufacturer's directions. Approximately 0.5 mL is placed in a test tube and inoculated with a loopful of the organism cultured on a noninhibitory medium, such as blood agar. The tube is incubated at 37° C and read hourly for 4 hours. A negative reaction is indicated by no clot formation, whereas a positive reaction is indicated by clots. If the test result remains negative, the sample is incubated again for 24 hours and then read.

The slide coagulase test is a commercially available rapid screening test that detects surface-bound coagulase or clumping factor. More than 95% of coagulase-producing staphylococci possess clumping factor. A loopful of staphylococci from a colony is first emulsified in a drop of water or saline solution to yield a thick suspension. A drop of fresh rabbit or human plasma is then added and stirred with a sterile loop. A positive reaction is indicated by clumping occurring within 5 to 20 seconds.

OXIDASE ACTIVITY

The oxidase test depends on the presence of cytochrome C oxidase in bacteria. A drop of 1% tetramethyl-p-phenylenediamine is added to a piece of filter paper in a Petri dish. The filter paper must be damp but not saturated. Prepared dry reagent slides are also available for performing the oxidase test and eliminate the need for reagent handling. A short streak of the sample is made on the filter paper or prepared slide using a glass rod or the end of a Pasteur pipette that has been bent into a hook. The sample should be applied with a gentle rubbing action. A nickel–chromium wire bacteriologic loop should not be used, because any traces of iron may give a false-positive result.

In a positive test, the reagent is reduced to a deep purple color within 60 seconds. If the color-change reaction takes longer than this, the result should be regarded as negative. Oxidase reagent tends to be unstable, and it becomes discolored with time. It should be discarded if it becomes dark purple. *Pseudomonas aeruginosa* can be used as an oxidase-positive control, and *Escherichia coli* can be used as an oxidase-negative control. A dry slide kit is available for this test (Fig. 47.3).

ACID PRODUCTION FROM GLUCOSE

A tube of 1% glucose in peptone broth that contains a pH indicator is inoculated and incubated for 24 to 48 hours at 37° C. For fastidious organisms such as *Streptococcus* species, approximately 5 drops of sterile serum should be added to the peptone water medium, or growth may not occur.

CALIFORNIA MASTITIS TEST

Mastitis may be caused by bacterial or mycotic organisms. Several laboratory tests are available to diagnose mastitis,

including the California Mastitis Test (CMT), the somatic cell count, and the milk culture. A quick check to detect bacteria can be performed by preparing a thin smear of mastitic milk. The smear is heat fixed and stained with Gram stain or methylene blue. The most common microorganisms involved with mastitis are *S. aureus*, *Streptococcus agalactiae*, *Streptococcus uberis*, *E. coli*, *Corynebacterium* species, and *Pseudomonas aeruginosa*.

The CMT is a qualitative screening test that can be used as a "cow-side" test. The test is based on gel formation when the test reagent reacts with DNA in somatic cells. As the cell count of the milk increases, the gelling action increases. Therefore, the test provides an indirect measure of the cell count. The degree of gel formation is scored as negative; trace; or 1, 2, or 3.

To perform the CMT, approximately 2 mL of milk is placed in each of the four cups on the CMT paddle, and an equal amount of reagent is added (Fig. 47.4). The paddle is gently rotated for approximately 10 seconds in a circular pattern to mix the milk and the reagent. A score is then assigned for each quarter according to the chart of grading and interpretation (Table 47.1).

Precautions to be considered when performing this test are as follows:

1. DNA in somatic cells deteriorates upon standing. If the test is to be used as a laboratory test, the milk samples should be kept refrigerated, but not for more than 48 hours. Unrefrigerated milk cannot be tested accurately after about 12 hours.
2. White blood cells tend to migrate with milk fat. Therefore, the thorough mixing of samples just before testing is essential.
3. CMT reaction must be scored 10 to 15 seconds after mixing starts. Weaker reactions fade thereafter.

Only positive milk samples that are identified by CMT or direct somatic cell count should be cultured (Fig. 47.5). The milk sample is inoculated on blood agar and MacConkey agar and then incubated at 37° C for 24 hours. Milk samples are also incubated simultaneously. If the cultures show minimal or no growth after 24 hours of incubation, a subculture is made on the blood and MacConkey agar plates from the incubated milk

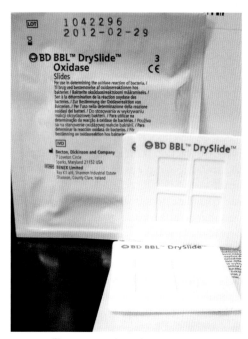

Fig. 47.3 DrySlide Oxidase Test.

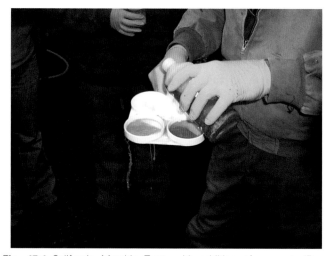

Fig. 47.4 California Mastitis Test, with addition of reagent. (From Holtgrew-Bohling K: *Large animal clinical procedures for veterinary technicians,* ed 2, St Louis, 2012, Mosby.)

TABLE 47.1   Grading of California Mastitis Test Results

Symbol	Meaning	Visible Reaction	Interpretation
–	Negative	The mixture remains liquid, with no evidence of a precipitate.	0–200,000 cells/mL 0%–25% PMNs
T	Trace	Slight precipitate forms and is seen to best advantage by tipping the paddle back and forth and observing the mixture as it flows over the bottom of the cup. Trace reactions tend to disappear with the continued movement of the fluid.	150,000–500,000 cells/mL 30%–40% PMNs
1	Weak positive	A distinct precipitate is present, but there is no tendency toward gel formation. With some samples, the reaction is reversible. With continued movement of the paddle, the precipitate may disappear.	400,000–1,500,000 cells/mL 40%–60% PMNs
2	Distinct positive	The mixture thickens immediately, with some suggestion of gel formation. As the mixture is swirled, it tends to move toward the center, leaving the bottom of the outer edge of the cup exposed. When the motion is stopped, the mixture levels out again and covers the bottom of the cup.	800,000–5,000,000 cells/mL 60%–70% PMNs
3	Strong positive	Gel formation causes the surface of the mixture to become convex. Usually a central peak remains projecting above the main mass after the motion of the paddle has been stopped. Viscosity is greatly increased, so there is a tendency for the mass to adhere to the bottom of the cup.	Cell number generally 5,000,000/mL 70%–80% PMNs

PMN, Polymorphonuclear leukocyte.

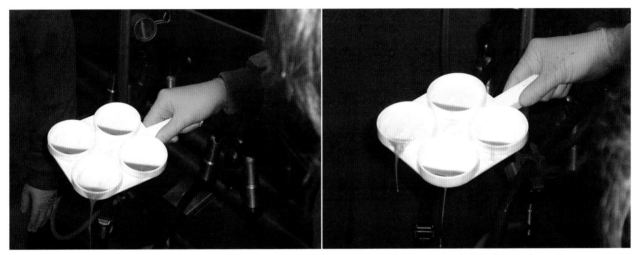

Fig. 47.5 Positive California Mastitis Test. (From Holtgrew-Bohling K: Large animal clinical procedures for veterinary technicians, ed 2, St Louis, 2012, Mosby.)

samples. The subcultured plates and the original culture plates are incubated for 24 hours at 37° C. A rapid but presumptive identification of the organism may be made on the basis of colonial morphologic characteristics, and this will be followed by confirmatory tests (e.g., triple sugar iron, lysine, SIM, methyl red, citrate, coagulase, catalase).

IMMUNOLOGIC EXAMINATION

Numerous immunologic tests are available for the identification of bacterial pathogens, particularly obligate intracellular bacteria. See Unit 9 for more information about immunologic testing.

KEY POINTS

- Additional testing is sometimes needed for the definitive identification of bacteria.
- The motility of bacteria can be evaluated with a wet mount, a hanging drop prep, or motility test media.
- Commonly performed biochemical tests performed on bacterial samples are the catalase, coagulase, and oxidase tests.
- The California Mastitis Test is a commonly used "cow-side" test that is used to detect mastitis.

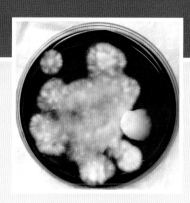

48

Mycology

LEARNING OBJECTIVES

After studying this chapter, you will be able to:

- Describe the procedure for preparing dermatophyte cultures.
- Describe the procedure for the microscopic evaluation of dermatophyte cultures.
- Describe the use of the Wood's lamp.

- Discuss the culture methods for nondermatophytes.
- List the characteristics of yeasts of veterinary importance.
- List the general characteristics of the systemic dimorphic fungi.
- Describe the microscopic appearance of fungi in clinical specimens.

OUTLINE

KEY TERMS

Dermatophyte test medium
Potassium hydroxide

Ringworm
Sabouraud agar

Wood's lamp

Supplies that are needed for the collection and examination of fungal samples are much the same as those used for bacterial samples—specifically, forceps, swabs, lactophenol cotton blue stain, potassium hydroxide solution, and culture media (e.g., dermatophyte test medium [DTM], Sabouraud agar). A Wood's lamp may prove helpful, and cellophane tape may also be used to collect certain types of samples for fungal analysis.

Ideally, a separate room and incubator should be used for fungal culture, because fungal spores may contaminate the plates that are used for bacteriologic culture. If an incubator is inadvertently contaminated with fungal spores, the interior should be swabbed thoroughly with 70% ethyl or isopropyl alcohol, or one bowl of water and one of alcohol should be placed at the bottom of the incubator and the incubator left empty of plates for 24 hours, with the door shut, at 37° C.

> **TECHNICIAN NOTE** A separate incubator for fungal samples will minimize the cross-contamination of bacterial samples with fungal spores.

Most fungal agents of clinical importance in the veterinary practice are the cutaneous mycotic organisms known as the dermatophytes. These organisms are often referred to as the ringworm fungi because of the characteristic circular lesions that they often cause on the skin of infected animals. The dermatophytes are saprophytic mycelial-forming fungi that

possess keratolytic properties that allow them to invade skin, nails, and hair. Some of these agents can infect human beings.

The dermatophytes comprise more than three dozen different organisms in the taxonomic genera *Microsporum* and *Trichophyton*. The most commonly seen species are *Microsporum canis*, *Microsporum gypseum*, and *Trichophyton mentagrophytes*. Dermatophytes can be classified by the habitat in which they are most likely to be found: anthropophilic (confined to human beings), zoophilic (parasites of animals), and geophilic (normally existing as free-living saprophytes in the soil). Of the 15 known geophilic species, five may occasionally be opportunist pathogens, and only one, *M. gypseum*, commonly causes lesions in animals. These geophilic species pose a certain difficulty with diagnosis, because they must be differentiated from zoophilic species. In approximately 98% of cats and 50% to 70% of dogs, infection is due to *Microsporum canis*.

DERMATOPHYTE TESTING

Most dermatophytes will grow on the outside of the hair shaft. In some cases, they can be visualized microscopically after mounting them in 10% potassium hydroxide (KOH) or a combination of KOH and dimethyl sulfoxide (DMSO). The DMSO eliminates the need to warm the slide and provides more rapid clearing of the sample. To examine for dermatophytes, a few hairs plucked from the periphery of the suspect lesion are placed on a slide with 1 or 2 drops of the clearing solution. A cover glass is applied, and the slide is warmed gently if just 10% KOH is used. After 2 to 10 minutes, small globular arthrospores attached to the hair shafts are visible and indicate a positive test result.

> **TECHNICIAN NOTE** Only about half of the cases of *M. canis* show evidence of fluorescence.

A Wood's lamp is an ultraviolet light source that may be used to screen suspect lesions for dermatophyte infection (Fig. 48.1), but results may be ambiguous. Hair samples from dogs and cats—or the animals themselves—can be examined under the Wood's lamp. Hairs that are infected with some species of *Microsporum* may fluoresce a clear apple-green under the Wood's lamp in a darkened room (Fig. 48.2). Fluorescence is only evident in approximately 50% of cases involving *M. canis*, apparently depending on whether the fungus has reached the right growth stage to produce fluorescence. A lack of

fluorescence with Wood's lamp examination does not rule out the possibility of ringworm infection. Always allow the Wood's lamp to warm up for 5 minutes before use.

> **TECHNICIAN NOTE** The Wood's lamp must be warmed up for at least 5 minutes before use.

Several products are available for culturing dermatophytes. The most common is standard DTM, which contains an indicator that turns red in the presence of most dermatophytes. The media is available in tube formats (Fig. 48.3) and in a variety of plate configurations. Plate configurations tend to allow for easier sampling of the colonies. Rapid sporulation medium (RSM) or enhanced sporulation media (ESM) with color indicators can be used in conjunction with standard DTM to accelerate the formation of macroconidia used for identification and confirmation (Fig. 48.4) (DermatoPlate, Vetlab Supply, Palmetto Bay, FL). Standard Sabouraud dextrose agar

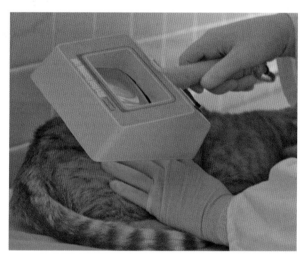

Fig. 48.1 Using the Wood's lamp to examine a patient in a darkened room. (From Taylor S: *Small animal clinical techniques,* St Louis, 2010, Saunders.)

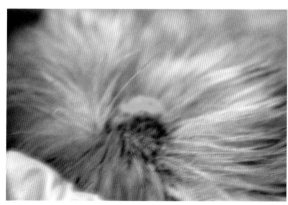

Fig. 48.2 Green fluorescence of the hairs around a skin lesion on a cat's neck caused by *Microsporum canis*. (From Taylor S: *Small animal clinical techniques,* St Louis, 2010, Saunders.)

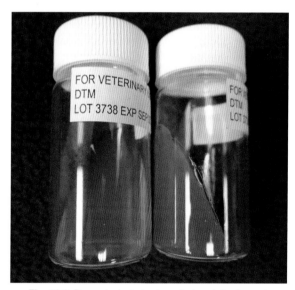

Fig. 48.3 Dermatophyte test media in a tube format.

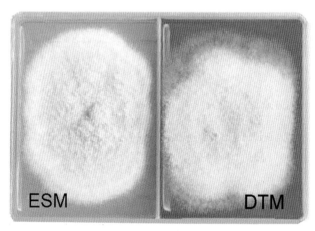

Fig. 48.4 Dermatophyte culture system with dual-chambered plate containing standard dermatophyte test medium (DTM) and enhanced sporulation medium (ESM). (Courtesy Vetlab Supply.)

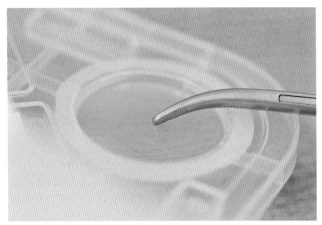

Fig. 48.5 The sample is placed onto the media and pressed slightly into and partly below the surface.

will also promote the earlier formation of macroconidia, but it contains no color indicator.

When collecting specimens for dermatophyte culture, clean the skin lesion to remove some of the surface contamination and collect specimens from the lesion periphery. Broken hair shafts and dry scale are most likely to contain viable organisms. Push the specimens into and partially below the surface of the media (Fig. 48.5). Incubate the culture at room temperature with the cap or plate cover loosened and observe daily for growth. At the first sign of color change, perform a wet prep using Fungi-Tape (Scientific Device Laboratory, Des Plaines, IL) or clear cellophane tape and lactophenol cotton blue stain to confirm the presence of pathogenic forms. Remember, the presence of red coloration (DTM) or teal coloration (ESM and other media) alone is not diagnostic of dermatophyte infection. Both bacterial contaminants and nonpathogenic fungi can, under certain conditions, cause positive color reactions. Therefore, a diagnosis must be supported by microscopic examination (Fig. 48.6).

> **TECHNICIAN NOTE** Confirm all dermatophyte infections by verifying the species with microscopic examination.

FUNGAL CULTURES

Cultures of nondermatophytes are usually streaked out on blood agar or Sabouraud dextrose agar, as is done for bacteria. For fungal organisms that do not produce spores, cultures may be prepared by cutting 1 cm² agar from the center of a Sabouraud dextrose agar plate with a sterile scalpel. A square of the same size is taken from the edge of the colony to be subcultured. This

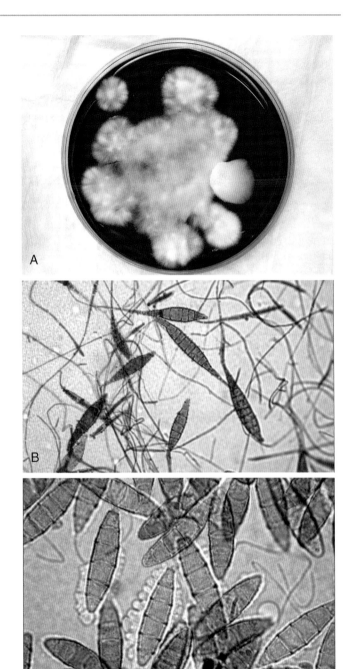

Fig. 48.6 Dermatophyte test medium fungal culture. **A,** *Microsporum canis* demonstrating the typical white, fluffy colony growth and red color change. The red color should develop as soon as colony growth becomes visible. **B,** Microscopic image of *M. canis* organisms as viewed with a 10× objective lens. Note the six or more cell divisions. **C,** Microscopic image of *Microsporum gypsum* as viewed with a 10× objective lens. Note the six or fewer cell divisions. (From Hnilica K: *Small animal dermatology,* ed 3, St Louis, 2011, Saunders.)

square is made to fit snugly into the hole in the agar. Taking material for subculture from the edge of a fungal colony is always advisable, because the old mycelia at the center of the colony may not be viable.

Fungi that can invade tissue grow at body temperature (37° C). This temperature for the incubation of primary cultures of nondermatophytes inhibits many contaminant saprophytic species. The exception to this is the examination of specimens for dimorphic fungi, such as *Blastomyces* and *Histoplasma* species. These organisms grow as yeasts when at body temperature and as molds at 25° C. Cultures should be incubated, in parallel, at both temperatures. Characteristics of the systemic dimorphic fungi of veterinary importance are given in Table 48.1.

Because many pathogenic fungi, such as *Candida albicans* and *Aspergillus fumigatus,* are ubiquitous, tissue sections showing invasion may be needed for the definitive diagnosis of a mycotic infection. Occasionally, mycelial fungi or yeasts may appear on blood agar plates that were prepared for bacteriology. These fungi or yeasts, of course, may be contaminants, but some of the original specimen should be submitted for histopathologic examination in 10% formalin. The examination of a KOH wet preparation for fungal elements is also useful. Table 48.2 summarizes the characteristics of common yeasts of veterinary importance.

After incubation, cultures can be examined to identify the types of spores that are present. This is done by taking about 2.5 inches of clear cellophane tape and pressing the center of the tape, sticky side down, onto the center of the colony. The tape, with hyphae and fruiting heads adhering to it, is placed with the sticky-side down on a microscope slide that has a drop of lactophenol cotton blue on it. The tape acts as its own coverslip. The slide preparation is examined under low power or with a high dry lens, if necessary. Additional information about the microscopic appearance of fungi is located in Table 48.3.

TABLE 48.1 Characteristics of the Systemic Dimorphic Fungi

Agent	Ecology	Saprobic Form	Parasitic Form
Blastomyces dermatitidis	Slightly acidic soils and wood; possible association with animal excreta, water sources, beaver dams	Hyphae; oval to pyriform terminal and lateral conidia, 2–10 μm in diameter	Unencapsulated yeasts with thick, refractile double walls, 5–20 μm in diameter
Coccidioides immitis	Alkaline desert soils with high levels of salt and carbonized organic materials	Hyphae with thick-walled or barrel-shaped arthroconidia alternating with thin-walled empty (disjunctor) cells	Spherules 10–100 μm in diameter with doubly refractile cell walls and containing endospores, 2–5 μm in diameter
Histoplasma capsulatum	Humid environments with highly nitrogenous soils, especially those contaminated with bird or bat droppings	Hyphae, globose microconidia, and tuberculate and nontuberculate macroconidia, 8–16 μm in diameter	Tiny, ovoid, budding yeasts with narrow bases, 2–4 μm in diameter

From Songer JG, Post KW: *Veterinary microbiology: bacterial and fungal agents of animal disease,* St Louis, 2005, Saunders.

TABLE 48.2 Characteristics of Yeasts of Veterinary Importance

Genus	Pseudohyphae	True Hyphae	Blastoconidia	Arthroconidia	Urease	Growth at 25° C With Cycloheximide	Growth at 37° C on Potato Dextrose Agar
Candida	+	+	+	−	−	Variable	+
Geotrichum	−	+	−	+	−	−	−
Malassezia	−	−	−	−	+	+	+
Trichosporon	+	−	+	+	+	+	+

From Songer JG, Post KW: *Veterinary microbiology: bacterial and fungal agents of animal disease,* St Louis, 2005, Saunders.

TABLE 48.3 Microscopic Appearance of Fungi in Clinical Specimens

Disease	Microscopic Examination Method	Appearance
Aspergillosis	Wet mount (lactophenol cotton blue or potassium hydroxide)	Septate hyphae with dichotomous branching; may see fruiting heads
Blastomycosis	Wet mount	Thick, double-walled budding yeasts with broad bases of attachment to mother cells
Candidiasis and other yeast infections	Wet mount	Budding and nonbudding yeasts; pseudohyphae may be present
Coccidioidomycosis	Wet mount	Spherules with and without endospores
Cryptococcosis	India ink	Encapsulated yeasts
Dermatophytosis	Wet mount	Hairs with arthrospores (endothrix or ectothrix); hyphae or sheath of spores around skin and nails
Histoplasmosis	Hematologic stain	Small yeasts with narrow necks of attachment to mother cells, often within macrophages
Mycetoma	Wet mount	Dark brown chlamydospores and hyaline hyphae in crushed granules
Phaeohyphomycosis	Wet mount	Dark hyphae
Pneumocystosis	Hematologic stain	Cysts and trophozoites
Protothecosis	Wet mount	Spherical to oval, nonbudding, small and large cells that contain two or more autospores
Rhinosporidiosis	Wet mount	Spherules (some large) with and without endospores
Sporotrichosis	Hematologic stain	Small oval to round to cigar-shaped yeasts
Zygomycosis	Wet mount	Broad, relatively nonseptate hyphae

From Songer JG, Post KW: *Veterinary microbiology: bacterial and fungal agents of animal disease*, St Louis, 2005, Saunders.

KEY POINTS

- Supplies that are needed for the collection and examination of fungal samples are much the same as those used for bacterial samples.
- Most fungal agents of clinical importance in the veterinary practice are the cutaneous mycotic organisms known as the dermatophytes.
- Fluorescence with the Wood's lamp is only evident in approximately half of the cases that involve *M. canis*.
- The most commonly encountered dermatophytes are *M. canis*, *M. gypseum*, and *T. mentagrophytes*.
- Dermatophyte diagnosis must be supported by microscopic examination.

Immunology

Unit Outline

Unit Objectives

Describe the physiology of the immune system.
List the components of the immune system.
Describe the functions of the various immune system components.
Describe commonly performed tests that are used to evaluate the immune system.
Discuss disorders of the immune system.

The science of the detection and measurement of antibodies or antigens is called serology or immunology. Detection depends on the binding of antibodies and antigens. Unfortunately, this binding phenomenon is ordinarily invisible. Visualization—and thus detection—of the antigen–antibody reaction depends on secondary events by which the union is easily detected and therefore of diagnostic use in the veterinary practice.

The commercial production of monoclonal antibodies to many different antigens has resulted in a variety of test kits for use in the veterinary laboratory. These specific antibodies to many different antigens can be produced and used in the laboratory for the rapid identification of disease-producing organisms.

Immunization with viruses, bacteria, or other entities stimulates antibody production in an animal. The antibody-secreting, transformed lymphocytes (plasma cells) may be isolated from the animal and chemically fused with a type of "immortal" cell that propagates indefinitely, such as mouse myeloma cells. The antibodies that these hybrid cells produce, which are called monoclonal antibodies, are collected. Because each monoclonal antibody attaches to only one specific part of one type of molecule (antigen), the use of these antibodies in diagnostic kits makes the tests specific and greatly reduces interpretation problems of the results. For example, the feline leukemia virus antigen only reacts with the feline leukemia virus antibody. A specific reaction is diagnostically significant for this complicated disease. In addition to their specificity, these procedures allow for the rapid identification of the pathogen.

Many serologic tests involve the use of monoclonal antibodies. Enzyme immunoassay, latex agglutination, immunodiffusion, and rapid immunomigration are methods that are used in veterinary laboratories. Methods such as complement fixation, immunofluorescence, immunoelectron microscopy, virus neutralization, and polymerase chain reaction DNA amplification are used in veterinary reference laboratories and research facilities.

Reference laboratories offer myriad serologic tests specifically developed for veterinary samples. Tests for blood typing, allergies, bovine leukemia virus, reproductive hormones, Lyme disease, and brucellosis just are a few of the diagnostic tests currently available.

49

Basic Principles of Immunity

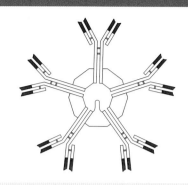

LEARNING OBJECTIVES

After studying this chapter, you will be able to:

- Differentiate between the innate immune system and the adaptive immune system.
- Describe the components of the innate immune system.
- Describe the sequence of events that comprise the immune system inflammatory response.
- Discuss the role of cytokines in the immune response.
- Differentiate between humoral immunity and cell-mediated immunity.

- List the five classes of immunoglobulins, and state the structure and primary role of each.
- Define *immunologic tolerance.*
- Describe the various populations of T lymphocytes and B lymphocytes, and explain the role of each in the immune system.
- Differentiate between passive and active immunity.

OUTLINE

KEY TERMS

Active immunity	Humoral immunity	Natural killer (NK) cells
Antigen	Immunoglobulin	Opsonization
Avidity	Immunologic tolerance	Passive immunity
Cell-mediated immune system	Inflammatory response	Phagocytosis
Complement system	Interferons	Vaccination

Vertebrate species have two major internal defense systems: the innate, or nonspecific, immune system and the adaptive, or specific, immune system (also called acquired immunity). Antigens are any substances that are capable of generating a response from the immune system.

INNATE IMMUNE SYSTEM

Foreign bodies such as bacteria, viruses, parasites, and fungi first encounter barriers of the innate immune system. These barriers include the skin; the physical and biochemical components in the nasopharynx, gut, lungs, and genitourinary tract; and the populations of commensal bacteria that compete with invading pathogens and the body's inflammatory response. The inflammatory response is a response to infection or tissue injury. Alerted by chemicals released from the infected site, blood vessels dilate and allow neutrophils to pass into

tissue, where they phagocytize bacteria and kill the pathogens with chemicals stored in their cytoplasm. The classic signs of inflammation are pain, heat, redness, swelling, and loss of function. Each of these is related to physiologic mechanisms taking place during the inflammatory process. Inflammation is a protective mechanism of the innate immune system, but it can overreact and actually cause tissue damage itself.

> **TECHNICIAN NOTE** The innate immune system involves physical and chemical barriers to prevent tissue injury and infection.

Monocytes also follow neutrophils to inflammatory sites. Here, like neutrophils, they ingest and destroy inert particles, viruses, bacteria, and cellular debris by phagocytosis. In the blood, they are called monocytes, but when they migrate to various tissues and organs and interact with specific cytokines, they become macrophages. Macrophages may also be derived from other tissues. They are located in the connective tissue, liver, brain, lung, spleen, bone marrow, and lymph nodes, and together they make up the mononuclear phagocytic system.

In addition to the phagocytic cells, natural killer (NK) cells, interferons, and the complement system are important components of the innate immune system. NK cells are not T or B lymphocytes, but rather, they are a small subset of lymphocytes found in the blood and the peripheral lymphoid organs. NK cells recognize and destroy host cells that are infected with microbes, such as viruses. They also activate phagocytes by releasing interferon-γ. Interferons are cytokines (soluble proteins secreted by cells to mediate immune responses) that elicit other cellular reactions, such as the prevention of viral replication, and they influence the actions of NK cells. They are also active in the adaptive immune response.

The complement system consists of a group of proteins found in the blood. Collectively they are referred to as complement, and they are integral in both the innate and adaptive systems. When activated, a series of chemical reactions known as the complement cascade occurs. The system can be activated through one of three pathways, but the later steps are the same for all pathways. The components of the complement system are numbered C1 through C9, with some having several subunits designated by letters.

The classical pathway, which is a mechanism of the adaptive immune system, is activated when C1 is bound to an antigen–antibody complex. The other pathways of complement activation are part of the innate immune system, and they are triggered by microbial surfaces and plasma lectins that bind to microbes (Fig. 49.1). All three initial pathways catalyze a series of reactions of other complement molecules that have numerous physiologic effects. These include opsonization of the microbes to promote phagocytosis. Opsonization refers to the binding of complement to the antigen. Complement activation can also result in the stimulation of inflammation and cell lysis by the formation of a membrane attack complex on the surface of the antigen.

ADAPTIVE IMMUNE SYSTEM

If foreign bodies evade the innate immune system, they then encounter the adaptive immune system, which is more sophisticated. The adaptive immune system is divided into two components: the humoral immune system and the cell-mediated immune system. The adaptive immune system has the ability to respond specifically to foreign substances. These substances, which are also called antigens, may be bacterial, viral, parasitic, or fungal, or they may be altered endogenous cells of the host's body. Their presence initiates humoral and cellular responses that neutralize, detoxify, and eliminate these foreign materials from the host.

Lymphocytes and their progeny are the cell types largely responsible for the adaptive immune system. However, this line of defense is not divorced from the innate immune system. Macrophages process antigens and present them to antigen-

committed lymphocytes. In other words, they act as antigen-presenting cells.

Lymphoid stem cells develop first in the yolk sac and then in the fetal liver. The bone marrow assumes this responsibility near parturition and serves as the source of these cells throughout postnatal life. The lymphoid stem cells are destined to further mature in one of two places: the bone marrow or the thymus. B lymphocytes mature in the bone marrow, whereas T lymphocytes mature in the thymus (Fig. 49.2).

> **TECHNICIAN NOTE** The primary function of B lymphocytes is the production of immunoglobulins as part of the humoral immune system.

Humoral Immune System

Lymphocytes that mature in the bone marrow (B cells) are concerned chiefly with the production and secretion of immunoglobulin (Ig) molecules, which are also known as

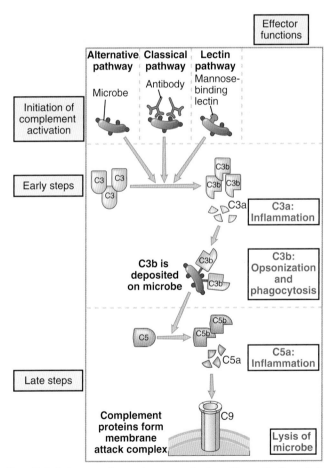

Fig. 49.1 Pathways of complement activation. The activation of the complement system may be initiated by three distinct pathways, all of which lead to the production of C3b (i.e., the early steps). C3b initiates the late steps of complement activation; these steps culminate in the production of numerous peptides and polymerized C9, which forms the membrane attack complex that has been so named because it creates holes in plasma membranes. (From Abbas AK: *Basic immunology updated edition: functions and disorders of the immune system,* ed 3, Philadelphia, 2011, Saunders.)

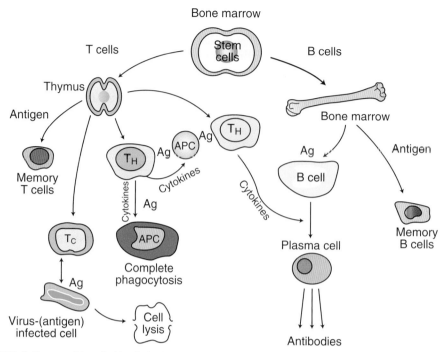

Fig. 49.2 Pathways of lymphoid cells in the immune response. Stem cells in the bone marrow give rise to T and B lymphocytes. Lymphocytes mature in the thymus and the bone marrow. Exposure to antigens causes lymphocytes to differentiate and proliferate into memory and effector cells. *Ag,* Antigen; *APC,* antigen-presenting cell; T_H, T-helper lymphocytes; T_C, T-cytotoxic lymphocytes.

antibodies. This is referred to as humoral immunity, because the antibodies are secreted into the body's fluids or "humors." Their maturation process consists of three stages: the lymphoblast, the prolymphocyte, and the mature lymphocyte. The mature cells leave the bone marrow to seed secondary lymphoid organs (chiefly the spleen and lymph nodes), where they encounter antigens. The humoral immune system can recognize billions of different antigens because, as B cells mature, each B cell develops a specific receptor molecule to a specific antigen. When an antigen enters the body, a mature B cell that is committed to that particular antigen will react with it. The stimulation of that B cell to produce antibodies is a complex process that requires the help of specialized T lymphocytes called helper T cells. Helper T cells produce proteins called cytokines that activate the B cells. The antigen-stimulated B cell then quickly divides and differentiates, thereby producing a clone of identical B cells that all produce the same type of antigen-specific antibody. These antibody-secreting B cells are now called plasma cells, which are a type of effector cell. An effector cell is a cell of the immune system that performs specific functions to destroy foreign antigens. Some of the antigen-stimulated B cells differentiate into memory B cells, which respond faster to a second exposure to that antigen (see Fig. 49.2).

Antibodies (immunoglobulins) are protein molecules that consist of two pairs of polypeptide chains configured in a Y shape (Fig. 49.3). Each Ig molecule contains two variable regions and one constant region. The variable regions (Fab regions) bind to the antigen, and the constant region (Fc region) is responsible for the unique functions of the different antibody classes.

Five distinct classes of immunoglobulins are produced: IgM, IgG, IgE, IgA, and IgD. The first antibody type produced in response to an antigen is IgM. IgM is a pentameric molecule (i.e., it contains five monomers), and it comprises approximately 5% of circulating immunoglobulin. IgM is relatively large and therefore unable to enter tissue spaces. As the first antibody produced in response to an antigen, IgM is often described as a high-titer, low-avidity antibody. It is abundant in the early stages following exposure to an antigen and then in lower amounts in later stages. Avidity refers to the strength of the binding of antigen and antibody and is partly the result of the affinity of the IgM for the specific antigen. The most abundant circulating immunoglobulin is IgG. It comprises approximately 75% of circulating immunoglobulin, and it remains in the circulation for the longest time. IgG is a relatively small monomer that is capable of entering tissue spaces, and it is usually produced during a secondary immune response. IgG is a low-titer, high-avidity antibody. IgE is usually present in very small amounts, and it is similar in structure to IgG. IgA comprises approximately 20% of circulating antibody, and IgD is a monomer that, when present, is in very low abundance.

> **TECHNICIAN NOTE** The most abundant circulating immunoglobulin is IgG.

Table 49.1 summarizes the functions of the classes of immunoglobulins.

Antibodies interact with antigens in different ways to prevent antigenic attachment or the invasion of body cells. A

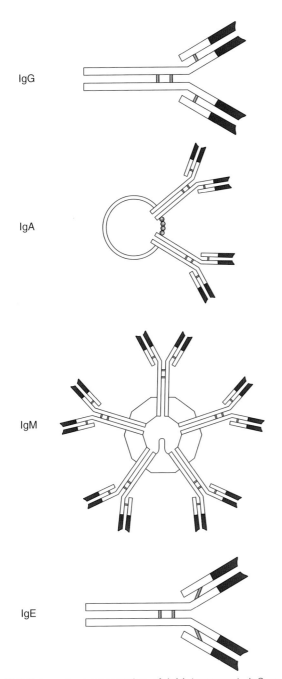

TABLE 49.1	Functions of the Classes of Immunoglobulins
Immunoglobulin Class	**Function**
IgG	• Neutralization of microbes and toxins • Opsonization of microbes for phagocytosis by macrophages and neutrophils • Activation of complement • Fetal and neonatal immunity by passive transfer across the placenta and in the colostrum
IgM	• Activation of complement
IgE	• Immediate hypersensitivity reactions, such as allergy and anaphylactic shock • Coating of helminth parasites for destruction by eosinophils
IgA	• Mucosal immunity • Protection of respiratory, intestinal, and urogenital tracts
IgD	• B lymphocyte surface antigen receptor in some species

Fig. 49.3 Schematic representation of IgM (pentamer), IgG and IgE (monomers), and IgA (dimer). (From Gershwin L, et al: *Immunology and immunopathology of domestic animals,* ed 2, St Louis, 1995, Mosby.)

neutralization antibody reaction occurs when antibody binds directly with the antigen. For example, if a foreign microbe or a microbial toxin is bound by antibody, it cannot infect or damage body cells. This essentially neutralizes the potential effect of the antigen. Sometimes antibodies coat microbes. The Fab region of the antibody attaches to receptors on the microbial surface. The Fc region of the antibody then binds to macrophages or neutrophils, and the microbe is phagocytized. If the antigenic material is a helminth parasite, IgE antibodies opsonize the worms; however, instead of phagocytosis, which

would be ineffectual against the large worms, eosinophils bind to and destroy the parasites. When complement is activated by some antibodies, the end result is antigenic cell lysis.

Precipitation reactions occur when antigens bind with antibodies and form an insoluble complex. This precipitate forms on surfaces, and the precipitant itself may cause pathology. For example, the precipitation of bacterial fragments in the glomerular membrane can result in glomerular nephritis, which is described in Chapter 54 as a type III hypersensitivity reaction.

Cell-Mediated Immune System

Lymphoid stem cells that mature in the thymus develop into T-cell lymphocytes. Like B cells, their maturation process consists of three morphologically distinct stages: lymphoblast, prolymphocyte, and lymphocyte. As these cells mature, they also develop receptors to specific antigens and become immunocompetent or antigen-committed T lymphocytes. Some references refer to T and B cells at this stage as naive lymphocytes. Then, after contact with their specific antigens, these cells proliferate and differentiate into either clones of memory cells or clones of effector cells against those antigens.

Memory cells recognize antigens to which they have previously been exposed. On a subsequent encounter, they elicit a more rapid immune response.

Different types of T-effector cells exist, such as helper T cells (CD4+ cells) and cytolytic T cells (CD8+ cells). The terms CD4+ and CD8+ refer to surface molecules or markers that are found on helper T and cytolytic T lymphocytes, respectively. Cytolytic T lymphocytes are also called cytotoxic T lymphocytes. Human immunodeficiency virus (HIV), which is the virus that causes the acquired immunodeficiency syndrome (AIDS), has a special affinity for the helper T lymphocytes.

Helper T lymphocytes recognize antigen that has been phagocytized by an antigen-presenting cell (APC) such as a macrophage. The APC displays a portion of the antigen on its surface and presents it to the helper T lymphocyte. This stimulates the helper lymphocyte to release cytokines. These cytokines then, in turn, are the chemical signals that help the APC to further phagocytize the ingested microbe. Helper T cells, when stimulated, also release cytokines that help B cells differentiate into antibody-producing cells.

Cytolytic T lymphocytes recognize antigen particles that are on the surface of infected body cells and that are able to lyse and kill the infected cells. Microbe-infected cells, tumor cells, and cells of foreign tissue graft all may be eliminated in this manner (see Fig. 49.2).

Immunologic Tolerance

One of the most important features of an animal's immune system is that it does not destroy its own cells. This may seem obvious, but it can actually happen. Maturing lymphocytes develop antigen receptors for foreign antigens but also for the animal's antigens on its own cells. Therefore, these self-reactive lymphocytes could attack the self-antigens. However, in a healthy animal, mechanisms normally are in place that prevent this self-destruction. The immune system can discriminate between self and non-self, which results in immunologic tolerance.

> **TECHNICIAN NOTE** Immunologic tolerance refers to the ability of the immune system to discriminate between self and non-self.

Invading microbes are typically immunogenic; they will interact with their specific naive lymphocytes, which then proliferate and differentiate into effector cells that destroy the foreign microbes. However, to tolerate self-antigens, the animal relies on mechanisms such as antigenic tolerance and ignorance. Self-antigens are normally tolerogenic; the lymphocytes are either unable to respond when they encounter self-antigens (anergy), or they die when they encounter self-antigens (apoptosis). Self-antigens may also be ignored by naive lymphocytes, in which case the self-antigens are called nonimmunogenic.

These mechanisms are elaborate. When naive lymphocytes are destroyed by apoptosis, the immune system is in effect selecting for the beneficial lymphocytes that have receptors for foreign antigens and eliminating the self-lymphocytes that would cause self-destruction. This is called negative selection, and it takes place in the bone marrow, thymus, and peripheral lymphoid tissues.

Another mechanism of immunologic tolerance occurs through the activity of regulatory lymphocytes. Some T lymphocytes, formerly called suppressor T cells, become regulatory lymphocytes. Regulatory T cells prevent self-reactive lymphocytes from differentiating into effector cells. They are unable to destroy self-antigens.

This is an oversimplification of the intricacies involved in the maintenance of immunologic tolerance. When these mechanisms fail, autoimmune disease results, and the animal's immune system is directed against itself.

PASSIVE IMMUNITY

Animals gain passive immunity to disease by receiving maternal antibodies in the colostrum or by receiving preformed antibodies by injection. These antibodies have been produced in a donor animal. A donor animal is vaccinated with a pathogen. When its serum antibodies reach a high concentration, the animal is bled, and the globulin portion that contains the antibodies is separated and purified. The protection that an animal receives from an injection of this immunoglobulin is short lived but immediate.

IMMUNIZATION

Animals become actively resistant to disease by having the disease and developing antibodies or by being vaccinated or immunized, in which case they also develop their own antibodies. This is referred to as active immunity. Immunization, or vaccination, is accomplished by injecting a suspension of microorganisms into an animal for the purpose of eliciting an antibody response but not causing the disease. The microorganisms may be either attenuated (weakened but still alive) or inactivated (killed). Attenuated vaccines normally cause a longer-lasting and more potent immune response. Inactivated vaccines are generally safer and have less ability to cause disease, although vaccine-associated sarcomas in cats have been an issue. An adjuvant may be added to the vaccine to enhance the normal immune response. Some adjuvants do this by simply slowing the rate of antigen elimination from the body so that the antigen is present longer to stimulate antibody production. Killed vaccines require more adjuvant, and the increased adjuvant has been implicated as one of the potential causes of the sarcomas.

Effective DNA vaccines are now being developed with the use of molecular genetics. They are expected to be safer and more stable than traditional vaccines, and they can be made more quickly. The DNA vaccines involve the direct introduction into the body tissues of a sequence of DNA representing an antigen to which an immune system response is desired.

Vaccines may be given subcutaneously or intramuscularly, depending on the vaccine. Other vaccines are aerosolized and given intranasally, and some vaccines are put in feed or drinking water. Veterinary technicians who work at fish hatcheries may vaccinate fish by putting vaccine in the water.

KEY POINTS

- Vertebrate species have two major internal defense systems: the innate or nonspecific immune system and the adaptive or specific immune system (also called acquired immunity).
- The innate immune system includes the skin; the physical and biochemical components in the nasopharynx, gut, lungs, and genitourinary tract; and the populations of commensal bacteria that compete with invading pathogens and the body's inflammatory response.
- Cytokines are chemical messengers produced by a variety of cells that interact with components of the immune system.

- Five classes of immunoglobulins are produced by B cells. Each class has a specific role in immunity.
- The complement system is made up of a series of chemicals that interact with the cells of the immune system.
- Passive immunity involves maternal antibodies in the colostrum or the injection of preformed antibodies.
- Active immunity involves the introduction of vaccines to stimulate an immune response to a specific antigen.

50

Common Immunologic Laboratory Tests

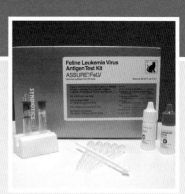

LEARNING OBJECTIVES

After studying this chapter, you will be able to:

- Discuss sensitivity and specificity as they relate to immunologic test kits.
- Describe sample collection and handling protocols for immunology testing.

- List the types of diagnostic test kits that are available for the in-house veterinary practice laboratory.
- Describe the principle of ELISA testing.
- Describe the principle of latex agglutination testing.
- Describe the principle of rapid immunomigration testing.

OUTLINE

KEY TERMS

Chemiluminescence
Competitive ELISA
Enzyme-linked immunosorbent
   assay

Immunochromatography
Immunodiffusion
Lateral flow immunoassay
Latex agglutination

Rapid immunomigration
Sensitivity
Specificity

Immunologic tests performed in the veterinary practice laboratory are designed to detect specific infectious agents. The tests are provided in a kit form that contains all of the reagents, pipettes, and reaction chambers needed to complete the evaluation rapidly and with minimal time and effort. However, careful attention to quality control is vital to ensuring the accuracy of results.

Tests kits are evaluated for their sensitivity and specificity. Sensitivity refers to the ability of the test to correctly identify all animals that are truly positive for a given reaction procedure. A large number of false negatives indicates a test with low sensitivity. Specificity is a measure of the numbers of false positives produced with the given reaction procedure. No test can provide 100% sensitivity and 100% specificity.

> **TECHNICIAN NOTE** Sensitivity refers to the ability of the test to correctly identify all animals that are truly positive for a given reaction procedure. Specificity is a measure of the numbers of false positives produced with the given reaction procedure.

SAMPLE COLLECTION AND HANDLING

Nearly all serologic tests require serum or plasma as the sample. Whole blood should not be sent to the diagnostic laboratory when serum or plasma is specified. The most practical method of collection is the Vacutainer System (Becton Dickinson, Franklin Lakes, NJ), which is commonly available from many veterinary and medical supply companies. A red-topped vacuum tube is used when serum is required, and a lavender-topped tube is used to collect plasma; if heparinized plasma is specifically requested, a green-topped tube is used.

> **TECHNICIAN NOTE** Most immunoassays involve the use of serum or plasma samples.

Reference laboratories have strict requirements concerning specimen type, quality, and handling. If any uncertainty exists, the laboratory should be contacted for specific details. For each test, the requirements should be read carefully, and exactly what is requested should be submitted. If a blood sample is to be collected in a syringe, then a 5-mL syringe and 20-gauge needle combination should be used, because it causes the least hemolysis.

HANDLING SEROLOGIC SAMPLES

When serum is to be submitted, the blood sample is allowed to clot for 20 to 30 minutes at room temperature, and it is then centrifuged for 10 minutes at a speed of no faster than 1500 rpm. If little serum has separated after centrifuging, "rimming" the tube with a wooden applicator stick to loosen the clot may help; however, this also may cause hemolysis. If plasma is desired, the sample may be centrifuged immediately after collection.

After centrifugation, a small pipette is used to aspirate the serum or plasma (i.e., the upper layer) off of the packed erythrocytes. The aspirate is placed into a transfer tube or another sealable test tube and clearly labeled. The serum or plasma may be tested immediately or frozen or refrigerated for later use. Once thawed, samples cannot be re-frozen for later testing without compromising the sample.

Samples for most serologic tests do not need to be frozen, but they should be shipped cold, especially during hot weather. The major problem with shipping tubes is breakage. The tubes must be packed firmly in place with packing material so that they do not move around when the package is jarred. Each sample must be clearly and correctly labeled and the pertinent paperwork enclosed to facilitate proper reporting of the results from the laboratory.

TESTS OF HUMORAL IMMUNITY

Enzyme immunoassay, latex agglutination, immunodiffusion, and rapid immunomigration are methods available for use in veterinary practice laboratories. These methods have been validated for testing to identify a large number of specific antigens. Additional immunoassays that incorporate these methods can detect certain blood components, such as coagulation factors,

Enzyme-Linked Immunosorbent Assay

The enzyme-linked immunosorbent assay (ELISA) has been adapted to many agents commonly tested for in the veterinary laboratory (Figs. 50.1 to 50.3). With monoclonal antibodies, the specificity of ELISA is high, meaning little cross-reactivity occurs with other agents. This phenomenon makes ELISA an accurate way to detect specific antigens (e.g., viruses, bacteria, parasites, hormones) in serum. ELISA may also be used to test for an antibody in the serum, in which case the test kit contains the specific antigen. Some of the available ELISA kits detect heartworms, feline leukemia virus, feline immunodeficiency virus, canine parvovirus, and progesterone (Procedures 50.1 to 50.3). For the ELISA antigen-detection system, monoclonal antibody is bound to the walls of the wells in a test tray, to a

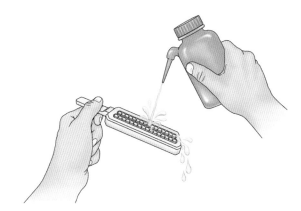

Fig. 50.1 A critical step in the Microwell enzyme immunoassay is washing away the unbound enzyme-labeled antibodies.

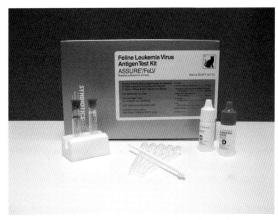

Fig. 50.2 A kit used to detect feline leukemia antigens in cat serum with the use of the enzyme-linked immunosorbent assay wand format. (Courtesy Zoetis Inc, Florham Park, NJ.)

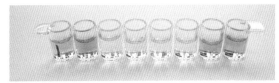

Fig. 50.3 With the enzyme-linked immunosorbent assay wells format for the determination of progesterone in canine serum (Ovuchek Premate), a positive reaction is indicated by color development. (Courtesy Zoetis Inc, Florham Park, NJ.)

PROCEDURE 50.1 Protocol for Microwell ELISA

1. Plastic wells come precoated with antibodies that are specific for the antigen being tested.
2. Add samples (that may contain antigen) and a second antibody, labeled with an enzyme, to the wells.
3. Antigen, if present, binds to both the solid phase (i.e., the wells) and the enzyme-labeled antibodies.
4. Unbound enzyme-labeled antibodies are washed away. Thorough washing is essential.
5. Add chromogenic substrate, which reacts with the enzyme and causes a color to develop.
6. The development of a color indicates the presence of the antigen in the sample.

PROCEDURE 50.2 Protocol for Membrane ELISA

1. Add sample to a membrane, which has been precoated with antibodies specific to the antigen being tested.
2. Any antigens in the sample are captured by the antibodies on the membrane.
3. Typically, positive control spots that contain the antigen have also been precoated on the membrane.
4. Add a second antibody (i.e., an enzyme labeled antibody) to the membrane. This antibody also binds to the captured patient antigen and the control antigen. The antigen is now "sandwiched" between two antibodies.
5. Wash the unbound enzyme-labeled antibodies away.
6. Add chromogen to the membrane. This reacts with the enzyme on the second antibody to produce a color.
7. Color appears where the positive control and patient antigens are present on the membrane.

PROCEDURE 50.3 Protocol for Wand ELISA

1. The bulbous ends of plastic wands come precoated with antibodies specific to the antigen being tested.
2. Any antigens in the sample are captured by the antibodies on the wand.
3. Incubate a second antibody (i.e., an enzyme-labeled antibody) with the sample and the wand. These antibodies also bind with the antigen.
4. Any unbound enzyme-labeled antibody is washed away, and a chromogenic reagent is added.
5. The reagent reacts with the enzyme-labeled antibodies that are bound to the antigens to produce a color reaction.

PROCEDURE 50.4 Protocol for CELISA

1. The test wells come precoated with monoclonal antibodies.
2. Patient samples that may contain antigen are added to the test wells.
3. Enzyme-labeled antigens are then added to the same test wells.
4. The two antigens compete for antibodies on the test wells. The antigen that has a higher concentration binds more antibodies.
5. After incubation, the wells are rinsed to wash away excess enzyme-labeled antigens.
6. Color developer is added, which reacts with the enzyme on the enzyme-labeled antigen.
7. If the sample contains low levels of patient antigen, most of the antigen bound to the antibodies on the test wells is enzyme-labeled antigen, and a deep color develops.
8. If the sample contains high levels of patient antigen, most of the antigen bound to the antibodies on the test wells is antigen from the patient, and little color develops.

membrane, or to a plastic wand. Antigen, if present in the sample, binds to this antibody and to a second enzyme-labeled antibody that is added to help with the detection of the antigen. This is followed by rinsing. This is a critical step in the process. If the wells are not thoroughly washed, false-positive results can occur. When a chromogenic (color-producing) substrate is added to the mixture, it reacts with the enzyme to develop a specific color, thereby indicating the presence of antigen in the sample. If the sample contained no antigen, the entire enzyme-labeled antibody would be washed away during the rinsing process, and no color reaction would develop.

> **TECHNICIAN NOTE** The ELISA method is the most common type of immunoassay used in the veterinary practice laboratory.

A similar procedure is used for ELISA antibody detection. During this procedure, antigen is bound to the wells, membrane, or wand, and the patient sample is assayed for the presence of a specific antibody.

Competitive Enzyme-Linked Immunosorbent Assay

The competitive ELISA (CELISA), when used to test for patient antigen, involves the use of an enzyme-labeled antigen as well as monoclonal antibodies. Patient antigen, if present, competes with enzyme-labeled antigens for the antibodies that coat the test wells. Color developer reacts with the enzyme to produce a color. The intensity of the color produced varies with the concentration of the patient antigen (Procedure 50.4). Equine infectious anemia antibodies may be detected in horse serum with a CELISA test.

Latex Agglutination

The latex agglutination test makes use of small, spherical, latex particles that are coated with antigen and suspended in water. If serum that contains the corresponding antibody is added to the mixture, the formation of antibody—antigen complexes causes agglutination (clumping). Agglutination changes the appearance of the latex suspension from smooth and milky to clumpy because the latex particles have clustered and cross-linked together. If no antibody is present in the sample, the mixture of latex and serum remains evenly dispersed. The strength of reaction can be graded (i.e., +1, +2, +3, or +4) to provide an indication of the amount of antigen present. One common test that uses this method is the test for bovine brucellosis antibodies (Fig. 50.4 and Procedure 50.5).

It is important to note that false negatives can occur when excessive amounts of antigen or antibody are present in the sample. In the presence of excess antibody, it is possible that each antibody molecule binds with only one or two antibodies and does not cross-link so that agglutination does not occur. This is known as the prozone phenomenon. Excess antigen can result in lack of cross-linking when the excess antigen surrounds any small clumps that may form. This is known as the postzone phenomenon. It is important to note that prozone and postzone phenomena can occur due to the characteristics of the patient sample or can occur due to errors in test performance such as improper pipetting techniques that result in inappropriate quantities of reagent added to the test system.

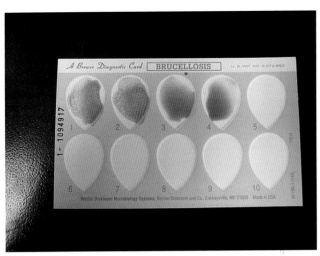

Fig. 50.4 Clumped latex particles representing antigen–antibody complexes. Samples 1 and 2 indicate a positive reaction. Samples 3 and 4, which show no clumping, indicate a negative reaction.

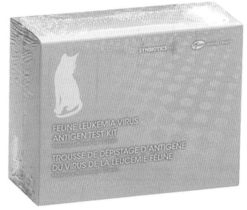

Fig. 50.5 The WITNESS FeLV test uses rapid immunomigration (a reliable one-way flow of sample and reagent) to aid in diagnosis of feline leukemia virus. (Courtesy Zoetis Inc, Florham Park, NJ.)

PROCEDURE 50.5 Protocol for Latex Agglutination

1. Use a dark glass slide to read the agglutination reactions.
2. Deposit the positive and negative reference sera (the positive sera contain the antibodies being tested) and the patient serum (with possible antibodies) separately on the glass slide.
3. Add a suspension of latex particles that have been coated with antigens and that will react with the test antibodies to each sample on the slide.
4. Rotate the slide, and observe for the appearance of visible agglutination. Agglutination indicates a positive result.

Lateral Flow Immunoassay Rapid Immunomigration and Immunochromatography

Lateral flow immunoassay has also been described as rapid immunomigration (RIM) or immunochromatography. The signal-generating components of these tests are colloidal gold, enzymes, and color reagent or agglutinated latex particles. All three types of components create a positive result.

In this type of procedure, the signal-generating component is conjugated to antibodies specific for the antigen being tested. These conjugated antibodies are present in the membrane of the test cassette where the patient sample is applied. If antigens are present in the patient sample, they bind to the conjugated antibodies, and the antibody–antigen complexes migrate along the membrane to another area of the cassette, where the results are read. Buffer may be added to help with the migrational flow of the antibody–antigen complexes. In the reading area, a second antibody is present in the membrane. If antigen is in the sample, it is captured—along with the first antibody and the conjugate—by the second antibody. The accumulation of conjugate in that area causes a color change. To ensure quality results, control antigen is present in another area of the membrane strip. The conjugated first antibody binds to the antigen in the control area. Its accumulation also causes a color

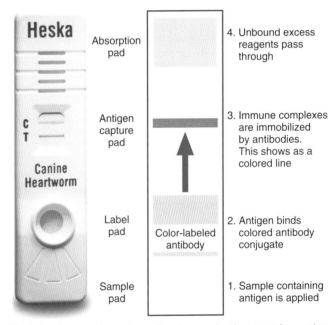

Fig. 50.6 Immunochromatography. A sample that contains antigen flows through a porous strip. Positive reactions are shown by the appearance of a colored band. (Courtesy Heska, Inc. In Tizard I: *Veterinary immunology*, ed 9, St Louis, 2013, Saunders.)

change and occurs whether or not antigen is present in the patient sample. A positive patient result shows two areas of color change: one for the patient and one for the quality control antigen. If the control antigen area does not change color, then the test is considered invalid, regardless of any color change in the patient area (Figs. 50.5 and 50.6 and Procedure 50.6).

IMMUNOLOGY ANALYZERS

Automated analyzers are available for use in the veterinary practice laboratory. In some cases, the analyzer is required to run certain tests. Large reference laboratories often have

1. Apply the patient sample to an area on the membrane that contains colloidal gold conjugated with antibodies to the test antigen.
2. If antigen is present in the patient sample, it binds to the conjugated antibodies and flows along the membrane to a reading area.
3. The reading area of the membrane contains capture antibodies to the test antigen.
4. If the patient sample contains antigen, it will be captured along with the bound conjugated antibody by the second antibody in the reading area.
5. The accumulation of colloidal gold (now complexed with the first antibody, the antigen, and the capture antibody) causes a color change.

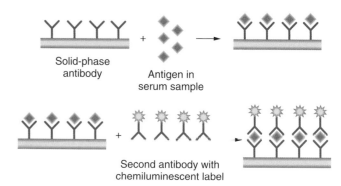

Fig. 50.7 Format for chemiluminescent immunoassays. (From Turgeon ML: *Immunology & serology in laboratory medicine,* ed 5, St Louis, 2014, Elsevier.)

automated analyzers for the performance of immunoassays. These analyzers are capable of performing tests on numerous patients simultaneously. Most are completely automated and require only the patient information entered in the analyzer's computer and the patient sample loaded. Small in-house immunology analyzers are generally of the type that only read test results. The technician prepares the sample and the test device and places the device on the analyzer. The results are read by the analyzer at the appropriate time.

Chemiluminescence

Many automated analyzers utilize the principles of chemiluminescence to detect and quantify specific antigens. The principle is similar to the ELISA method except that the test uses a substrate that reacts to produce light rather than an enzyme that reacts to produce color (Fig. 50.7). The light produced can be detected by a photomultiplier, and the amount of light produced can be quantified. The chemiluminescent immunoassay (ChLIA) has many applications both in medicine and in other industries. In addition to immunology testing, ChLIA has been used for detection and quantification of other substances, including thyroid hormones, cortisol, pancreatic lipase, progesterone, and testosterone.

▮ KEY POINTS

- Sensitivity refers to the ability of the test to correctly identify all animals that are truly positive for a given reaction procedure.
- Specificity is a measure of the numbers of false positives produced with the given reaction procedure.
- Serum or plasma samples are required for most immunoassays.
- Many of the immunoassays used in the veterinary practice laboratory utilize the ELISA method.

- The latex agglutination test makes use of small, spherical latex particles coated with antigen and suspended in water to detect antibody in samples.
- Lateral flow immunoassay is also referred to as immunochromatography or RIM.
- With the lateral flow assay methods, a sample that contains antigen flows through a porous strip, and positive reactions are shown by the appearance of a colored band.

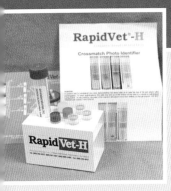

51

Blood Groups and Immunity

LEARNING OBJECTIVES

After studying this chapter, you will be able to:

- Describe the various blood group antigens of small and large animals.
- State the major blood groups of dogs.
- State the blood group of cats.
- Discuss aspects of blood typing related to large animals.
- Describe the tube method of blood typing.
- Describe the card agglutination method of blood typing.
- Describe the immunochromatographic method of blood typing.
- Describe the procedures for major and minor crossmatching.

OUTLINE

KEY TERMS

Alloantibodies
Blood group antigens

Crossmatching
Dog erythrocyte antigen

Neonatal isoerythrolysis

Red blood cell (RBC) antigens are structures on RBC surfaces in one animal that may react with antibodies in the plasma of another animal. The specific surface markers in an individual animal are genetically determined and are referred to as blood group antigens. The number of blood groups varies among species. Antigen–antibody reactions can occur with blood transfusions as a result of variations in blood group antigens between the recipient and the donor. These reactions usually result in the clumping or agglutination of RBCs, or they may manifest clinically as RBC lysis.

Some species of domestic animals (e.g., cats, cattle, sheep, pigs) have naturally occurring antibodies (alloantibodies) against the RBC antigens that they do not possess. In the absence of alloantibodies, a mismatched transfusion given to an animal results in antibodies forming against the RBC antigen in the transfused sample (immune antibodies). Breeding females should always be given properly matched blood to minimize the potential for the production of antibodies that can result in the destruction of a neonate's RBCs.

> **TECHNICIAN NOTE** RBC antigens may react with antibodies in the plasma of another animal.

The increased availability of blood components such as packed RBCs and platelet-rich plasma has improved treatment for some patients in emergency and critical care settings. Veterinary blood banks provide blood components, and most also perform blood typing and crossmatching. These procedures can also be performed in in-house veterinary practice laboratories. Veterinary technicians must understand the concepts of blood component transfusion and its related procedures to help ensure that transfusion therapy is safe.

BLOOD TYPES

Dogs

More than a dozen different canine blood groups have been described. Nomenclature for the blood group systems is designated with DEA (which stands for dog erythrocyte antigen), followed by a number. For DEA systems, the erythrocytes are designated as positive or negative for the specific antigen. The DEA 1 group was once considered to have three subgroups, but recent research has documented that these reflected varying degrees of expression of the same gene. DEA 3, DEA 4, DEA 5, and DEA 7 designate other major blood groups. The blood groups considered to be clinically significant are DEA 1 and DEA 7. DEA 1 elicits the greatest antigen response and causes the most serious transfusion reactions. Approximately 50% of dogs are positive for DEA 1. Transfusion reactions to the other blood groups are less likely to cause clinical signs. Dal, another canine antigen, has also been described. Because naturally occurring anti-DEA1 antibodies are not known to exist, the first transfusion of DEA 1—positive blood into a DEA 1—negative recipient may not result in an immediate reaction. However, antibodies can develop and result in a delayed transfusion reaction within a week of the original mismatched transfusion. If a DEA 1—negative dog previously received DEA 1—positive blood, a severe reaction can occur in less than 1 hour if the dog is subsequently transfused with DEA 1—positive blood.

> **TECHNICIAN NOTE** Administration of mismatched DEA 1 blood elicits the greatest antigen response and causes the most serious transfusion reactions.

Cats

One blood group system has been identified in cats, and it has been designated the AB system. The blood groups of cats are A, B, and AB. Few cats have group AB blood. The vast majority of cats in the United States have group A blood, which probably accounts for the low incidence of transfusion reactions in cats. Type B blood is found in certain purebred breeds (e.g., Devon Rex, British shorthair) and certain geographic areas (e.g., Australia). Unlike dogs, cats have naturally occurring antibodies to the erythrocyte antigen that they lack. Type B cats have strong anti-A antibodies, whereas type A cats have weak anti-B antibodies. Transfusing type B cats with type A blood may result in a serious transfusion reaction and death. Thus, blood for transfusions in purebred cats should be selected by typing or crossmatching. Mik, which is another blood cell antigen, has also been described in cats. Neonatal isoerythrolysis has been documented in type A and type AB kittens of type B queens with naturally occurring anti-A antibodies.

> **TECHNICIAN NOTE** Transfusing type B cats with type A blood may result in a serious transfusion reaction and death.

Cattle

Eleven blood groups have been described in cattle, and these have been designated A, B, C, F, J, L, M, R, S, T, and Z. Group B is polymorphic, with more than 60 different antigens. Anti-J antibodies are the only common natural antibodies in cattle.

J-negative donors may be used to minimize transfusion reactions.

Sheep and Goats

Seven blood group systems have been identified in sheep, and these have been designated A, B, C, D, M, R, and X. Similar to cattle, the B system is highly polymorphic. Naturally occurring R antibodies may be present. Neonatal isoerythrolysis may occur in lambs that are administered bovine colostrum. This is caused by the presence of antibodies to sheep erythrocytes in bovine colostrum. Five major systems have been identified in goats and designated A, B, C, M, and J. Naturally occurring J antibodies may be present.

Horses

More than 30 blood groups have been described in eight major blood group systems in horses; the major groups have been designated A, C, D, K, P, Q, T, and U. Naturally occurring antibodies do exist, but antibodies may be present as a result of vaccinations that contain equine tissue or transplacental immunization. Crossmatching should be done before the first transfusion in a horse, because transfusion reactions in horses are commonly fatal.

The mare—foal incompatibility test is a crossmatching procedure that detects the presence of antibodies in mare serum (or colostrum) to foal erythrocytes to confirm or prevent neonatal isoerythrolysis.

BLOOD TYPING

Methods of identifying some canine and feline blood groups are available for use in veterinary practice. These methods include an immunochromatography assay and a card/slide agglutination assay. The tube method is the gold standard for blood typing, but it is primarily used in reference laboratories.

The Tube Method

The tube method for determining blood type requires the use of antisera, which consist of antibodies specific for each possible blood type of a given species. Commercial antisera for canine and feline group testing are available for a few canine and feline blood groups (Box 51.1). The tube method requires

---

BOX 51.1 Canine and Feline Blood Types*

Dogs
- DEA 1
- DEA 3
- DEA 4
- DEA 5
- DEA 7

Cats
- Type A
- Type B
- Type AB

*Typing antisera are available for these blood types.

the collection of a whole blood sample using ethyl-enediaminetetraacetic acid (EDTA), heparin, or acid—citrate—dextrose anticoagulant. The blood is centrifuged at 1000 *g* for 10 minutes. After the removal of the plasma and buffy coat, the erythrocytes are washed three times in a saline solution, centrifuged, and resuspended. The RBC suspension is distributed among as many tubes as required for the number of blood type antisera being tested. A small amount (usually 0.1 mL) of the antisera is added to the appropriately labeled tube. The tubes are incubated for 15 minutes at room temperature and then recentrifuged for 15 seconds at 1000 *g*. Each tube is examined macroscopically and microscopically for evidence of hemolysis or agglutination. Weak positive results may require repeat testing.

The blood typing of large animals is impractical for routine analysis before transfusion. Literally thousands of different antisera would be required because of the large number of different blood groups in the sheep, cow, and horse.

The Card Agglutination Test

Blood samples used to perform the card-based assay must not already show evidence of autoagglutination, which is usually visible as clumps in the blood sample. Washing the RBCs with phosphate-buffered saline may help to salvage a sample that is showing evidence of agglutination. The RapidVet-H Canine DEA 1 (DMS Laboratories) is a blood-typing test card that is used to classify dogs as positive or negative for DEA 1 (Fig. 51.1). The typing card contains a monoclonal antibody specific to DEA 1. Each card has visually defined wells for the patient test and controls. One drop of EDTA-anticoagulated whole blood and one drop of phosphate-buffered saline are mixed on the lyophilized reagents within each well. In the

DEA 1—positive test well, the monoclonal antibody forms an antiserum, which is then mixed with whole blood from the patient. If present, DEA 1—positive erythrocytes react with the antiserum to cause agglutination. The antiserum in the patient test well does not react with DEA 1—negative erythrocytes.

RapidVet-H (feline) is a similar blood-typing test card for classifying feline blood as type A, B, or AB. The assay uses test wells that contain lyophilized reagent, which represents an antibody to the A antigen, and an anti-B antigen, which consists of a lectin. Erythrocytes from type A cats agglutinate with anti-A monoclonal antibodies (the A well on the card), and erythrocytes from type B cats agglutinate with anti-B solution (the B well on the card). Erythrocytes from type AB cats agglutinate with both anti-A and anti-B reagents. The third well on the card serves as an autoagglutination saline screen and must be negative for results to be valid. Samples are first screened for autoagglutination. If autoagglutination is present, the RBCs may be washed with phosphate-buffered saline and the autoagglutination screen repeated. If the autoagglutination result is negative, the typing test may be performed.

> **TECHNICIAN NOTE** The card agglutination and immunochromatographic assays are rapid and accurate blood typing tests for use in the veterinary practice laboratory.

Immunochromatographic Assay

Several commercial test kits make use of the immunochromatographic test principle rather than agglutination (Figs. 51.2 and 51.3). The control band detects a separate antigen on the RBCs. The canine test uses a paper strip impregnated with monoclonal anti—DEA 1 antibody and a second antibody to a universal RBC antigen as a control. An RBC solution diffuses up the strip, and if the cells express DEA 1, they concentrate in the area of antibody impregnation. The cells also concentrate in the area of the control antigen, thereby demonstrating that cells

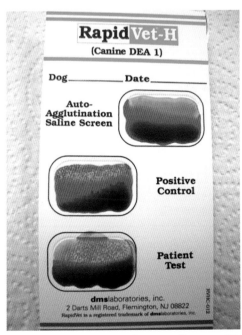

Fig. 51.1 Card agglutination blood-typing test. (Courtesy DMS Laboratories, Tempe, Arizona.)

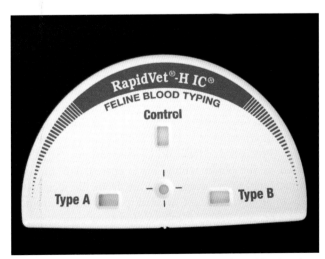

Fig. 51.2 An immunochromatographic test for feline blood typing.

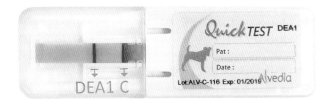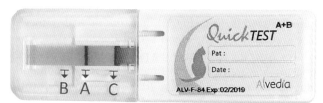

Fig. 51.3 Blood typing tests. (Courtesy Alvedia.)

PROCEDURE 51.1   Crossmatching

Materials
- Normal saline
- Plastic, conical bottom, 12-mL tubes
- Centrifuge
- Microscope
- Slide/coverslip

Procedure
1. Obtain whole blood samples (in ethylenediaminetetraacetic acid [EDTA] anticoagulant) from the donor and the recipient.
   a. Samples may also be obtained from stored whole blood or packed red blood cells (pRBCs).
2. Centrifuge the EDTA tubes at 1000 g for 10 minutes. Remove the plasma, and place it in labeled tubes.
3. Place three to five drops of the pRBCs from each EDTA tube into the labeled conical centrifuge tubes.
4. Add 5 to 10 mL of saline to the pRBCs.
5. Centrifuge the tubes that contain the pRBCs for 2 to 5 minutes.
6. Pour off the supernatant and discard it.
7. Resuspend the pRBCs in saline and centrifuge them.
   a. Repeat Steps 6 and 7 one to three times until the supernatant is clear.
8. Add a few drops of saline to resuspend the pRBCs.

9. **Major crossmatch:** Label a plain tube with the donor name and the word "Major."
   a. Add two drops of the recipient plasma and two drops of donor cell suspension.
10. **Minor crossmatch:** Label a tube with the donor number and the word "Minor."
    a. Add two drops of the donor plasma and two drops of the recipient cell suspension.
11. **Controls:** Label two control tubes.
    a. Add two drops of donor plasma and two drops of donor RBCs to the first tube.
    b. Add two drops of recipient plasma and two drops of recipient RBCs to the second tube.
12. Incubate all four tubes at 37° C (98.6° F) for 15 to 30 minutes.
    a. Room-temperature incubation is sometimes performed and generally yields accurate results.
13. Centrifuge all four tubes for 5 minutes.
14. Examine all four tubes macroscopically for evidence of hemolysis or agglutination.
15. Grade any agglutination reactions, and examine the samples microscopically.
16. Positive reactions in the donor control tubes indicate unsuitable donors.

---

have successfully diffused up the length of the strip. The feline test works the same way; however, it has an area that contains an anti-A monoclonal antibody, an area that contains an anti-B monoclonal antibody, and a control antibody for a common feline RBC antigen, thereby allowing for the identification of blood type A, B, or AB.

CROSSMATCHING

In the absence of commercial antisera, crossmatching a blood donor and a recipient reduces the possibility of a transfusion reaction. The two-part procedure (i.e., major and minor crossmatching) requires a serum sample and a whole blood sample (Procedure 51.1). RBC suspensions, which are collected as for blood typing, are prepared. For the major crossmatching, a few drops of serum from the recipient are added to a few drops of washed packed RBCs from the donor. The mixture is incubated and then centrifuged. The macroscopic or microscopic presence of hemolysis or agglutination indicates a blood-type mismatch. The minor crossmatch is similar except that donor serum and recipient RBCs are used. Both procedures should be performed for all animals with unknown blood types that require transfusion. Two controls are used for the test, which consists of using donor cells with donor serum as well as recipient cells with recipient serum. Commercial test kits for crossmatching are also available (Fig. 51.4).

> **TECHNICIAN NOTE** Critically ill patients should undergo blood typing and crossmatching before a transfusion.

Agglutination reactions are sometimes graded. Several classification schemes are used for this purpose. Table 51.1 shows one type of grading scale. The clinician determines whether evidence of agglutination constitutes an unsuitable transfusion.

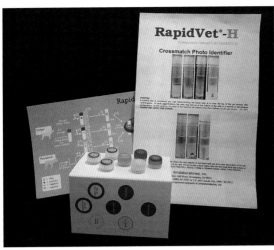 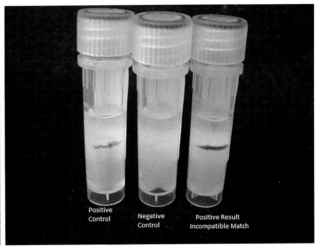

Fig. 51.4 RapidVet-H test kits are available for in-house canine and feline blood crossmatching. (Courtesy DMS Laboratories, Tempe, Arizona.)

TABLE 51.1	**Grading Crossmatch Reactions**
Grade	**Description**
0	No evidence of agglutination or hemolysis
1	Many small agglutinates and some free cells
2	Large agglutinates and smaller clumps of cells
3	Many large agglutinates
4	Solid aggregate of cells

KEY POINTS

- Proper blood typing and crossmatching can minimize problems in critically ill patients.
- Dogs have more than a dozen different blood groups.
- Cats have one blood group antigen system.
- The most clinically significant blood group in dogs is DEA 1.
- The majority of cats have type A blood.
- Type A cats have naturally occurring antibodies to type B antigens; type B cats have naturally occurring antibodies to type A antigens.
- Dozens of blood groups have been identified in large animal species.
- Blood typing with the tube method is performed in the reference laboratory.
- Blood typing of dogs and cats can be performed in the veterinary practice laboratory with either agglutination or immunochromatographic methods.
- The crossmatching of blood before transfusion helps to minimize potential reactions.
- Both major and minor crossmatching are needed before transfusion.

Intradermal Testing

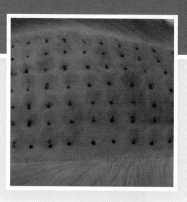

TESTS OF CELL-MEDIATED IMMUNITY

Tests of humoral immunity involve the detection of circulating antibodies; the evaluation of cell-mediated immunity is much more difficult. The commonly performed intradermal tests are used to evaluate patients with allergic (hypersensitivity) reactions and to detect the presence of the tuberculosis antigen.

Intradermal Tests

Skin tests are used to diagnose various allergies to allergens in the environment. Allergies are mediated by immunoglobulin E (IgE) antibody molecules. They can be detected by using allergenic extracts of grasses, trees, weed pollens, molds, dust, insects, and other possibly offending antigens. The extracts are injected intradermally, and the injection sites are monitored for allergic reactions. A positive reaction appears as a raised welt and means that the animal is allergic to that antigen.

Patients with hypersensitivity reactions may manifest with urticaria (hives), wheals, or angioedema (edema of the dermis and subcutaneous tissues). These reactions are triggered when basophils or mast cells release their histamine-containing granules and trigger the inflammatory response. Many substances and environmental parameters have been demonstrated to cause urticaria (Fig. 52.1 and Box 52.1) and angioedema.

> **TECHNICIAN NOTE** Allergic dogs frequently have reactions to more than one allergen.

Allergens are chosen on the basis of the patient's history and geographic area. Common allergens include dust mites, house dust, human dander, feathers, molds, weeds, grasses, and trees. Intradermal skin testing for food allergens has not been well validated. Dogs are frequently allergic to more than one substance. False-positive and false-negative reactions can occur for a variety of reasons (Boxes 52.2 and 52.3).

When performing the test, the patient is placed in lateral recumbency, and the hair is shaved from the lateral thorax. The skin is not scrubbed. A felt-tip marker is used to mark the injection sites, which should be 2 cm apart. A 26-gauge needle is used to inject a small volume (generally 0.05 mL) of suspected individual allergens. Most patients tolerate the injections well and do not require sedation.

An intradermal injection of saline is used as a negative control, and an injection of a histamine product is used as a positive control. The injection sites are then evaluated at 15 and 30 minutes after the injection, and the reactions, if any, are graded. The saline injection is graded as 0, and the positive control is graded as +4. The test sites are scored in relation to the two controls. Each test site is evaluated for the presence of

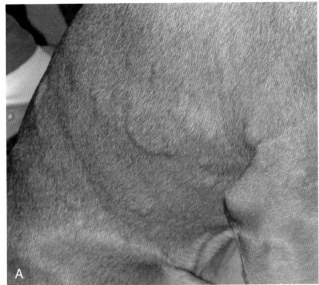

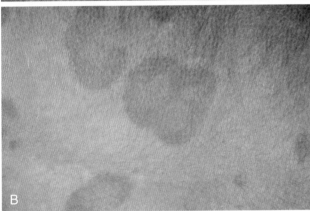

Fig. 52.1 Urticaria. **A,** Tufts of raised hair in a short-coated dog. **B,** Erythematous wheals. (From Miller WH, Griffin CE, Campbell KL: *Muller and Kirk's small animal dermatology*, ed 7, St Louis, 2013, Saunders.)

---

erythema. The diameter of each wheal should be measured (Fig. 52.2).

> **TECHNICIAN NOTE** The test sites are compared with the positive and negative control sites and graded accordingly.

An enzyme-linked immunosorbent assay (ELISA) test is also available for the determination of allergen-specific IgE antibodies in dogs, cats, and horses (ALLERCEPT, Heska, Loveland, Colorado). The test uses a high-affinity IgE receptor and is available for testing dozens of grasses, trees, weeds, mites, insects, and fungi.

Tuberculin Skin Test

The tuberculin skin test correlates with a specific cell-mediated immune reaction. Animals infected with *Mycobacterium* spp. bacteria develop characteristic delayed hypersensitivity reactions when exposed to purified derivatives of the organism called tuberculin. The test is commonly performed on cattle

---

BOX 52.1 Factors Reported to Have Caused Urticaria and Angioedema in Dogs and Cats

- Foods
- Drugs
- Penicillin, cephalexin, ampicillin, tetracycline, vitamin K, propylthiouracil, amitraz, ivermectin, moxidectin, radiocontrast agents, vincristine, azathioprine
- Antisera, bacterins, and vaccines
- Panleukopenia, leptospirosis, distemper-hepatitis, rabies, feline leukemia
- Stinging and biting insects
- Bees, hornets, mosquitoes, black flies, spiders, ants
- Hairs from processionary caterpillars
- Allergenic extracts
- Blood transfusions
- Plants
- Nettles, buttercups
- Intestinal parasites
- Ascarids, hookworms, tapeworms
- Infections
- Staphylococcal pyoderma, canine distemper*
- Sunlight*
- Excessive heat or cold*
- Estrus*
- Dermatographism*
- Atopy*
- Psychogenic factors*
- Vasculitis, food allergy induced*

*Reported in dogs only.
From Miller WH, Griffin CE, Campbell KL: *Muller and Kirk's small animal dermatology*, ed 7, St Louis, 2013, Saunders.

BOX 52.2 Reasons for False-Negative Intradermal Skin Test Reactions

- Subcutaneous injections
- Too little allergen
- Testing with mixes
- Outdated allergens
- Allergens too dilute (1000 PNU/mL recommended)
- Too small volume of allergen injected
- Drug interference
- Glucocorticoids
- Antihistamines
- Tranquilizers
- Progestational compounds
- Any drugs that significantly lower blood pressure
- Anergy (testing during peak of hypersensitivity reaction)
- Inherent host factors
- Estrus, pseudopregnancy
- Severe stress (systemic diseases, fright, struggling)
- Endoparasitism or ectoparasitism? ("blocking" of mast cells with antiparasitic immunoglobulin E?)
- Off-season testing (testing more than 1 to 2 months after clinical signs have disappeared)
- Histamine "hyporeactivity"

From Miller WH, Griffin CE, Campbell KL: *Muller and Kirk's small animal dermatology*, ed 7, St Louis, 2013, Saunders.

BOX 52.3   Reasons for False-Positive Intradermal Skin Test Reactions

- Irritant test allergens (especially those that contain glycerin; also, some house dust, feathers, wool, mold, and all food preparations)
- Contaminated test allergens (bacteria, fungi)
- Skin-sensitizing antibody only (prior clinical or present subclinical sensitivity)
- Poor technique (traumatic placement of needle, dull or burred needle, too large a volume injected, air injected)
- Substances that cause nonimmunologic histamine release (narcotics)
- "Irritable" skin (large reactions seen to all injected substances, including saline control)
- Dermatographism
- Mitogenic allergen

From Miller WH, Griffin CE, Campbell KL: *Muller and Kirk's small animal dermatology*, ed 7, St Louis, 2013, Saunders.

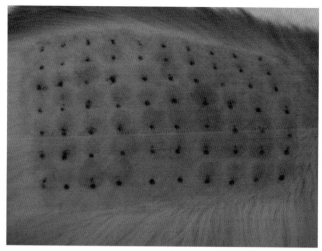

Fig. 52.2 Positive intradermal test in a cat. Note the large number of wheal and flare reactions. Unlike what is commonly reported in cats, this cat had strong and easily identified skin test reactions. (Photo Courtesy University of Wisconsin, School of Veterinary Medicine. In Little S: *The cat*, St Louis, 2012, Saunders.)

and primates. For the tuberculin skin test, tuberculin is injected intradermally at a site in the cervical region or in a skinfold at the base of the tail in large animals. A delayed local inflammatory reaction is observed if the animal has been exposed to *Mycobacterium*. The reaction to injection is delayed because a day or more passes before the T lymphocytes migrate to the foreign antigen injected into the dermis.

▌ KEY POINTS

- Intradermal testing is performed to identify IgE-mediated allergic responses and to detect the presence of *Mycobacterium* antigens.
- Intradermal testing for allergies requires extracts of common antigens.
- Lesions that result from intradermal testing are evaluated for erythema and sized to grade the reaction.
- Allergic reactions result when basophils or mast cells release their histamine-containing granules and trigger the inflammatory response.

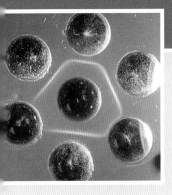

Reference Laboratory Immunoassays

COOMBS TESTING

The presence of inappropriate antibodies (i.e., antibodies against the body's own tissues) are detected with the Coombs test (Fig. 53.1). The direct Coombs reaction is used to detect antibody that has attacked the body's own erythrocytes. There are commercially available Coombs tests that can be performed in the in-house practice laboratory, but the test is more commonly performed at the reference lab (Fig. 53.2).

A positive direct Coombs test provides evidence of immune-mediated hemolytic disease. The procedure involves incubating the suspect sample with antisera, which reacts with the species' immunoglobulins. If the erythrocytes in the sample are coated with immunoglobulin (self-antibody), then the antisera and immunoglobulin on the erythrocytes will react and result in visible agglutination of the erythrocytes.

> **TECHNICIAN NOTE** The Coombs test detects autoantibodies.

Indirect Coombs testing detects circulating antibody. A positive indirect Coombs test result indicates the presence of circulating antibodies against the body's own tissues. To visualize the reaction, patient serum is incubated with erythrocytes from a normal animal of the same species. If antibody is present in the patient serum, it will bind to these erythrocytes just like it would to its own. The subsequent addition of an anti–gamma globulin for the species being tested results in hemagglutination.

IMMUNODIFFUSION

For immunodiffusion, patient serum samples that possibly contain antibodies and the antigen to these antibodies, which is supplied in the test kit, are placed in separate wells in an agar gel plate. Both components diffuse into the agar and form a visible band of precipitation when they combine. If no band forms, no antibody exists in the patient's serum sample, or the patient's antibody levels are insufficient to cause precipitation in the gel. Diseases that may be detected by immunodiffusion are equine infectious anemia and Johne disease (Fig. 53.3 and Procedure 53.1).

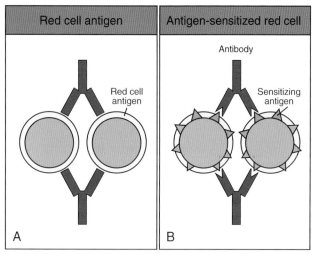

Fig. 53.1 Principles of the Coombs reaction. **A,** Direct Coombs test. **B,** Indirect Coombs test.

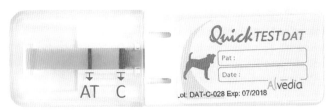

Fig. 53.2 A commercially available Coombs test for the in-house veterinary practice laboratory. (Courtesy Alvedia, France.)

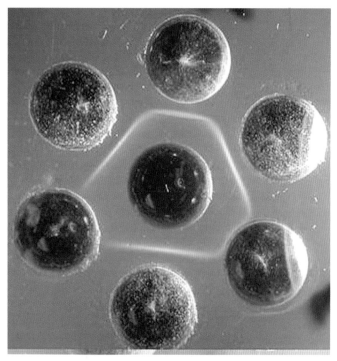

Fig. 53.3 Agar plate showing lines of precipitation. No lines of precipitation are evident near negative patient wells. (LAB-EZ/EIA immunodiffusion. Courtesy Zoetis Inc, Florham Park, NJ.)

> **PROCEDURE 53.1   Protocol for Immunodiffusion**
>
> 1. Use an agar plate with one central well and multiple surrounding wells.
> 2. Place the antigens from the test kit in the center well.
> 3. Place the patient serum samples with possible antibodies and positive controls with antibodies in alternating surrounding wells. The control samples are used for comparison.
> 4. Antigen from the center well and antibodies from the surrounding wells migrate through the agar toward each other.
> 5. Where the antigens and antibodies meet, a line of visible precipitation forms. A line of precipitate in front of a patient well indicates that antibodies are present in the patient serum.

RADIOIMMUNOASSAY

A competitive form of radioimmunoassay has primarily been used in research and diagnostic laboratories for many years. The test principle is similar to the competitive enzyme-linked immunosorbent assay (CELISA) technique except that a radioisotope is used in place of the enzyme. The assay typically consists of an antigen that is labeled with a radioisotope and an antibody. When combined with patient serum that contains the same antigen, both antigens compete for the antibody. With increasing amounts of patient antigen, more labeled antigen is displaced from the antibody. The remaining amount of radioactivity is measured and compared with a standard curve to determine the concentration of antigen in the patient's serum.

FLUORESCENT ANTIBODY TESTING

Although it is not commonly performed in veterinary practices, fluorescent testing is available at most veterinary reference laboratories. These test procedures are frequently used to verify a tentative diagnosis that has been made by the veterinarian. Two methods are available: direct antibody testing and indirect antibody testing. Both of these detect the presence of specific antibody in a sample (Fig. 53.4). In the direct procedure, the patient sample is added to a test slide that has been precoated with a fluorescent-dye—conjugated antigen. The dye combines with a specific antibody if it is present in the patient sample. The slide is then examined with a special microscope that has been designed for fluorescent microscopy. For cellular antigens, the cell will appear to be outlined with fluorescent material.

With an indirect fluorescent antibody (IFA) technique, the patient sample is incubated on a slide that contains the specific test antigen. The slide is then washed to remove any unbound antibody. Fluorescent-labeled antiantibody is added to the system, and the slide is then microscopically examined. Any fluorescence indicates a positive test result. Fluorescent techniques exist for antigen detection as well.

ANTIBODY TITERS

Although they are not routinely performed in all veterinary practice laboratories, antibody titer tests may be needed by the

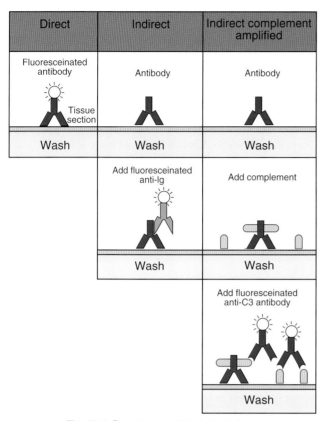

Fig. 53.4 Fluorescent antibody technique.

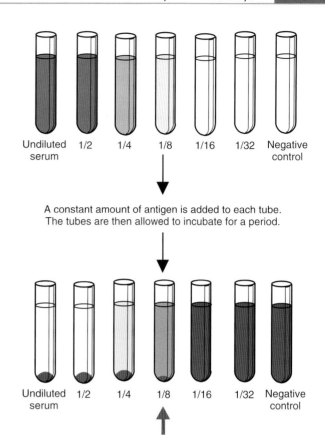

Fig. 53.5 The principle of antibody titration. Serum is first diluted in a series of tubes. A constant amount of antigen is then added to each tube, and the tubes are incubated. At the end of the incubation period, the last tube in which a reaction has occurred is identified. In this example, agglutination has occurred in all tubes up to a serum dilution of 1:8. The agglutination titer of the serum is said to be 8. (From Tizard I: *Veterinary immunology*, ed 9, St Louis, 2013, Saunders.)

clinician to distinguish between active infection and prior exposure to certain antigens. This is particularly important when no reliable antigen test is available. Titer refers to the greatest dilution at which a patient sample no longer yields a positive result for the presence of a specific antibody.

TECHNICIAN NOTE Antibody titers are performed to differentiate active infection from prior exposure and to evaluate the need for revaccination.

The test as it is performed in the reference laboratory requires the making of serial dilutions of a sample. Each dilution is then examined for the presence of the antibody (Fig. 53.5). The reciprocal of the greatest dilution that still elicits a positive test result is the titer. A high titer often indicates active infection. Low titers usually indicate previous exposure to the specific antigen.

Recently, a number of titer kits have been made available for use in the in-house veterinary practice laboratory. The tests primarily use enzyme-linked immunosorbent assay (ELISA) technology, and they provide rapid and accurate results. Some clinicians will request these tests when determining the need to revaccinate a patient.

MOLECULAR DIAGNOSTICS

Leptospira spp., which are slow-growing bacteria on a culture plate, are one of many bacteria that can now be identified with

the use of molecular diagnostic testing. The DNA molecule of this bacteria, which contains its genetic information, is the molecule of interest for the test. Molecular diagnostic testing is based on the analysis of DNA or RNA. Veterinarians can send samples out to be tested in a short amount of time via methods that are too sophisticated for use in veterinary practices. Many of the state veterinary diagnostic laboratories now offer several molecular tests. The obvious use for the veterinarian is to identify the presence of pathogens such as viruses, fungi, or bacteria, but there are many other uses for this technology (Tables 53.1 and 53.2).

The branches of medicine and science that use these types of DNA tests include microbiology, genetics, immunology, pharmacology, forensics, biology, food science, agriculture, archaeology, and ecology. DNA tests are available to classify cancers, detect genetic defects, verify animal pedigrees, and determine bacterial contaminants in food science applications, to name but a few uses.

The advantages of these kinds of tests are increased sensitivity and increased specificity. The amount of specimen needed for the test can be exceedingly small. The tests are safe, and many factors that influence other procedures—such as the age

TABLE 53.1 Molecular Diagnostic Tests for Veterinary Pathogens

Organism	Suggested Samples
Bacillus anthracis	Blood
Bovine viral diarrhea virus 1 and 2	Lymph nodes, spleen, serum
Chlamydia spp.	Placenta, liver
Clostridium perfringens	Isolated colony from bacterial culture
Escherichia coli virulence typing panel	Isolated colony from bacterial culture
Leptospira spp.	Urine, liver, kidney
Mycobacterium paratuberculosis	Intestinal mucosa, mesenteric lymph nodes
Porcine reproductive and respiratory syndrome virus	Serum, spleen, lung
Salmonella spp.	Intestinal mucosa, feces, other tissues
West Nile virus	Kidney, heart, brain, liver, spleen

TABLE 53.2 Selected Veterinary DNA Tests

Animal	Test	Test Sample
Avian	Bird sexing	Blood or freshly plucked feathers
Canine	DNA banking and profiling	Buccal swab (for animal identification)
Canine	Inherited disease screening	Buccal swab
Canine	Parentage verification	Buccal swab
Equine	DNA banking (for animal identification)	15–20 hairs pulled from the mane, including the hair root bulbs
Equine	Hyperkalemic periodic paralysis screening	15–20 hairs pulled from the mane, including the hair root bulbs
Feline	DNA banking and profiling	Buccal swab (for animal identification)
Feline	Parentage verification	Buccal swab
Feline	Polycystic kidney disease	Buccal swab

BOX 53.1 Interesting Polymerase Chain Reaction Facts

During the 1960s, bacteriologist Thomas Brock from the University of Wisconsin was studying bacteria in a hot stream at Yellowstone National Park. As he approached the hot spring that fed the stream, he was still finding bacteria—bacteria that were living in water that nearly reached boiling temperatures of 100° C. He named one of these bacteria *Thermus aquaticus*. It was later discovered that *T. aquaticus* produces an enzyme that can catalyze chemical reactions at high temperatures, which is just what was needed for the polymerase chain reaction.

During the 1980s, Kary Mullis, a biochemist for Cetus Corporation, was driving along a highway in northern California one night when he had a sudden flash of insight. It was while driving on this mountain road that he conceived the concept that became the basis for the polymerase chain reaction. Mullis won the Nobel Prize in chemistry for the polymerase chain reaction in 1993.

are making these tests available to clinical diagnostic laboratories.

Many varieties of molecular diagnostic tests are available, but perhaps the most familiar—if not most widely used—is the polymerase chain reaction (PCR). This test detects the DNA segment of interest in the specimen submitted and amplifies its amount (Box 53.1).

Reverse Transcriptase Polymerase Chain Reaction

Sometimes RNA is the nucleic acid used for the molecular test, such as when testing for RNA viruses. The process used is called reverse transcriptase PCR. It is similar to PCR, but the single-stranded RNA must first be converted to double-stranded DNA before the PCR process can continue.

Real-Time Polymerase Chain Reaction

Another significant test is real-time PCR. Compared with PCR, this method decreases the risk of contamination, is more easily automated, and is generally faster and easier to run. A fluorescent probe is added to the sample mix. This probe attaches to the DNA segments; as the quantity of segments is amplified, fluorescence increases. At a set amount of fluorescence, the sample is considered positive.

Polymerase Chain Reaction

PCR is called an amplification assay because a small amount of a DNA segment detected in the sample is amplified to run the test better and to determine the results. In other words, a PCR test produces many copies of a small, select region of the DNA molecule. Before performing the test, the nucleotide sequence of this section of DNA must be known so that the proper reagents are used. The region of the DNA that will identify the virus or bacterium is predetermined.

The amplification process consists of three basic steps: denaturation, annealing, and extension. After amplification, the

and condition of the sample, fastidious growth requirements, and the viability of the organism—are not as crucial with molecular diagnostic tests. The newer techniques also have faster turnaround times. Whereas the traditional identification of a bacterium may take 2 or 3 days or more, molecular diagnostic testing can be accomplished in a matter of hours, depending on the test.

Disadvantages include contamination that leads to false-positive results, the high level of technical expertise needed to run the tests, the need for more than one room in which to perform the tests, and high costs. Many of these problems are being solved, and commercial kits and automated instruments

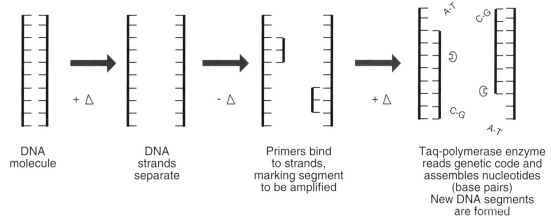

Fig. 53.6 Polymerase chain reaction showing the denaturation of DNA into two strands, the annealing of primers to single strands, and the extension of the DNA molecule with nucleotides via the enzymatic action of Taq polymerase.

DNA segments are separated on an electrophoretic gel for identification. The sample mixture contains the specimen with the original DNA in question (if present), primers, nucleotides, and Taq DNA polymerase (Fig. 53.6).

Denaturation

The sample is heated to break apart the double-stranded DNA molecule into two separate strands. Each strand serves as a template to which new nucleotides will attach.

Annealing

The temperature is lowered to cause the primers to bind (anneal) to the separated strands. Primers mark the beginning and the end of the section of DNA to be copied. This will only happen if DNA is present in the sample that is complementary to the primers.

Extension

The temperature is raised once more, and the Taq DNA polymerase (the enzyme that can read the DNA code and assemble the nucleotide bases to form new complementary strands) causes new DNA segments to be produced (extended). Portions of two DNA molecules have been obtained, each with two strands. They are not the complete DNA molecule, but they do contain the desired segment.

This process is repeated 25 to 30 times in an automated thermal cycler (Fig. 53.7). The timing, temperature, and number of cycles are regulated by the instrument. The amount of DNA segments produced is far greater than the original amount of DNA in the specimen. This is why PCR is useful for

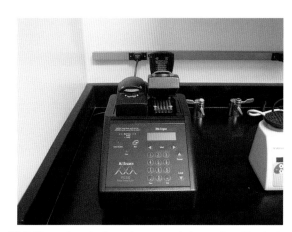

Fig. 53.7 Thermal cycler for polymerase chain reaction. The instrument automatically controls the temperature and timing. (Courtesy Bio-Rad Laboratories, Inc., ©2019. Hercules, CA.)

detecting minute quantities of the unknown in a mixed specimen.

Finally, to see if the microbe was present in the specimen, agarose gel electrophoresis is used. The DNA segments are negatively charged particles and will move along the gel toward the positive electrode when a current is applied. The segments separate according to size, and they appear as separate bands on the gel. Controls are run at the same time as the test samples. By knowing the identity of the control bands, the test bands can be compared and identified.

The interpretation of PCR tests must be done carefully. A microbe may be present in the sample but may not be the cause of the patient's disease. As with any laboratory test, the results must be evaluated along with all of the other information from the clinical case.

KEY POINTS

- Molecular diagnostic testing (e.g., PCR) makes use of DNA or RNA analysis to identify pathogens, classify cancers, detect genetic defects, verify animal pedigrees, and determine bacterial contaminants in food science applications.
- Coombs testing is performed to identify autoantibodies.
- Fluorescent antibody testing can be performed via a direct or indirect method.

- Antibody titers are performed to differentiate active infection from prior exposure and to evaluate the need for revaccination.
- During the immunodiffusion test, patient serum samples diffuse through agar on a gel plate and react with diffusing antigen from other wells if antibody is present.

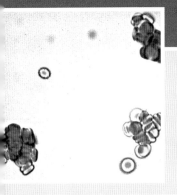

Disorders of the Immune System

Some immune responses have an adverse effect on the host animal. If the immune responses are uncontrolled or hypersensitive, they can cause tissue injury. Immune responses in which the body's own tissues are attacked by the body's own antibodies also occur. In addition to hypersensitivity reactions, the immune system also may show deficiencies. A deficiency may exist in phagocytes or in immunoglobulins. A condition called combined immunodeficiency affects animals during early life, after serum levels of maternally derived antibodies have declined. Arabian foals with this disease often die from opportunistic infection that results from an absence or deficiency of immunoglobulins.

HYPERSENSITIVITY

Four types of hypersensitivity diseases have been categorized on the basis of the immunologic mechanism involved (Fig. 54.1). Type I hypersensitivity is an immediate hypersensitivity that occurs when chemical mediators from mast cells are released. Allergies (atopy) and anaphylactic shock (a severe reaction that may occur within seconds after an antigen enters the circulation) are type I hypersensitivity diseases. These disorders occur when immunoglobulin E (IgE) antibodies are formed in response to a previously encountered antigen. When the antigen is re-encountered, the IgE binds to receptors on mast cells, which results in the cross-linking of IgE and the release of mast cell mediators. Mast cell mediators cause smooth muscle contraction and increase the permeability of the vasculature

within minutes. Mast cell mediators are also cytokines that attract cells of the inflammatory response (i.e., neutrophils and eosinophils) to the area. A variety of clinical signs are evident, depending on the location of the hypersensitivity reaction (Fig. 54.2).

> **TECHNICIAN NOTE** Atopy and anaphylaxis are type I hypersensitivity disorders.

Antibody-mediated diseases in which the antibodies are directed against the animal's own cells or components of the extracellular matrix are type II hypersensitivity disorders. Immune-mediated hemolytic anemia (IMHA), which is a condition that causes the destruction of red blood cells by the host itself, and immune-mediated thrombocytopenia (IMT), which results in platelet destruction, are type II hypersensitivity disorders. Type II hypersensitivity disorders are mediated by IgG binding to receptors on the cell surfaces. IgM may also be involved, and the resulting immune complexes will serve to activate the complement system. The activation of complement leads to the initiation of the inflammatory response. In the case of IMHA, the antibodies bind to several surface receptors on the red blood cell membrane, where they undergo opsonization and are subsequently phagocytized. A similar mechanism occurs with IMT.

Neonatal isoerythrolysis is an IMHA of neonates that occurs most often in foals and cats. The disorder results from the

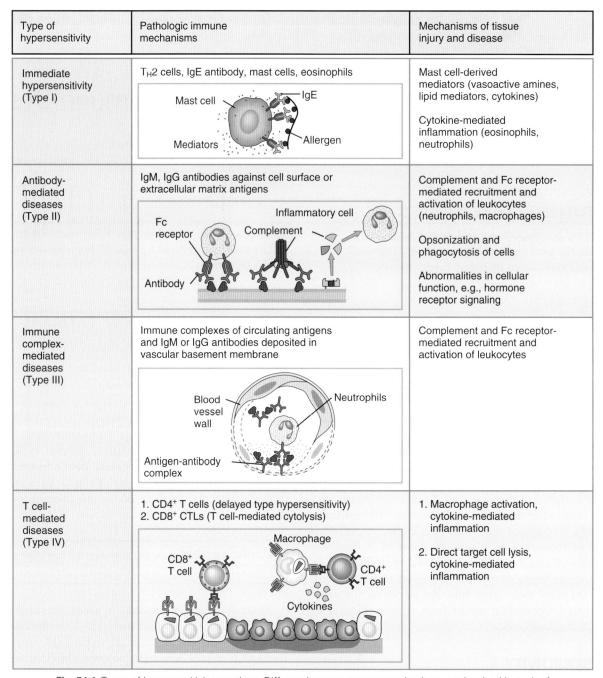

Type of hypersensitivity	Pathologic immune mechanisms	Mechanisms of tissue injury and disease
Immediate hypersensitivity (Type I)	T_H2 cells, IgE antibody, mast cells, eosinophils Mast cell — IgE — Allergen — Mediators	Mast cell-derived mediators (vasoactive amines, lipid mediators, cytokines) Cytokine-mediated inflammation (eosinophils, neutrophils)
Antibody-mediated diseases (Type II)	IgM, IgG antibodies against cell surface or extracellular matrix antigens Fc receptor — Complement — Inflammatory cell — Antibody	Complement and Fc receptor-mediated recruitment and activation of leukocytes (neutrophils, macrophages) Opsonization and phagocytosis of cells Abnormalities in cellular function, e.g., hormone receptor signaling
Immune complex-mediated diseases (Type III)	Immune complexes of circulating antigens and IgM or IgG antibodies deposited in vascular basement membrane Blood vessel wall — Neutrophils — Antigen-antibody complex	Complement and Fc receptor-mediated recruitment and activation of leukocytes
T cell-mediated diseases (Type IV)	1. CD4+ T cells (delayed type hypersensitivity) 2. CD8+ CTLs (T cell-mediated cytolysis) CD8+ T cell — Macrophage — CD4+ T cell — Cytokines	1. Macrophage activation, cytokine-mediated inflammation 2. Direct target cell lysis, cytokine-mediated inflammation

Fig. 54.1 Types of hypersensitivity reactions. Different immune system mechanisms are involved in each of the four major types of hypersensitivity reactions. (From Abbas AK: *Basic immunology updated edition: functions and disorders of the immune system*, ed 3, Philadelphia, 2011, Saunders.)

ingestion of colostrum that contains maternal antibodies against the fetal erythrocytes (Fig. 54.3). Transfusion reactions are also mediated by antibodies.

Immune-complex disease or type III hypersensitivity occurs when antibodies and antigens form complexes that are deposited in various blood vessels. Glomerulonephritis, which is caused by the deposition of antibody–antigen complexes in the kidney, is an example of type III hypersensitivity. Systemic lupus erythematosus is an immune-complex disorder characterized by the production of a large amount of autoantibodies

to a diverse population of cells and tissues. Its causes are not clear.

Type IV hypersensitivity is T-cell–mediated disease caused by the reaction of T lymphocytes against self-antigens in tissues. Contact hypersensitivity reactions, such as those that may occur in dogs after contact with plastic in food dishes and collars or in human beings after contact with poison ivy, cause tissue injury with a delayed response. The chemicals from these substances react with skin proteins, and the immune system recognizes this chemical–protein complex as foreign, thereby resulting in

Clinical syndrome	Clinical and pathologic manifestations
Allergic rhinitis, sinusitis (hay fever)	Increased mucus secretion; inflammation of upper airways, sinuses
Food allergies	Increased peristalsis due to contraction of intestinal muscles
Bronchial asthma	Bronchial hyperresponsiveness caused by smooth muscle contraction; inflammation and tissue injury caused by late phase reaction
Anaphylaxis (may be caused by drugs, bee sting, food)	Fall in blood pressure (shock) caused by vascular dilation; airway obstruction due to laryngeal edema

Fig. 54.2 Clinical manifestations of type I hypersensitivity reactions. (From Abbas AK: *Basic immunology updated edition: functions and disorders of the immune system*, ed 3, Philadelphia, 2011, Saunders.)

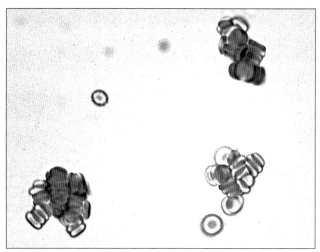

Fig. 54.3 Microscopic agglutination in an unstained wet mount preparation of saline-washed erythrocytes from a foal with neonatal isoerythrolysis. (From Harvey J: *Veterinary hematology*, St Louis, 2012, Saunders.)

dermatitis. Type 1 diabetes, rheumatoid arthritis, and chronic infections such as tuberculosis are all T-cell—mediated autoimmune diseases.

> **TECHNICIAN NOTE** T-cell—mediated immune system disorders are classified as type IV hypersensitivities.

Lymphoma, which is a type of tumor characterized by the uncontrolled proliferation of lymphocytes, is another abnormality of the immune system. The immune system normally recognizes and destroys cancer cells before they become established in the body, but sometimes the cancer seems to become resistant and escapes the immune defense mechanisms.

▌ KEY POINTS

- Immune responses that cause tissue injury are called hypersensitivity reactions.
- Type I hypersensitivity is also called immediate hypersensitivity.
- Atopy is a type I hypersensitivity disorder.
- Type II hypersensitivity includes a number of antibody-mediated diseases.
- IMHA, IMT, neonatal isoerythrolysis, and transfusion reactions are antibody-mediated type II hypersensitivity reactions.
- Immune-complex disorders are type III hypersensitivities that result in the deposition of immune complexes in various tissues.

Cellular Development Identification

Cell Type	Photo
Metarubricyte	Fig. A.1 From Turgeon M: *Clinical hematology*, ed 5, Philadelphia, 2011, Lippincott Williams & Wilkins: 94, Fig. 5.2.

Rubricyte
(polychromatic normoblast)

Cell Type	Photo
Polychromatophil	Fig. A.2 From Pincus, MR, McPherson RA: *Henry's clinical diagnosis and management by laboratory methods*, ed 24, 2022, Elsevier Inc.

Cell Type	Photo
Red Blood Cell	Fig. A.3 From Turgeon M: *Clinical hematology*, ed 5, Philadelphia, 2011, Lippincott Williams & Wilkins: 94, Fig. 5.2.

Mature erythrocyte

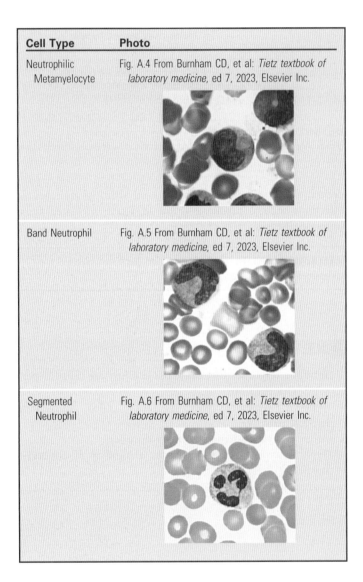

Cell Type	Photo
Neutrophilic Metamyelocyte	Fig. A.4 From Burnham CD, et al: *Tietz textbook of laboratory medicine*, ed 7, 2023, Elsevier Inc.
Band Neutrophil	Fig. A.5 From Burnham CD, et al: *Tietz textbook of laboratory medicine*, ed 7, 2023, Elsevier Inc.
Segmented Neutrophil	Fig. A.6 From Burnham CD, et al: *Tietz textbook of laboratory medicine*, ed 7, 2023, Elsevier Inc.

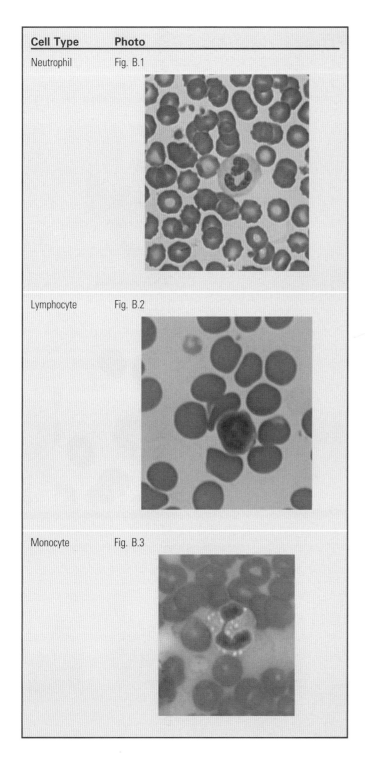

Cell Type	Photo
Neutrophil	Fig. B.1
Lymphocyte	Fig. B.2
Monocyte	Fig. B.3

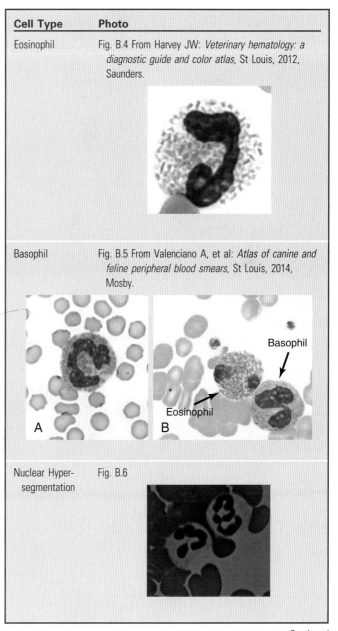

Cell Type	Photo
Eosinophil	Fig. B.4 From Harvey JW: *Veterinary hematology: a diagnostic guide and color atlas*, St Louis, 2012, Saunders.
Basophil	Fig. B.5 From Valenciano A, et al: *Atlas of canine and feline peripheral blood smears*, St Louis, 2014, Mosby.
Nuclear Hyper-segmentation	Fig. B.6

Continued

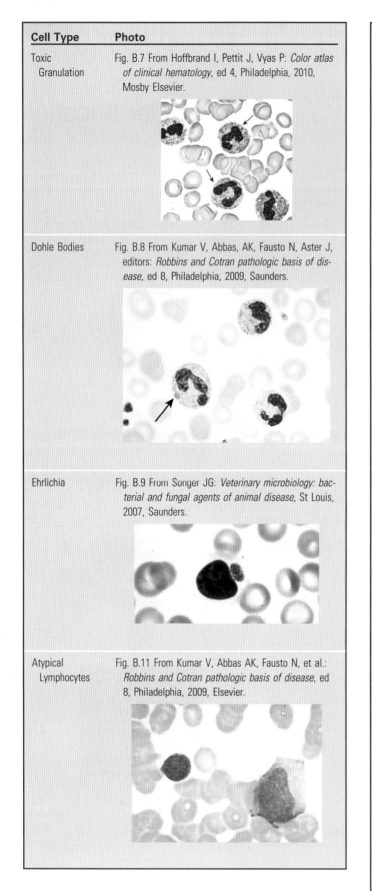

Cell Type	Photo
Toxic Granulation	Fig. B.7 From Hoffbrand I, Pettit J, Vyas P: *Color atlas of clinical hematology*, ed 4, Philadelphia, 2010, Mosby Elsevier.
Dohle Bodies	Fig. B.8 From Kumar V, Abbas, AK, Fausto N, Aster J, editors: *Robbins and Cotran pathologic basis of disease*, ed 8, Philadelphia, 2009, Saunders.
Ehrlichia	Fig. B.9 From Songer JG: *Veterinary microbiology: bacterial and fungal agents of animal disease*, St Louis, 2007, Saunders.
Atypical Lymphocytes	Fig. B.11 From Kumar V, Abbas AK, Fausto N, et al.: *Robbins and Cotran pathologic basis of disease*, ed 8, Philadelphia, 2009, Elsevier.

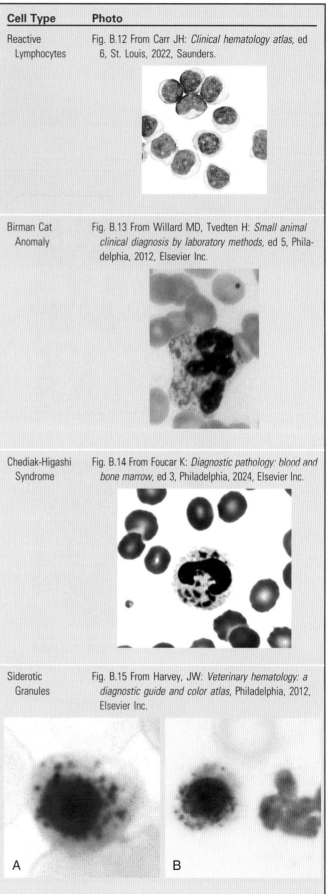

Cell Type	Photo
Reactive Lymphocytes	Fig. B.12 From Carr JH: *Clinical hematology atlas,* ed 6, St. Louis, 2022, Saunders.
Birman Cat Anomaly	Fig. B.13 From Willard MD, Tvedten H: *Small animal clinical diagnosis by laboratory methods*, ed 5, Philadelphia, 2012, Elsevier Inc.
Chediak-Higashi Syndrome	Fig. B.14 From Foucar K: *Diagnostic pathology: blood and bone marrow*, ed 3, Philadelphia, 2024, Elsevier Inc.
Siderotic Granules	Fig. B.15 From Harvey, JW: *Veterinary hematology: a diagnostic guide and color atlas*, Philadelphia, 2012, Elsevier Inc.

A   B

Cell Type	Photo
Karyorrhexis	Fig. B.16 From Meyer DJ, et al: *Canine and feline cytopathology: a color atlas and interpretation guide,* ed 4, Philadelphia, 2022, Elsevier Inc.

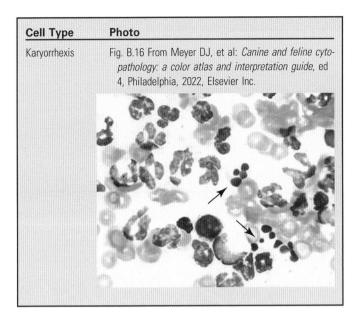

RBC Identification

Name	Photo	Differentials
Rouleaux	Fig. C.1	Normal in cats & horses IMHA
Autoagglutination	Fig. C.2 From Carr JH: *Clinical hematology atlas*, ed 6, Philadelphia, 2022, Elsevier Inc.	IMHA
Anisocytosis	Fig. C.3 From Pincus MR, McPherson RA: *Henry's clinical diagnosis and management by laboratory methods*, ed 24, Philadelphia, 2022, Elsevier Inc.	Anemia

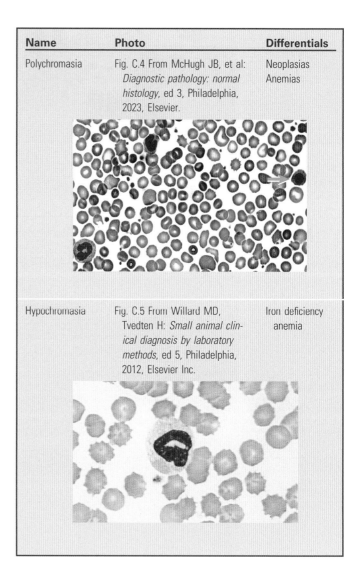

Name	Photo	Differentials
Polychromasia	Fig. C.4 From McHugh JB, et al: *Diagnostic pathology: normal histology*, ed 3, Philadelphia, 2023, Elsevier.	Neoplasias Anemias
Hypochromasia	Fig. C.5 From Willard MD, Tvedten H: *Small animal clinical diagnosis by laboratory methods*, ed 5, Philadelphia, 2012, Elsevier Inc.	Iron deficiency anemia

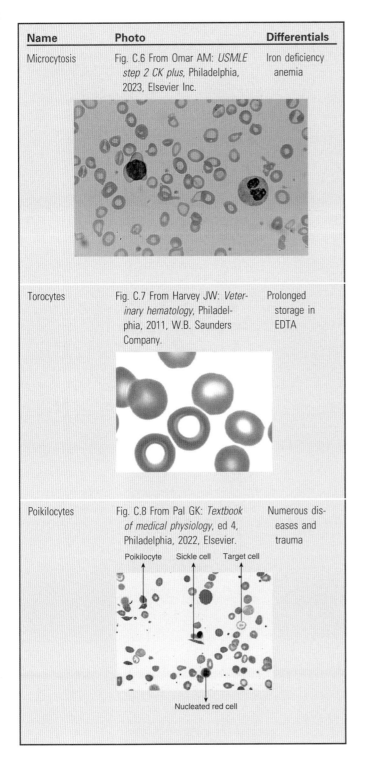

Name	Photo	Differentials
Microcytosis	Fig. C.6 From Omar AM: *USMLE step 2 CK plus*, Philadelphia, 2023, Elsevier Inc.	Iron deficiency anemia
Torocytes	Fig. C.7 From Harvey JW: *Veterinary hematology*, Philadelphia, 2011, W.B. Saunders Company.	Prolonged storage in EDTA
Poikilocytes	Fig. C.8 From Pal GK: *Textbook of medical physiology*, ed 4, Philadelphia, 2022, Elsevier.	Numerous diseases and trauma

Poikilocyte Sickle cell Target cell

Nucleated red cell

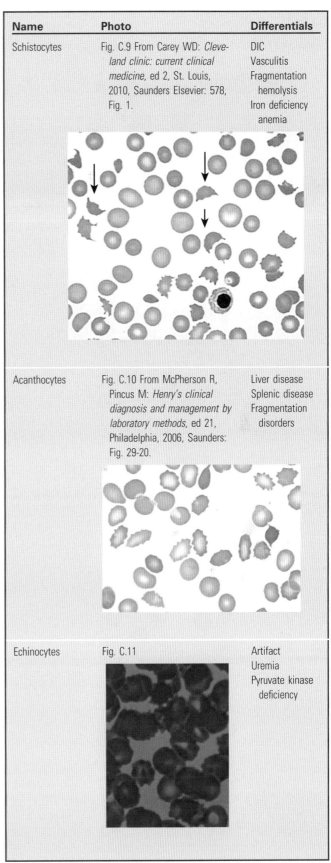

Name	Photo	Differentials
Schistocytes	Fig. C.9 From Carey WD: *Cleveland clinic: current clinical medicine*, ed 2, St. Louis, 2010, Saunders Elsevier: 578, Fig. 1.	DIC Vasculitis Fragmentation hemolysis Iron deficiency anemia
Acanthocytes	Fig. C.10 From McPherson R, Pincus M: *Henry's clinical diagnosis and management by laboratory methods*, ed 21, Philadelphia, 2006, Saunders: Fig. 29-20.	Liver disease Splenic disease Fragmentation disorders
Echinocytes	Fig. C.11	Artifact Uremia Pyruvate kinase deficiency

Continued

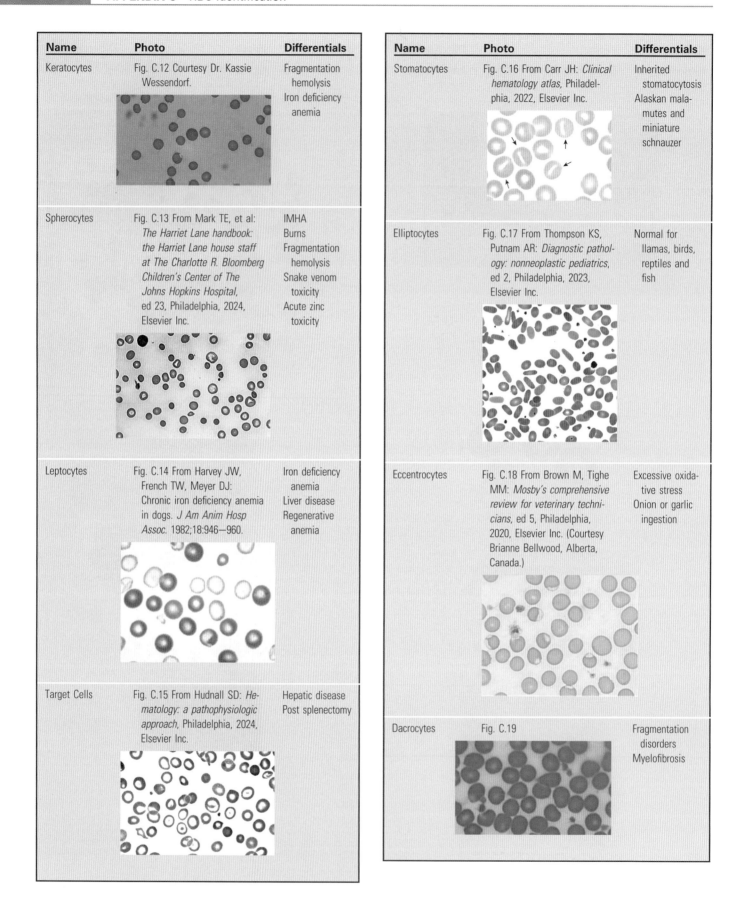

Name	Photo	Differentials
Keratocytes	Fig. C.12 Courtesy Dr. Kassie Wessendorf.	Fragmentation hemolysis Iron deficiency anemia
Spherocytes	Fig. C.13 From Mark TE, et al: *The Harriet Lane handbook: the Harriet Lane house staff at The Charlotte R. Bloomberg Children's Center of The Johns Hopkins Hospital*, ed 23, Philadelphia, 2024, Elsevier Inc.	IMHA Burns Fragmentation hemolysis Snake venom toxicity Acute zinc toxicity
Leptocytes	Fig. C.14 From Harvey JW, French TW, Meyer DJ: Chronic iron deficiency anemia in dogs. *J Am Anim Hosp Assoc*. 1982;18:946–960.	Iron deficiency anemia Liver disease Regenerative anemia
Target Cells	Fig. C.15 From Hudnall SD: *Hematology: a pathophysiologic approach*, Philadelphia, 2024, Elsevier Inc.	Hepatic disease Post splenectomy

Name	Photo	Differentials
Stomatocytes	Fig. C.16 From Carr JH: *Clinical hematology atlas*, Philadelphia, 2022, Elsevier Inc.	Inherited stomatocytosis Alaskan malamutes and miniature schnauzer
Elliptocytes	Fig. C.17 From Thompson KS, Putnam AR: *Diagnostic pathology: nonneoplastic pediatrics*, ed 2, Philadelphia, 2023, Elsevier Inc.	Normal for llamas, birds, reptiles and fish
Eccentrocytes	Fig. C.18 From Brown M, Tighe MM: *Mosby's comprehensive review for veterinary technicians*, ed 5, Philadelphia, 2020, Elsevier Inc. (Courtesy Brianne Bellwood, Alberta, Canada.)	Excessive oxidative stress Onion or garlic ingestion
Dacrocytes	Fig. C.19	Fragmentation disorders Myelofibrosis

Name	Photo	Differentials
Basophilic stippling	Fig. C.20 From McPherson R et al: *Henry's clinical diagnosis and management by laboratory methods*, ed 22, Philadelphia, 2011, Saunders: 526.	Lead poising Some anemias
Howell-Jolly Bodies	Fig. C.21 From Carr JH, Rodak BF: *Clinical hematology atlas*, ed 3, St Louis, 2009, Saunders.	Post-splenectomy Sepsis Congenital disorders
Heinz Bodies	Fig. C.22 Heinz bodies (arrows) are seen on a feline blood film stained with Wright's stain.	Hemolytic anemia Hereditary defects
Reticulocyte	Fig. C.23 Coutesy Dr. Kassie Wessendorf.	Anemia

Name	Photo	Differentials
Nucleated Erythrocytes	Fig. C.24 From Nelson RW, Couto G: *Small animal internal medicine*, ed 5, Philadelphia, 2014, Elsevier Inc.	Anemia
Mycoplasma	Fig. C.25 From Sykes JE: *Greene's infectious diseases of the dog and cat*, ed 5, Philadelphia, 2023, Elsevier Inc.	Parasite
Dirofilaria immitis	Fig. C.26 From *Greene's infectious diseases of the dog and cat*, ed 5, Philadelphia, 2023, Elsevier Inc. (Courtesy Byron Blagburn, Auburn University, Auburn, AL.)	Parasite
Eperythrozoa	Fig. C.27	Parasite

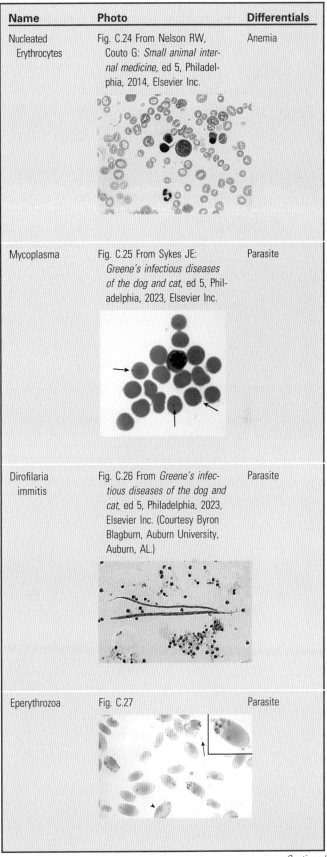

Continued

Name	Photo	Differentials
Babesia	Fig. C.28 From Valenciano A, Cowell R: *Cowell and Tyler's diagnostic cytology and hematology of the dog and cat*, ed 4, St Louis, 2014, Mosby.	Parasite

Urinalysis Identification

Urine Crystals	Photo
Crystal	
Calcium Oxalate Monohydrate	Fig. D.1 From Brunzel NA: *Fundamentals of urine & body fluid analysis*, ed 5, 2023, Elsevier Inc. (Courtesy Michel Daudon, Service d'Explorations Fonctionelles, Hôpital Tenon in Paris, France.)
Calcium Oxalate Dihydrate	Fig. D.2 From Brunzel NA: *Fundamentals of urine & body fluid analysis*, ed 5, 2023, Elsevier Inc.
Ammonium Urate	Fig. D.3 From Brunzel NA: *Fundamentals of urine & body fluid analysis*, ed 5, 2023, Elsevier Inc.

Urine Crystals	Photo
Cystine	Fig. D.4 From Brunzel NA: *Fundamentals of urine & body fluid analysis*, ed 5, 2023, Elsevier Inc.
Bilirubin	Fig. D.5 From Bhattacharya GK: *Concise pathology for exam preparation*, ed 4, 2021, Elsevier Ltd.
Cholesterol	Fig. D.6 From Johnson RJ, Feehally J: *Comprehensive clinical nephrology*, ed 3, St. Louis, 2007, Mosby.

Continued

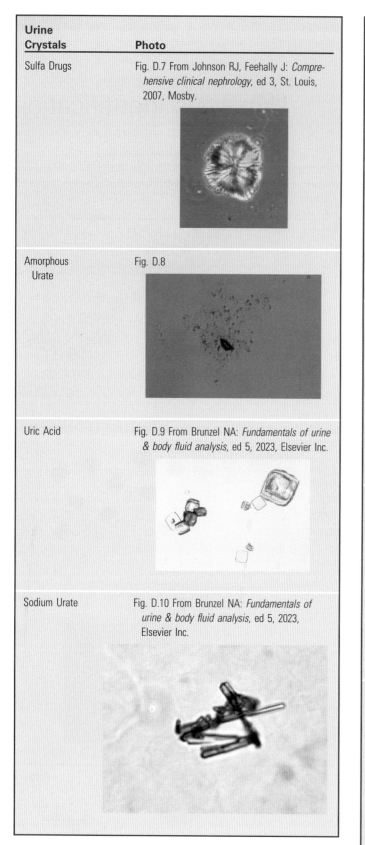

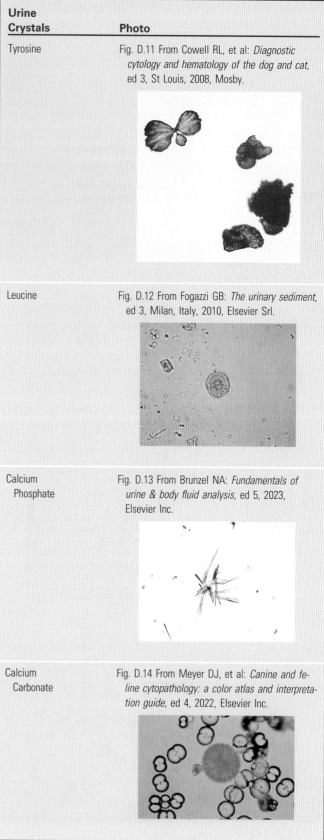

Urine Crystals	Photo
Sulfa Drugs	Fig. D.7 From Johnson RJ, Feehally J: *Comprehensive clinical nephrology*, ed 3, St. Louis, 2007, Mosby.
Amorphous Urate	Fig. D.8
Uric Acid	Fig. D.9 From Brunzel NA: *Fundamentals of urine & body fluid analysis*, ed 5, 2023, Elsevier Inc.
Sodium Urate	Fig. D.10 From Brunzel NA: *Fundamentals of urine & body fluid analysis*, ed 5, 2023, Elsevier Inc.

Urine Crystals	Photo
Tyrosine	Fig. D.11 From Cowell RL, et al: *Diagnostic cytology and hematology of the dog and cat*, ed 3, St Louis, 2008, Mosby.
Leucine	Fig. D.12 From Fogazzi GB: *The urinary sediment*, ed 3, Milan, Italy, 2010, Elsevier Srl.
Calcium Phosphate	Fig. D.13 From Brunzel NA: *Fundamentals of urine & body fluid analysis*, ed 5, 2023, Elsevier Inc.
Calcium Carbonate	Fig. D.14 From Meyer DJ, et al: *Canine and feline cytopathology: a color atlas and interpretation guide*, ed 4, 2022, Elsevier Inc.

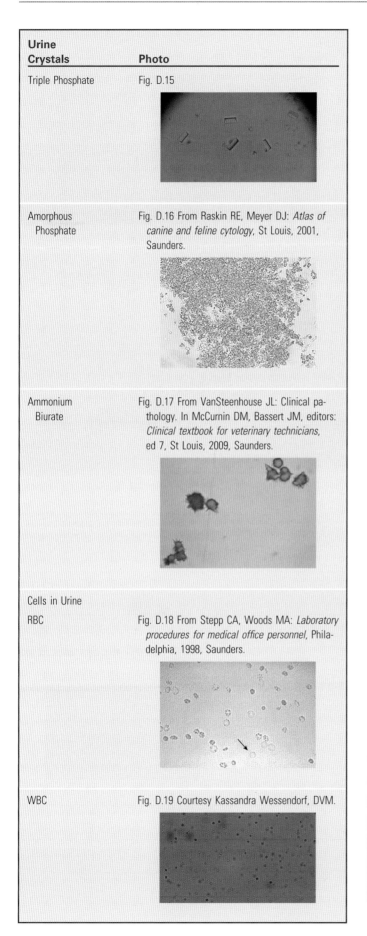

Urine Crystals	Photo
Triple Phosphate	Fig. D.15
Amorphous Phosphate	Fig. D.16 From Raskin RE, Meyer DJ: *Atlas of canine and feline cytology*, St Louis, 2001, Saunders.
Ammonium Biurate	Fig. D.17 From VanSteenhouse JL: Clinical pathology. In McCurnin DM, Bassert JM, editors: *Clinical textbook for veterinary technicians*, ed 7, St Louis, 2009, Saunders.
Cells in Urine	
RBC	Fig. D.18 From Stepp CA, Woods MA: *Laboratory procedures for medical office personnel*, Philadelphia, 1998, Saunders.
WBC	Fig. D.19 Courtesy Kassandra Wessendorf, DVM.

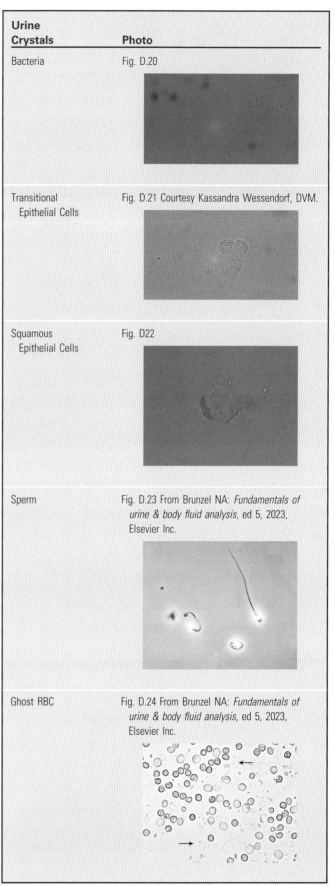

Urine Crystals	Photo
Bacteria	Fig. D.20
Transitional Epithelial Cells	Fig. D.21 Courtesy Kassandra Wessendorf, DVM.
Squamous Epithelial Cells	Fig. D22
Sperm	Fig. D.23 From Brunzel NA: *Fundamentals of urine & body fluid analysis*, ed 5, 2023, Elsevier Inc.
Ghost RBC	Fig. D.24 From Brunzel NA: *Fundamentals of urine & body fluid analysis*, ed 5, 2023, Elsevier Inc.

Continued

Urine Crystals	Photo
Casts in Urine	
Hyaline Casts	Fig. D.25 From Brunzel NA: *Fundamentals of urine & body fluid analysis*, ed 5, 2023, Elsevier Inc.
Fatty Casts	Fig. D.26 From Brunzel NA: *Fundamentals of urine & body fluid analysis*, ed 5, 2023, Elsevier Inc.
Granular Casts	Fig. D.27 From Brunzel NA: *Fundamentals of urine & body fluid analysis*, ed 5, 2023, Elsevier Inc.
Waxy Cast	Fig. D.28 From Brunzel NA: *Fundamentals of urine & body fluid analysis*, ed 5, 2023, Elsevier Inc.

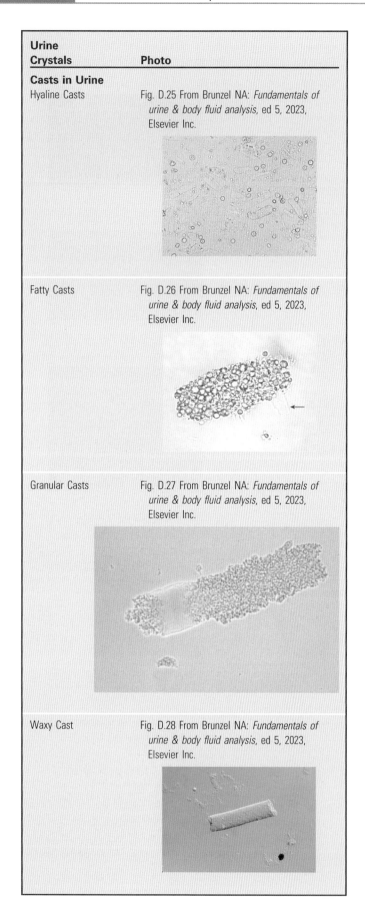

Urine Crystals	Photo
White Cell Casts	Fig. D.29 From Gilbert S, et al: *National Kidney Foundation primer on kidney diseases*, ed 8, 2023, Elsevier Inc.
RBC Casts	Fig. D.30 From Brunzel NA: *Fundamentals of urine & body fluid analysis*, ed 5, 2023, Elsevier Inc.
Renal Epithelial Cast	Fig. D.31 From Brunzel NA: *Fundamentals of urine and body fluid analysis*, ed 3, Philadelphia, 2013, Saunders.
Fat	Fig. D.32 Courtesy Dr. Kassandra Wessendorf.

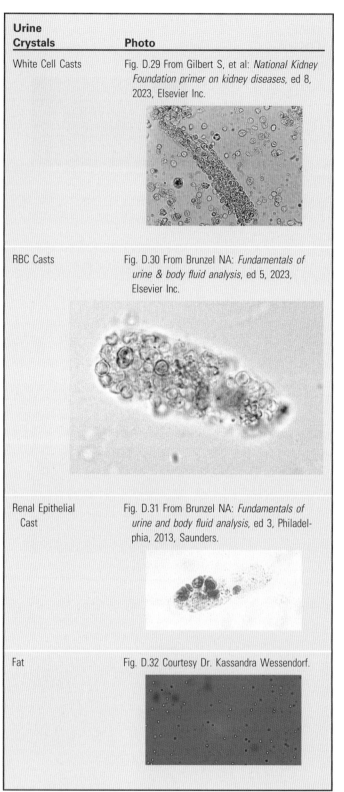

Parasites of Dogs

Species	Common Name and Egg Size	Photo	Treatment
Toxocara canis & Toxascaris leonina ZOONOTIC	Roundworms or ascarids 80 μm × 75 μm	Fig. E.1	Fenbendazole: 50 mg/kg PO q24h × 3d Pyrantel: 5–10 mg/kg PO
Trichuris vulpis	Whipworm 75 μm × 40 μm	Fig. E.2 From Samples OM et al: *McCurnin's clinical textbook for veterinary technicians and nurses*, ed 10, Philadelphia, 2022, Elsevier Inc.	Fenbendazole: 50 mg/kg PO q24h × 3d Ivermectin: 0.1 mg/kg SC PO
Ancylostoma caninum & Uncinaria stenocephala ZOONOTIC	Hookworms 60 μm × 40 μm	Fig. E.3 From *Organ-specific parasitic diseases of dogs and cats*, Philadelphia, 2023, Elsevier Inc.	Fenbendazole: 50 mg/kg PO q24h × 3d Ivermectin: 0.1 mg/kg SC PO Pyrantel: 5–10 mg/kg PO
Strongyloides stercoralis ZOONOTIC	Threadworm 55 μm × 30 μm	Fig. E.4 Courtesy World Health Organization.	Ivermectin: 0.2 mg/kg PO

Continued

Species	Common Name and Egg Size	Photo	Treatment
Physaloptera	Stomach worm 40 μm × 30 μm	Fig. E.5 From Wulcan JM, Little SE, Ketzis JK: *Greene's infectious diseases of the dog and cat*, ed 5, Philadelphia, 2023, Elsevier Inc. (Courtesy J. Ketzis.) 	Fenbendazole: 50 mg/kg PO q24h × 5d Ivermectin: 0.05–0.5 mg/kg SC or PO
Nanophyetus salmincola	Salmon poisoning fluke 70 μm × 40 μm	Fig. E.6 From Sykes JE: *Greene's infectious diseases of the dog and cat*, ed 5, Philadelphia, 2023, Elsevier Inc. 	Oxytetracycline: 7 mg/kg IV q12h × 3d Doxycycline: 10 mg/kg IV q12h × 7d Praziquantel: 2.5–5 mg/kg PO or SQ
Paragonimus kellicotti	Lung fluke 90 μm × 50 μm	Fig. E.7 From Hendrix CM, Robinson E: *Diagnostic parasitology for veterinary technicians*, ed 6, Philadelphia, 2023, Elsevier Inc. 	Albendazole: 25–50 mg/kg PO q24h × 14–21d Fenbendazole: 50 mg/kg PO q24h × 10–14d Praziquantel: 25 mg/kg PO q24h × 2d
Alaria sp.	Intestinal fluke 134 μm × 70 μm	Fig. E.8 From Bowman DD: *Georgis' parasitology for veterinarians*, ed 11, Philadelphia, 2021, Elsevier Inc. (Specimen courtesy Dr. Jay Stewart, Aumsville Animal Clinic, Aumsville, OR.) 	Praziquantel: 10 mg/kg PO or SQ

Species	Common Name and Egg Size	Photo	Treatment
Taenia pisiformis	Tapeworm 38 μm × 32 μm	Fig. E.9 From Bowman DD: *Georgis' parasitology for veterinarians*, ed 11, Philadelphia, 2021, Elsevier Inc. 	Fenbendazole: 50 mg/kg PO q24h × 3d Praziquantel: 2.5–5 mg/kg PO
Dipylidium caninum ZOONOTIC	Flea tapeworm 200 μm × 150 μm	Fig. E.10 From Hendrix CM, Robinson E: *Diagnostic parasitology for veterinary technicians*, ed 6, Philadelphia, 2023, Elsevier Inc. 	Praziquantel: 2.5–5 mg/kg PO
Echinococcus granulosus ZOONOTIC	Hydatid tapeworm 35 μm × 30 μm	Fig. E.11 Photo from the Centers for Disease Control and Prevention website. 	Praziquantel: 25–50 mg/kg
Cystoisospora spp. *(Isospora spp.)*	Coccidia 13 μm × 10 μm 24 μm × 21 μm 36 μm × 30 μm	Fig. E.12 From Bowman DD: *Georgis' parasitology for veterinarians*, ed 9, St Louis, 2009, Saunders. 	Amprolium: 100–200 mg/kg q24h × 7d

Continued

Species	Common Name and Egg Size	Photo	Treatment
Sarcocystis spp. ZOONOTIC	16 μm × 11 μm	Fig. E.13 From Moré G, Rambeaud M, Braun F, Campero L, Walkoski A, Venturini MC: *Isolation of Sarcocystis neurona from an opossum (Didelphis albiventris) in Argentina. J Equine Vet Sci.* 2016;39: S53, Fig. 1. 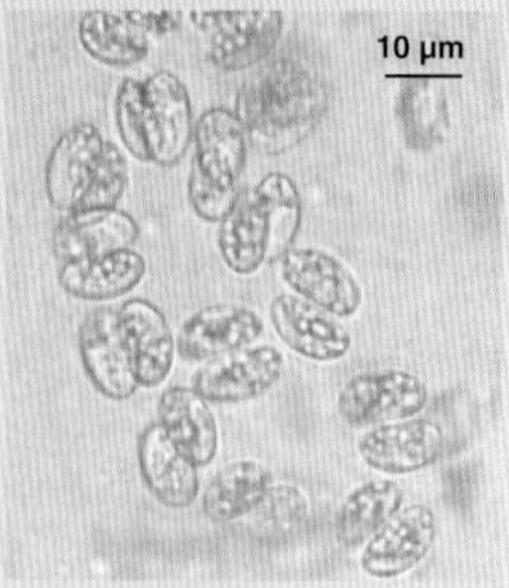 	None
Giardia spp.*(canis)* ZOONOTIC	None 18 μm × 10 μm	Fig. E.14 From Sykes JE: *Greene's infectious diseases of the dog and cat,* ed 5, Philadelphia, 2023, Elsevier Inc. 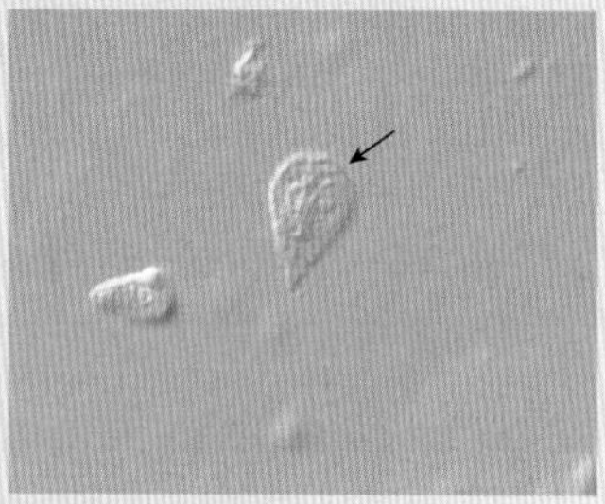 	Metronidazole: 50–70 mg/kg PO q24h × 5d Albendazole: 25 mg/kg q 12h × 2d Fenbendazole: 50 mg/kg q24h × 3d
Taenia hydatigenia, Taenia multiceps, Taenia krabbei	Tapeworms 38 μm × 32 μm	Fig. E.15 From Kang G, et al: *Manson's tropical diseases,* ed 24, Philadelphia, 2024, Elsevier Ltd. (Courtesy Dr. J. Jimenez.) 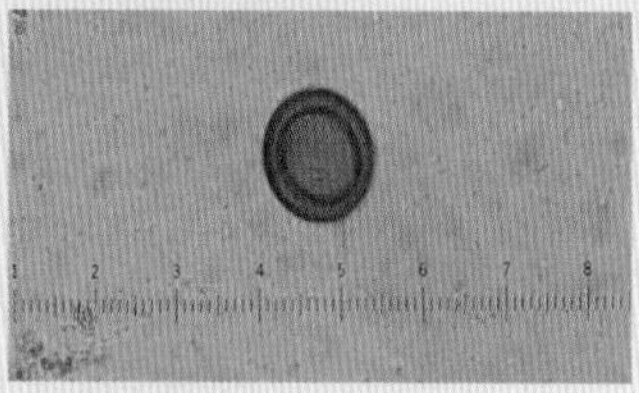 	Fenbendazole: 50 mg/kg PO q24h × 3d Praziquantel: 2.5–5 mg/kg PO
Capillaria aerophila	Fox lungworm 70 μm × 35 μm	Fig. E.16 From Hendrix CM, Robinson E: *Diagnostic parasitology for veterinary technicians,* ed 6, Philadelphia, 2023, Elsevier Inc. 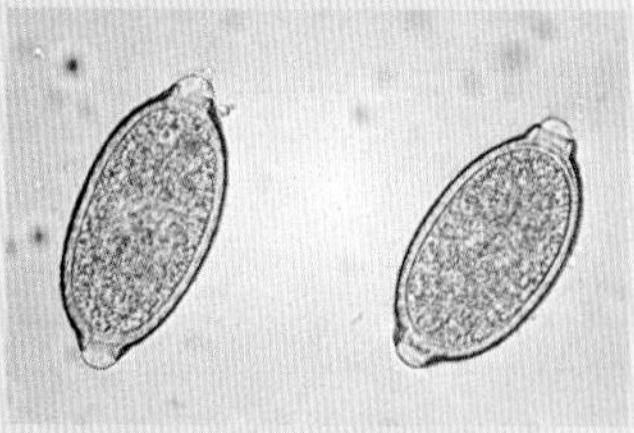 	Ivermectin: 0.2 mg/kg PO or SQ
Diphyllobothrium latum	Broad fish tapeworm 75 μm × 45 μm	Fig. E.17 From Connie R. Mahon, Donald C. Lehman: *Textbook of Diagnostic Microbiology,* ed 7, Philadelphia, 2023, Elsevier Inc. 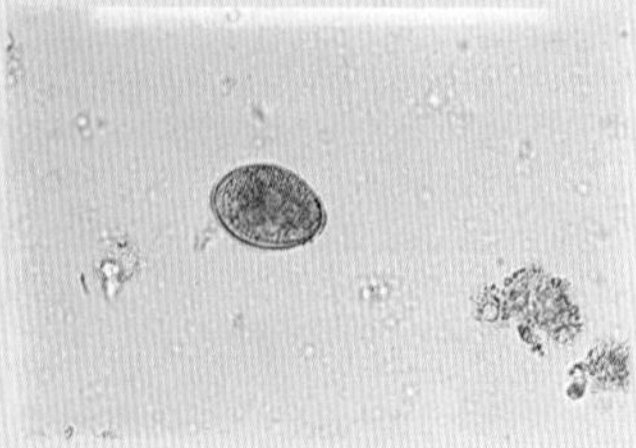 	Praziquantel: 5–20 mg/kg PO

Species	Common Name and Egg Size	Photo	Treatment
Spirocerca lupi	Esophageal worm 40 µm × 12 µm	Fig. E.18 From Hendrix CM, Robinson E: *Diagnostic parasitology for veterinary technicians*, ed 6, Philadelphia, 2023, Elsevier Inc.	
Dioctophyma renale	Giant kidney worm 65 µm × 42 µm	Fig. E.19 From Hendrix CM, Robinson E: *Diagnostic parasitology for veterinary technicians*, ed 6, Philadelphia, 2023, Elsevier Inc.	Surgical removal

Parasites of Cats

Species	Common Name and Egg Size	Photo	Treatment
Toxocara cati & *Toxocara leonina* ZOONOTIC	Roundworms or ascarids 75 μm × 65 μm	Fig. F.1 From Hendrix CM, Robinson E: *Diagnostic parasitology for veterinary technicians*, ed 6, Philadelphia, 2023, Elsevier Inc.	Fenbendazole: 50 mg/kg PO q24h × 3d Pyrantel: 10–20 mg/kg PO
Ancylostoma tubaeforme ZOONOTIC	Hookworm 60 μm × 40 μm	Fig. F.2 From Rana T: *Organ-specific parasitic diseases of dogs and cats*, Philadelphia, 2023, Elsevier Inc.	Fenbendazole: 100 mg/kg PO Pyrantel: 20–30 mg/kg PO Selamectin: 7–13 mg/kg topically
Capillaria aerophile	Cat lungworm or bladderworm 60 μm × 30 μm	Fig. F.3 From Hendrix CM, Robinson E: *Diagnostic parasitology for veterinary technicians*, ed 6, Philadelphia, 2023, Elsevier Inc.	Fenbendazole: 100 mg/kg PO
Dipylidium caninum ZOONOTIC	Tapeworm 200 μm × 150 μm	Fig. F.4 From Bowman DD: *Georgi Parasitología para veterinarios*, ed 11, Barcelona, 2022, Elsevier España, S.L.U.	Fenbendazole: 50 mg/kg PO q24h × 3d Praziquantel: 2.5–5 mg/kg PO or SC

Species	Common Name and Egg Size	Photo	Treatment
Spirometra ZOONOTIC	Tapeworm 70 μm × 35 μm	Fig. F.5 From Bowman DD: *Georgis' parasitology for veterinarians*, ed 11, Philidelphia, 2021, Elsevier Inc.	Praziquantel: 5 mg/kg PO or SC
Taenia taeniaeformis	Tapeworm 50 μm × 50 μm	Fig. F.6 From Bowman DD: *Georgis' parasitology for veterinarians*, ed 11, Philidelphia, 2021, Elsevier Inc.	Fenbendazole: 50 mg/kg PO q24h × 3d Praziquantel: 2.5–5 mg/kg PO or SC
Paragonimus kellicotti	Lung fluke 90 μm × 50 μm	Fig. F.7 From Hendrix CM, Robinson E: *Diagnostic parasitology for veterinary technicians*, ed 6, Philidelphia, 2023, Elsevier Inc.	Albendazole: 50–100 mg/kg PO q24h × 14–21d Fenbendazole: 50 mg/kg PO q24h × 10–14d Praziquantel: 25 mg/kg PO q24h × 3d

Continued

Species	Common Name and Egg Size	Photo	Treatment
Giardia sp. & *Giardia canis* ZOONOTIC	None 10 μm × 18 μm	Fig. F.8 From Sykes JE: *Greene's Infectious diseases of the dog and cat,* ed 5, Philidelphia, 2023, Elsevier Inc.	Fenbendazole: 50 mg/kg q 24h × 3d Albendazole: 25 mg/kg q 12h × 2d Metronidazole: 25 mg/kg PO q12h × 5d
Toxoplasma gondii ZOONOTIC	Toxo 12 μm × 11 μm	Fig. F.9 From Bowman DD: *Georgis' parasitology for veterinarians,* ed 11, Philidelphia, 2021, Elsevier Inc.	Clindamycin: 8–17 mg/kg × 14d
Sarcocystis sp. ZOONOTIC	None 18 μm × 15 μm	Fig. F.10 Courtesy www.cdc.gov/dpdx. A B	None
Cystoisospora spp. *(Isospora* spp.*).*	Coccidia 13 μm × 10 μm 42 μm × 31 μm 23 μm × 19 μm	Fig. F.11 From Hendrix CM, Robinson E: *Diagnostic parasitology for veterinary technicians,* ed 6, Philidelphia, 2023, Elsevier Inc.	Sulfadimethoxine: 55 mg/kg q24h, then 27.5 mg/kg q24h × 5d Amprolium: 60–100 mg/kg q24h × 7d

Parasites of Cattle, Sheep, and Goats (Ruminants)

Species	Common Name and Egg Size	Photo	Treatment
HOT Complex *Haemonchus contortus,* *Ostertagia ostertagi,* *Trichostrongylus axei*	Barber's pole worm Brown stomach worm Bankrupt worm 80 μm × 45 μm	Fig. G.1 From Silva CR, Lifschitz AL, Macedo SRD, Campos NRCL, Viana-Filho M, Alcântara ACS, Araújo JG, Alencar LMR, Costa-Junior LM: Combination of synthetic anthelmintics and monoterpenes: assessment of efficacy, and ultrastructural and biophysical properties of Haemonchus contortus using atomic force microscopy. *Vet Parasitol.* 2021;290:109345. 	Albendazole: 10 mg/kg PO Doramectin: 0.2 mg/kg IM or SQ Eprinomectrin: 0.5 mg/kg Pour on Ivermectin: 0.2 mg/kg SC Fenbendazole: 5 mg/kg PO Morantel tartrate: 9.7 mg/kg PO Moxidectin: 0.5 mg/kg Pour on
Nematodirus spp.	Thin-necked intestinal worm 200 μm × 90 μm 175 μm × 75 μm	Fig. G.2 From Bowman DD: *Georgis' parasitology for veterinarians*, ed 10, Philadelphia, 2014, Elsevier Inc. 	Albendazole: 10 mg/kg PO Eprinomectrin: 0.5 mg/kg Pour on Ivermectin: 0.2 mg/kg SC Fenbendazole: 5 mg/kg PO Morantel tartrate: 9.7 mg/kg PO Moxidectin: 0.5 mg/kg Pour on
Strongyloides papillosus	Threadworm 50 μm × 22 μm	Fig. G.3 From Bowman D: *Georgis' parasitology for veterinarians*, ed 10, St Louis, Saunders, 2014. 	Eprinomectrin: 0.5 mg/kg Pour on Ivermectin: 0.2 mg/kg SC

Continued

Species	Common Name and Egg Size	Photo	Treatment
Oesophagostomum columbianum	Nodular worm 80 μm × 40 μm	Fig. G.4 From Bowman DD: *Georgis' parasitology for veterinarians*, ed 11, Philadelphia, 2021, Elsevier Inc. 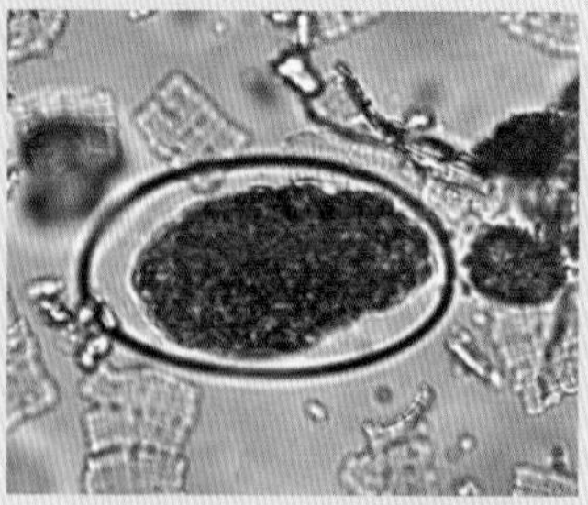	Albendazole: 10 mg/kg PO Doramectin: 0.2 mg/kg IM or SQ Eprinomectin: 0.5 mg/kg Pour on Morantel tartrate: 9.7 mg/kg PO Moxidectin: 0.5 mg/kg Pour on
Coperia spp.	Cattle bankrupt worm 77 μm × 34 μm	Fig. G.5 From Buchmann K, Christiansen L-L, Kania PW, Thamsborg SM: Introduced European bison (*Bison bonasus*) in a confined forest district: A ten year parasitological survey. *Int J Parasitol Parasites Wildl.* 2022;18:292–299, Fig. 1. 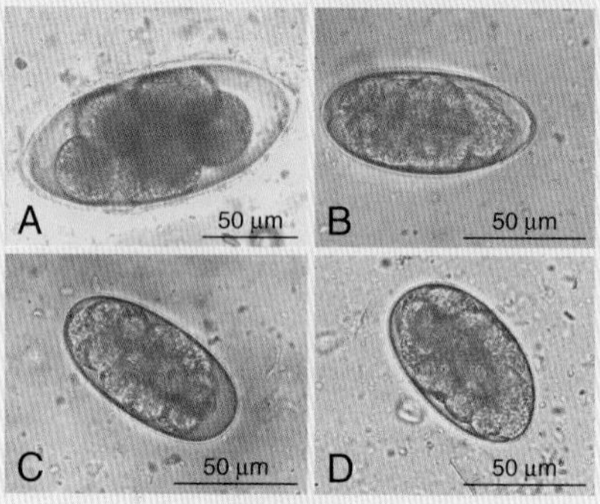	Albendazole: 10 mg/kg PO Doramectin: 0.2 mg/kg IM or SQ Eprinomectin: 0.5 mg/kg Pour on Ivermectin: 0.2 mg/kg SC Fenbendazole: 5 mg/kg PO Morantel tartrate: 9.7 mg/kg PO Moxidectin: 0.5 mg/kg Pour on
Bunostomum sp.	Hookworm 95 μm × 50 μm	Fig. G.6 From Thilakarathne SS, Rajakaruna RS, Fernando DD, Rajapakse RPVJ, Perera PK: Gastro-intestinal parasites in two subspecies of toque macaque (*Macaca sinica*) in Sri Lanka and their zoonotic potential. *Vet Parasitol Reg Stud Reports.* 2012;24:100558, Fig. 2. 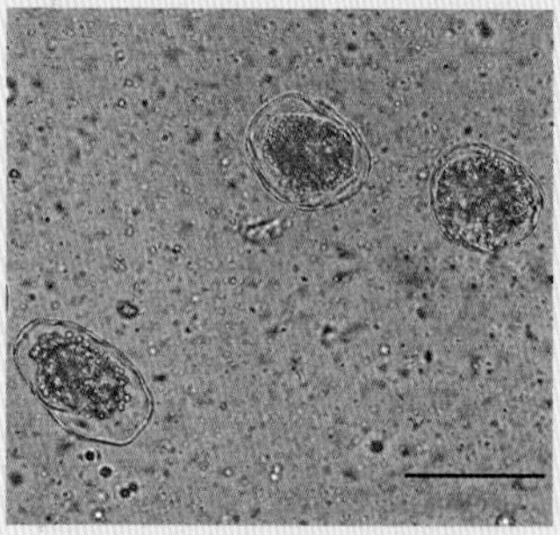	Albendazole: 10 mg/kg PO Doramectin: 0.2 mg/kg IM or SQ Ivermectin: 0.2 mg/kg SC Eprinomectin: 0.5 mg/kg Pour on Fenbendazole: 5 mg/kg PO Moxidectin: 0.5 mg/kg Pour on
Trichuris ovis	Whipworm 75 μm × 35 μm	Fig. G.7 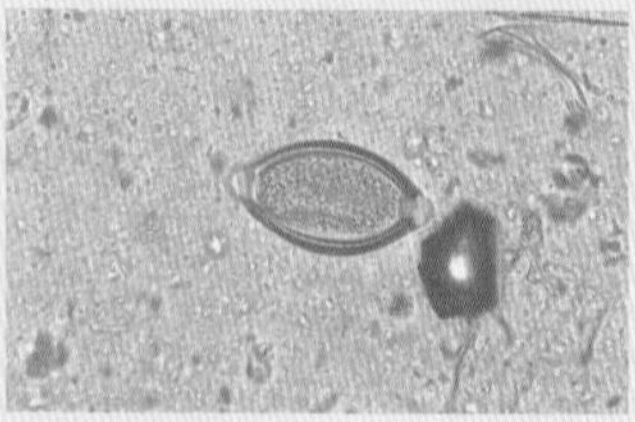	Doramectin: 0.2 mg/kg IM or SQ Eprinomectin: 0.5 mg/kg Pour on Fenbendazole: 5 mg/kg PO Ivermectin: 0.2 mg/kg SC

Species	Common Name and Egg Size	Photo	Treatment
Capillaria sp.	Capillary worm 50 μm × 30 μm	Fig. G.8 From Nath TC, Eom KS, Choe S, Islam S, Sabuj SS, Saha E, Tuhin RH, Ndosi BA, Kang Y, Kim S, Bia MM, Park H, Lee, D: Insights to helminth infections in food and companion animals in Bangladesh: Occurrence and risk profiling. *Parasite Epidemiol Control.* 2022;17:e00245, Fig. 1. 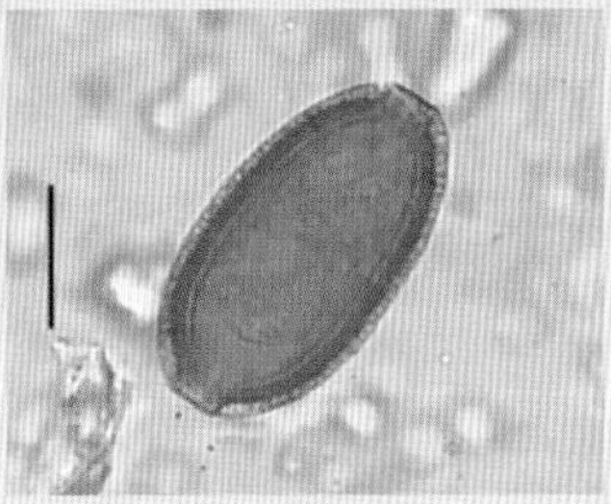	Doramectin: 0.2 mg/kg IM or SQ Ivermectin: 0.2 mg/kg SC Eprinomectrin: 0.5 mg/kg Pour on Fenbendazole: 5 mg/kg PO
Moniezia benedeni	Tapeworm 60 μm	Fig. G.9 Courtesy [C] Yoko Nagamori, DVM, MS, DACVM, Stillwater, OK; and [D] Paul Gajda, University of Calgary. 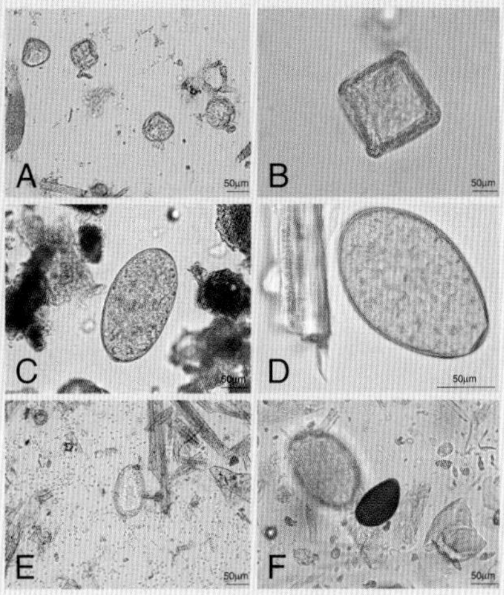	Albendazole: 10 mg/kg PO Fenbendazole: 10 mg/kg PO
Fasciola hepatica	Common liver fluke 140 μm × 80 μm	Fig. G.10 From Bowman DD: *Georgis' parasitology for veterinarians*, ed 11, Philadelphia, 2021, Elsevier Inc. 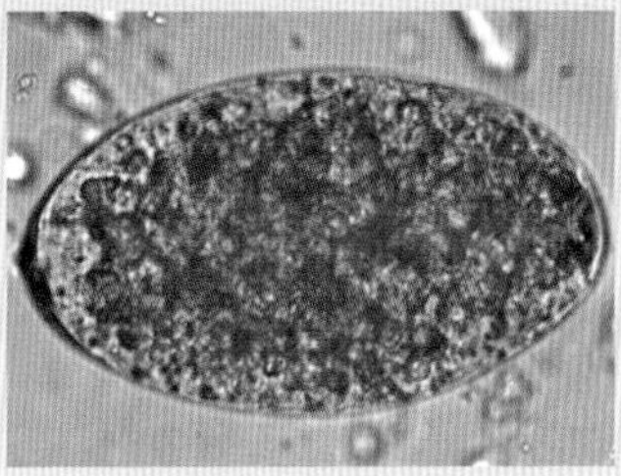	Albendazole: 10 mg/kg for Cattle 15 mg/kg for Sheep Nitroxynil: 10 mg/kg SC

Continued

Species	Common Name and Egg Size	Photo	Treatment
Eimeria spp.	Coccidia 16–47 µm × 13–47 µm	Fig. G.11 From Bowman DD: *Georgi Parasitología para veterinarios*, ed 11, Barcelona, 2022, Elsevier España, S.L.U. 	Decoquinate: 0.5 mg/kg PO q24h × 28d Lasalocid: 1 mg/kg PO q24h × 31d Monensin: 0.25 mg/kg PO in feed q24h × 31d Sulfaquanidine: 0.2% of feed Amprolium: As directed on feed or bottle
Cryptosporidium ZOONOTIC	Crypto 6 µm × 6 µm	Fig. G.12 From Hendrix CM, Robinson E: *Diagnostic parasitology for veterinary technicians*, ed 6, Philadelphia, 2023, Elsevier Inc. 	Supportive care

Parasites of Horses

Species	Common Name and Egg Size	Photo	Treatment
Strongylus vulgaris	Large strongyle 90 μm × 50 μm	Fig. H.1 NOTE: You can't differentiate small from large strongyles by ovum.	Ivermectin: 0.2 mg/kg PO Moxidectin: 0.4 mg/kg PO Fenbendazole: 5 mg/kg PO
Cyathostomum, Cylicocyclus, Cylicocephalus, Gyalocephalus	Small strongyles 90 μm × 50 μm	Fig H.2 From Hendrix CM, Robinson E: *Diagnostic parasitology for veterinary technicians*, ed 6, 2023, Elsevier Inc. NOTE: You can't differentiate small from large strongyles by ovum.	Ivermectin: 0.2 mg/kg PO Moxidectin: 0.4 mg/kg PO Pyrantel: 6.6 mg/kg PO

Continued

Species	Common Name and Egg Size	Photo	Treatment
Oxyuris equi	Pinworm 90–100 μm × 40–50 μm	Fig. H.3 From Hendrix CM, Robinson E: *Diagnostic parasitology for veterinary technicians*, ed 6, 2023, Elsevier Inc. 	Moxidectin: 0.4 mg/kg PO Pyrantel: 12.5 mg/kg PO
Parascaris equorum	Roundworm 100 μm	Fig. H4 From Hendrix CM, Robinson E: *Diagnostic parasitology for veterinary technicians*, ed 6, 2023, Elsevier Inc. 	Fenbendazole: 5 mg/kg PO Pyrantel: 6.6 mg/kg PO Ivermectin: 0.2 mg/kg PO Moxidectin: 0.4 mg/kg PO
Habronema spp.	Stomach worm 50–80 μm × 10–20 μm	Fig. H.5 From Devi CN, Borthakur SK, Patra G, Singh NS, Tolenkhomba TC, Ravindran R, Ghosh S: Incidence of cutaneous habronemosis in Manipuri ponies in India. *Vet Parasitol Reg Stud Reports.* 2019;17:100295. 	Ivermectin: 0.2 mg/kg PO Moxidectin: 0.4 mg/kg PO
Strongyloides westeri	Threadworm 50 μm	Fig. H.6 From Sellen DC, Long MT: *Equine infectious diseases*, ed 2, 2014, Elsevier Inc. 	Ivermectin: 0.2 mg/kg PO
Anoplocephala spp.	Tapeworm 80 μm × 50 μm	Fig. H.7 From Bohórquez A, Meana A, Pato NF, Luzón M: Coprologically diagnosing Anoplocephala perfoliata in the presence of A. magna. *Vet Parasitol.* 2014;204(3-4):396–401. 	Albendazole: 25 mg/kg PO Pyrantel: 13 mg/kg PO Praziquantel: 1 mg/kg PO

Parasites of Llamas and Alpacas

Species	Common Name and Egg Size	Photo	Treatment
HOT Complex Camelostrongylous *Cooperia* *Haemonchus* *Oesophagostomum* *Ostertagia* *Trichostrongylus*	Strongyles 77 μm × 45 μm	Fig. I.1 From Busari IO, Soetan KO, Aiyelaagbe OO, Babayemi OJ: Phytochemical screening and in vitro anthelmintic activity of methanolic extract of Terminalia glaucescens leaf on Haemonchus contortus eggs. *Acta Trop.* 2021;223:106091, Fig. 2. 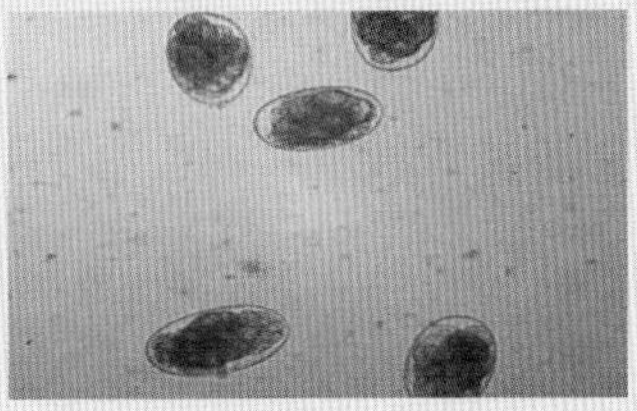 	Albendazole: 10 mg/kg PO Fenbendazole: 10 mg/kg q24h × 3d PO Ivermectin or doramectin: 0.2 mg/kg SC or IM Pyrantel: 18 mg/kg q24 × 1–3d PO
Trichuris tenuis	Whipworm 64 μm × 32 μm	Fig. I.2 From Bassert J: *Images for veterinary technician educators*, Summer 2001. 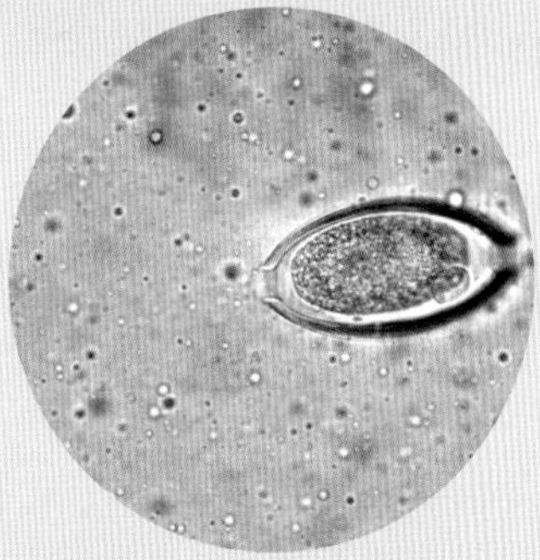 	Albendazole: 10 mg/kg PO Doramectin: 0.2 mg/kg SC or IM Fenbendazole: 10–15 mg/kg q24h × 3d PO Ivermectin: 0.2 mg/kg SC
Capillaria spp.	Capillary worm 50 μm × 30 μm Or 75 μm × 40 μm	Fig. I.3 Courtesy Antoinette Marsh. From Valenciano AC, Cowell RL: *Cowell and Tyler's diagnostic cytology and hematology of the dog and cat*, ed 5, 2020, Elsevier Inc. 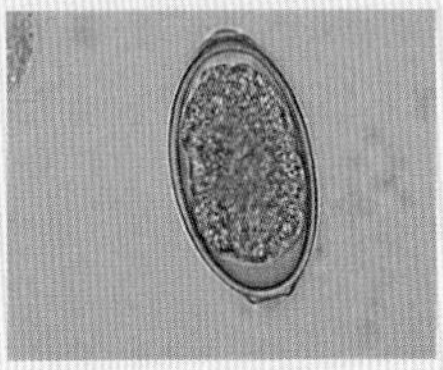 	Albendazole: 10 mg/kg PO Doramectin: 0.2 mg/kg SC or IM Fenbendazole: 10–15 mg/kg q24h × 3d PO Ivermectin: 0.2 mg/kg SC

Continued

Species	Common Name and Egg Size	Photo	Treatment
Nematodirus battus, Nematodirus helvetianus	Thin-necked intestinal worm 200 μm × 90 μm	Fig. I.4 From Hendrix CM, Robinson E: *Diagnostic parasitology for veterinary technicians*, ed 6, 2023, Elsevier Inc.	Albendazole: 10 mg/kg PO Doramectin: 0.2 mg/kg SC or IM Fenbendazole: 10–15 mg/kg q24h × 3d PO Ivermectin: 0.2 mg/kg SC Pyrantel: 18 mg/kg q24h × 1–3d PO
Eimeria lamae, Eimeria alpacae, Eimeria macusaniensis, Eimeria punoensis	Coccidia 38 μm x 28 μm	Fig. I.5 From Van Saun RJ, et al: *Llama and alpaca care: medicine, surgery, reproduction, nutrition, and herd health*, 2014, Elsevier Inc.	Decoquinate: 0.5 mg/kg PO q24h × 28d Lasalocid: 1 mg/kg PO q24h × 30d Monensin: 0.25 m/kg PO in feed q24h × 31d
Cryptosporidium sp. ZOONOTIC	Crypto 5 μm × 6 μm	Fig. I.6 From Goering R, Dockrell H, Wakelin D, et al: *Mims' medical microbiology*, ed 4, Philadelphia, 2007, Elsevier. (Courtesy S. Tzipori.)	None

Parasites of Swine

Species	Common Name & Egg Size	Photo	Treatment
Ascaris suum ZOONOTIC	Roundworm 85 μm × 80 μm	Fig. J.1 From *Diagnostic parasitology for veterinary technicians*, ed 6, 2023, Elsevier Inc. 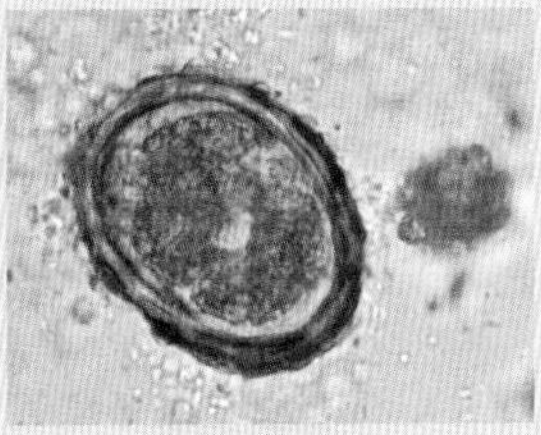	Doramectin: 0.3 mg/kg IM Fenbendazole: 3 mg/kg q24h × 3d Ivermectin: 0.3 mg/kg IM, SC, or in the feed
Trichuris suis	Whipworm 55 μm × 25 μm	Fig. J.2 From Gertzell E, Magnusson U, Ikwap K, Dione M, Lindström L, Eliasson-Selling L, Jacobson M: Animal health beyond the single disease approach – A role for veterinary herd health management in low-income countries? *Res Vet Sci.* 2021;136:453–463, Fig. 4. 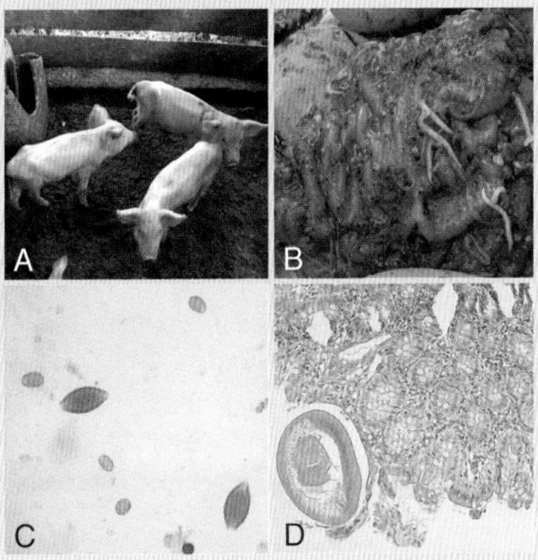	Fenbendazole: 3 mg/kg q24h × 3d Ivermectin: 0.3 mg/kg IM, SC, or in the feed
Oesophago-stomum dentatum	Nodular worm 70 μm × 40 μm	Fig. J.3 From Bowman DD: *Georgis' parasitology for veterinarians*, ed 11, 2021, Elsevier Inc. 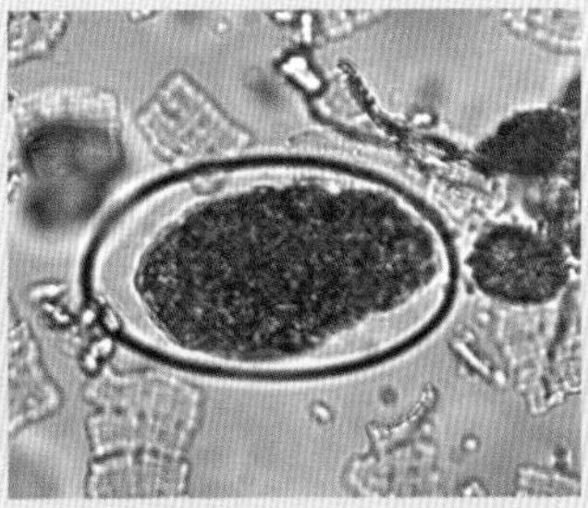	Doramectin: 0.3 mg/kg IM Fenbendazole: 3 mg/kg q24h × 3d Ivermectin: 0.3 mg/kg IM, SC, or in the feed Pyrantel: 800 g/ton feed for 1 feeding per day

Continued

Species	Common Name & Egg Size	Photo	Treatment
Metastrongylus spp.	Lungworm 55 μm × 40 μm	Fig. J.4 From Hendrix CM, Robinson E: *Diagnostic parasitology for veterinary technicians*, ed 6, 2023, Elsevier Inc.	Doramectin: 0.3 mg/kg IM Fenbendazole: 3 mg/kg q24h × 3d Ivermectin: 0.3–0.5 mg/kg IM, SC, or in the feed
Ascarops strongylina	Stomach worm 20 μm × 40 μm	Fig. J.5 From Hendrix CM, Robinson E: *Diagnostic parasitology for veterinary technicians*, ed 6, 2023, Elsevier Inc.	Doramectin: 0.3 mg/kg IM Ivermectin: 0.3 mg/kg IM, SC, or in the feed
Isospora suis	Coccidia 16–20 μm × 19–22 μm	Fig. J.6 From Hendrix CM, Robinson E: *Diagnostic parasitology for veterinary technicians*, ed 6, 2023, Elsevier Inc.	Decoquinate: 1 mg/kg q24h × 21d to sows before and after farrowing Sulfamethazine: 0.5% in feed or 130 mg/kg PO, then 65 mg/kg q12d × 4d

Parasites of Birds

Species	Common Name & Egg Size	Photo	Treatment
Ascaridia galli	Roundworm 85 μm × 50 μm	Fig. K.1 From Lebram von Sohsten A, Vieira da Silva A, Rubinsky-Elefant G, Santana ISF, Correia JE, Alves da Cruz L, Santos EMR, Oliveira PMV: Chickens bred extensively as sentinels from soil contamination by Toxocara. *Exp Parasitol.* 2020;211:107852. 	Fenbendazole: 10–50 mg/kg once, repeat in 10d
Heterakis gallinarium	Cecal worm 70 μm × 40 μm	Fig. K.2 Reproduced with permission from *BSAVA Manual of Backyard Poultry Medicine and Surgery.* © BSAVA 2019. 	Metronidazole: 25 mg/kg q12h × 5d
Capillaria spp.	None 50 μm × 25 μm	Fig. K.3 From Nath TC, Eom KS, Choe S, Islan S, Sabuj SS, Saha E, Tuhin RH, Ndosi BA, Kang Y, Kim S, Bia MM, Park H, Lee D: Insights to helminth infections in food and companion animals in Bangladesh: Occurrence and risk profiling. *Parasite Epidemiol Control.* 2022;17:e00245, Fig. 1. 	Fenbendazole: 10–50 mg/kg q24h × 5d Ivermectin: 0.4 mg/kg PO or IM

Continued

Species	Common Name & Egg Size	Photo	Treatment
Syngamus trachea	Gapeworm 90 μm × 50 μm	Fig. K.4 From Meister SL, Wenker C, Wyss F, Zühlke I, Veiga IB, Basso WU: *Syngamus trachea* in free-ranging white stork (*Ciconia ciconia*) nestlings in Switzerland. *Int J Parasitol Parasites Wildl.* 2022;18:76–81.	Fenbendazole: 30 mg/kg × 5d
Eimeria	Coccidia 16–32 μm × 14–24 μm	Fig. K.5	Amprolium: 0.012–0.024% in water q24h × 3–5d Sulfadimethoxine: 0.006–0.05% q24h × 6d Sulfonamides (enteric): 55 mg/kg PO q24h PRN

Parasites of Exotics

RABBITS
Nematodes
Passalurus ambiguous
Obeliscoides cuniculi

Cestodes
Cittotaenia variabilis
Cittotaenia ctenoides
Mosgovoyia spp.
Monoecocestus americana

Trematodes
Hasstilesia tricolor
Fasciola hepatica

Arthropods
Cheyletiella
Psoroptes cuniculi
Listrophorus spp.

HAMSTERS
Nematodes
Syphacia spp.

Cestodes
Hymenolepis nana
Hymenolepis diminuta
Larval tapeworms

Protozoan
Spironucleus muris
Giardia
Tritrichomonas spp.
Balantidium spp.
Cryptosporidium

Arthropods
Demodex
Notoedres
Ornithonyssus bacoti
Liponyssus bacoti

GERBILS
Nematodes
Dentostomella translucida
Syphacia

Cestodes
Hymenolepis spp.

Protozoan
Giardia

Arthropods
Demodex
Liponyssoides spp.

MICE
Nematodes
Syphacia obvelata
Aspiculuris tetraptera

Cestodes
Hymenolepis diminuta
Hymenolepis nana
Hymenolepis microstoma
Taenia taeniaeformis

Protozoan
Trypanosoma musculi
Toxoplasma gondii
Sarcocystis muris
Klossiella muris
Encephalitozoan cuniculi
Pneumocystis carinii
Giardia muris
Spironucleus muris
Tritrichomonas muris
Eimeria falciformis
Cryptosporidium muris
Cryptosporidium parvum

Arthropods
Xenopsylla cheopis

Nosopsyllus fasciatus
Leptopsylla segnis
Polyplax serrata
Hoplopleura spp.
Ornithonyssus bacoti
Ornithonyssus sylviarum
Liponyssoides sanguineous
Haemogamasus pontiger
Eulaelaps stabularis
Laelaps echidnus
Haemolaelaps spp.
Myobia musculi
Radfordia affinis
Psorergates simplex
Notoedres musculi
Demodex musculi
Myocoptes musculinus

RATS

Nematodes

Syphacia muris
Aspiculuris tetraptera
Heterakis spumosa

Cestodes

Hymenolepis nana
Hymenolepis diminuta

Protozoa

Trypanosoma lewisi
Toxoplasma gondii
Sarcocystis muris
Encephalitozoon cuniculi
Pneumocystis carinii
Giardia muris
Spironucleus muris
Eimeria nieschultzi
Entamoeba muris

Arthropods

Polyplax spinulosa
Radfordia ensifera
Notoedres muris
Laelaps echidninus

GUINEA PIGS

Nematodes

Praspidodera uncinate

Protozoan

Cryptosporidium wrairi
Giardia caviae

Eimeria caviae
Toxoplasma gondii
Sarcocystis caviae

Arthropods

Gliricola lindolphi
Gliricola porcelli
Gyropus ovalis
Trimenopon hispidum
Nosopsyllus fasciatus
Pulex irritans
Ctenocephalides felis
Rhopalopsylla clavicula
Demodex caviae
Chirodiscoides caviae
Myocoptes musculinus
Notoedres muris
Trixacarus caviae

HEDGEHOGS

Nematodes

Capillaria aerophila

Arthropods

Crenosoma
Capillaria hepatica
Archaeopsylla erinacei
Caparini
Chorioptes
Otodectes cynotis
Ornithonyssus
Ixodes hexagonus
Amblyomma nuttalli

SNAKES AND LIZARDS

Cestodes

Pseudophyllideans
  Bothridium
  Bothriocephalus
  Spirometra
Sparganum larvae
Mesocestoides larvae
Protocaephalus
Acanthotaenia
Crepidobothrium
Ophiotaenia

Trematodes

Lechriochis
Dasymetra
Ochetostoma
Stomatrema

Zeugorchis
Styphylodora
Spirorchis

Protozoan

Entamoeba invadens
Emeria
Isopora
Cryptosporidium
Haemoproteus
Hepatozoon
Plasmodium
Trichomonas
Leishmania
Trypanosoma
Balantidium

TURTLES

Nematodes

Augusticaecum

Camallanus
Spionura
Spiroxys
Kalicephalus
Proatractis

Cestodes

Neoechinorhychus

Trematodes

Dictyangium
Heronimus
Neopolystoma
Telorchis

Protozoan

Entamoeba invadens
Eimeria
Balantidium

Arthropod Identification

Species	Common Name	Photo
Ctenocephalides felis, Ctenocephalides canis, Pulex irritans, Xenopsylla cheopis, Echidnophaga gallinacea	Fleas	Fig. M.1 From Bowman DD: *Georgis' parasitology for veterinarians*, ed 11, Philadelphia, 2021, Elsevier Inc.
Anoplura	Sucking louse	Fig. M.2 From Bowman DD: *Georgis' parasitology for veterinarians*, ed 11, Philadelphia, 2021, Elsevier Inc.
Mallophaga	Biting louse	Fig. M.3
Culicoides	Biting midges or "no-see-ums"	Fig. M.4 From Bowman DD: *Georgis' parasitology for veterinarians*, ed 11, Philadelphia, 2021, Elsevier Inc.

Species	Common Name	Photo
Simulium	Blackflies or buffalo gnats	Fig. M.5 From Bowman DD: *Georgis' parasitology for veterinarians*, ed 11, Philadelphia, 2021, Elsevier Inc.
Phlebotomus and Lutzomyia	Sandflies	Fig. M.6 From Dolin R, et al: *Mandell, Douglas, and Bennett's principles and practice of infectious diseases: 2-volume set*, ed 9, Philadelphia, 2020, Elsevier Inc. (Courtesy Dr. Ed Rowton, Silver Spring, MD.)
Haematobia irritans	Horn flies	Fig. M.7 From Mullen GR, Durden LA: *Medical and veterinary entomology*, ed 3, Philadelphia, 2019, Elsevier Inc. (Original drawings by Fritz Gregor, and published in Greenburg, 1971, reprinted by permission of Princeton University Press).
Stomoxys calcitrans	Biting housefly or stable fly	Fig. M.8 From Mullen GR, Durden LA: *Medical and veterinary entomology*, ed 3, Philadelphia, 2019, Elsevier Inc. (Original drawings by Fritz Gregor, and published in Greenburg, 1971, reprinted by permission of Princeton University Press).

Continued

Species	Common Name	Photo
Musca domestica	Common housefly	Fig. M.9 From Mullen GR, Durden LA: *Medical and veterinary entomology*, ed 3, Philadelphia, 2019, Elsevier Inc. (Original drawings by Fritz Gregor, and published in Greenburg, 1971, reprinted by permission of Princeton University Press).
Tabanus	Horse flies	Fig. M.10 From Hendrix CM, Robinson E: *Diagnostic parasitology for veterinary technicians*, ed 6, Philadelphia, 2023, Elsevier Inc.
Melophagus ovinus	Sheep ked	Fig. M.11 From Rezaei N: *Encyclopedia of infection and immunity*, Philadelphia, 2022, Elsevier Inc.
Gastrophilus spp. *Hypoderma* spp. *Cuterebra, Oestrus ovis*	Botflies	Fig. M.12 From Hendrix CM, Robinson E: *Diagnostic parasitology for veterinary technicians*, ed 6, Philadelphia, 2023, Elsevier Inc.
Anopheles, Aedes, Culex	Mosquitoes	Fig. M.13 Hendrix CM, Robinson E: *Diagnostic parasitology for veterinary technicians*, ed 6, Philadelphia, 2023, Elsevier Inc.

Species	Common Name	Photo
Dermacentor andersoni	Rocky Mountain wood tick	Fig. M.14 Tille P: *Bailey & Scott's diagnostic microbiology*, ed 15, Philadelphia, 2022, Elsevier Inc.
Dermacentor occidentalis	Pacific Coast tick	Fig. M.15 From Shapiro MR, Fritz CL, Tait K, et al.: Rickettsia 364D: a newly recognized cause of eschar-associated illness in California. *Clin Infect Dis.* 2010;50:541–548; and Centers for Disease Control and Prevention, Atlanta, GA. (Photographs courtesy James Gathany).
Dermacentor variabilis	American dog tick	Fig. M.16 (A) Female. (B) Male.
Rhipicephalus sanguineus	Brown dog tick	Fig. M.17 From Public Health Image Library. Image 7646. Atlanta, GA: Centers for Disease Control and Prevention.

Continued

Species	Common Name	Photo
Dermacentor albipictus	Winter tick or moose tick	Fig. M.18 From Duncan K, Clow KM, Sundstrom KD, Saleh MN, Reichard MV, Little SE: Recent reports of winter tick, Dermacentor albipictus, from dogs and cats in North America. *Vet Parasitol Reg Stud Rep.* 2020;22:100490.
Ixodes scapularis Lyme disease transmission	Deer tick or blacklegged tick	Fig. M.19 From Rifai N: *Tietz textbook of clinical chemistry and molecular diagnostics*, ed 6, Philadelphia, 2018, Elsevier Inc.
Ixodes pacificus Lyme disease transmission	Western blacklegged tick	Fig. M.20 From Biggs HM, Behravesh CB, Bradley KK, et al.: Diagnosis and management of tickborne rickettsial diseases: Rocky Mountain spotted fever and other spotted fever group rickettsioses, ehrlichioses, and anaplasmosis — United States. *MMWR Recomm Rep.* 2016;65(No. RR-2):1—44. DOI: https://dx.doi.org/10.15585/mmwr.rr6502a1
Amblyomma americanum & Amblyomma maculatum	Lonestar tick	Fig. M.21 From Public Health Image Library. Image 8683. Centers for Disease Control and Prevention.
Rhipicephalus annulatus	Cattle tick	Fig. M.22 From Senbill H, Tanaka T, Karawia D, Rahman S, Zeb J, Sparagano O, Baruah A: Morphological identification and molecular characterization of economically important ticks (Acari: Ixodidae) from North and North—Western Egypt. *Acta Trop.* 2022;231:106438.

Species	Common Name	Photo
Otobius megnini	Spinose ear tick	Fig. M.23
Ornithodoros	Soft ticks	Fig. M.24 From Tickborne Diseases of the United States. Soft tick. Centers for Disease Control and Prevention. https://www.cdc.gov/ticks/tickbornediseases/tickID.html.
Dermanyssus gallinae	Red poultry mite	Fig. M.25 From Speer BL: *Current therapy in avian medicine and surgery*, Philadelphia, 2016, Elsevier Inc. (Photo courtesy Dr. Heather Walden, University of Florida.)
Ornithonyssus bacoti	Tropical rat mite	Fig. M.26 From Powderly WG, et al: *Infectious diseases*, ed 4, Philadelphia, 2017, Elsevier Ltd.
Notoedres cati	Notoedric mange	Fig. M.27 Courtesy National Center for Veterinary Parasitology.

Continued

Species	Common Name	Photo
Knemidokoptes spp.	Scaley leg mites	Fig. M.28 From Mullen GR, Durden LA: *Medical and veterinary entomology*, ed 2, Philadelphia, 2009, Elsevier Inc.
Demodex	Demodectic mange	Fig. M.29
Psoroptes	Psoroptic mange	Fig. M.30 From Bowman DD: *Georgis' parasitology for veterinarians*, ed 11, Philadelphia, 2021, Elsevier Inc.
Chorioptes	Chorioptic mange	Fig. M.31 From Hendrix CM, Robinson E: *Diagnostic parasitology for veterinary technicians*, ed 6, Philadelphia, 2023, Elsevier Inc.
Otodectes cynotis	Ear mites	Fig. M.32

Species	Common Name	Photo
Cheyletiella	Walking dandruff	Fig. M.33
Linguatula serrata	Tongue worm	Fig. M.34 From Shamsi S, Halajian A, Barton DP, Zhu X, Smit WJ, Roux F, Luus-Powell WJ: Occurrence and characterisation of tongue worms, *Linguatula* spp., in South Africa. *Int J Parasitol Parasites Wildl.* 2020;11:268–281.

Cytology Identification

Photo	Tumor Type	Cell Description	Examples
Fig. N.1 From Cowell RL, Valenciano AC: *Cowell and Tyler's diagnostic cytology and hematology of the dog and cat*, ed 4, St Louis, 2014, Mosby. 	Epithelial	Large, round to polygonal cells Distinct cell borders Tightly adherent to each other Round to oval nuclei that can be basilar in columnar cells or eccentric in other cell shapes	Benign=(adenoma) Malignant=(carcinoma)
Fig. N.2 From Cowell RL, Valenciano AC: *Cowell and Tyler's diagnostic cytology and hematology of the dog and cat*, ed 4, St Louis, 2014, Mosby. 	Mesenchymal	Spindle, oval or stellate-shaped cells Indistinct cell borders that taper into the background Round to oval to elongate nuclei that are usually centrally located Cells are scattered individually or in aggregates, usually within matrix Less cellular than the other tumors due to matrix Matrix can be present in the background as well as within aggregates	Benign=("..oma") Malignant=("sarcoma")
Fig. N.3 From Johnston, SA, Tobias, KM: *Veterinary surgery: Small animal*, ed 2, Philadelphia, 2018, Elsevier. 	Round Cell Mast Cell Tumor	These are readily recognized by the presence of purple cytoplasmic granules They also have round eccentric nuclei with smooth chromatin	Mast Cell Tumor

Photo	Tumor Type	Cell Description	Examples
Fig. N.4 From Cowell RL, Valenciano AC: *Cowell and Tyler's diagnostic cytology and hematology of the dog and cat*, ed 5, Philadelphia, 2020, Elsevier.	Round Cell Histiocytoma	Round to oval with variably distinct cytoplasmic borders Moderate to abundant amounts of clear to light blue cytoplasm Nuclei are eccentric and round to oval to indented Nuclei have finely stippled chromatin and nucleoli are not apparent Cells are often found dispersed within a moderately blue background Minimal cellular atypia, uniform cell size and morphology—they have a bland appearance	Histiocytoma
Fig. N.5 From Cowell RL, Valenciano AC: *Cowell and Tyler's diagnostic cytology and hematology of the dog and cat*, ed 5, Philadelphia, 2020, Elsevier.	Round Cell Plasmacytoma	Round to slightly oval cells Distinct cell borders Variable amounts of blue cytoplasm (often deep blue), some have perinuclear clear zones Nuclei are round, occasionally oval, and eccentric Nuclei have clumped chromatin and nucleoli are not apparent More atypia (anisocytosis and anisokaryosis) than histiocytic tumors Binucleation and, occasionally, multinucleation is common Multinucleated cells may show marked intracellular anisokaryosis Amyloid may be present in skin tumors	Plasmacytoma

Continued

Photo	Tumor Type	Cell Description	Examples
Fig. N.6 From Cowell RL, Valenciano AC: *Cowell and Tyler's diagnostic cytology and hematology of the dog and cat*, ed 5, Philadelphia, 2020, Elsevier.	Round Cell Lymphoma	Lymphoma is most easily recognized when it consists of large cells or cells that are not expected in inflammatory lesions, such as many granular lymphocytes It is far harder to recognize when the cells are intermediate to small; however, the lack of other immune cells (plasma cells) or inflammatory cells can lead to a suspected diagnosis of lymphoma Lymphoid cells have the highest nuclear to cytoplasmic ratios of all the round cells They can rupture easily and one can see cytoplasmic fragments ("lymphoglandular" bodies) in the background, which can be a helpful but not definitive finding	Lymphoma
Fig. N.7 From Cowell RL, Valenciano AC: *Cowell and Tyler's diagnostic cytology and hematology of the dog and cat*, ed 5, Philadelphia, 2020, Elsevier.	Round Cell Transmissible Venereal Tumor	Monomorphic population of round cells Medium to large round nucleus that is eccentric or central Nuclear chromatin is clumped, and mitotic figures are common Can see binucleation or multinucleation as well as nucleoli The cytoplasm is characteristic: Abundant light blue to gray with moderate to many discrete margined vacuoles Can have infiltrates of small lymphocytes	Transmissible Venereal Tumor
Fig. N.8	Lipoma	Fails to dry once smeared out on the slide	Lipoma

Photo	Sample Type	Description
Fig. N.9 From Raskin RE, Meyer DJ: *Atlas of canine and feline cytology*, St Louis, 2001, Saunders.	Suppurative Inflammation	Suppurative inflammation as evidenced by the large number of neutrophils Note the presence of karyorrhexis in the center cell
Fig. N.10 From Cowell RL, Valenciano AC: *Cowell and Tyler's diagnostic cytology and hematology of the dog and cat*, ed 4, St Louis, 2014, Mosby.	Pyogranulomatous Inflammation	Pyogranulomatous inflammation in the eyelid of a dog Note neutrophils and epithelioid macrophages, including binucleate forms Lymphocytes and low numbers of red blood cells also are present
Fig. N.11 From Cowell RL, Valenciano AC: *Cowell and Tyler's diagnostic cytology and hematology of the dog and cat*, ed 4, St Louis, 2014, Mosby.	Septic Inflammation	Septic neutrophilic inflammation Many neutrophils are present, some of which contain phagocytized bacterial rods *(arrows)*
Fig. N.12 From Raskin RE, Meyer DJ: *Atlas of canine and feline cytology*, St Louis, 2001, Saunders.	Pyogranulomatous Lymphadenitis	
Fig. N.13 From Cowell RL, Valenciano AC: *Cowell and Tyler's diagnostic cytology and hematology of the dog and cat*, ed 4, St Louis, 2014, Mosby.	Mesothelial Cells	A small cluster of mesothelial cells

Continued

Photo	Sample Type	Description
Fig. N.14 From Cowell RL, Valenciano AC: *Cowell and Tyler's diagnostic cytology and hematology of the dog and cat*, ed 4, St Louis, 2014, Mosby.	Plasma Cells	Numerous plasma cells in a scraping of the third eyelid from a German Shepherd with plasmacytic conjunctivitis
Fig. N.15 From Raskin, RE, Meyer, DJ, Boes, KM: *Canine and feline cytopathology: a color atlas and interpretation guide*, ed 4, St Louis, 2023, Elsevier.	Small Lymphocytes	Similar in appearance to the small lymphocyte seen on a peripheral blood film Slightly larger than an RBC Scanty cytoplasm, dense nucleus
Fig. N.16 From Raskin, RE, Meyer, DJ, Boes, KM: *Canine and feline cytopathology: a color atlas and interpretation guide*, ed 4, St Louis, 2023, Elsevier.	Intermediate Lymphocytes	Nucleus approximately twice as large as an RBC; abundant cytoplasm
Fig. N.17 From Raskin RE, Meyer DJ: *Canine and feline cytology*, ed 3, St. Louis, 2016, Elsevier.	Lymphoblasts	Two to four times as large as the RBC Usually contains a nucleolus Diffuse nuclear chromatin
Fig. N.18 From Cassarino D: *Diagnostic pathology: Neoplastic dermatopathology*, ed 3, Philadelphia, 2022, Elsevier.	Plasmablasts	Similar to lymphoblasts with more abundant, basophilic cytoplasm May contain vacuoles

Photo	Sample Type	Description
Fig. N.19 From Raskin, RE, Meyer, DJ, Boes, KM: *Canine and feline cytopathology: a color atlas and interpretation guide*, ed 4, St Louis, 2023, Elsevier. 	Histiocytes	Large, pleomorphic, single or multinuclear; nuclei are round to oval
Fig. N.20 From Raskin, RE, Meyer, DJ, Boes, KM: *Canine and feline cytopathology: a color atlas and interpretation guide*, ed 4, St Louis, 2023, Elsevier. 	Mast Cells	Round cells that are usually slightly larger than lymphoblasts Distinctive purple staining granules may not stain adequately with Diff Quick
Fig. N.21 From Miller WH, Griffin CE, Campbell KL: *Muller and Kirk's small animal dermatology*, ed 7, St Louis, 2013, Mosby. 	Malassezia	
Fig. N.22 From Kradin RL: *Diagnostic pathology of infectious disease*, ed 1, Philadelphia, 2010, Elsevier. 	Bacteria	Bacteria

Photo	Cells	Interpretation
Fig. N.23 From Cowell RL, Valenciano AC: *Cowell and Tyler's diagnostic cytology and hematology of the dog and cat*, ed 4, St Louis, 2014, Mosby.	Parabasal Cells	Parabasal cells in a vaginal smear from a dog in anestrus
Fig. N.24 From Cowell RL, Valenciano AC: *Cowell and Tyler's diagnostic cytology and hematology of the dog and cat*, ed 4, St Louis, 2014, Mosby.	Intermediate Vaginal Epithelial Cells	Degenerating superficial vaginal epithelial cells with vacuolated cytoplasm in a canine vaginal smear
Fig. N.25 From Cowell RL, Valenciano AC: *Cowell and Tyler's diagnostic cytology and hematology of the dog and cat*, ed 4, St Louis, 2014, Mosby.	Squamous Cell	Mature squamous cells have cornified cytoplasm that has sharp angular borders Mature squamous cells may be nucleated or anucleate A, Mature nucleated squamous cells have abundant light blue–gray cytoplasm that has an angular appearance. B, Mature squamous cell with a pyknotic nucleus *(lower left)* and anucleate, mature squamous cells.
Fig. N.26 From Cowell RL, Valenciano AC: *Cowell and Tyler's diagnostic cytology and hematology of the dog and cat*, ed 4, St Louis, 2014, Mosby.	Cornified Cells = 80% or greater reveals cytological estrus Confirm appropriate breeding time with progesterone Natural breeding: should occur 3 days after progesterone reaches 2.5 ng/ml Chilled semen insemination: breed 48 hours after the progesterone reaches 5 ng/ml Frozen semen insemination breed 72 hours after the progesterone reaches 5 ng/ml	Mature, cornified cells from a canine vaginal swab Low-magnification image shows that these cells tend to exfoliate individually rather than in cohesive clusters Individual cells show angular cytoplasmic borders Nuclei become pyknotic *(arrow)* and eventually disappear, leaving anucleate cells

Bacterial Pathogens of Veterinary Importance

The following table is a summary of characteristics of and diseases produced by microbial pathogens seen in mammals and birds. A comprehensive bacteriology text should be consulted for additional characteristics used to identify these species definitively and for additional information about less common species.

Organism	Primary Species Affected	Disease or Lesion	Characteristics
Actinobacillus Species			
A. arthritidis	Horses	Arthritis, septicemia	• Gram-negative bacilli and coccobacilli
A. equuli equuli	Foals, pigs, calves	"Sleepy foal" disease; diarrhea, meningitis, pneumonia, purulent nephritis, septic polyarthritis	• Facultative anaerobe; requires carbon dioxide
A. equuli haemolyticus	Horses	Endocarditis, meningitis, metritis, abortion	• Pus may contain club-shaped structures that represent bacterial colonies surrounded by spicules of calcium phosphate <1 mm in diameter
A. lignieresii	Cattle, sheep	Granulomatous/pyogranulomatous lesions; commonly affects tongue (wooden tongue); may also cause pyogranulomatous lesions in soft tissues of the head, neck, limbs, lungs, pleura, udder, and subcutaneous tissue	• Identification/differentiation • Growth on MacConkey agar • CAMP test • Esculin hydrolysis • Acid production in carbohydrate substrates
A. pleuropneumoniae	Pigs	Pleuropneumonia; pleuritis, pulmonary abscess in pigs <5 months old	• Oxalase test
A. rossii	Pigs	Abortion, metritis	• Catalase test
A. seminis	Sheep	Epididymitis in rams; purulent polyarthritis in lambs	• Urease test
A. salpingitidis	Chickens	Salpingitis and peritonitis in chickens of layer type	
A. suis	Young pigs, foals	Fatal septicemia in animals <6 weeks old, arthritis, pneumonia, pericarditis, abscesses in older animals	
Actinomyces Species			
A. bovis	Cattle, horses	Lumpy jaw and lung abscesses in cattle, chronic fistulous withers and chronic poll evil in horses	• Gram-positive, non–acid-fast bacilli • Non–spore-forming • Poor growth on Sabouraud dextrose agar
A. hordeovulneris	Dogs	Localized abscesses, pleuritis, peritonitis, visceral abscesses, septic arthritis	• Facultative anaerobe; requires carbon dioxide
A. hyovaginalis	Pigs	Vaginitis, abortion	• Usually filamentous
A. suis	Pigs	Pyogranulomatous mastitis	• Often contains yellowish granules
A. viscosus	Dogs, hamsters	Chronic pneumonia, pyothorax, localized subcutaneous abscesses	• Identification/differentiation • Colony characteristics • Hemolysis pattern • Esculin hydrolysis test • Acid production in carbohydrate substrates • Nitrate reduction test • Catalase test • Urease test

Organism	Primary Species Affected	Disease or Lesion	Characteristics
Anaplasma Species			• Gram-negative, coccoid to ellipsoid forms
A. bovis	Cattle	Anemia, weight loss	• Located within cytoplasmic vacuoles of myeloid cells, neutrophils, erythrocytes, or thrombocytes
A. caudatum	Ruminants	Anemia, icterus, splenomegaly, erythrophagocytosis	• Identification/differentiation
A. centrale	Ruminants	Fever, anemia	• Demonstration of organisms on blood film
A. marginale	Ruminants	Fever, anorexia, weight loss, lethargy	• Immunology
A. ovis	Sheep, goats	Anemia, depression, fever, anorexia	
A. phagocytophilum	Horses, small ruminants	Granulocytic ehrlichiosis	
A. platys	Dogs	Infectious thrombocytopenia	
Arcobacter Species			• Gram-negative, curved or spiral bacilli
A. cryaerophilus	Cattle, horses, pigs, sheep, dogs	Abortion, mastitis	• Microaerophilic

A. butzleri	Horses, cattle, pigs, nonhuman primates	Diarrhea	• Identification/differentiation
			  • Colony characteristics
			  • Nitrate reduction test

A. skirrowii	Cattle, pigs	Abortion, diarrhea (lambs and calves)	• Catalase test • Growth on MacConkey agar • Hydrogen sulfide production
Arcanobacterium Species			• Gram-positive, nonmotile, coccoid bacilli

A. pyogenes	Cattle, goats, sheep, pigs	Liver abscess, endocarditis, abortion, endometriosis, suppurative mastitis, pneumonia, septic arthritis, umbilical infections, seminal vesiculitis	• Identification/differentiation
			  • Colony characteristics
			  • Hemolysis pattern

A. hippocoleae	Horses	Vaginitis	
Bacillus Species			• Gram-positive, spore-forming bacilli
B. anthracis	Ruminants, dogs, cats, horses	Septicemia, pharyngitis (dogs and cats)	• Identification/differentiation • Colony characteristics
B. cereus	Cattle, sheep, horses	Gangrenous mastitis, abortion	• Hemolysis pattern • Motility test
B. licheniformis	Cattle	Abortion	• Nitrate reduction test • PCR testing
Bacteroides Species			• Gram-negative, non–spore-forming bacilli
B. asaccharolyticus	Dogs, cats, horses, cattle	Osteomyelitis	• Anaerobic

B. fragilis	Cattle, sheep, goats, horses, pigs, dogs, cats	Neonatal diarrhea, abortion, mastitis, soft tissue abscess (dogs and cats)	• Identification/differentiation
			  • Cellular morphology
			  • Colony characteristics
			  • Bile sensitivity test

B. levii	Cattle	Mastitis	• Esculin hydrolysis test • Indole production test • Fermentation of sugars
Bordetella Species			• Gram-negative bacilli

B. bronchiseptica	Dogs, cats, horses, pigs, nonhuman primates, rodents, rabbits	Sinusitis, pneumonia, rhinitis, tracheobronchitis, conjunctivitis, endocarditis, meningitis, peritonitis	• Identification/differentiation
			  • Colony characteristics
			  • Growth on MacConkey and blood agar

B. avium	Birds	Turkey coryza	• Slide agglutination test • Urease test • Oxidase test • Nitrate reduction test • Citrate utilization test • Motility test

Organism	Primary Species Affected	Disease or Lesion	Characteristics
Borrelia Species			
B. anserina	Birds	Fatal septicemia	• Coiled spirochetes
B. burgdorferi	Dogs, cats, horses, cattle	Lyme disease	• Microaerophilic or anaerobic • Identification/differentiation
B. coriaceae	Cattle	Abortion	• Demonstration of organisms on blood films, smears of spleen or liver tissue
B. theileri	Cattle, sheep, horses	Relapsing fever, anemia	• Immunologic testing
Brachyspira Species			
B. aalborgi	Nonhuman primates	Colonic spirochetosis	• Gram-negative, slender spirochetes
B. alvinipulli	Poultry	Colonic spirochetosis	• Identification/differentiation
B. hyodysenteriae	Pigs	Dysentery	• Cellular morphology
B. intermedia	Poultry	Colonic spirochetosis	• Colony characteristics
B. pilosicoli	Pigs, chickens	Colonic spirochetosis	• Hemolysis pattern • Indole production test
Brucella Species			
B. abortus	Cattle, pigs, sheep, goats, dogs	Abortion, orchitis, epididymitis, chronic bursitis, fistulous withers	• Gram-negative bacilli and coccobacilli • Nonmotile
B. canis	Dogs	Abortion, epididymitis, osteomyelitis, meningitis, glomerulonephritis	• Facultative intracellular parasites • Identification/differentiation
B. melitensis	Sheep, goats	Abortion, mastitis, orchitis, lameness	• Hemolysis pattern • Indole production test
B. ovis	Sheep	Epididymitis, orchitis, infertility, nephritis, abortion, vaginitis	• Oxidase test • Catalase test
B. suis	Pigs	Abortion, arthritis, infertility, orchitis, posterior paralysis	• Nitrate reduction test • Urease test
Burkholderia Species			
B. mallei	Horses	Glanders	• Gram-negative bacilli

B. pseudomallei	Dogs, carnivores	Pseudoglanders, fever, myalgia, dermal abscess, epididymitis	• Identification/differentiation
			  • Cellular morphology
			  • Colony characteristics
			  • Growth on MacConkey agar
			  • Motility
			  • Oxidase test
			  • Catalase test
			  • Nitrate reduction test
			  • Carbohydrate metabolism

Campylobacter Species			
C. fetus fetus	Cattle, sheep	Abortion	• Gram-negative slender, spiral, or curved bacilli
C. fetus venerealis	Cattle	Abortion, infertility	• Microaerophilic

C. jejuni jejuni	Dogs, cats, pigs, cows, sheep	Diarrhea in young animals, abortion	• Motile
			• Identification/differentiation
			  • Colony characteristics
			  • Hydrogen sulfide production
			  • Oxidase test
			  • Catalase test
			  • Nitrate reduction test
			  • Carbohydrate metabolism

Chlamydia Species			
C. muridarum	Mice, hamsters	Pneumonitis	• Gram-negative intracellular bodies
C. psittaci	Birds	See *Chlamydophila psittaci*	• Identification/differentiation

C. suis	Pigs	Conjunctivitis, pneumonia, pericarditis, enteritis, rhinitis, pneumonia	• Cytology impression smears
			  • Immunology (fluorescent antibody test, PCR)
			  • Cell culture

Organism	Primary Species Affected	Disease or Lesion	Characteristics
***Chlamydophila* Species**			
C. abortus	Ruminants, pigs	Abortion	• Gram-negative intracellular bodies
C. caviae	Guinea pigs	Conjunctivitis	• Identification/differentiation
C. felis	Cats	Conjunctivitis, rhinitis, pneumonitis	• Cytology impression smears
C. pecorum	Ruminants, pigs	Abortion, infertility, arthritis, conjunctivitis, cystitis, encephalitis, enteritis, pneumonia	• Immunology (fluorescent antibody test, PCR)
C. psittaci	Birds	Conjunctivitis, encephalitis, enteritis, pneumonia, hepatitis	• Cell culture
***Citrobacter* Species**			

C. rodentium	Mice, gerbils, guinea pigs	Transmissible murine colonic hyperplasia	• Identification/differentiation
			  • Colony characteristics
			  • Hydrogen sulfide production
			  • Motility
			  • Acid production in carbohydrate substrates

***Clostridium* Species**			
C. botulinum	Ruminants, horses, swine, carnivores	Botulism	• Gram-positive, spore-forming bacilli
C. chauvoei	Cattle, sheep	Blackleg	• Oxygen tolerant or anaerobic
C. colinum	Chickens, quail, turkeys	Quail disease	• Produce toxins • Identification/differentiation
C. difficile	Horses, dogs, rodents, pigs	Diarrhea, colitis	• Colony characteristics • Hemolysis pattern
C. novyi	Sheep, goats	Infectious hepatitis, myonecrosis	• Immunology (ELISA)
C. perfringens	Warm-blooded animals	Myonecrosis, gas gangrene	• Histology • Cytology
C. piliforme	Mammals	Tyzzer's disease	
C. septicum	Sheep, cattle	Myonecrosis, malignant edema, gangrenous dermatitis, enteritis, braxy	
C. sordellii	Sheep, cattle	Myonecrosis, enteritis	
C. spiroforme	Rabbits, rodents	Enterotoxemia	
C. tetani	Horses, cattle, pigs, carnivores	Tetanus	
***Corynebacterium* Species**			
C. auriscanis	Dogs	Otitis, dermatitis, vaginitis	• Gram-positive, non–spore-forming pleomorphic bacilli
C. cystitidis	Cattle	Bladder and kidney infection	• Aerobic or facultative anaerobes
C. diphtheriae	Cattle, horses	Mastitis, dermatitis, wound infection (equine)	• Most are nonmotile • Non–acid-fast
C. equi	Horses, pigs	See *Rhodococcus equi*	• Identification/differentiation
C. kutscheri	Rats, mice	Abscesses of lung, liver, lymph node, kidney	• Colony characteristics • Catalase test
C. pilosum	Cattle	Bladder and kidney infection	• Hemolysis pattern
C. pseudotuberculosis	Cattle, sheep, goats	Abscesses, lymphadenitis, abortion, arthritis	• Nitrate reduction test • Esculin hydrolysis test
C. renale	Cattle, sheep, pigs	Bladder and kidney infection	• Acid production in carbohydrate substrates
C. ulcerans	Cattle, rodents	Mastitis, abscesses, gangrenous dermatitis (rodents)	• Urease test

Organism	Primary Species Affected	Disease or Lesion	Characteristics
Dermatophilus Species			

D. congolensis	Cattle, horses, goats, sheep, pigs, dogs, cats	Exudative dermatis, alopecia	• Gram-positive, filamentous bacilli
			• Aerobic
			• Motile zoospores
			• Non—acid-fast
			• Identification/differentiation
			  • Cellular morphology
			  • Colony characteristics
			  • Catalase test
			  • Hemolysis pattern
			  • Acid production from glucose
			  • Nitrate reduction test

Dichelobacter Species			

D. nodosus	Sheep, cattle, pigs, goats	Foot rot	• Gram-negative, pleomorphic, slightly curved bacilli
			• Anaerobic
			• Identification/differentiation
			  • Cellular morphology
			  • Colony characteristics
			  • Esculin hydrolysis test
			  • Acid production in carbohydrate substrates
			  • Indole production test

Ehrlichia Species			

E. bovis	Cattle	See *Anaplasma bovis*	• Gram-negative, coccoid to ellipsoid forms
			• Located within cytoplasmic vacuoles of endothelium, myeloid cells, granulocytes, or thrombocytes
			• Identification/differentiation
			  • Demonstration of organisms on blood film
			  • Immunology

E. canis	Dogs, other canids	Monocytic ehrlichiosis	
E. chaffeensis	Dogs	Monocytic ehrlichiosis	
E. ewingii	Dogs	Granulocytic ehrlichiosis	
E. muris	Mice	Ehrlichiosis	
E. platys	Dogs	See *Anaplasma platys*	
E. ruminantium	Ruminants	Heartwater	
Enterobacter Species			

E. aerogenes	Most mammals	Mastitis, neonatal septicemia, metritis, urinary tract infection, wound infection	• Gram-negative, motile bacilli
			• Identification/differentiation
			  • Colony characteristics
			  • Cellular morphology
			  • Citrate utilization test
			  • Hydrogen sulfide production
			  • Acid and gas production from lactose

E. cloacae	Birds		
Eperythrozoon Species			
See *Mycoplasma*			
Erysipelothrix Species			

E. rhusiopathiae	Cattle, pigs, sheep, turkeys	Diamond skin disease, arthritis, endocarditis	• Gram-positive, non—spore-forming bacilli
			• Facultative anaerobes
			• Nonmotile
			• Identification/differentiation
			  • Cellular morphology
			  • Colony characteristics
			  • Hemolysis pattern
			  • Catalase test
			  • Esculin hydrolysis test
			  • Acid production from carbohydrates
			  • Hydrogen sulfide production
			  • CAMP test
			  • Immunology (agglutination)

Organism	Primary Species Affected	Disease or Lesion	Characteristics
Escherichia Species			

E. coli (numerous pathotypes)	Most vertebrates	Enteritis, septicemia, ruminant mastitis, canine pyometra, cystitis, calf scours	• Gram-negative bacilli
			• Most are motile
			• Identification/differentiation
			  • Cellular morphology
			  • Colony characteristics
			  • Hemolysis pattern
			  • Growth on MacConkey agar
			  • Catalase test
			  • Oxidase test
			  • Acid and gas production from glucose
			  • Hydrogen sulfide production
			  • Immunology (agglutination, ELISA, PCR)
			  • Histology

Francisella Species			

F. tularensis	Rabbits, most other mammals	Pneumonia, fever, lymphadenitis, ulcerative dermatitis	• Gram-negative coccobacilli
			• Identification/differentiation
			  • Cellular morphology with fluorescent antibody stain
			  • Immunology (agglutination, ELISA, antibody titer)
			  • Histology

Fusobacterium Species			

F. equinum	Horses	Lower respiratory tract disease	• Gram-negative, non–spore-forming fusiform bacilli
			• Identification/differentiation
			  • Cellular morphology
			  • Colony characteristics
			  • Hemolysis pattern
			  • Catalase test
			  • Nitrate reduction test
			  • Esculin hydrolysis test
			  • Fermentation of glucose
			  • Indole production test

F. necrophorum	Cattle, sheep, horses, pigs, rabbits	Foot rot, mastitis, liver abscess, metritis, calf diphtheria, thrush (equine), abortion, ulcerative stomatitis, "bull nose"	
F. nucleatum	Cattle, sheep	Abortion	
Haemobartonella Species			
H. canis	Dogs	See *Mycoplasma haemocanis*	
H. felis	Cats	See *Mycoplasma haemofelis*	
Haemophilus Species			

H. felis	Cats	Rhinitis, conjunctivitis	• Gram-negative, pleomorphic bacilli or coccobacilli
			• May form filaments
			• Nonmotile
			• Facultative anaerobes
			• Growth on chocolate agar
			• Identification/differentiation
			  • Catalase test
			  • Indole production test
			  • CAMP test
			  • Acid production in carbohydrate substrates
			  • Urease test
			  • Immunology (immunohistochemistry, PCR)

H. haemoglobinophilus	Dogs	Vaginitis, cystitis	
H. influenzaemurium	Rodents	Respiratory disease, ocular disease	
H. paragallinarum	Chickens	Infectious coryza	
H. parasuis	Pigs	Glasser's disease, meningitis, myositis, pneumonia, septicemia	

Organism	Primary Species Affected	Disease or Lesion	Characteristics
Helicobacter Species			
H. bilis	Mice	Hepatitis	• Gram-negative helical, curved, or unbranched bacilli
H. canis	Dogs	Gastroenteritis	• Motile
H. cholecystus	Hamsters	Cholecystitis, pancreatitis	• Microaerophilic
H. felis	Cats, dogs	Gastritis	• Identification/differentiation
H. hepaticus	Mice, rats	Hepatitis	• Colony characteristics
H. muridarum	Mice, rats	Gastritis	• Catalase test
H. mustelae	Ferrets	Gastritis	• Oxidase test
H. nemestrinae	Macaques	Gastritis	• Urease test
H. pullorum	Poultry	Gastroenteritis, hepatitis	
H. pylori	Monkeys, cats	Gastritis	
H. rappini	Mice, rats, dogs, sheep	Abortion	
Histophilus Species			

H. somni	Cattle	Bronchopneumonia, "honker syndrome," myocarditis, otitis, conjunctivitis, myelitis, vaginitis, orchitis, thromboembolic meningoencephalitis	• Gram-negative, nonmotile, pleomorphic bacilli
			• Capnophilic
			• Identification/differentiation
			  • Colony characteristics
			  • Hemolysis pattern
			  • Catalase test
			  • Oxidase test
			  • Nitrate reduction test
			  • Immunology

Klebsiella Species			
K. pneumoniae pneumoniae	Cattle, horses, sheep, dogs, birds	Metritis, mastitis, neonatal septicemia	• Gram-negative, nonmotile, encapsulated bacilli • Identification/differentiation
K. oxytoca	Horses	Vaginitis, metritis, abortion, infertility	• Colony characteristics • Cellular morphology • Citrate utilization test • Hydrogen sulfide production • Acid and gas production from lactose • Urease test • Indole production test
Lawsonia Species			

L. intracellularis	Pigs, hamsters, cats, dogs, horses, ferrets	Proliferative enteritis, "wet tail," ileitis	• Gram-negative, curved intracellular body
			• Motile
			• Identification/differentiation
			  • Cellular morphology with silver staining
			  • Immunology (ELISA, immunofluorescence)

Leptospira Species			
L. bratislava	Horses, pigs	Abortion	• Spiral bacteria
L. canicola	Cattle, pigs, dogs	Uremia, abortion	• Aerobic
L. grippotyphosa	Cattle, pigs, horses	Fever, jaundice, uremia	• Motile
L. hardjo	Cattle	Abortion, infertility	• Identification/differentiation
L. icterohaemorr-hagiae	Dogs, cattle, rats	Septicemia, abortion	• Cellular morphology with dark field microscopy
L. kennewicki	Horses	Abortion	• Immunology (agglutination, PCR, fluorescent antibody stain)
L. pomona	Pigs, cattle, horses	Abortion	

Organism	Primary Species Affected	Disease or Lesion	Characteristics
Listeria Species			
L. monocytogenes	Cattle, sheep, goats, horses, birds, dogs, rodents, pigs	Central nervous system infection, abortion, mastitis, septicemia	• Gram-positive, non–spore-forming bacilli • Facultative anaerobes • Motile • Identification/differentiation • Cellular morphology • Colony characteristics • Hemolysis pattern • Catalase test • Esculin hydrolysis test • Acid production from carbohydrates • Hydrogen sulfide production • CAMP test
Mannheimia Species			
M. haemolytica	Cattle, sheep	Pneumonia, septicemia, mastitis	• Gram-negative bacilli and coccobacilli • Nonmotile • Facultative anaerobes • Identification/differentiation • Colony characteristics • Hemolysis pattern • Oxidase test • Acid production from glucose • Nitrate reduction test
M. granulomatis	Cattle	Panniculitis	
M. varigena	Cattle	Pneumonia, septicemia, mastitis	
Moraxella Species			
M. bovis	Cattle	Infectious keratoconjunctivitis	• Gram-negative coccobacilli • Nonmotile • Identification/differentiation • Colony characteristics • Growth on MacConkey agar • Hemolysis pattern • Oxidase test • Catalase test • Nitrate reduction test • Immunology (fluorescent antibody stain, ELISA)
M. canis	Dogs	Bite-wound infections	
M. ovis	Small ruminants	Pinkeye	
Morganella Species			
M. morganii	Dogs	Otitis externa, cystitis	• Gram-negative bacilli • Identification/differentiation • Colony characteristics • Oxidase test • Indole production test
Mycobacterium Species			
M. avium avium	Birds	Tuberculosis	• Gram-positive, non–spore-forming bacilli • Nonmotile • Aerobic • Acid fast • Identification/differentiation • Colony characteristics • Cellular morphology • Intradermal skin test • Carbohydrate utilization test
M. avium paratuberculosis	Ruminants	Johne's disease	
M. bovis	Ruminants, dogs, cats, pigs, goats, nonhuman primates	Tuberculosis	
M. fortuitum	Cattle, cats, dogs, pigs	Mastitis; joint, lung, and skin disease	
M. intracellularae	Pigs, cattle, nonhuman primates	Tuberculosis, granulomatous enteritis	
M. lepraemurium	Cats, rats	Leprosy	
M. porcinum	Pigs	Lymphadenitis	
M. smegmatis	Cattle, cats	Mastitis, ulcerative skin disease	
M. vaccae	Cattle	Skin disease	
M. xenopi	Cats, pigs	Nodular skin lesions, lymphadenitis	

Organism	Primary Species Affected	Disease or Lesion	Characteristics
Mycoplasma Species			
Nonhemotropic Mycoplasmas			
M. agalactiae	Goats, sheep	Contagious agalactia	• Identification/differentiation
M. alkalescens	Cattle	Arthritis, mastitis	• Colony characteristics
M. bovigenitalium	Cattle	Infertility, mastitis	• Colony stain with Diene stain
M. bovis	Cattle	Arthritis, mastitis, pneumonia, abortion, abscesses, otitis media, genital infections	• Urease test • Immunology (immunodiffusion, immunofluorescent assay, agglutination, ELISA)
M. bovoculi	Cattle	Conjunctivitis	
M. californicum	Cattle	Mastitis	
M. canadense	Cattle	Abortion, mastitis	
M. capricolum	Goats	Abortion, mastitis, septicemia, polyarthritis, pneumonia	
M. conjunctivae	Sheep	Infectious keratoconjunctivitis	
M. cynos	Dogs	Pneumonia	
M. dispar	Cattle	Respiratory disease	
M. felis	Cats, horses	Conjunctivitis, pneumonia	
M. gallisepticum	Chickens, turkeys	Airsacculitis, sinusitis	
M. gatae	Cats	Arthritis	
M. hyopneumoniae	Pigs	Pneumonia	
M. hyorhinis	Pigs	Polyarthritis	
M. meleagridis	Turkeys	Airsacculitis, skeletal abnormalities	
M. mycoides capri	Goats	Arthritis, mastitis, pleuropneumonia, septicemia	
M. mycoides mycoides	Cattle, goats, sheep	Pleuropneumonia, mastitis, septicemia, polyarthritis, pneumonia	
M. ovipneumoniae	Goats, sheep	Pleuropneumonia	
M. pulmonis	Rats, mice	Murine respiratory mycoplasmosis	
M. synoviae	Chickens, turkeys	Infectious synovitis	
Hemotropic Mycoplasmas			
M. haemocanis	Dogs	Haemobartonellosis	• Coccoid organisms
M. haemofelis	Cats	Haemobartonellosis, feline infectious anemia	• Obligate intracellular parasites • Attach to red blood cell surface
M. haemomuris	Rats, mice	Haemobartonellosis	• Identification/differentiation
M. ovis	Sheep, goats	Eperythrozoonosis	• Cellular morphology
M. suis	Pigs	Eperythrozoonosis	• Immunology (PCR)
M. wenyonii	Cattle	Eperythrozoonosis	
Neisseria Species			
N. canis	Dogs	Bite-wound infections	• Gram-negative coccobacilli

N. weaveri	Dogs	Bite-wound infections	• Nonmotile
			• Identification/differentiation
			  • Colony characteristics
			  • Hemolysis pattern
			  • Oxidase test
			  • Catalase test
			  • Acid production from carbohydrates

Neorickettsia Species			
N. helminthoeca	Dogs, other canids	"Salmon poisoning"	• Gram-negative, coccoid to ellipsoid forms

N. risticii	Horses	Potomac horse fever, monocytic ehrlichiosis	• Located within cytoplasmic vacuoles of myeloid cells or enterocytes
			• Identification/differentiation
			  • Demonstration of organisms on blood film
			  • Immunology

Organism	Primary Species Affected	Disease or Lesion	Characteristics
Nocardia Species			
N. asteroides	Dogs, cats, cattle, horses, pigs	Lymphadenitis, subcutaneous abscess, stomatitis, mastitis, pleuritis, peritonitis, abortion	• Gram-positive, pleomorphic, non—spore-forming bacilli • Nonmotile • Aerobic
N. brasiliensis	Horses	Pneumonia, pleuritis	• Acid-fast

N. otitidiscaviarum	Cattle, guinea pigs	Ear infections, mastitis	• Identification/differentiation
			  • Colony characteristics
			  • Cellular morphology
			  • Nitrate reduction test
			  • Esculin hydrolysis test
			  • Urease test

Pasteurella Species			
P. caballi	Horses	Respiratory infection, metritis	• Gram-negative bacilli and coccobacilli
P. canis	Dogs	Puppy septicemia	• Nonmotile
P. gallinarum	Chickens, turkeys	Fowl cholera, salpingitis	• Aerobes
P. haemolytica	Cattle, sheep	See *Mannheimia haemolytica*	• Identification/differentiation
P. lymphangitidis	Cattle	Lymphangitis	• Colony characteristics
P. mairii	Pigs	Abortion, septicemia	• Hemolysis pattern
P. multocida	Ruminants, pigs, rodents, dogs, cats, cattle	Pneumonia, fowl cholera, rhinitis, mastitis, hemorrhagic septicemia, bite-wound infections	• Growth on chocolate agar and MacConkey agar • Catalase test • Urease test
P. pneumotropica	Rodents, rabbits	Pneumonia	• Indole production test
P. trehalosi	Sheep	Septicemia, pneumonia	• Oxidase test • Acid and gas production from carbohydrates • Nitrate reduction test
Porphyromonas Species			
P. levii	Cattle, most mammals	Bovine summer mastitis, pleuritis	• Non—spore-forming, pleomorphic bacilli

P. gingivalis	Numerous	Periodontitis, gingivitis	• Nonmotile
			• Obligate anaerobes
			• Identification/differentiation
			  • Colony characteristics
			  • Hemolysis pattern
			  • Acid production on carbohydrate substrates
			  • Indole production test

Prevotella Species			
P. melaninogenica	Cattle	Foot rot	• Non—spore-forming, pleomorphic bacilli

P. heparinolytica	Horses	Lower respiratory tract disease	• Nonmotile
			• Obligate anaerobes
			• Identification/differentiation
			  • Colony characteristics
			  • Hemolysis pattern
			  • Acid production on carbohydrate substrates
			  • Indole production test

Proteus Species			
P. mirabilis	Dogs, horses, calves	Cystitis, pyelonephritis, prostatitis, otitis externa	• Gram-negative bacilli

P. vulgaris			• Motile
			• Identification/differentiation
			  • Colony characteristics
			  • Oxidase test
			  • Hydrogen sulfide production
			  • Indole production test

Organism	Primary Species Affected	Disease or Lesion	Characteristics
Pseudomonas Species			
P. aeruginosa	Cattle, dogs, horses, sheep	Mastitis, otitis externa, metritis, corneal ulcer, fleece rot	• Gram-negative, non–spore-forming bacilli
P. fluorescens	Cattle	Mastitis	• Aerobic

P. mallei		See *Burkholderia mallei*	• Identification/differentiation
			  • Colony characteristics
			  • Oxidase test
			  • Growth on MacConkey agar

Rhodococcus Species			

R. equi	Horses, pigs	Bronchopneumonia, cervical lymphadenitis	• Gram-positive, pleomorphic coccobacillus
			• Aerobic
			• Partially acid-fast
			• Identification/differentiation
			  • Colony characteristics
			  • Catalase test
			  • Hemolysis pattern
			  • CAMP test
			  • Immunology (immunodiffusion, ELISA)

Rickettsia Species			
R. felis	Cats	Flea typhus	• Intracellular coccobacilli
R. rickettsii	Dogs	Rocky Mountain spotted fever	• Located in endothelial cells and smooth muscle cells
R. typhi	Rats	Murine typhus	• Identification/differentiation • Immunology (fluorescent antibody tests, PCR)
Salmonella Species			
S. ser. abortusovis	Sheep	Abortion	• Gram-negative, non–spore-forming bacilli
S. ser. anatum	Sheep, goats, horses	Peracute septicemia; acute, subacute, or chronic enteritis	• Most are motile
S. ser. choleraesuis	Pigs		• Nearly 2500 serovars
S. ser. dublin	Cattle, sheep, goats		• Organisms are referred to by the genus name and serovar
S. ser. enteritidis	Horses		• Identification/differentiation
S. ser. newport	Cattle		• Colony characteristics
S. ser. pullorum	Poultry		• Growth on MacConkey agar

S. ser. typhimurium	Cattle, sheep, goats, horses, pigs		• Growth on Simmons citrate
			  • Urease test
			  • Indole production test
			  • Hydrogen sulfide production

Staphylococcus Species			
S. aureus	Mammals	Wound infections, mastitis, skin infections, vaginitis	• Gram-positive cocci
S. epidermidis	Cattle, other mammals	Mastitis, skin abscess	• Aerobic • Identification/differentiation • Colony characteristics
S. felis	Cats	Otitis externa, cystitis, abscesses, wound infections	• Hemolysis pattern • Catalase test
S. intermedius	Dogs, cattle	Skin and ear infections, mastitis	• Coagulase test • Fermentation of sugars

Organism	Primary Species Affected	Disease or Lesion	Characteristics
Streptococcus Species			
S. agalactiae	Cattle, horses	Mastitis	• Gram-positive, non–spore-forming cocci
S. canis	Dogs, cats	Genital, skin, and wound infections; metritis, mastitis, kitten septicemia	• Facultative anaerobes
S. dysgalactiae dysgalactiae	Cattle, dogs	Mastitis, dermatitis, abortion, septicemia	• Identification/differentiation • Colony characteristics
S. equi equi	Horses	Strangles, genital infection, mastitis	• Hemolysis pattern
S. zooepidemicus equi	Rats, cattle, goats, sheep, chickens	Mastitis, lymphadenitis, wound infections, pneumonia, septicemia	• Catalase test • Esculin hydrolysis test
S. porcinus	Pigs	Abscesses, lymphadenitis	• CAMP test
S. suis	Pigs	Encephalitis, meningitis, arthritis, septicemia, abortion, endocarditis	• Fermentation of sugars
Taylorella Species			

T. equigenitalis	Horses	Contagious equine metritis	• Gram-negative coccobacilli
			• Identification/differentiation
			  • Colony characteristics
			  • Growth on chocolate agar
			  • Indole production test
			  • Oxidase test
			  • Catalase test
			  • Esculin hydrolysis test
			  • Immunology (PCR)

Treponema Species			
T. brennaborense	Cattle, horses	Digital dermatitis, "hairy foot warts"	• Tight spiral bacteria
T. paraluiscuniculi	Rabbits	Rabbit syphilis	• Motile • Identification/differentiation • Cellular morphology with silver staining
Ureaplasma Species			

U. diversum	Cattle	Abortion, vulvitis, pneumonia	• Small mycoplasmas
			• Identification/differentiation
			  • Colony characteristics
			  • Urea hydrolysis
			  • Immunology (PCR, immunofluorescence assay)

Yersinia Species			
Y. enterocolitica	Rabbits, dogs, pigs, horses	Ileitis, gastroenteritis	• Gram-negative bacilli

Y. pestis	Dogs, cats, goats	Plague	• Facultative anaerobes
			• Identification/differentiation
			  • Cellular morphology
			  • Colony characteristics
			  • Oxidase test
			  • Catalase test
			  • Fermentation of sugars

Y. pseudotuberculosis	Rodents, guinea pigs, cats, cattle, goats	Pseudotuberculosis, abortion, epididymitis, orchitis	

Abdominocentesis Paracentesis of the abdomen.

Absolute value The number of each type of leukocyte in peripheral blood; this is calculated by multiplying the relative percentage from the differential count by the total white blood cell count.

Acanthocyte An erythrocyte with spiny projections of varying lengths distributed irregularly over its surface.

Acariasis Infestation with mites.

Accuracy The closeness with which test results agree with the true quantitative value of the constituent.

Acid–base balance A state of equilibrium between the acidity and alkalinity of the body fluids; also called the hydrogen ion (H^+) balance.

Acid-fast stain A staining procedure for demonstrating the presence of microorganisms that are not readily decolorized by acid after staining; this is a characteristic of certain bacteria, particularly *Mycobacterium* and *Nocardia*.

Acidosis A pathologic decrease in the pH of blood or body tissues as a result of the accumulation of acids or a decrease in bicarbonate.

Acinar Pertaining to or affecting an acinus or acini. This term refers specifically to glandular tissue with a structure that is often described as grapelike clusters.

ACTH stimulation test A test designed to test the response of the hormone that stimulates adrenocortical growth and secretion.

Activated clotting time A test of the intrinsic and common pathways of blood coagulation that involves the use of a diatomaceous earth or kaolin tube to initiate clotting.

Activated partial thromboplastin time A test of intrinsic and common coagulation pathways. An intrinsic pathway activator is added to plasma, and the time taken for clot formation is measured.

Active immunity An animal's production of antibody as a result of infection with an antigen or immunization.

Acute-phase proteins Proteins, including serum amyloid A and C-reactive protein, that are produced by hepatocytes immediately following injury or inflammation.

Addison's disease See *Hypoadrenocorticism*.

Adrenocorticotropic hormone A hormone secreted by the anterior pituitary gland that has a stimulating effect on the adrenal cortex. Also referred to as corticotropin and abbreviated as ACTH.

Agar A seaweed extract that is used to solidify culture media.

Agranulocytes The white blood cell group that has no visible cytoplasmic granules.

Alanine transaminase Cytoplasmic enzyme of hepatocytes released when hepatocytes are damaged.

Albumin A group of plasma proteins that comprises the majority of protein in plasma.

Alkaline phosphatase A group of enzymes that functions at an alkaline pH and that catalyzes the reactions of organic phosphates.

Alkalosis A condition in which the blood pH is higher than 7.45.

Allantoin A crystalline substance produced by the oxidation of uric acid by uricase and present in the urine of most mammals, except primates and Dalmatian dogs (which lack uricase).

Allergen An allergen is a substance that can cause an allergic reaction.

Alloantibodies A naturally occurring antibody that is produced by an individual and that reacts with antigens of another individual of the same species.

Alpha-hemolysis Characterized by the partial destruction of blood cells on blood agar, which is evident as a greenish zone around the bacterial colony.

Amastigote A protist cell that does not have visible external flagella or cili.

Ammonium biurate Brownish crystals seen in the urine of animals with severe liver disease.

Amylase An enzyme derived primarily from the pancreas that functions in the breakdown of starch.

Amyloclastic A method of measuring serum amylase by evaluating the disappearance of starch substrate.

Anaphylactic shock A severe, life-threatening allergic reaction.

Anemia A problem of not having enough healthy red blood cells or hemoglobin to carry oxygen to the body's tissues.

Angiodema Angioedema is swelling that is similar to hives, but the swelling is under the skin instead of on the surface.

Anion A negatively charged ion.

Anion gap A method that is used to evaluate a patient's acid–base status; the calculation is based on subtracting the sum of measured major serum anions ($Cl^- + HCO_3^-$) from the sum of measured major serum cations ($Na^+ + K^+$).

Anisocytosis Describes red blood cells that are of different sizes.

Anisokaryosis Variation in the size of the nuclei of cells in a sample.

Anisonucleoliosis Variation in the size of nucleoli.

Antibody titer The level of a specific antibody that is present in serum. This is calculated as the reciprocal of the highest dilution at which a sample no longer exhibits a positive reaction for the presence of the antibody. It is often used to help differentiate active infection from prior exposure to an antigen.

Anticoagulant Any substance that inhibits or prevents clotting.

Antigen Any substances that are capable of generating a response from the immune system.

Antimicrobial disks Paper disks impregnated with antibiotic agents and used during the performance of the antimicrobial sensitivity test.

Antimicrobial susceptibility test An in vitro test of the effectiveness of selected antimicrobial agents against microorganisms.

Anulocyte Ring-shaped monoconcave erythrocytes with a white center and a thin dark staining ring containing hemoglobin.

Anuria Absence of urine.

Aplastic anemia A rare but serious blood condition that occurs when your bone marrow cannot make enough new blood cells for your body to work normally.

Apoptosis The death of single cells by a process involving shrinkage, rapid fragmentation, and the engulfment of the fragments by neighboring cells and macrophages.

Arachnid A member of the class Arachnida, which includes mites and ticks.

Arthrocentesis The removal of fluid from a joint.

Ascarid Any of the nematodes of the superfamily Ascaridoidea, which includes the genera *Ascaris*, *Parascaris*, *Toxocara*, and *Toxascaris*.

Ascospores The sexual spore of *Ascomycetes*.

Aspartate transaminase An enzyme that is present in body serum and in certain body tissues that catalyzes the transfer of an amino group from aspartic acid to alpha-ketoglutaric acid, thereby forming glutamic acid and oxaloacetic acid. Also referred to as aspartate aminotransferase.

Aspiration The removal of fluids or gases from a cavity with the aid of suction.

Aspiration biopsy The removal of cells and tissue fluid from a lesion with the use of suction from a needle and syringe.

Atypical lymphocyte A general term used to describe a lymphocyte with morphologic abnormalities, including azurophilic granules, increased cytoplasmic basophilia, overly abundant cytoplasm, or a larger and more convoluted nucleus than seen in normal lymphocytes.

Autoagglutination The clumping or agglutination of an individual's cells by that individual's own serum, usually because of the presence of autoantibodies.

Avidity Refers to the strength of the binding of antigen and antibody.

Azotemia The increased retention of urea in the blood.

Bacilli Rod-shaped bacteria.

Baermann technique A parasitology test that is used to recover larvae.

Base excess The amount of acid or base required to titrate a sample of whole arterial blood to the normal pH of 7.4.

Basidiospores The sexual spore of basidiomycetes.

Basophil   A granular leukocyte with an irregularly shaped, relatively pale-staining nucleus that is partially constricted into two lobes and with cytoplasm that contains coarse bluish-black granules of variable size.

Basophilic stippling   Erythrocytes that are characterized by small, blue-staining granules; this represents the presence of residual RNA.

Beer's law   A principle that describes the relationship between light absorbance, transmission, and the concentration of a substance in solution.

Bence Jones protein   A light chain protein of immunoglobulin molecules that readily passes through the glomerulus and into the urine.

Benign   A term used to describe a tumor or growth that is not malignant; this word can refer to any condition that is not life threatening.

Beta-hemolysis   The complete destruction of red blood cells on blood agar that creates a clear zone around the bacterial colony.

Beta-lactamase   Enzyme produced by bacteria that are resistant to beta-lactam antibiotics.

Bicarbonate (HCO₃)   An electrolyte in plasma; part of the bicarbonate–carbonic acid buffer system that maintains the blood pH in equilibrium.

Bile acids   A group of compounds that are synthesized by hepatocytes from cholesterol that help with fat absorption.

Bilirubin   An insoluble pigment derived from the breakdown of hemoglobin, which is processed by hepatocytes.

Bilirubinuria   An abnormal increase in the concentration of bilirubin in the urine.

Binocular   Having two eyepieces (e.g., a type of microscope).

Biohazard   Biological substances that contain infectious agents that pose a threat to human health.

Bladder expression   The manual compression of the urinary bladder to cause the release of urine through the urethra.

Blood agar   An enriched medium that supports the growth of most bacterial pathogens; usually composed of sheep's blood.

Blood group antigens   The antigens that are present on the surface of erythrocytes and antibodies that may be present in serum.

Blood urea nitrogen   The principal end product of amino acid breakdown in mammals.

Bloodborne pathogens   Infectious agents that are present in the bloodstream.

Bothria   Two longitudinal grooves or sucker-like expansions on the scolex of members of the cestode orders Bothriocephalidea, Diphyllidea, Diphyllobothriidea, and Trypanorhyncha.

Buccal mucosa bleeding time   A test that uses a standardized shallow incision into the buccal mucosa of the upper lip to evaluate primary hemostasis.

Buffer   A substance that increases the amount of acid or alkali necessary to produce a unit change in pH.

Buffy coat   The layer of material above the packed erythrocytes after centrifugation; it consists primarily of leukocytes and thrombocytes.

Bradyzoites   A slowly multiplying cell form in the life cycle of certain Apicomplexans.

Calcium   The most abundant mineral in the body. Calcium is an important cation in intracellular and extracellular fluid. It is essential to the normal clotting of blood, the maintenance of a normal heartbeat, and the initiation of neuromuscular and metabolic activities.

Calcium carbonate   A type of crystal that is commonly seen in the urine of rabbits and horses.

Calcium oxalate   A crystal that is found in acidic and neutral urine; commonly seen in small amounts in dogs and horses.

California Mastitis Test   An indirect test for bovine mastitis that is based on the presence of a high leukocyte count in mastitic milk.

Candle jar   A method of producing anaerobic conditions for the growth of anaerobic bacteria.

Capnophilic   An organism that requires high levels of carbon dioxide for growth or for the enhancement of growth.

Capsule stain   A differential stain that is used to identify the cell capsules of pathogenic bacteria.

Carcinoma   A term that describes tumors of epithelial cell origin.

Casts   Structures that are formed from the protein precipitates of degenerating kidney tubule cells; may contain embedded materials.

Catalase   An enzyme that catalyzes the breakdown of hydrogen peroxide into oxygen and water.

Catheterization   The placement of a catheter in the urethra or the placement of an indwelling catheter in a blood vessel.

Cation   A positively charged ion.

Cell-mediated immunity   An immune system mechanism that involves actions of the cells of the immune system rather than antibodies.

Cellophane tape preparation   A test using cellophane tape to collect ectoparasites.

Cellular cast   A formed element in urine that consists of a hyaline cast that contains blood cells or epithelial cells.

Centesis   The act of puncturing a body cavity or organ with a hollow needle to draw out fluid.

Centrifugal flotation   A method of processing fecal samples for the detection of parasite ova and cysts. It recovers more eggs and cysts in a sample and takes less time than standard flotation.

Centrifuge   A piece of equipment that spins samples at high speed.

Cercaria   The life-cycle stage of trematodes that develops in the intermediate host.

Cestode   An organism in the order Cestoda; a type of tapeworm.

Chemical hygiene plan   A document that contains details about the specific chemical hazards present in the workplace.

Chemiluminescence   Describes a chemical reaction that results in the emission of light.

Chloride   The principal anion in extracellular fluid and gastric juice.

Cholesterol   A plasma lipoprotein that is produced primarily in the liver as well as ingested in food; used in the synthesis of bile acids.

Chronic granulomatous inflammation   Special type of chronic inflammation characterized by often focal collections of macrophages, epithelioid cells, and multinucleated giant cells.

Chronic inflammation   Slow, long-term inflammation lasting for prolonged periods of several months to years.

Chronic pyogranulomatous inflammation   A chronic inflammatory response of both macrophages and neutrophils that can result from a variety of causes.

Cilia   A short microscopic hairlike vibrating structure found in large numbers on the surface of certain cells, either causing currents in the surrounding fluid, or, in some protozoans and other small organisms, providing propulsion.

Citrate   Any salt of citric acid; citrate salts are used as temporary anticoagulants for studies of blood coagulation.

Clot retraction   A crude but simple test that allows for the evaluation of platelet number and function and intrinsic and extrinsic pathways.

Coagulase   A molecule produced by some bacteria that allows for the adhesion of fibrinogen to the cell surface.

Cocci   Bacteria with a round shape.

Coccidiosis   A disease of birds and mammals that chiefly affects the intestines, caused by coccidia.

Codocyte   An erythrocyte that is characterized by an increased membrane surface area relative to the cell's volume.

Competitive ELISA   An immunoassay. Patient antigen, if present, competes with enzyme-labeled antigens for the antibodies that are coating the test wells.

Complement system   A group of plasma proteins that function to enhance the activities of the immune system.

Complete blood count   A blood test. It's used to look at overall health and find a wide range of conditions.

Compound light microscope   A microscope that generates an image by using a combination of lenses.

Compression smear   This technique is most commonly used to spread FNA samples expelled onto glass slides and can be used for semi-solid, mucus-like, or pelleted material.

Condenser   The part of the microscope that consists of two lenses that focus light from the light source on the object being viewed. Light is focused by raising or lowering the condenser.

Conidia   An asexual fungal spore that is deciduous (shed at maturity) and formed by budding or splitting off from the summit of a conidiophore. Also called a conidiospore.

Conjugated bilirubin   Bilirubin that has been taken up by the liver cells and conjugated to form the water-soluble compound bilirubin diglucuronide.

Control   A biological solution of known values that is used for the verification of the accuracy and precision of test results.

Coombs test   An immunologic test designed to detect antibodies on the surface of erythrocytes (direct Coombs test) or antibodies against erythrocytes in plasma (indirect Coombs test).

Coracidium   The individual free-swimming or free-crawling, spherical, ciliated embryo of tapeworms of the order Pseudophyllidea.

Core biopsy   The removal of a tissue sample with a wide needle for examination under a microscope.

Cornified   Keratinized; used to describe vaginal epithelial cells as seen in a vaginal cytology smear from a patient in estrus.

Cortisol   A steroid hormone produced by the adrenal glands.

Coverslip smear   A method of preparing a blood film with the use of two coverslips.

Creatine kinase   An enzyme that is found predominantly in cells of the heart, brain, and skeletal muscle; released when cells are damaged.

Creatinine   A waste product that is formed during normal muscle cell metabolism.

Crossmatching   A blood test designed to identify compatibility between donor and recipient samples before transfusion.

Crystalluria   The presence of crystals in the urine

Culture medium   A substrate for the growth of microbiology samples.

Culturette   The trade name for a sterile swab in transport media that is used for collection of microbiology samples.

Curschmann's spirals   The coiled mucinous fibrils that are sometimes found in cytology preparations of bronchial samples.

Cushing's disease   See *Hyperadrenocorticism*.

Cuticle   The outer layer or covering of epithelium.

Cystine   An amino acid that may be present in the form of hexagonal crystals in the urine.

Cystocentesis   The aspiration of fluid from the urinary bladder.

D-Dimer   A protein fragment that is formed from the breakdown of fibrin.

Dacryocyte   An abnormal erythrocyte that is shaped like a teardrop.

Dark-field microscope   A type of microscope that is used primarily in reference laboratories, especially for the viewing of unstained specimens.

Definitive host   The host that harbors the adult, mature, or sexual stages of a parasite.

Dermatophyte test medium   A differential culture medium designed to support the growth of cutaneous fungal organisms and to inhibit bacterial growth.

Dexamethasone suppression test   An endocrine system test designed to detect hyperadrenocorticism.

Differential media   A bacterial culture method that allows bacteria to be differentiated into groups on the basis of their biochemical reactions on the medium.

Dilution   The process of making a solution weaker or less concentrated.

Direct life cycle   The life cycle of an organism that does not require an intermediate host.

Direct sensitivity testing   An antimicrobial sensitivity test that involves the application of undiluted samples (e.g., urine) directly to the Mueller-Hinton plate.

Direct smear   A test that can be utilized using a small amount of specimen.

Discrete round cell tumors   A neoplasia that is characterized by cells with discrete round shapes. Examples of round cell neoplasms include mast cell tumors, histiocytomas, lymphomas, plasmacytomas, and transmissible venereal tumors.

Disseminated intravascular coagulation   An acquired secondary coagulation disorder that is characterized by the depletion of thrombocytes and coagulation factors. Also referred to as consumption coagulopathy and defibrination syndrome.

Dog erythrocyte antigen (DEA)   A naming convention for canine blood types.

Döhle bodies   Small, gray-blue areas that represent ribosomes and that are seen in the cytoplasm of some immature and toxic granulocytes.

Drepanocyte   A morphologic abnormality of erythrocytes that is characterized by sickle-shaped cells.

Echinocyte   An erythrocyte with multiple small projections that are evenly spaced over the cell circumference.

Ectoparasite   A parasite that resides on the surface of its host.

Effective renal plasma flow   The effective rate of blood flow through the kidneys; the determining factor relative to the rate of glomerular filtration.

Electrolyte   Any substance that dissociates into ions when in solution.

End-point assay   A chemical reaction that proceeds to a stable end point.

Endocrine   A term that refers to the system of glands and other structures that secrete hormones directly into the circulatory system.

Endoparasite   A parasite that resides within a host's tissues.

Endospore   The dormant form of a bacterium; intracellular refractile bodies that are resistant to heat, desiccation, chemicals, and radiation; formed by some bacteria when environmental conditions are poor.

Endospore stain   A differential stain that has been designed to identify the presence, location, and shape of spores in bacterial samples.

Engineering controls   Safety procedures focused on changing the work environment to eliminate or minimize exposure to a hazard.

Enriched media   A type of culture media that has been formulated to meet the requirements of the most fastidious pathogens.

Enterotubes   A commercially available modular system of culture media that contains media and reagents for numerous bacteriologic tests that can be performed simultaneously.

Enzyme-linked immunosorbent assay (ELISA)   An enzyme immunoassay that makes use of an enzyme-labeled immunoreactant (antigen or antibody) and an immunosorbent (antigen or antibody bound to a solid support).

Enzymuria   The presence of specific enzymes in urine.

Eosin   A type of pink to red acid dye that is a component of differential stains; primarily used for the routine staining of blood films.

Eosinophil   A granulocyte with granules that have an affinity for the acidic components of stains.

Eosinophilic   A term that refers to an increase in circulating eosinophils or a reddish appearance of cells or components of cells that have a high affinity for stains with acid pH.

Epithelial cell tumors   A type of neoplasm associated with a clustered arrangement of cells into ball shapes or monolayer sheets. Examples include lung adenocarcinoma, perianal adenoma, basal cell tumor, sebaceous adenoma, transitional cell carcinoma, and mesothelioma.

Erythrocyte indices   Calculated values that provide the average volume and hemoglobin concentrations of erythrocytes in a peripheral blood sample.

Erythrocyte sedimentation rate   A test measures how quickly red blood cells settle to the bottom of a test tube.

Erythropoiesis   The production of erythrocytes.

Erythropoietin   The hormone that stimulates erythropoietic activity in the bone marrow.

Ethylene glycol   A solvent with a sweet, acrid taste that is found in many products, such as antifreeze, drying agents, and inks. Ingestion or excessive skin exposure can be toxic.

Ethylenediaminetetraacetic acid   An anticoagulant that binds calcium.

Exudate   A fluid accumulation that results from inflammatory processes; characterized by increased cellularity and protein concentration.

Facultative anaerobes   Bacteria that do not require oxygen for metabolism but that can survive in the presence of oxygen.

Fastidious   A term used to describe a bacterial species with complex growth or nutritional requirements.

Fatty casts   Formed elements that may be found in urine and that consist of a hyaline cast with embedded globules of fat.

Fecal loop   A long narrow wand with a loop at the end is inserted into the rectum to collect fecal samples.

Fecal sedimentation   A procedure that is used to prepare samples for examination for parasites; it demonstrates objects that are too heavy or too delicate to evaluate with standard fecal flotation.

Fibrin degradation products   Protein fragments formed from the breakdown of fibrin.

Fibrinous inflammation   A form of inflammation that is characterized by fibrin deposition.

Fibrometer   An instrument used for the hemostatic evaluation of samples.

Filamentous   Thin in diameter; resembling a thread.

Fine-needle biopsy   A sample collection method in which tissue is obtained by puncture of a lesion.

Fixative   A chemical substance used to preserve or stabilize biological material prior to microscopy or other examination.

Flagella   Long, thin, helical structures that function in cell motility.

Flagella stain   A differential stain to detect and characterize flagella if present on bacterial cells.

Flea-bite dermatitis   The inflammatory lesions and self-trauma caused by a hypersensitivity to flea bites.

Flocculent Having a loosely clumped texture.

Fluorescent antibody A specific antibody that has been labeled with a fluorochrome and that is used in immunoassays.

Fluorescent microscope A type of microscope that is capable of viewing fluorescent particles, such as an antibody labeled with specific fluorescent dye.

Fractional excretion of electrolytes A mathematical manipulation that describes the excretion of specific electrolytes relative to the glomerular filtration rate.

Free catch A method of collecting a urine sample by collecting the sample as the animal voids naturally.

Fructosamine A molecule formed as a result of the irreversible reaction of glucose bound to protein.

Gamma-glutamyltransferase An intracellular enzyme found in high concentrations in liver, pancreatic, and renal tubular cells.

Gamma-hemolysis A term that describes a bacterial sample that produces no hemolysis on blood agar.

Giemsa stain A differential stain that is used for blood and bone marrow smears. Also used to visualize fungal organisms and mast cell granules.

Globulins A complex group of plasma proteins that have been designated as alpha, beta, or gamma; this group includes immunoglobulins, complement, and transferrin.

Glomerular filtration rate The rate at which substances are filtered through the glomerulus and excreted in the urine.

Glomerulus A tuft of capillaries located in the renal cortex.

Glucagon A hormone secreted by the alpha cells of the islets of Langerhans in response to hypoglycemia.

Glucose A monosaccharide that represents the end product of carbohydrate metabolism.

Glucose tolerance test A metabolic test of carbohydrate tolerance.

Glucosuria The presence of glucose in the urine.

Glutamate dehydrogenase A mitochondrial-bound enzyme that is found in high concentrations in the hepatocytes of cattle, sheep, and goats.

Glycosylated hemoglobin The irreversible reaction of hemoglobin bound to glucose.

Gram A metric unit of mass equal to one thousandth of a kilogram.

Gram stain A differential stain that is used to classify bacterial samples on the basis of the chemical structure of their cell walls.

Granular casts A structure that is formed from the protein precipitate of degenerating kidney tubule cells that contain granular material derived from the breakdown of cells incorporated into the cast.

Granulocytes Any cell with distinct cytoplasmic granules.

Granulomatous A term that refers to an inflammatory condition that is characterized by high numbers (more than 70%) of macrophages.

Hanging drop A method of preparing specimens to evaluate motility.

Heinz bodies Round structures of erythrocytes that represent denatured hemoglobin and that appear as a pale area when stained with Wright's stain.

Hematochezia The presence of blood in the feces.

Hematopoiesis The production of blood cells and platelets.

Hematuria The presence of intact erythrocytes in the urine.

Hemoglobin The oxygen-carrying pigment of erythrocytes, which is formed by developing erythrocytes in the bone marrow. It is a type of hemoprotein that contains four heme groups and globin.

Hemoglobinuria The presence of free hemoglobin in urine.

Hemolysis The destruction of erythrocytes.

Hemolyzed Red appearance of a fluid sample (e.g., serum, urine) as a result of the destruction of erythrocytes.

Hemophilia A genetic abnormality of hemostasis that results from the deficient production of certain coagulation factors.

Hemoprotozoa Unique unicellular protists that have developed sophisticated life cycles alternating between development in the tissues and blood of a range of vertebrate hosts and the gut and tissues of various blood feeding invertebrate vectors.

Heparin An acid mucopolysaccharide that is present in many tissues, especially the liver and lungs, and that has potent anticoagulant properties.

Hepatoencephalopathy Severe hepatic insufficiency that may induce a syndrome of excitability, tremor, compulsive walking, head pressing, and apparent blindness, followed by coma and convulsions.

Heterophil A leukocyte of avian, reptile, and some fish species that contains prominent eosinophilic granules; functionally equivalent to the mammalian neutrophil.

Hexacanth The infective stage of some cestodes.

Hirudiniasis Infestation with leeches.

Histamine A substance that has many effects in the body. It is released from some types of white blood cells during allergic reactions. It causes small blood vessels to dilate (widen) and become leaky, which can cause tissues to swell.

Histiocytoma A tumor that contains histiocytes (macrophages).

Histogram A graphic display of a frequency distribution that is represented by a series of rectangles that divide the data into classes. The height of a rectangle indicates the number of values that are contained in that class (class frequency), and the width of each base represents the size of the intervals into which the classes have been divided.

Howell-Jolly bodies Basophilic inclusions of young erythrocytes that represent nuclear remnants.

Humoral immunity An immune response that involves the production of specific antibody.

Hyaline casts The structures that are formed from protein precipitates of degenerating kidney tubule cells with no embedded materials.

Hyperadrenocorticism The abnormally increased secretion of adrenocortical hormones, as with conditions such as Cushing's syndrome.

Hypercalcemia An increased plasma calcium level.

Hypercapnia An excess of carbon dioxide in the blood that is indicated by an elevated PCO_2 level as determined by blood gas analysis and that results in respiratory acidosis. Also known as hypercarbia or hypercarbemia.

Hypercellular The state of having abnormally numerous cells.

Hyperchromatophilic A term that refers to a cell that appears darker than normal on a peripheral blood sample.

Hypercoagulable Characterized by abnormally increased coagulability.

Hyperglycemia An abnormally increased glucose level in the blood.

Hyperkalemia An increased plasma potassium level.

Hyperlipoproteinemia A condition characterized by excess lipids in the blood. Also referred to as hyperlipidemia and hyperlipemia.

Hypernatremia An increased plasma sodium level.

Hyperphosphatemia An excessive amount of phosphates in the blood.

Hyperproteinemia An increased protein level in the blood.

Hypersegmented A term that refers to a neutrophil with more than five nuclear lobes.

Hypersthenuria Increased urine specific gravity.

Hyperthyroidism A condition that is caused by the excessive production of iodinated thyroid hormones.

Hyphae The body of a fungus that is created as a result of the linear arrangements of cells and that forms multicellular or multinucleate growth.

Hypoadrenocorticism A deficiency in the production of mineralocorticoid or glucocorticoid steroid hormones.

Hypocalcemia A decreased plasma calcium level.

Hypocapnia A deficiency of carbon dioxide in the blood. Also called hypocarbia.

Hypocellular Containing less than the normal number of cells.

Hypochromasia The presence of erythrocytes with decreased staining intensity as a result of a decrease in hemoglobin concentration.

Hypocoagulable Characterized by abnormally decreased coagulability.

Hypoglycemia A decreased plasma glucose level.

Hypokalemia A decreased plasma potassium level.

Hyponatremia A decreased plasma sodium level.

Hypophosphatemia A decreased amount of phosphates in the blood.

Hypoproteinemia A condition characterized by an abnormally low level of protein in the blood.

Hyposegmentation A term that is used to describe the nucleus of a leukocyte with fewer than the normal number of nuclear lobes.

Hyposthenuria Decreased urine specific gravity.

Hypostome The penetrating, anchor-like sucking organ of the tick.

Icteric Affected by jaundice that causes yellowing of skin.

Icterus Abnormal yellowish discoloration of skin, mucous membranes, or plasma as a result of an increased concentration of bile pigments.

Iditol dehydrogenase An enzyme of the oxidoreductase class that catalyzes the oxidation of l-iditol to l-fructose; it occurs in significant quantities only in the liver, and its increased activity in serum is used as an indicator of parenchymal liver damage. Also referred to as sorbitol dehydrogenase.

Illinois sternal needle Helps ensure safe and simple marrow aspiration from the iliac crest or sternum by effectively penetrating the bone.

Immune-complex disease Describes a state in which circulating antigen–antibody complexes, formed by coexisting immune reactants, induce vascular injury.

Immune-mediated hemolytic anemia An autoimmune disease in dogs in which the body attacks its own red blood cells.

Immunochromatography A testing method for detecting a disease by dropping the sample containing an analyte onto a test strip.

Immunodiffusion An immunologic test that is performed by placing reactants in an agar plate and allowing them to migrate through the gel toward each other.

Immunoglobulins Antibodies; plasma proteins produced against specific antigens.

Immunologic tolerance A state of non-responsiveness to antigens, whether self or foreign.

Impedance analyzer A type of analyzer that counts particles based on their displacement of electrolyte solution when the particles pass through an aperture. The magnitude of the displacement creates an electrical signal that allows particles (e.g., cells) to be classified on the basis of their size.

Impression smear Used to collect the surface material so that it can be examined more closely.

Imprint A mark made by pressing something onto a softer substance so that its outline is reproduced.

Incubator A piece of equipment that is used to maintain a constant and suitable temperature for the development of cultures of microorganisms or other living cells.

Indirect life cycle The life cycle of an organism that requires one or more intermediate hosts.

Indirect sensitivity testing An antimicrobial sensitivity test that involves the application of diluted samples (e.g., urine) directly to the Mueller-Hinton plate.

Indole a crystalline organic compound with an unpleasant odor, present in coal tar and in feces.

Infectious enterohepatitis A destructive disease of turkeys and related birds caused by a protozoan of the genus *Histomonas* (*H. meleagridis*) that invades the intestinal ceca and liver.

Inflammatory response The defensive response of body tissues that is initiated by the release of histamine from damaged cells.

Inoculating loops A tool usually made of platinum or nichrome wire in which the tip forms a small loop with a diameter of about 5 mm, used to smear, streak, or take an inoculum from a culture of microorganisms.

Inorganic phosphorus Inorganic phosphate (Pi) is an essential nutrient to living organisms.

Instar Any stage of an arthropod between molts.

Insulin A protein hormone that is secreted by the beta cells of the pancreatic islets in response to elevated blood levels of glucose and amino acids.

Interferons Small soluble proteins that enhance the function of the immune system.

Intermediate host The host that harbors the larval, immature, or asexual stages of a parasite.

International System of Units The Système International (SI) set of basic units, which is based on the metric system.

Ion-selective electrode An analytical technique used to determine the activity of ions in aqueous solution by measuring the electrical potential.

Isosthenuria Occurs when the urine-specific gravity approaches that of glomerular filtrate (1.008 to 1.012).

Jamshidi needle A trephine needle for performing bone marrow biopsy, whereby a cylindrical sample of tissue, a core biopsy specimen, is obtained.

Jaundice A condition that is characterized by hyperbilirubinemia and the deposition of bile pigments in the skin, mucous membranes, and sclera.

Karyolysis The degeneration or dissolution of a cell nucleus.

Karyorrhexis The fragmentation of a cell nucleus.

Keratocyte In hematology, an abnormally shaped erythrocyte that appears to have horns.

Ketones Found in urine, indicating diabetes mellitus, ketosis in cows, and pregnancy disease in ewes. Urine has a characteristic sweet or fruity odor.

Ketonuria The presence of detectable ketone bodies in urine.

Kinetic assay A chemical test that measures the rate of change of a substance in the test system.

Kirby-Bauer test A type of antimicrobial susceptibility test in which agar plates are inoculated with a standardized suspension of a microorganism, and then antibiotic-containing disks are applied to the agar surface.

Kovac's reagent A substance used in bacteriology to detect the ability of bacteria to produce indole.

Lactate The anionic form of lactic acid; a salt of lactic acid.

Lactophenol cotton blue A preparation of phenol, lactic acid, glycerin, distilled water, and cotton blue dye that is used to stain fungi in wet preparations.

Laser flow cytometry A technology that provides rapid multi-parametric analysis of single cells in solution.

Lateral flow immunoassay A paper-based platform for the detection and quantification of analytes in complex mixtures, where the sample is placed on a test device and the results are displayed within 5 to 30 min.

Latex agglutination A test done in a lab to check for certain antibodies or antigens in body fluids, including saliva, urine, cerebrospinal fluid, or blood.

Left shift The presence of increased numbers of immature cells in a peripheral blood sample.

Leptocyte An erythrocyte that is characterized by an increased membrane surface area relative to the cell volume.

Leucine Crystals that are wheel or "pincushion" shaped and yellow or brown in color and may be present in animals with liver disease.

Leukemia A condition characterized by the presence of neoplastic cells in the blood or bone marrow.

Leukemoid response The exhibition of blood counts (particularly leukocytosis) and sometimes other clinical findings that resemble those of leukemia.

Leukocytosis The presence of increased numbers of leukocytes in the blood.

Leukopoiesis The production of leukocytes.

Line smear A technique "concentrates" the cells in a "line" at the end of the smear.

Lipase A pancreatic enzyme that functions in the breakdown of fats.

Lipemia The presence of fatty material in plasma or serum.

Liter A metric unit of capacity, formerly defined as the volume of one kilogram of water under standard conditions, now equal to 1000 cubic centimeters (about 1.75 pints).

Lymphocyte A leukocyte that is involved in the inflammatory process and that also has roles in humoral and cell-mediated immunity.

Lymphoma A neoplastic disorder of the lymphoid tissue.

Lymphopenia The presence of decreased numbers of leukocytes in a peripheral blood sample.

Lymphoproliferative disease A heterogeneous group of diseases characterized by uncontrolled production of lymphocytes that cause monoclonal lymphocytosis, lymphadenopathy, and bone marrow infiltration.

MacConkey agar An agar medium that contains peptone, lactose bile salts, sodium chloride, neutral red, and crystal violet that is used to differentiate lactose fermenters (coliforms) from non–lactose fermenters among the enteric bacilli.

Macrocytosis A condition in which a cell is abnormally large.

Magnesium The chemical element of atomic number 12, a silver-white metal of the alkaline earth series. It is used to make strong lightweight alloys, especially for the aerospace industry, and is also used in flashbulbs and pyrotechnics because it burns with a brilliant white flame.

Malignant Very virulent or infectious.

Mange A dermatologic condition produced by obligate parasites, which spend their entire life cycle on the host.

Mast cell tumors   A benign local aggregation of mast cells that forms a nodular tumor that occurs in the skin of most species (most commonly dogs).

Material Safety Data Sheet (MSDS)   Informational material that contains detailed product safety information about hazardous materials found in a particular place of a business; an OSHA mandate.

McFarland suspension   Used as a reference to adjust the turbidity of bacterial suspensions so that the number of bacteria will be within a given range to standardize microbial testing.

McMaster technique   A flotation test that separates parasite eggs from debris based on density.

Mean corpuscular hemoglobin (MCH)   An expression of the average hemoglobin content of a single cell in picograms that is obtained by multiplying the amount of hemoglobin (in grams) by 10 and then dividing that number by the number of erythrocytes (in millions).

Mean corpuscular hemoglobin concentration   Measures the average hemoglobin concentration in a given volume of red blood cells. Hemoglobin is an iron-rich protein that carries oxygen to tissues.

Mean corpuscular volume   An expression of the average volume of individual red cells in cubic microns that is obtained by multiplying the hematocrit percentage by 10 and then dividing that number by the number of erythrocytes (in millions).

Mean platelet volume   An expression of the average size of individual platelets.

Megathrombocytes   Abnormally large platelets that are usually newly formed; seen in greater numbers during an increase in platelet production.

Melanoma   A tumor that arises from melanocytes of the skin or other organs.

Melena   Dark sticky feces containing partly digested blood.

Merozoites   A cell developed from a schizont that parasitizes a red blood cell in the host.

Mesenchymal cell tumors   Tumors of mixed mesenchymal tissues with two or more cellular elements that are not commonly associated (not counting fibrous tissue as one of the elements).

Mesophiles   Organisms with optimal growth temperatures of between 25° C and 40° C.

Metacercaria   The encysted resting or maturing stage of a trematode parasite in the tissues of an intermediate host or on vegetation.

Methanol   Methyl alcohol.

Methemoglobin   The form of hemoglobin that contains oxidized iron; inefficient at oxygen transport.

Methylene blue   A salt used as a dye and as a medication.

Metric system   The decimal measuring system based on the meter, liter, and gram as units of length, capacity, and weight or mass.

Microcytosis   A cell that appears much smaller than normal.

Microfilaria   The larval offspring of the group of filarial worms in the phylum Nematoda.

Microhematocrit   A term that refers to use of a capillary tube and a high-speed centrifuge to determine the packed cell volume.

Microparticles   A microscopic particle.

Micturition   The action of urinating.

Minimum inhibitory concentration   The smallest concentration of an antibiotic that regularly inhibits the growth of a bacterium in vitro.

Miracidium   The ciliated larval stage of a digenetic trematode.

Modified compression preparation   A method of preparing samples for observation under the microscope.

Modified Knott's test   The method is used for the detection of microfilariae in the blood.

Modified transudate   A transudate with additional protein, cells, or both; it may be a transitional stage that ultimately progresses into an exudate.

Monocyte   A precursor cell representing a stage in the development of the tissue macrophage; after a monocyte leaves the bloodstream and enters tissue at a site of inflammation, it becomes an activated macrophage.

Monovette   A blood collection system combining two blood collection techniques.

Motility media   A media that provides an easy method for determining motility.

Mucin clot test   The adding of acetic acid to normal synovial fluid, which causes clot formation; the compactness of the clot and the clarity of the supernatant fluid are the criteria on which the result is based.

Mucoid   Forming large moist sticky colonies.

Mueller-Hinton medium   A standard culture material that is used to evaluate the susceptibility of microorganisms to antimicrobial agents.

Myeloproliferative disease   A type of disease in which the bone marrow makes too many red blood cells, platelets, or certain white blood cells.

Myiasis   An infestation with the larvae (maggots) of dipterans.

Myoglobinuria   Urine that contains myoglobulin and may be brown when voided.

Natural killer (NK) cells   A subpopulation of lymphocytes that is capable of the direct lysis of cells that have been infected with antigen.

Nematode   A multicellular parasitic animal of the phylum Nematoda.

Neonatal isoerythrolysis   Hemolytic anemia of the newborn.

Neoplasia   A generic term that is used to describe any growth; often used to describe a tumor, which may be malignant or benign.

Nephron   A structural and functional unit of the kidney that resembles a microscopic funnel with a long stem and two convoluted tubular sections.

Neubauer rulings   A specific pattern of precise markings on a hematocytometer slide that facilitates the counting of leukocytes, erythrocytes, and platelets in the blood and of all cells in other fluids.

Neutrophil   A leukocyte that functions to phagocytize infectious agents and cellular debris; plays a major role in the inflammatory process.

Neutrophilia   An abnormal increase in the number of neutrophils seen in a peripheral blood sample.

New methylene blue (NMB)   An organic compound of the thiazine class of heterocycles. It is used as a stain and as an antimicrobial agent.

Nits   The egg stage of lice, which binds to the hair or feather shaft of the host.

Nonregenerative anemia   Occurs when the bone marrow is unable to produce sufficient new red blood cells to replace cells that naturally die off as they age.

Nuclear molding   A deformation of nuclei by other nuclei within the same cell or adjacent cells.

Nucleated erythrocyte   An immature red blood cell that still contains a nucleus.

Numerical aperture   A measure of the efficiency of a microscope objective lens; it is proportional to the square root of the amount of light that enters the instrument.

Nymph   A developmental stage of certain arthropods between the larval form and the adult; resembles the latter in appearance.

Objective lens   A lens that accepts light from the output phosphor of an image intensifier tube and converts it into a parallel beam to record the image on film.

Obligate aerobes   An organism that requires oxygen to grow.

Obligate anaerobes   Organisms that cannot grow in the presence of oxygen.

Occupational Safety and Health Administration (OSHA)   A U.S. government agency that mandates specific laboratory practices that must be incorporated into a laboratory's safety policy.

Ocular   Pertaining to the eye.

Oliguria   A decrease in the volume of urine produced.

Oocyst   A cyst containing a zygote formed by a parasitic protozoan such as the malaria parasite.

Opsonization   The complement-mediated adherence of phagocytes to antigens that enhances the phagocytosis of the antigen.

Optical density   The degree to which light is transmitted through a medium.

Oxalate   An anion of oxalic acid.

Oxidase   An enzyme that is present in some groups of bacteria and that is involved with the reduction of oxygen during normal bacteria metabolism.

Oxyhemoglobin   The normal, oxygen-carrying form of hemoglobin in which iron is in the reduced (ferrous) state.

Packed cell volume   The ratio of red blood cells to total plasma volume.

Pancreatic lipase immunoreactivity   Measures the concentration of pancreatic lipase in a biological sample.

Pancytopenia   A condition in which there is a lower-than-normal number of red and white blood cells and platelets in the blood.

Parabasal   Beyond the base.

Paracentesis   The removal of fluid from a body cavity.

Parthenogenetic   A condition in which female organisms produce eggs that develop without fertilization.

Passive immunity   A condition that involves receiving antibodies from colostrum or synthesized antibodies.

Pediculosis   The term used to describe an infestation with lice.

Pelger-Huët anomaly   An inherited anomaly that is characterized by the appearance of bilobed neutrophils in a peripheral blood sample.

Periodic parasite   A parasite that lives part of its life cycle on its host and part of its life off of its host.

Peritoneal fluid   A naturally produced fluid in the abdominal cavity that lubricates surfaces, thereby preventing friction between the peritoneal membrane and the internal organs.

Personal protective equipment   Items such as eye protection and other protective clothing, shields, and barriers that are designed to minimize exposure to hazards in the workplace.

pH   A measure of the hydrogen ion concentration of a solution.

Phagocytosis   The ingestion of bacteria or other material by phagocytes and amoeboid protozoans.

Phase-contrast microscope   A type of light microscope that involves a special condenser and objective lens with a phase-shifting ring; it is used to visualize small differences in refractive index as differences in intensity or contrast.

Phosphatidylserine   A phospholipid that protects the cells in your brain. This fatty substance transmits messages in your brain to help your memory and cognitive function. Phosphatidylserine is available as a supplement.

Pipette   A calibrated, transparent, open-ended tube made out of glass or plastic that is used to measure or transfer small quantities of a liquid or gas. This word can also be used to refer to the use of a pipette to dispense liquid.

PIVKA   Proteins induced by vitamin K deficiency or antagonists; the nonfunctional precursor forms of vitamin-K–dependent coagulation factors.

Planachromatic   A type of achromatic lens, also referred to as flat field lens, provides a more uniform field of focus from the center to the periphery of the microscopic image.

Plasma   The fluid portion of the blood.

Plasma cell tumor   An extramedullary myeloma; this type of tumor occurs outside of the bone marrow, and it usually affects the visceral organs or the nasopharyngeal and oral mucosa.

Platelet distribution width   Reflects variability in platelet size and is considered a marker of platelet function and activation.

Plateletcrit   Measures total platelet mass as a percentage of volume occupied in the blood.

Platelet–large cell ratio   The percentage of platelets that exceed the normal value of platelet volume of 12 fL in the total platelet count.

Platelets   Irregular, disc-shaped fragments of megakaryocytes in the blood that assist with blood clotting.

Pleomorphism   A term that refers to something that takes a variety of shapes and forms or that has multiple morphologies.

Pleural fluid   A pleural fluid analysis is a group of tests that examine a sample of abnormal fluid that builds up in the space between the lungs and chest.

Plumbism   A chronic form of lead poisoning that is caused by the absorption of lead or lead salts.

Pluripotent stem cell   A cell capable of differentiating into one of many cell types.

Poikilocytosis   Any abnormal cell shape.

Pollakiuria   Frequent urination.

Polycythemia   An abnormally high number of red blood cells in the blood, as a primary disease or secondary condition (usually associated with lung or heart disease or living at high altitude).

Polydipsia   An increase in water consumption.

Polymerase chain reaction   A method that is used to replicate and amplify DNA molecules in a sample.

Polyuria   An increase in the total volume of urine produced.

Pooled sample   A screening approach that combines samples from some number of people into one test.

Potassium   A mineral that your body needs to work properly. It is a type of electrolyte.

Potassium hydroxide   An odorless, white or slightly yellow, flakey or lumpy solid that is often in a water solution.

Preanalytic variables   Occur prior to specimen testing and may include variables involving the process of obtaining a specimen.

Precision   The magnitude of random errors and the reproducibility of measurements.

Prepatent period   The time interval between infection with a parasite and the demonstration of that infection.

Presumptive identification   Identification by the colony morphology, growth on selective media, gram stains.

Proglottid   A segment that comprises the body of a cestode.

Prokaryotic   Any organism that lacks a distinct nucleus and other organelles due to the absence of internal membranes.

Promastigote   The motile, elongated, extracellular form in the life cycle of some protozoans.

Protein   Highly complex substance that is present in all living organisms.

Proteinuria   The abnormal presence of protein in the urine.

Prothrombin time tests   A one-stage test for detecting certain plasma coagulation defects that are caused by a deficiency of factors V, VII, or X.

Protozoa   A phylum or group of phyla that comprises the single-celled microscopic animals, which include amoebas, flagellates, ciliates, sporozoans, and many other forms. They are now usually treated as a number of phyla belonging to the kingdom Protista.

Pseudocoelom   A body cavity filled with fluid that lies between the mesoderm layer of the external body wall and the endoderm layer of the gut in invertebrates.

Pseudopodia   A temporary protrusion of the surface of an amoeboid cell for movement and feeding.

Psychrophiles   Organisms that demonstrate optimal growth at cold temperatures (i.e., between 15° C and 20° C).

Punch biopsy   The removal of living tissue for microscopic examination with the use of a punch.

Pupa   The second stage in the life cycle of certain insects, which occurs between the larval and adult stages. A pupa shows the basic external features of the adult form, but it does not have expanded wings.

Pyknosis   The presence of condensed nuclear chromatin in a degenerating cell.

Pyogranulomatous   A term used to describe a cytology sample that is characterized by the presence of macrophages representing more than 15% of total nucleated cells in the sample.

Quadrant streak   A technique for microbial inoculation in which a single colony is isolated on a culture plate and divided into four sections.

Quality assurance   Any evaluation of services provided and the results achieved as compared with accepted standards.

Quantitative buffy coat analysis   A technique for a method of diagnosing malarial parasites based on micro-centrifugation, fluorescence, and density gradient of infected red blood cells.

Radioimmunoassay   A technique that is used to determine the concentration of an antigen, antibody, or other protein in the serum. A radioactively labeled substance that is known to react in a certain way with the suspected protein is injected, and any reaction is monitored.

Rapid immunomigration   Also known as immunochromatography, one of the fastest and most practical techniques for detecting antibody–antigen interactions.

Ratio   The relationship of one quantity to one or more other quantities that is expressed as a proportion of one to the others and written either as a fraction or linearly.

Reactive lymph node   When lymph glands respond to infection by becoming swollen.

Reactive lymphocyte   Large, immune-stimulated lymphocytes with dark-blue cytoplasm and irregular, scalloped, or cleaved nuclei.

Red cell distribution width test   Measures the differences in the volume and size of red blood cells (erythrocytes).

Redia   A secondary larval form of some digenetic trematodes that develops within a mollusk intermediate host.

Reference range   A set of values that includes upper and lower limits of a lab test based on a group of otherwise healthy people.

Reflectometer   An instrument for measuring quantities associated with reflection, in particular (also *time domain reflectometer*) an instrument for locating discontinuities (e.g., faults in electric cables) by detecting and measuring reflected pulses of energy.

Refractive index   A measure of the degree that light bends as it passes from one medium to another.

Refractometer   A device that measures the refractive index of a solution.

Regenerative anemia   The bone marrow responds appropriately to the decreased number of red blood cells by increasing production of new blood cells.

Reliability   The ability of a method to be accurate and precise.

Renal epithelial cells   Originate in the renal tubules and are the smallest epithelial cells observed in urine.

Renal threshold   The concentration level up to which a substance (as glucose) in the blood is prevented from passing through the kidneys into the urine.

Resolution   The ability of an imaging process to distinguish adjacent structures in the object; an important measure of image quality.

Reticulocyte production index   Also called a corrected reticulocyte count (CRC), a calculated value used in the diagnosis of anemia.

Reticulocytes   Immature red blood cells (RBCs) produced in the bone marrow and released into the peripheral blood, where they mature into RBCs within 1 to 2 days.

Rhizoid   Resembling a root or serving to anchor.

Rickettsia   Any of a group of very small bacteria that includes the causative agents of typhus and various other febrile diseases in humans. Like viruses, many of them can only grow inside living cells, and they are frequently transmitted by mites, ticks, or lice.

Ringworm   A group of fungal skin diseases that are caused by dermatophytes of several kinds.

Romanowsky stain   Stains made from water-soluble eosin, methylene blue, and methanol.

Rosenthal needle   For use in bone marrow biopsy.

Rostellum   The anterior of a tapeworm scolex, which commonly features hooklike jaws.

Rouleaux   An arrangement of erythrocytes that appears as a column or stack.

Sabouraud dextrose agar   A type of agar growth medium containing peptones.

Sarcoma   A generic term that is used to describe any cancer that arises from cells of the connective tissues.

Schistocytes   Fragmented erythrocytes that are usually formed as a result of shearing of the red cell by intravascular trauma.

Scolex   The anterior portion of a cestode by which it attaches to its host.

Selective media   A type of culture media that contains antibacterial substances that inhibit or kill all but a few types of bacteria.

Sensitivity   The probability of a positive test result, conditioned on the individual truly being positive.

Serial dilution   A laboratory technique in which a substance (e.g., serum) is decreased in concentration in a series of proportional amounts.

Serum   The fluid portion of blood after it has clotted; it does not contain cells or coagulation proteins.

Simple fecal flotation   A routine veterinary test used to diagnose internal parasites or worms.

Simple stain   Involves directly staining the bacterial cell with a positively charged dye in order to see bacterial detail.

Skin scraping   A common diagnostic procedure that is used to evaluate animals with suspected external parasites.

Slant tube   An agar slant tube (or simply an agar slant) is a screw-capped culture tube partly filled with an agar mix such as nutrient agar.

Smudge cell   A leukocyte that has ruptured.

Sodium   The chemical element of atomic number 11, a soft silver-white reactive metal of the alkali metal group.

Sodium fluoride   An inorganic compound with the formula NaF. It is a colorless or white solid that is readily soluble in water.

Specific gravity   The weight (density) of a quantity of liquid as compared with that of an equal amount of distilled water.

Specificity   The ability of a test to evaluate a given parameter correctly.

Spectrophotometer   A piece of equipment designed to measure the amount of light that is transmitted through a solution.

Spherocyte   An intensely stained erythrocyte that has reduced or no central pallor.

Spirochete   Any bacterium of the genus *Spirochaeta* that is motile and spiral-shaped, with flexible filaments.

Sporangiospores   The spores that are encapsulated in the sporangium (a special cell that contains spores).

Sporocyst   The larval stage of a digenetic trematode that develops in a mollusk intermediate host.

Standard operating procedures   A set of written instructions that describes the step-by-step process that must be taken to properly perform a routine procedure.

Standards   A level of quality or attainment.

Starfish smear   Involves dragging the ejected material on the slide peripherally in several directions using a needle.

Stomatocyte   An erythrocyte with a linear area of central pallor.

Strobila   The segmented part of the body of a tapeworm that consists of a long chain of proglottids.

Struvite   A common crystal that is seen in alkaline to slightly acidic urine. Also referred to as triple phosphate crystals or magnesium ammonium phosphate crystals.

Supernatant   The fluid portion of a sample that is present after centrifugation.

Suppurative   Containing, discharging, or causing the production of pus; cytology sample characterized by the presence of neutrophils representing more than 85% of total nucleated cells in the sample. May also be described as purulent.

Swabbing   Take a specimen of tissue or secretions (from a person or part of the body) for examination.

Synovial fluid   A transparent, viscous fluid that is secreted by synovial membranes and that acts as a lubricant for many joints, bursae, and tendons. It contains mucin, albumin, fat, and mineral salts.

Tachyzoites   Refers to the rapidly growing life stage of *T. gondii* that has also been called endozoites or trophozoites.

Target cell   A leptocyte with a peripheral ring of cytoplasm surrounded by a clear area and a dense, central, rounded area of pigment.

Thermophiles   Organisms that undergo optimal growth at elevated temperatures.

Thioglycollate   A salt or ester of thioglycolic acid.

Thoracocentesis   The removal of fluid from the thoracic cavity.

Thrombin   An enzyme that is formed from prothrombin, calcium, and thromboplastin in plasma during the clotting process. Thrombin causes fibrinogen to change to fibrin, which is essential during the formation of a clot.

Thrombocrit   The percentage of blood volume occupied by platelets; an assessment of circulating platelet mass.

Thrombocytes   Platelets; cytoplasmic fragments of bone marrow megakaryocytes.

Thrombocytopenia   A condition that involves a decrease in the number of circulating platelets.

Thrombocytosis   A condition that involves an increase in the number of circulating platelets.

Thromboelastography   A graphical image of the recorded amplitude of movement of the pin as a function of time.

Thrombopathia   A condition in which there is a deficiency of clotting ability for reasons other than thrombocytopenia.

Thrombopoiesis   The production of platelets.

Thrombopoietin   A hormone that regulates blood platelet production by promoting the proliferation and maturation of megakaryocyte progenitor cells and the development of megakaryocytes into blood platelets.

Thyroid-stimulating hormone   A substance secreted by the anterior lobe of the pituitary gland that controls the release of thyroid hormone and that is necessary for the growth and function of the thyroid gland.

Thyroxine   A hormone of the thyroid gland that is derived from tyrosine and that influences the metabolic rate.

Tick paralysis   A condition that results from the introduction of a neurotoxin into the body during the attachment of and feeding by the female of several tick species.

Tom cat catheter   Used for aid in treatment of urinary tract disease.

Torocyte   These have a thickened peripheral rim «< donut-cell »» and may arise from desiccation of the thick portion at the beginning of a smear.

Toxic granulation   The term used to describe an increase in staining density and possibly number of granules that occurs regularly with bacterial infection and often with other causes of inflammation.

Transitional epithelial cells   Cells that come from the bladder, the ureters, the renal pelvis, and the proximal urethra.

Transmissible venereal tumors   Tumors that arise from the dysregulated growth of cells called histiocytes.

Transport media   Essentially buffer solutions containing carbohydrates, peptones, and other nutrients (excluding growth factors) designed to preserve the viability of bacteria during transport without allowing them to multiply.

Transtracheal wash   Minimally invasive procedures that allow for blind sampling of the larger airways for cytologic and culture.

Transudate   An effusion that is characterized by a low protein concentration and a low total nucleated cell count.

Trematode   An organism in the phylum Trematoda; commonly referred to as a fluke.

Trophozoite   A growing stage in the life cycle of some sporozoan parasites, when they are absorbing nutrients from the host.

Trypomastigote   The developmental stage or the morphological form in the life cycle of trypanosomatids in which the characteristic morphological form is a flagellum that arises from a posteriorly located kinetoplast and emerges from the side of the body, with an undulating membrane running along the length of the body.

Trypsin   A proteolytic digestive enzyme that is produced by the exocrine pancreas and that catalyzes the breakdown of dietary proteins into peptones, peptides, and amino acids in the small intestine.

Trypsinogen   The inactive precursor form of trypsin; it is secreted in pancreatic juice and converted into active trypsin through the action of enterokinase in the intestine.

Tuberculin skin test   The Mantoux tuberculin skin test (TST) is one method of determining whether a person is infected with *Mycobacterium tuberculosis*. Reliable administration and reading of the TST requires standardization of procedures, training, supervision, and practice.

Tyrosine   An amino acid that is synthesized in the body from the essential amino acid phenylalanine; it is found in most proteins and is a precursor of melanin and several hormones, including epinephrine and thyroxin.

Tzanck preparation   A simple and cheap test that relies on viewing and interpretation of single cells (cytology).

Undulate   To have wavelike fluctuations or oscillations.

Undulatory ridges   Undulatory waves in the surface of some protozoa, probably aided by sub-pellicular micro-tubules; the means of locomotion in some species.

Urease   A naturally occurring enzyme that hydrolyzes urea into ammonium carbonate.

Uric acid   A metabolic by-product of nitrogen catabolism.

Urinometer   A small hydrometer for determining the specific gravity of urine.

Urochromes   Pigments present in urine giving it a light yellow to amber color.

Uroliths   Calculi (stones) composed of various minerals that are found anywhere in the urinary tract.

Urticaria   A rash of round, red welts on the skin that itch intensely, sometimes with dangerous swelling, caused by an allergic reaction, typically to specific foods.

Vaccination   Any injection of attenuated microorganisms (e.g., bacteria, viruses, rickettsiae) that is administered to induce immunity or to reduce the effects of associated infectious diseases.

Vacutainer   A glass tube with a rubber stopper from which air can be removed to create a vacuum; usually used to draw blood.

Vacuum collection   A method of collecting samples using a vacuum.

von Willebrand disease   An inherited disorder that is characterized by the abnormally slow coagulation of the blood as well as spontaneous epistaxis and gingival bleeding. It is caused by a deficiency of a component of factor VIII. Excessive bleeding is common after injury or surgery.

von Willebrand factor   Glycoprotein crucial to primary hemostasis through platelet and subendothelial collagen adhesion, and the intrinsic coagulation cascade, through factor VIII stabilization.

Warbles   The common name for the larva of some species of flies; they are often in swollen, cyst-like subcutaneous sites, with a fistula or pore that communicates with the outside environment.

Wave motion   Propagation of disturbances—that is, deviations from a state of rest or equilibrium.

Waxy casts   Probably represent the last stage of granular cast degeneration. Waxy casts are nonspecific and can be observed in a wide variety of acute and chronic kidney diseases. However, they indicate a certain degree of slowing in urine formation and, therefore, possibly more advanced kidney disease.

Wedge biopsy   A surgical procedure in which a small, wedge-shaped portion of tissue is removed from an organ,

Wedge smear   A sample of blood that is spread on a glass slide that is treated with a special stain.

Wheals   A raised, itchy (pruritic) area of skin that is sometimes an overt sign of allergy.

Wood's lamp   An illuminating device with a nickel oxide filter that holds back all light except for a few violet rays of the visible spectrum and ultraviolet wavelengths of about 365 nm. It is used extensively to help diagnose fungal infections.

Wright-Giemsa stain   Mixtures of basic dyes (methylene blue) that stain as blue and acidic dyes (eosin) that stain as red.

Wright's stain   A hematologic stain that facilitates the differentiation of blood cell types. It is classically a mixture of eosin (red) and methylene blue dyes.

Yeast   Any unicellular (usually oval) nucleated fungus that reproduces by budding.

Ziehl-Neelsen stain   One of the most widely used methods of acid-fast staining; it is commonly used during the microscopic examination of a smear of sputum that is suspected of containing *Mycobacterium tuberculosis*.

Zinc sulfate   A crystalline salt ($ZnSO_4$) used especially in making a white paint pigment, in printing and dyeing, in sprays and fertilizers, and in medicine as an astringent, emetic, and weak antiseptic.

Zone of inhibition   An area of no bacterial growth around an antimicrobial disc that indicates some sensitivity of the organism to the particular antimicrobial.

Zoonoses   Diseases that can be transmitted between animals and humans.

Zygospores   The spores that result from the conjugation of two isogametes, as occurs with certain fungi and algae.

RESOURCES

UNIT 1 THE VETERINARY PRACTICE LABORATORY

Recommended Reading

Bishop M, Fody E, Schoeff L: *Clinical chemistry: principles, techniques, and correlations*, ed 8, Philadelphia, 2017, Lippincott Williams & Wilkins.

Kroll M, McCudden C: *Endogenous interferences in clinical laboratory tests*, Berlin, 2012, deGruyter.

Lake T, Green N: *Essential calculations for veterinary nurses and technicians*, ed 3, St Louis, 2016, Elsevier.

U.S. Department of Labor, Occupational Safety and Health Administration: *Laboratory safety guidance*, 2012.

Internet Resources

https://www.osha.gov/law-regs.html

https://www.osha.gov/shpguidelines

https://www.osha.gov/Publications/laboratory/OSHA3404laboratory-safety-guidance.pdf

http://www.vetlabassoc.com

http://www.asvcp.org/pubs/qas/index.cfm

http://vetlab.com/newqa.htm

http://www.sosmath.com/algebra/fraction/frac7/frac7.html

http://mathforum.org/alejandre/numerals.html

http://www.algebrahelp.com/lessons/proportionbasics

http://www.factmonster.com/ipka/A0769547.html

http://www.mapharm.com/roman_numbers.htm

http://www.sosmath.com/algebra/fraction/frac3/frac3.html

http://www.sosmath.com/algebra/fraction/frac4/frac4.html

http://www.sosmath.com/algebra/fraction/frac5/frac5.html

http://www.factmonster.com/ipka/A0881929.html

http://www.vendian.org/envelope/dir0/exponential_notation.html

http://www.mathsisfun.com/measure/metric-system.html

UNIT 2 HEMATOLOGY

Recommended Reading

Harvey JW: *Veterinary hematology: a diagnostic guide and color atlas*, St Louis, 2012, Saunders.

Meyer DJ, Harvey JW: *Veterinary laboratory medicine: interpretation and diagnosis*, ed 3, St Louis, 2004, Saunders.

Thrall MA, Weiser G, Allison R, Campbell T: *Veterinary hematology and clinical chemistry*, ed 2, Ames, IA, 2012, Wiley-Blackwell.

Valenciano AC, Cowell RL: *Cowell and Tyler's diagnostic cytology and hematology of the dog and cat*, ed 4, St Louis, 2014, Mosby.

Internet Resources

https://www.idexxlearningcenter.com/idexx/user_taxonomy_training.aspx?id=them&SSOTOKEN=0

http://www.vetstream.com/canis/Content/Lab_test/lab00113.asp

http://www.merckmanuals.com/vet/circulatory_system/hematopoietic_system_introduction/overview_of_hematopoietic_system.html?qt=&sc=&alt=

http://www.merckmanuals.com/vet/circulatory_system/hematopoietic_system_introduction/red_blood_cells.html?qt=&sc=&alt=

http://www.merckmanuals.com/vet/circulatory_system/hematopoietic_system_introduction/white_blood_cells.html?qt=&sc=&alt=

http://www.ephlebotomytraining.com/phlebotomy-order-draw-explained

https://ahdc.vet.cornell.edu/Sects/ClinPath/sample/test/hema.cfm#Bloodsmear

UNIT 3 HEMOSTASIS

Recommended Reading

Ford RB, Mazzaferro E: *Kirk & Bistner's handbook of veterinary procedures and emergency treatment*, ed 9, St Louis, 2012, Saunders.

Harvey JW: *Veterinary hematology: a diagnostic guide and color atlas*, St Louis, 2012, Saunders.

Jandrey K, Brainard B: Thromboelastography. In Bonagura JD, Twedt D, editors: *Kirk's current veterinary therapy XV*, St Louis, 2014, Saunders.

Meyer DJ, Harvey JW: *Veterinary laboratory medicine: interpretation and diagnosis*, ed 3, St Louis, 2004, Saunders.

Murphy M: Rodenticide toxicoses. In Bonagura JD, Twedt D. (Eds.): *Kirk's current veterinary therapy XV*, ed 14, St Louis, 2014, Saunders.

Internet Resources

https://www.idexxlearningcenter.com/idexx/user_taxonomy_training.aspx?id=them&SSOTOKEN=0

http://www.merckmanuals.com/vet/circulatory_system/hematopoietic_system_introduction/platelets.html?qt=&sc=&alt=

http://www.eclinpath.com/hemostasis

http://vetlab.com/slideshow2

http://www.eclinpath.com/hemostasis/tests

http://www.ncbi.nlm.nih.gov/pmc/articles/PMC2378355

https://ahdc.vet.cornell.edu/Sects/Coag/clinical/bleeding.cfm

http://www.petplace.com/cats/bruising-and-bleeding-in-cats/page1.aspx

UNIT 4 CLINICAL CHEMISTRY

Recommended Reading

Karselis I: *The pocket guide to clinical laboratory instrumentation*, Philadelphia, 1994, FA Davis.

Meyer DJ, Harvey JW: *Veterinary laboratory medicine: interpretation and diagnosis*, ed 3, St Louis, 2006, Saunders.

Sodikoff C: *Laboratory profiles of small animal diseases: a guide to laboratory diagnosis*, St Louis, 2001, Mosby.

Thrall MA, Baker DC, Lassen ED: *Veterinary hematology & clinical chemistry*, ed 2, Baltimore, 2012, Lippincott Williams & Wilkins.

Willard MD, Tvedten H: *Small animal clinical diagnosis by laboratory methods*, ed 5, St Louis, 2011, Saunders.

Internet Resources

http://www.eclinpath.com/chemistry/

http://www.asvcp.org/pubs/pdf/RI%20Guidelines%20For%20ASVCP%20website.pdf

https://www.idexxlearningcenter.com/mod/scorm/view.php?id=1044

https://www.idexxlearningcenter.com/mod/scorm/view.php?id=1046

UNIT 5 URINALYSIS

Recommended Reading

Meyer DJ, Harvey JW: *Veterinary laboratory medicine interpretation and diagnosis*, ed 3, St Louis, 2004, Saunders.

Modern urine chemistry, Elkhart, 1993, Miles Laboratories.

Mundt L, Shanahan K: *Graff's textbook of urinalysis and body fluids*, 3e, Philadelphia, 2015, Lippincott.

Osborne CA, Stevens JB: *Urinalysis: a clinical guide to compassionate patient care*, Shawnee Mission, KS, 1999, Bayer.

Raskin RE, Meyer DJ: *Canine and feline cytology: a color atlas and interpretation guide*, ed 3, St Louis, 2015, Saunders.

Valenciano AC, Cowell RL: *Cowell and Tyler's diagnostic cytology and hematology of the dog and cat*, ed 4, St Louis, 2014, Mosby.

Internet Resources

http://www.merckmanuals.com/vet/clinical_pathology_and_procedures/diagnostic_procedures_for_the_private_practice_laboratory/urinalysis.html

http://www.vet.ohio-state.edu/assets/courses/vcs753/case9/dogurin.html

https://www.idexxlearningcenter.com/course/view.php?id=2349

https://www.purinaproplanvets.com/media/1315/pur-urinalysis-clinical-handbook.pdf

http://35.169.230.41/sites/default/files/attachments/ASK_Urinalysis_Interpretation_.pdf

http://www.eclinpath.com/urinalysis/cellular-constituents/

UNIT 6 PARASITOLOGY

Recommended Reading

Bowman D: *Georgis' parasitology for veterinarians*, ed 10, St Louis, 2013, Saunders.

Foreyt W: *Veterinary parasitology reference manual*, ed 6, Ames, IA, 2017, Wiley-Blackwell.

Hendrix CM, Robinson E: *Diagnostic parasitology for veterinary technicians*, ed 5, St Louis, 2016, Mosby.

Zajac AM, Conboy G: *Veterinary clinical parasitology*, ed 8, Ames, IA, 2012, Wiley-Blackwell.

Internet Resources

http://www.capcvet.org/expert-articles/whats-your-risk/

http://www.cdc.gov/parasites/animals.html

http://www.who.int/zoonoses/en/

https://www.capcvet.org/articles/avoiding-common-pitfalls-in-fecal-examinations/

https://www.idexxlearningcenter.com/mod/resource/view.php?id=3255

https://www.idexxlearningcenter.com/mod/video/view.php?id=3913

UNIT 7 CYTOLOGY

Recommended Reading

Ford RB, Mazzaferro E: *Kirk & Bistner's handbook of veterinary procedures and emergency treatment*, ed 9, Philadelphia, 2011, Saunders.

Latimer KS, Prasse KW, Mahaffey EA: *Duncan and Prasse's veterinary laboratory medicine: clinical pathology*, ed 5, Ames, IA, 2011, Blackwell.

Raskin RE, Meyer DJ: *Canine and feline cytology: a color atlas and interpretation guide*, ed 3, St Louis, 2016, Saunders.

Taylor SM: *Small animal clinical techniques*, St Louis, 2010, Saunders.

Valenciano AC, Cowell RL: *Cowell and Tyler's diagnostic cytology and hematology of the dog and cat*, ed 4, St Louis, 2014, Mosby.

Internet Resources

https://www.merckvetmanual.com/clinical-pathology-and-procedures/diagnostic-procedures-for-the-private-practice-laboratory/cytology

http://veterinarymedicine.dvm360.com/vetmed/article/articleDetail.jsp?id=748260

https://www.banfield.com/getmedia/3c0c9853-d9d8-450a-983d-1ce0208682bc/1_5-inside-the-ear

https://www.cliniciansbrief.com/article/image-gallery-ear-cytology

https://www.wormsandgermsblog.com/2012/11/articles/animals/dogs/fecal-cytology-in-dogs-what-does-it-mean/

http://todaysveterinarypractice.navc.com/common-neoplastic-skin-lesions-dogs-catscytologic-diagnosis-treatment-options/

http://todaysveterinarypractice.navc.com/cytology-of-neoplasia-an-essential-component-of-diagnosis/

https://www.mspca.org/angell_services/cytologic-diagnosis-of-canine-gastrointestinal-neoplasia-via-ultrasound-guided-fine-needle-aspiration/

UNIT 8 MICROBIOLOGY

Recommended Reading

Latimer KS, Prasse KW, Mahaffey EA: *Duncan and Prasse's veterinary laboratory medicine: clinical pathology*, ed 5, Ames, IA, 2011, Blackwell.

McVey D, Kennedy M, Chengappa M: *Veterinary microbiology*, ed 3, Ames, IA, 2013, Wiley-Blackwell.

Quinn P, et al.: *Veterinary microbiology and microbial disease*, ed 2, Ames, IA, 2011, Wiley-Blackwell.

Songer J, Post K: *Veterinary microbiology: bacterial and fungal agents of animal disease*, St Louis, 2005, Saunders.

Internet Resources

http://helid.digicollection.org/en/d/Jwho01e/4.10.7.html

https://www.merckvetmanual.com/clinical-pathology-and-procedures/diagnostic-procedures-for-the-private-practice-laboratory/clinical-microbiology

https://www.wormsandgermsblog.com/2018/03/articles/animals/other-animals/turtles-and-salmonella/

https://veteriankey.com/introduction-to-veterinary-mycology/

UNIT 9 IMMUNOLOGY

Recommended Reading

Abbas AK: *Basic immunology updated edition: functions and disorders of the immune system*, ed 3, Philadelphia, 2011, Saunders.

Harvey JW: *Veterinary hematology: a diagnostic guide and color atlas*, St Louis, 2012, Saunders.

Quinley E: *Immunohematology: principles and practice*, ed 3, Philadelphia, 2017, Lippincott Williams & Wilkins.

Tizard IR: *Veterinary immunology*, ed 9, St Louis, 2013, Saunders.

Turgeon ML: *Immunology & serology in laboratory medicine*, ed 5, St Louis, 2013, Mosby.

Internet Resources

http://www.nlm.nih.gov/medlineplus/ency/article/003332.htm
http://jeeves.mmg.uci.edu/immunology/Assays/ELISA.htm
http://www.nlm.nih.gov/medlineplus/ency/article/003334.htm
http://www.maxanim.com/genetics/PCR/PCR.htm
http://www.vetfolio.com/emergency-medicine/transfusion-medicine
https://www.merckvetmanual.com/immune-system

Page numbers followed by "*f*" indicate figures, "*t*" indicate tables, and "*b*" indicate boxes.